PHYSICAL THERAPIST ASSISTANT EXAM

PHYSICAL THERAPIST ASSISTANT EXAM

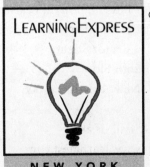

LEARNINGEXPRESS ®

NEW YORK

Library of Congress Cataloging-in-Publication Data

Physical therapist assistant exam.
    p.; cm.
 Includes bibliographical references.
 ISBN-13: 978-1-57685-754-0 (pbk.: alk. paper)
 ISBN-10: 1-57685-754-9 (pbk.: alk. paper)
 1. Physical therapy assistants—Examinations—Study guides. I. LearningExpress (Organization)
 [DNLM: 1. physical therapy modalities—Examination questions. 2. Physical therapy (specialty)—
Examination questions. WB 18.2 P57789 2010]
 RM701.6.P55 2010
 615.8'2076—dc22
                                2009051206

Printed in the United States of America

9 8 7 6 5 4 3 2 1

First Edition

For information on LearningExpress, other LearningExpress products, or bulk sales, please write to us at:
  LearningExpress
  2 Rector Street
  26th Floor
  New York, NY 10006

Or visit us at:
  www.learnatest.com

CONTENTS

This book is dedicated to all the students who have facilitated my learning through their original, insightful questions and honest feedback.

ACKNOWLEDGMENTS

I would like to acknowledge Lauren Fedorko for her skilled mentoring and patient support throughout this project and Barney Poole for going above and beyond in the editing department. Eternal gratitude goes to my husband, Tim, and my daughter, Meghan, for their tolerance of my many projects and their endless love.

CONTRIBUTORS

General Editor   Susan Griffin, PT, DPT, MS, GCS
Lead Instructor/Physical Therapist Assistant Program
Blackhawk Technical College
Janesville, Wisconsin

Contributors   Wendy D. Bircher, PT, EdD
Director/Physical Therapist Assistant Program
San Juan College
Farmington, New Mexico

Susan Griffin, PT, DPT, MS, GCS
Director/Physical Therapist Assistant Program
Blackhawk Technical College
Janesville, Wisconsin

Norman Johnson, PT, DPT, DEd, MSS, MBA
Professor, Director/Physical Therapist Assistant Program
Community College of Allegheny County
Monroeville, Pennsylvania

Michael S. Krackow, PhD, ATC, PTA, CSCS
Director/Physical Therapist Assistant Program
Jefferson College of Health Sciences
Roanoke, Virginia

Karey Ledbetter, PT, DPT, GTC, GCS
Manager/Physical Therapist Assistant Program
Florida State College
Jacksonville, Florida

Peggy DeCelle Newman, PT, MHR
Director/Clinical Education Program
University of Oklahoma Health Sciences Center
Oklahoma City, Oklahoma

Claire Olney, PT, ABDA
Instructor/Physical Therapist Assistant Program
ECPI—Medical Careers Institute
Newport News, Virginia

Robert M. Barney Poole, PT, DPT, MEd, ATC
President, Director/Performance Physical Therapy, PC
Outpatient Orthopaedic Physical Therapy Private Practice
Atlanta, Georgia

Karen Stephens, PT, DPT
Professor/Physical Therapist Assistant Program
Orange County Community College
Middletown, New York

Lisa Weaver, PTA, CMT
Instructor/Physical Therapist Assistant Program
Northeast Wisconsin Technical College
Green Bay, Wisconsin

PHYSICAL THERAPIST ASSISTANT EXAM

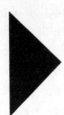

CHAPTER

1 ▶ PHYSICAL THERAPIST ASSISTANT CAREERS

CHAPTER SUMMARY

Congratulations on your decision to join the rewarding healthcare profession of physical therapy and to become a physical therapist assistant (PTA)! If you are considering a career in physical therapy, continue reading and learn what is required to become a PTA. Or, if you have recently completed your course work and clinical internship, one last hurdle awaits you—the National Physical Therapy Examination for Physical Therapist Assistants (NPTE for PTAs).

The NPTE for PTAs is a national exam developed by the Federation of State Boards of Physical Therapy (FSBPT) to test entry-level clinical and didactic knowledge of the PTA candidate for licensure. You can use this book to understand the structure and content of the exam and learn test-taking skills and strategies designed to help you translate your knowledge into a successful performance on the test. Practice and hone your skills by completing test questions that are similar in format and content to those found on the NPTE for PTAs.

If you are in the investigation phase of considering a career in physical therapy as a PTA, this book will help you with resources and a listing of schools that will prepare you to become a PTA. Included in these pages are job requirements, special skills you may need for the job, and ways to find the specific practice type for the state or states where you will be working.

History and Future of the PTA Profession

Initial discussions regarding the need for a trained assistant to work with the physical therapist began in the 1940s. At that time, the emphasis was on training, not education, which placed the PTA in a technically trained personnel category. The 1970s saw a period of PTA-program growth as Congress approved financial assistance and basic improvement grants for junior colleges with allied health curricula. The decade began with just 9 PTA programs, but ended with 47 accredited programs. The growth continued into the 1980s with 60 accredited programs by 1985.

Today, a physical therapist assistant continues to be a technically educated healthcare provider who may assist the physical therapist in the provision of many types of physical therapy interventions. PTAs are graduates of accredited programs and earn an associate's degree. PTA programs are accredited by the Commission on Accreditation in Physical Therapy Education (CAPTE).

In her 1980 guest commentary in *Physical Therapy*, Betty Canan, MEd, then director of the PTA program at University of Alabama at Birmingham, predicted a bright future for the physical therapist assistant. At that time, PTA educational accreditation and criteria were less than 20 years old. Canan did not rely solely on her prediction, however; she expressed the need for critical analysis and careful planning in the use of a skilled technician on the physical therapy team. She further opined that efficiency in the delivery of quality care would require the PTA to gain a greater role in physical therapy.

Now more than two decades later, as the population ages and reimbursement rates decline, the need for even greater efficiency may lead to further development of the role of the PTA in the delivery of care. The role of the physical therapist has become more managerial with physical therapists providing the overall direction of physical therapy management and completing the initial examination and skilled interventions requiring ongoing evaluation, such as manual manipulation mobilization of the spine. The PTA, under the direction and supervision of the PT, carries out more of the hands-on components of the daily plan of care, such as oversight of exercise programs and application of modalities including ultrasound and moist heat.

Emphasis on a Healthy Lifestyle

The future for physical therapy is indeed a bright one. As the baby boomer population ages, this more active and interactive group will seek ways to remain viable in sports and healthy lifestyles. Physical therapy will be on the leading edge of evidence-based healthcare (i.e., plans of care and interventions based on published and reviewed research) to maintain wellness and fitness and restore strength and functional activity. Also, insurance companies, Medicare, and proposed federal healthcare reform have begun to place a greater emphasis on prevention and the individual's maintaining a healthy lifestyle. The hope is that these changes will positively impact the healthcare system by prolonging the onset of systemic health issues such as obesity, diabetes, and emphysema. As the providers of choice for musculoskeletal issues, the PT/PTA team plays a vital part in providing programs to educate and improve the overall health of the population through outcomes driven by exercise-based wellness and fitness programs.

Demographics and Salaries of the PTA Profession

According to the U.S. Bureau of Labor Statistics, employment of physical therapist assistants is expected to increase 29% over the next decade. The age range of PTAs in the United States is between 20 and 65+.

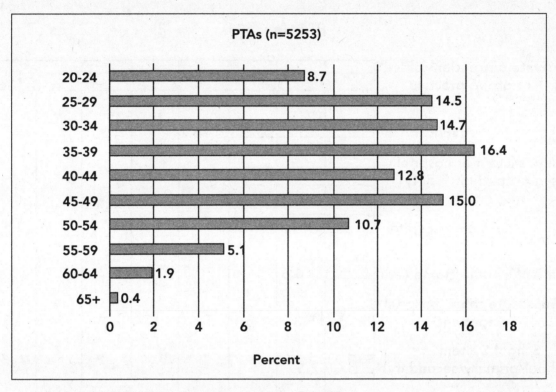

The majority of active full-time PTAs are between the ages of 35 and 39.

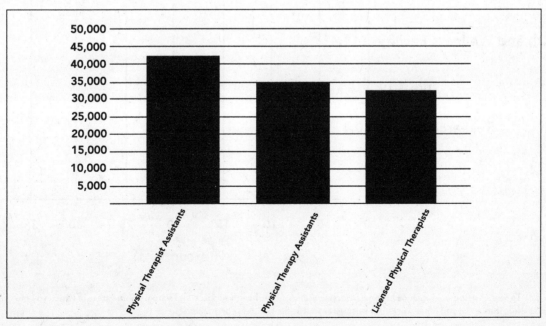

The average annual salary of a full-time PTA is between $30,000 and $40,000. However, the range goes as high as $80,000+.

While the profession of physical therapy as a whole is predominantly female, males are showing a slight gain in numbers. As of June 2007, 78.5% of PTAs were female, and 21.5% were male. Although PTAs may be found in a variety of work settings, the majority of PTAs work in private outpatient practice facilities.

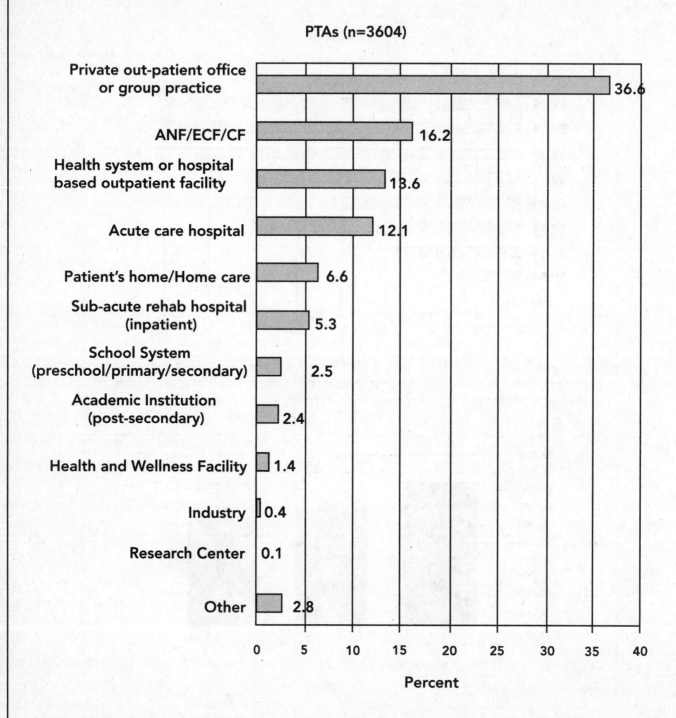

PTAs (n=3604)

Work Setting	Percent
Private out-patient office or group practice	36.6
ANF/ECF/CF	16.2
Health system or hospital based outpatient facility	13.6
Acute care hospital	12.1
Patient's home/Home care	6.6
Sub-acute rehab hospital (inpatient)	5.3
School System (preschool/primary/secondary)	2.5
Academic Institution (post-secondary)	2.4
Health and Wellness Facility	1.4
Industry	0.4
Research Center	0.1
Other	2.8

Other popular PTA work settings may include hospitals, nursing homes, home health services, and schools. Some areas in which you may be surprised to find PTAs include industrial and other workplace settings as well as fitness and sports facilities.

Scope of Work of a PTA

Physical therapists and physical therapist assistants have a responsibility to deliver quality services in an efficient and effective manner and with a constant eye on the safety of the consumer. PTs are responsible for all aspects of the plan of care, including those that may be delegated to the physical therapist assistant. The PTA, under the direction and supervision of a PT, is the only individual permitted to assist in selected physical therapy interventions. These may include exercises for strength, coordination, balance, and proprioception; training in the use of assistive devices (crutches, canes, and walkers) and activities of daily living; and the application of physical modalities, such as electrical stimulation, hot or cold packs, and ultrasound. Other important responsibilities of the PTA include collecting and documenting patient progress and communicating ongoing information concerning the patient to the physical therapist.

Supervision

In determining the needed level of supervision of the PTA, the PT will consider the PTA's education, skill level, and experience. The severity and complexity of the patient's case, the frequency of reexamination needed by the patient, and the setting in which care is delivered are also important factors. Additionally, federal and state laws and regulations, policies and positions of the APTA, and liability and risk management concerns are carefully considered.

The physical therapist is at all times directly responsible for the care delivered by the physical therapist assistant. The PT must provide at least general supervision of the PTA on an ongoing basis with documented interaction and communication by both practitioners according to individual state practice acts. General supervision may be provided in the room or facility or off-site by telecommunication. The PTA may modify selected interventions when working with a patient as directed by the supervising PT or to ensure patient safety and comfort.

Job Requirements

The job requirements for a PTA include leadership and communication skills, decision-making skills, and a modicum of physical coordination. Whether assuming control of a single patient or a group of patients, the PTA must be a good leader. The PTA is required to manage episodes of care based on instruction and supervision from the PT. PTAs must be good teachers, as much of their time is spent instructing patients on correct techniques for gait, exercise, and use of equipment, in addition to precautions to prevent re-injury or exacerbation of existing injury.

Communication is essential between the PTA and supervising PT and other health professionals as indicated by the PT. A PTA may communicate information regarding a patient's exercise session that may indicate a need for modification of the frequency, duration, or intensity of the exercise program. Enthusiasm for the job and empathy for the patient as well as a sense of good customer service are all pluses when dealing with the healthcare consumer.

The PTA must be able to accept direction from the supervising PT and use his or her judgment and decision-making skills when interacting with patients. As previously noted, the severity and complexity of the patient's condition should be considered when making a decision on the level of supervision the PTA needs to provide during treatment.

Resources

There is a wealth of information available on the APTA website at www.apta.org, including which PTA school to attend or if a career as a PTA is appropriate for you. From this Web page, choose the "Membership & Leadership" then "Students" headings on the left navigation bar. This will take you to a page containing information for current PTA, high school and undergraduate, and recently graduated PTA students. Membership in the APTA is not necessary to access these pages. Additionally, there are links to all the accredited PT and PTA programs in the United States. You also may access APTA information using Facebook and Twitter; here, you will also find links to the APTA website.

Under the current "Students" link, you will find further information for students, including a link to other resources and even an e-community where PT/PTA students can join in discussions and share and develop ideas. Other available information includes how to be involved in the APTA and a listing of upcoming events and opportunities in which to participate. The "High School and Undergraduate Students" link will take you to career decision-making information, including a video presentation entitled "Why should I become a PT/PTA?" You will also find a history of physical therapy. Additionally, these pages include scholarship information and a link to the centralized application service website. There are links on the website to other resources, such as ExploreHealthCareers.org, and you may even personally contact a current PTA student to learn first-hand what the process of application and a particular school are like.

The "Recent PT/PTA School Graduates" page will give you information about upcoming events in physical therapy and how to become more involved with the professional association. Finally, "Job Search Resources" and a "FSBPT Jurisdictional Licensure Reference Guide" are available on the website. Also, there is a summary of the benefits of membership in the APTA, with links to programs such as Hooked on Evidence (www.hookedonevidence.com), a research database on the effectiveness of physical therapy interventions.

NATIONAL PHYSICAL THERAPIST EXAMINATION FOR PHYSICAL THERAPIST ASSISTANTS

CHAPTER SUMMARY

Familiarizing yourself with the purpose and format of the National Physical Therapy Examination for Physical Therapist Assistants will help you prepare for the exam. In this chapter, you will find a thorough description of the exam format, including detailed information on each topic covered. You will also find information about the application and testing processes.

First formed in 1986, the FSBPT is responsible for developing, maintaining, and administering the NPTE for PTAs. It is used by the physical therapy licensing boards in all 50 states, the District of Columbia, Puerto Rico, and the U.S. Virgin Islands. The purpose of the exam is to determine if candidates for licensure possess the knowledge and skills required for safe and effective function as a physical therapist assistant under the direction and supervision of a physical therapist. Since all jurisdictions accept the same passing score, the NPTE for PTAs provides for a common national standard for physical therapist assistants. In other words, once the exam has been successfully completed, the PTA graduate may use those results to apply for credentialing anywhere in the United States, District of Columbia, Puerto Rico, or U.S. Virgin Islands.

Purpose of the Exam

The purpose of the Federation of State Boards of Physical Therapy is to protect the public by providing service and leadership that promote safe and competent physical therapy practice. As an organization, the federation strives to protect the public by setting a strong foundation of laws and regulations that govern the practice of physical therapy, standards that are consistent from state to state. These laws and regulatory standards are used to assess entry level and continued competency of physical therapists and physical therapist assistants and provide resources for public protection.

Format of the Exam

The NPTE for PTAs has 200 multiple-choice questions. Fifty of those questions are items that are in development and are not counted in the scoring of the exam. The developers of the exam do not provide a breakdown of how many of these items in development are in each of the major content areas. The remaining 150 items are divided among three major content areas—Clinical Application of Physical Therapy Principles and Foundational Sciences; Data Collection/Interventions/ Equipment and Devices/Therapeutic Modalities; and Safety, Protection, and Professional Roles, Teaching and Learning, and Evidence-Based Practice. The focus of the exam is the clinical application of knowledge, concepts, and principles necessary for the provision of safe and effective patient care consistent with the principles of best practice. It is important to note that you, as a test taker, will not be able to distinguish an unscored item that is in development from a scored item. So you should do your best on all 200 questions.

Clinical Application of Physical Therapy Principles and Foundational Sciences

The clinical application of physical therapy principles and foundational sciences content area is designed to assess the candidate's knowledge of the essential scientific principles, pathologies, diseases, and conditions that serve as the foundation for physical therapy treatment of patients of all ages. Questions in this content area cover anatomy, physiology, pathophysiology (physiology of abnormal states), diseases and conditions, medical management of diseases and conditions, and the effects of activity and exercise on the various body systems. This section is composed of 59 test questions, which is approximately 40% of the scored questions on the test. Ten items in the section cover the cardiac, vascular, and pulmonary systems. The section also contains 15 questions related to the musculoskeletal system and 14 questions that relate to the neuromuscular and nervous systems. In addition, there are 4 questions about the integumentary system (skin) and 16 related to the metabolic, the endocrine, and the gastrointestinal systems, and to multisystem involvement.

Data Collection

Data collection questions concern the types and applications of tests and measures used by physical therapist assistants, as well as the body's response to data collection activities. Twenty-three questions comprise the data collection section. This is 15% of the exam. Four questions pertain to the cardiac, vascular, and pulmonary systems, nine to the musculoskeletal system, seven to the neuromuscular and nervous systems, two to the integumentary system (skin), and one question pertains to other systems in the body.

Interventions

Questions in the intervention section of the exam refer to the types, applications, responses, and potential complications of physical therapy interventions. The impact on one system from interventions applied to other systems is also examined. For example, a question might refer to or ask about strengthening exercises applied to the musculoskeletal system and their impact on the cardiovascular system. There are 27 questions related to interventions, which constitutes 18% of the exam. There are five questions regarding interventions applied to the cardiac, vascular, and pulmonary systems; eight for the musculoskeletal system; nine for the neuromuscular and nervous systems; three for the integumentary system (skin); and two for the other bodily systems.

Equipment and Devices

The equipment and devices content area of the exam covers all factors involved in the application of equipment and devices related to physical therapy management for patients of all ages. The types of equipment include assistive and adaptive devices, prosthetics and orthotics, and bariatric equipment. The exam contains nine questions, accounting for 6% of the exam.

Therapeutic Modalities

The 13 questions in the therapeutic modalities content area examine the underlying principles for the use of physical therapy, as well as the indications, precautions, and contraindications for their use. The application of physical agents, mechanical modalities, and electrical stimulation is also covered. This section is 9% of the exam.

Safety, Protection, and Professional Roles

The content area of safety, protection, and professional roles refers to the responsibilities of healthcare providers to ensure that patient management and healthcare decisions take place in a secure and trustworthy environment. Factors influencing patient safety, such as a patient's fall risk and the use of restraints, are included in this category. Emergency preparedness is covered,

Therapeutic Modalities

PHYSICAL AGENTS	MECHANICAL MODALITIES	ELECTRICAL STIMULATION
Nonthermal agents, such as massage	Compression therapies	Functional electrical stimulation (FES)
Cryotherapy	Continuous passive motion	Transcutaneous electrical nerve stimulation (TENS)
Heat therapy, such as hot pack, paraffin bath, shortwave diathermy	Traction	Interferential current
Hydrotherapy		Iontophoresis
Light agents, such as infrared or ultraviolet		Electrical stimulation for wound healing
Ultrasound		

The table highlights specific examples of therapeutic modalities that are covered on the NPTE for PTAs.

which includes first aid, disaster response, and cardio-pulmonary resuscitation (CPR). Injury prevention and proper body mechanics also fall under this category, as well as infection control procedures.

Patient rights as delineated by laws and regulations, such as the Americans with Disabilities Act (ADA), the Health Insurance Portability and Accountability Act (HIPAA), and the Individuals with Disabilities Education Act (IDEA), are in this section. There may be questions about standards of documentation and risk reduction strategies. Finally, the role of the PTA in relation to the PT is covered in this section; the roles of other healthcare professionals may be examined as well. There are 12 questions about safety, protection, and professional roles which constitute 8% of the exam.

Teaching and Learning

Theories of teaching and learning, including verbal and nonverbal forms of communication and the application of strategies and techniques to create an effective learning environment for patients and care-givers, are covered in this section of the exam. Effective communication is essential to ensure appropriate patient management and decision making. There are four questions on the topic of teaching and learning.

Evidence-Based Practice

The purpose of the evidence-based practice section of the exam is to assess the candidate for licensure's ability to use his or her knowledge of basic research concepts and outcome measures to interpret information from a variety of sources. This information can then be used to support choices regarding the evidence-based management of physical therapy patients. There are three questions in this section.

Content of the NPTE for PTAs by Topic

CONTENT AREA	NUMBER OF ITEMS	PERCENT OF ITEMS
PT principles and foundational sciences	59	40%
Data collection	23	15%
Interventions	27	18%
Equipment and devices	9	6%
Therapeutic modalities	13	9%
Safety, protection, and professional roles	12	8%
Teaching and learning	4	3%
Evidence-based practice	3	2%

This table describes the relative emphasis of various areas on the NPTE for PTAs.

Content of the NPTE for PTAs by Body System

BODY SYSTEM	PERCENTAGE OF NPTE FOR PTAS
Musculoskeletal	21%
Neuromuscular	20%
Cardiac/vascular/pulmonary	13%
Integumentary	6%
Other	13%

This table describes the relative distribution of questions by body system.

Administration of the Exam

The NPTE for PTAs is a multiple-choice exam that is offered in a computer-based testing format. Prometric is the name of the company that supplies computer-based testing services to the FSBPT (visit www.prometric.com for more information about Prometric).

Computer skills are not necessary to take the exam. There is a five- to ten-minute tutorial that allows test takers to practice moving from question to question and selecting answers. The tutorial can be repeated; the time needed to complete it does NOT count against the examination time.

Duration of the Exam

Candidates are allowed a total of 30 minutes to complete the tutorial for the exam and four hours to complete the 200 questions on the exam itself. The exam is divided into four sections of 50 questions each. Once you complete a section, you cannot return to that or a previously completed section. Each section is a "mini-exam" that follows the same basic outline as the larger exam and will contain both scored and unscored items. (Remember, because you cannot distinguish scored items from unscored items, you need to do your best on all 200 questions.) Exam scores are based on the number of correct answers and there is no penalty for answering a question incorrectly, so no questions should be left blank. Candidates are also allowed a 15-minute break. This break is scheduled after completion of the second section of the test. This time does not count in the four hours allotted for exam completion. Candidates may also take up to two unscheduled breaks between the sections of the exam. However, the timer will continue to run during these unscheduled breaks.

Navigating the Exam

Candidates select answers using either the keyboard or the mouse. Questions can be marked for later review, and the test taker can move forward or backward through the exam. However, once a section is completed, the questions in that section are no longer available for review, and the answers to those questions cannot be changed. There is only one correct or best answer to each question. Candidates may not bring scratch paper or writing utensils into the testing center; however, each candidate will be issued an erasable board to use for jotting notes. These boards are returned to the testing center at the completion of the examination.

Security Issues

There are a number of security procedures that are put into place at the Prometric testing center. Each candidate must bring a photo ID and another preprinted card bearing his or her signature (e.g., a credit card) to the testing center. The name on both of these pieces of identification must match exactly the name the person used to register for the examination. The photo ID will be scanned. The candidate will have a digital record of his or her fingerprint taken when he or she enters or leaves the examination room. The examination is also videotaped. As mentioned earlier, writing utensils and paper are not allowed in the testing room. Nor are electronic devices such as digital watches, cell phones, and iPods.

The FSBPT also has security policies in place. Each candidate is required to sign an agreement stating, in part, that he or she has not received any information about specific test questions from others who have taken the exam. (For more information about this agreement, see page 15 of the FSBPT candidate handbook.) Candidates agree not to use or take notes during the examination. Candidates also agree not to communicate specific information about test questions to those who have not yet taken the exam. Anyone who violates any of the security procedures will have his or her score invalidated and will be prosecuted by the FSBPT.

Scoring of the Exam

Scoring of the examination is done electronically. The number of questions a candidate answers correctly is converted, through a mathematical formula, into a score on a scale from 200 to 800. This is done because different versions of the NPTE for PTAs are used, and these versions vary in difficulty. A candidate taking a more difficult exam will have to answer fewer questions to achieve a passing scaled score than one taking an easier exam. This ensures that no one is being unfairly advantaged or penalized. The passing scaled score is 600. Exam results will be sent to the licensure entity through which the candidate registered for the exam; the licensure entity will then notify the candidate.

From 2004 to 2008, the percentage of people passing the NPTE for PTAs on the first attempt was 71, 73, 74, 80, and 82%, respectively. The pass rate on the exam after all attempts is around 90%. If a candidate fails to pass the exam, he or she may retake it. The FSBPT limits the number of retakes to three in one year. Normally, there is at least one month between exam attempts.

How to Apply for the Exam

The candidate must apply for and receive registration materials to take the exam from the licensing authority in the state or jurisdiction in which he or she hopes to obtain a credential. Passing the NPTE for PTAs is only one of several components that are required in order to be credentialed as a PTA. Each jurisdiction has its own requirements, and each candidate must contact the jurisdiction in which he or she hopes to become credentialed in order to find out the exact requirements.

Registration materials and fees must be returned to the credentialing authority. Fees vary by state. Currently, the fee to take the NPTE for PTAs is $400. Of this, $350 goes to the FSBPT and $50 goes to the Prometric testing center. The licensing authority makes sure each candidate is eligible to sit for the exam and sends the registration information and fees to the FSBPT. The FSBPT then sends each candidate an Authorization to Test letter containing information on how to make an appointment at a Prometric center. There are approximately 300 testing centers throughout the country that administer the NPTE for PTAs. A candidate may take the exam in any center; the exam does not have to be taken in the jurisdiction in which the candidate is pursuing credentialing. For example, if a candidate completed his or her schooling in Washington, but was planning to apply for a credential in California, he or she may still take the test in Washington if that is more convenient. An appointment must be made within the 60-day period indicated on the Authorization to Test letter.

Obtaining a State Credential

Since physical therapy is regulated by the state, each state or jurisdiction has its own requirements for PTA credentialing. It is called *credentialing* because only 39 states and Puerto Rico grant a license to the PTA. In Arizona, Indiana, Kansas, Kentucky, Nebraska, and New York, PTAs are granted a certificate. In Pennsylvania and Wyoming, they are registered. Colorado, Hawaii, Michigan, Utah, and the Virgin Islands do not credential the PTA.

As noted earlier, each jurisdiction establishes its own criteria for credentialing. Maine, Tennessee, and Washington do not require passage of the NPTE for PTAs in order to become credentialed, but all other jurisdictions in which the PTA is credentialed do require a passing score on this exam as a requirement to become credentialed. Other requirements may include graduation from a CAPTE-accredited PTA program, a criminal background check, submission of your Social Security number, and successful completion of a jurisprudence exam. The candidate for licensure must contact the licensing authority in the jurisdiction in which he or she hopes to obtain his or her credential for details regarding credentialing requirements.

A Final Word

The organization of the NPTE for PTAs can be looked at in many ways. One way is to look at the percentage of items in each of the different content areas. Another is to look at the percentage of items in each of the body systems. Yet another is simply to view the exam as four sections of 50 questions, with questions covering all content areas and body systems in each section. Remember that each of the 200 questions is important, and you should try to determine the best answer for each. Understanding the format, content, scoring, and application process of the NPTE for PTAs will help alleviate the fear of the unknown and assist the candidate in adequately preparing for the exam.

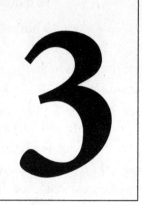

THE LEARNINGEXPRESS TEST PREPARATION SYSTEM

CHAPTER SUMMARY

Taking the National Physical Therapy Examination for Physical Therapist Assistants is tough. It demands a lot of preparation if you want to achieve a top score. Your career depends on your passing the exam. The LearningExpress Test Preparation System, developed exclusively for LearningExpress by leading test experts, gives you the discipline and attitude you need to succeed.

First, the bad news: Taking the physical therapist assistants exam is no picnic, and neither is getting ready for it. Your future career as a physical therapist assistant depends on your getting a passing score, and there are all sorts of pitfalls that can keep you from doing your best on this all-important exam. Here are some of the obstacles that can stand in the way of your success:

- being unfamiliar with the format of the exam
- being paralyzed by test anxiety
- leaving your preparation to the last minute
- not preparing at all!
- not knowing vital test-taking skills (i.e., how to pace yourself through the exam, how to use the process of elimination, and when to guess)
- not being in tip-top mental and physical shape
- arriving late at the test site

- having to work on an empty stomach
- shivering through the exam because the room is cold

What's the common denominator in all these test-taking pitfalls? One word: control. Who's in control, you or the exam?

Now the good news: The LearningExpress Test Preparation System puts you in control. With our simple, easy-to-follow steps, you will learn everything you need to know to make sure that you are in charge of your preparation and your performance on the exam. Other test takers may let the test get the better of them, other test takers may be unprepared or out of shape, but not you. You will have taken all the steps you need to get a high score on the physical therapist assistants exam.

The LearningExpress Test Preparation System—Nine Easy Steps

Here's how the LearningExpress Test Preparation System works: Nine easy steps lead you through everything you need to know and do to get ready to master your exam. Each of the steps listed below includes both reading and one or more related activities. (It's important that you do the activities along with the reading, or you won't be getting the full benefit of the system.) Each step tells you approximately how much time it will take you to complete.

Step 1:	Get Information	50 minutes
Step 2:	Conquer Test Anxiety	20 minutes
Step 3:	Make a Plan	30 minutes
Step 4:	Learn to Manage Your Time	10 minutes
Step 5:	Learn to Use the Process of Elimination	20 minutes

Step 6:	Know When to Guess	20 minutes
Step 7:	Reach Your Peak Performance Zone	10 minutes
Step 8:	Get Your Act Together	10 minutes
Step 9:	Do It!	10 minutes
Total		**3 hours**

We estimate that working through the entire system will take you approximately three hours, though it's perfectly okay if you work faster or slower than the time estimates suggest. If you can take a whole afternoon or evening, you can work through the entire LearningExpress Test Preparation System in one sitting. Otherwise, you can break it up, and do just one or two steps a day for the next several days. It's up to you—remember, you're in control.

Step 1: Get Information

Time to complete: 50 minutes
Activities: Read Chapter 1, Physical Therapist Assistant Careers.

Knowledge is power. The first step in the LearningExpress Test Preparation System is finding out everything you can about the physical therapist assistants exam. Once you have your information, the next steps in the LearningExpress Test Preparation System will show you what to do about it.

Part A: Straight Talk about the National Physical Therapy Examination

The NPTE for PTAs exam is just one part of a whole series of evaluations you have to go through to show that you are prepared to perform the many, varied tasks of a physical therapist assistant. The exam attempts to measure acquired knowledge of your field and the clinical reasoning skills that you have developed as you have studied to be a PTA. According to the candidate handbook for the National Physical Therapy Examination for Physical Therapist Assistants, the purpose of the exam is to provide examination services to the regulatory authorities charged with regulating physical therapist assistants and to provide a common element that can be used in the evaluation of candidates from different jurisdictions.

It's important for you to remember that your score on the physical therapist assistants exam does not determine how smart you are or even whether you will make a good physical therapist assistant. There are all kinds of things an exam like this can't test: whether you are likely to show up late or call in sick a lot; whether you have the interpersonal skills necessary to build the trusting, comfortable relationships that will keep your clients coming back; and whether you have an enthusiastic dedication to learning and performing your skills well. Those kinds of things are hard to evaluate, while selecting the best answer choice on a computer-based exam is easier to evaluate.

This is not to say that choosing the best answer is not important! The knowledge and clinical reasoning skills tested on the exam are the types of knowledge and skills that you will need to do your job. And your ability to enter the profession you've trained for depends on your passing this exam. And that's why you're here—using the LearningExpress Test Preparation System to achieve control over the exam.

Part B: What's on the Test

If you haven't already done so, stop here and read Chapter 1 of this book, which gives you an overview of the typical National Physical Therapy Examination for Physical Therapist Assistants exam.

Turn to Chapter 2 for more information about the test and for a breakdown of topics on the exam. If you haven't already gotten the full rundown on credentialing procedures as part of your training program, you can contact the Federation of State Boards of Physical Therapy agency listed in the Appendix for details.

Step 2: Conquer Test Anxiety

Time to complete: 20 minutes
Activity: Take the Test Stress Test.
Having complete information about the exam is the first step in getting control of the exam. Next, you have to overcome one of the biggest obstacles to test success: test anxiety. Test anxiety can not only impair your performance on the exam itself, it can keep you from even preparing! In Step 2, you'll learn stress management techniques that will help you succeed on your exam. Learn these strategies now, and practice them as you work through the exams in this book, so they'll be second nature to you by test day.

Combating Test Anxiety

The first thing you need to know is that a little test anxiety is a good thing. Everyone gets nervous before a big exam—and if that nervousness motivates you to prepare thoroughly, so much the better. It's said that Sir Laurence Olivier, one of the foremost British actors of the twentieth century, threw up before every performance. His stage fright didn't impair his performance; in fact, it probably gave him a little extra edge—just the kind of edge you need to do well, whether on a stage or in an examination room.

Following is the Test Stress Test. Answer the questions to find out whether your level of test anxiety is something you should worry about.

Test Stress Test

You only need to worry about test anxiety if it is extreme enough to impair your performance. The following questionnaire will provide a diagnosis of your level of test anxiety. In the blank before each statement, write the number that most accurately describes your experience.

0 = Never
1 = Once or twice
2 = Sometimes
3 = Often

___I have gotten so nervous before an exam that I simply put down the books and didn't study for it.

___I have experienced disabling physical symptoms such as vomiting and severe headaches because I was nervous about an exam.

___I have simply not showed up for an exam because I was scared to take it.

___I have experienced dizziness and disorientation while taking an exam.

___I have had trouble filling in the little circles because my hands were shaking too hard.

___I have failed an exam because I was too nervous to complete it.

___Total: Add up the numbers in the blanks above.

Your Test Stress Score

Here are the steps you should take, depending on your score. If you scored:

- **below 3**, your level of test anxiety is nothing to worry about; it's probably just enough to give you that little extra edge.
- **between 3 and 6**, your test anxiety may be enough to impair your performance, and you should practice the stress management techniques listed in this section to try to bring your test anxiety down to manageable levels.
- **above 6**, your level of test anxiety is a serious concern. In addition to practicing the stress management techniques listed in this section, you may want to seek additional, personal help. Call your local high school or community college and ask for the academic counselor. Tell the counselor that you have a level of test anxiety that sometimes keeps you from being able to take the exam. The counselor may be willing to help you or may suggest someone else you should talk to.

Stress Management before the Test

If you feel your level of anxiety getting the best of you in the weeks before the test, here is what you need to do to bring the level down again:

- **Get prepared.** There's nothing like knowing what to expect and preparing for it to put you in control of test anxiety. That's why you're reading this book. Use it faithfully, and remind yourself that you're better prepared than most of the people taking the test.
- **Practice self-confidence.** A positive attitude is a great way to combat test anxiety. This is no time to be humble or shy. Stand in front of the mirror and say to your reflection, "I'm prepared. I'm full of self-confidence. I'm going to do my best on this test. I know I can do well." Say it into an MP3 player and play it back once a day. If you hear it often enough, you'll believe it.
- **Fight negative messages.** Every time someone starts telling you how hard the exam is or how it's almost impossible to get a high score, start telling them your self-confidence messages above. If the person with the negative messages is you telling yourself "you don't do well on exams, you just can't do this", don't listen. Turn on your MP3 player and listen to your self-confidence messages.
- **Visualize.** Imagine yourself reporting for duty on your first day as a physical therapist assistant. Think of yourself with a patient, assessing his or her open wound—you're part of a very important decision-making process. Visualizing a positive outcome can help make it happen—and it reminds you of why you're going through all this work in preparing for the exam.
- **Exercise.** Physical activity helps calm your body down and focus your mind. Besides, being in good physical shape can actually help you do well on the exam. Go for a run, lift weights, go swimming—and do it regularly.

Stress Management on Test Day

There are several ways you can bring down your level of test anxiety on test day. They'll work best if you practice them in the weeks before the test so you know which ones work best for you.

- **Deep breathing.** Take a deep breath while you count to five. Hold it for a count of one, then let it out on a count of five. Repeat several times.
- **Move your body.** Try rolling your head in a circle. Rotate your shoulders. Shake your hands from the wrist. Many people find these movements very relaxing.
- **Visualize again.** Think of the place where you are most relaxed: lying on the beach in the sun, walking through the park, or whatever. Now close your eyes and imagine you're actually there. If you practice in advance, you'll find that you only need a few seconds of this exercise to experience a significant increase in your sense of well-being.

When anxiety threatens to overwhelm you right there during the exam, there are still things you can do to manage the stress level:

- **Repeat your self-confidence messages.** You should have them memorized by now. Say them quietly to yourself, and believe them!
- **Visualize—one more time.** This time, visualize yourself moving smoothly and quickly through the test answering every question right and finishing just before time is up. Like most visualization techniques, this one works best if you've practiced it ahead of time.
- **Find an easy question.** Skim over the test until you find an easy question, and answer it. Getting even one question answered gets you into the test-taking groove.
- **Take a mental break.** Everyone loses concentration once in a while during a long test. It's normal,

so you shouldn't worry about it. Instead, accept what has happened. Say to yourself, "Hey, I lost it there for a minute. My brain is taking a break." Stop what you're doing, close your eyes, and do some deep breathing for a few seconds. Then you're ready to go back to work.

Try these techniques ahead of time, and see if they don't work for you!

Step 3: Make a Plan

Time to complete: 30 minutes
Activity: Construct a study plan.

Maybe the most important thing you can do to get control of yourself and your exam is to make a study plan. Too many people fail to prepare simply because they fail to plan. Spending hours on the day before the exam poring over sample test questions not only raises your level of test anxiety, it also is simply no substitute for careful preparation and practice over time.

Don't fall into the cram trap. Take control of your preparation time by mapping out a study schedule. On the following pages are two sample schedules, based on the amount of time you have before you take the physical therapist assistants exam. If you're the kind of person who needs deadlines and assignments to motivate you for a project, here they are. If you're the kind of person who doesn't like to follow other people's plans, you can use the suggested schedules here to construct your own.

Even more important than making a plan is making a commitment. You can't review everything you learned in your physical therapist assitant program in one night. You have to set aside some time every day for study and practice. Try for at least 20 minutes a day. Twenty minutes daily will do you much more good than two hours on Saturday.

Don't put off your study until the day before the exam. Start now. A few minutes a day, with half an hour or more on weekends, can make a big difference in your score.

Schedule A: the 30-Day plan

If you have at least a month before you take the National Physical Therapy Examination for Physical Therapist Assistants, you have plenty of time to prepare—as long as you don't waste it! If you have less than a month, turn to Schedule B.

TIME	PREPARATION
Days 1–4	Skim over the written materials from your training program, particularly noting (1) areas you expect to be emphasized on the exam and (2) areas you don't remember well. On Day 4, concentrate on those areas.
Day 5	Take the diagnostic exam in Chapter 4.
Day 6	Score the diagnostic exam. Use the information on the test given in Chapter 2 to help you identify which are your strongest and weakest areas. Select two areas on which you will concentrate before you take the first practice exam in Chapter 9.
Days 7–10	Study the two areas you identified as your weak points.
Day 11	Take the second practice exam in Chapter 9.
Day 12	Score the first practice exam. Identify one area to concentrate on before you take the second practice exam.
Days 13–18	Study the one area you identified for review.
Day 19	Take the second exam in Chapter 10.
Day 20	Refine your study plan. Once again, identify one area to review, based on

your score on the second practice exam.

Days 20–21 Study the one area you identified for review.

Days 22–25 Take an overview of all your training materials, consolidating your strengths and improving on your weaknesses.

Days 26–27 Review all the areas that have given you the most trouble on the practice exams you've taken so far.

Day 28 Take the second practice exam in Chapter 10 again. Note how much you've improved!

Day 29 Review one or two weak areas, doing any sample questions in these areas that you haven't already done.

Day before the exam Relax. Do something unrelated to the exam, and go to bed at a reasonable hour.

Schedule B: The Ten-Day Plan

If you have two weeks or less before you take the exam, you may have your work cut out for you. Use this ten-day schedule to help you make the most of your time.

TIME	PREPARATION
Day 1	Take the diagnostic exam in Chapter 4 and score it using the answer key. Turn to the list of subject areas on the exam in Chapter 2, and find out in which areas you need the most work, based on your exam score.
Day 2	Review one area that gave you trouble on the diagnostic exam in Chapter 4.
Day 3	Review another area that gave you trouble on the diagnostic exam.
Day 4	Take the first practice exam in Chapter 9 and score it.

Day 5 If your score on the first practice exam doesn't show improvement in the two areas you studied, review them again. If you did improve in those areas, choose a new weak area to study today.

Day 6 Take the second practice exam in Chapter 10 and score it.

Day 7 Choose your weakest area from the second practice exam to review.

Day 8 Review any areas that you have not yet reviewed on this schedule.

Day 9 Take the second practice exam in Chapter 10 again and score it.

Day 10 Use your last study day to brush up on any areas that are still giving you trouble. Do any sample questions in those areas from Lesson 4 that you haven't already done.

Day before the exam Relax. Do something unrelated to the exam, and go to bed at a reasonable hour.

Step 4: Learn to Manage Your Time

Time to complete: Ten minutes to read, many hours of practice!

Activities: Practice these strategies as you take the sample tests in this book.

Steps 4, 5, and 6 of the LearningExpress Test Preparation System put you in charge of your exam by showing you test-taking strategies that work. Practice these strategies as you take the sample tests in this book, and then you'll be ready to use them on test day.

First, you'll take control of your time on the exam. The National Physical Therapy Examination for Physical Therapist Assistants has a time limit of four hours, which may give you more than enough time to complete

Physical Preparation Checklist

For the week before the test, write down (1) what physical exercise you engaged in and for how long and (2) what you ate for each meal. Remember, you're trying for at least half an hour of exercise every other day (preferably every day) and a balanced diet that's light on junk food.

Exam minus seven days

Exercise: _____ for _____ minutes

Breakfast: _____

Lunch: _____

Dinner: _____

Snacks: _____

Exam minus six days

Exercise: _____ for _____ minutes

Breakfast: _____

Lunch: _____

Dinner: _____

Snacks: _____

Exam minus five days

Exercise: _____ for _____ minutes

Breakfast: _____

Lunch: _____

Dinner: _____

Snacks: _____

Exam minus four days

Exercise: _____ for _____ minutes

Breakfast: _____

Lunch: _____

Dinner: _____

Snacks: _____

Exam minus three days

Exercise: _____ for _____ minutes

Breakfast: _____

Lunch: _____

Dinner: _____

Snacks: _____

Exam minus two days

Exercise: _____ for _____ minutes

Breakfast: _____

Lunch: _____

Dinner: _____

Snacks: _____

Exam minus one day

Exercise: _____ for _____ minutes

Breakfast: _____

Lunch: _____

Dinner: _____

Snacks: _____

all the questions—or may not. It's a terrible feeling to hear the examiner say, "Five minutes left," when you're only three-quarters of the way through the test. Here are some tips to keep that from happening to you:

- **Follow directions.** If the directions are given orally, listen to them. Before the exam begins, a simple introductory lesson, or tutorial, is presented. It explains the process of moving from question to question and selecting answers. Most candidates take five to ten minutes to complete the tutorial. Please be sure to carefully complete the tutorial and to repeat it, if you wish to do so. You will be given scratch paper—an erasable note board supplied at the testing center. (You are not allowed to bring your own scratch paper.) Use the erasable board to write down the beginning time and the ending time of the exam.
- **Ask questions.** If there's anything you don't understand, ask questions before the exam begins.
- **Pace yourself.** The exam consists of four sections, which have 50 questions each (although only 150 questions are ultimately scored). Glance at your watch every few minutes, and compare the time to how far you've gotten in the section of the test that you are working on. When one-quarter of the time for a section has elapsed, you should be one-quarter of the way through that section, and so on. If you're falling behind, pick up the pace a bit.
- **Keep moving.** Don't dither around on one question. If you don't know the answer, skip the question and move on. The testing software allows you to mark questions that you want to review before the end of a section. You may mark a question regardless of whether or not you have answered it. (Also, you do not have to unmark a question in order for it to be scored. It will be scored whether it is marked or unmarked.) You may move back and forth through the section and review questions, whether the questions are marked or unmarked, but you may find it helpful to mark questions you want to return to in case you have time to come back to them later.

- **Don't rush.** Though you should keep moving, rushing won't help. Try to keep calm and work at an efficient and effective pace.

Step 5: Learn to Use the Process of Elimination

Time to complete: 20 minutes
Activity: Complete worksheet on Using the Process of Elimination.

After time management, your next most important tool for taking control of your exam is using the process of elimination wisely. It's standard test-taking wisdom that you should always read all the answer choices before choosing your answer. This helps you find the right answer by eliminating wrong answer choices. And, sure enough, that standard wisdom applies to your exam, too.

Let's say you're facing a question that goes like this:

1. Which of the following is the best indicator of venous circulation?
   a. ankle-brachial index
   b. blood pressure
   c. girth measurement
   d. temperature assessment

You should always use the process of elimination on a question like this, even if the right answer jumps out at you. Sometimes the answer that jumps out isn't right after all. Let's assume, for the purpose of this exercise, that you're a little rusty on your terminology, so you need to use a little intuition to make up for what you don't remember. Proceed through the answer choices in order.

So you start with answer **a.** *Ankle-brachial index* sounds familiar, but you can't remember what it is used for exactly. Is it for arterial or venal circulation? Put a question mark next to choice **a,** meaning "well, maybe."

On to the next. *Blood pressure* looks okay, since blood pressure is a measure that is useful for a lot of things. But you just aren't sure about this choice. Put a question mark next to **b**, meaning "well, maybe."

Choice **c** looks good. You remember that venous insufficiency results in edema formation in the lower extremity and/or skin abnormalities and ulcerations. Girth measurement would be an appropriate way to assess edema formation.

Choice **d** seems unlikely. What does temperature assessment have to do with venous circulation? Put an X next to this one so that you never look at it again.

Now your question looks like this:

1. Which of the following is the best indicator of venous circulation?
? **a.** ankle-brachial index
? **b.** blood pressure
✓ **c.** girth measurement
✗ **d.** temperature assessment

You've got just one check mark, for a good answer. If you're pressed for time, you should simply mark answer **c** on your answer sheet. If you've got the time to be extra careful, you could compare your check-mark answer against your question-mark answers to make sure that it's better.

It's good to have a system for marking good, bad, and maybe answers. We're recommending this one:

✓ = good
✗ = bad
? = maybe

If you don't like these marks, devise your own system. Just make sure you do it long before test day—while you're working through the practice exams in this book—so you won't have to worry about it during the test.

Even when you think you're absolutely clueless about a question, you can often use process of elimination to get rid of one answer choice. If so, you're better prepared to make an educated guess, as you'll see in Step 6. More often, the process of elimination allows you to get down to only two possibly right answers. Then you're in a strong position to guess. And sometimes, even though you don't know the right answer, you find it simply by getting rid of the wrong ones, as you did in the previous example.

Try using your powers of elimination on the questions in the worksheet Using the Process of Elimination beginning on the next page. The questions aren't about physical therapist assitant work; they're just designed to show you how the process of elimination works. The answer explanations for this worksheet show one possible way you might use the process to arrive at the right answer.

The process of elimination is your tool for the next step, which is knowing when to make an educated guess.

Use the process of elimination to answer the following questions:

1. Ilsa is as old as Meghan will be in five years. The difference between Ed's age and Meghan's age is twice the difference between Ilsa's age and Meghan's age. Ed is 29. How old is Ilsa?
   a. 4
   b. 10
   c. 19
   d. 24

2. "All drivers of commercial vehicles must carry a valid commercial driver's license whenever operating a commercial vehicle."

   According to this sentence, which of the following people need NOT carry a commercial driver's license?
   a. a truck driver idling his engine while waiting to be directed to a loading dock
   b. a bus operator backing her bus out of the way of another bus in the bus lot
   c. a taxi driver driving his personal car to the grocery store
   d. a limousine driver taking the limousine to her home after dropping off her last passenger of the evening

3. What has smoking tobacco been linked to?
   a. increased risk of stroke and heart attack
   b. all forms of respiratory disease
   c. increasing mortality rates over the past ten years
   d. juvenile delinquency

4. Which of the following words is spelled correctly?
   a. incorrigible
   b. outragous
   c. domestickated
   d. understandible

Answers

Here are the answers, as well as some suggestions as to how you might have used the process of elimination to find them.

1. d. You should have eliminated choice **a** off the bat. Ilsa can't be four years old if Meghan is going to be Ilsa's age in five years. The best way to eliminate other answer choices is to try plugging them in to the information given in the problem. For instance, for choice **b**, if Ilsa is 10, then Meghan must be 5. The difference between their ages is 5. The difference between Ed's age, 29, and Meghan's age, 5, is 24. Is 24 two times 5? No. Then choice **b** is wrong. You could eliminate choice **c** in the same way and be left with choice **d**.

2. c. Note the word *not* in the question, and go through the answers one by one. Is the truck driver in choice **a** operating a commercial vehicle? Yes, idling counts as operating, so he needs to have a commercial driver's license. Likewise, the bus operator in choice **b** is operating a commercial vehicle; the question doesn't say the operator has to be on the street. The limo driver in choice **d** is operating a commercial vehicle, even if it doesn't have passenger in it. However, the cabbie in choice **c** is not operating a commercial vehicle, but his own private car.

3. **a.** You could eliminate choice **b** simply because of the presence of the word *all*. Such absolutes hardly ever appear in correct answer choices. Choice **c** looks attractive until you think a little about what you know—aren't fewer people smoking these days, rather than more? So how could smoking be responsible for a higher mortality rate? (If you didn't know that mortality rate means the rate at which people die, you might keep this choice as a possibility, but you would still be able to eliminate two answers and have only two to choose from.) And choice **d** is plain silly, so you could eliminate that one, too. You are left with the correct choice, **a**.

4. **a.** How you used the process of elimination here depends on which words you recognized as being spelled incorrectly. If you knew that the correct spellings were *outrageous*, *domesticated*, and *understandable*, then you were home free. Surely you knew that at least one of those words was wrong!

Step 6: Know When to Guess

Time to complete: 20 minutes
Activity: Complete worksheet on Your Guessing Ability.

Armed with the process of elimination, you're ready to take control of one of the big questions in test taking: Should I guess? The first and main answer is "Yes." Some exams have what's called a guessing penalty, in which a fraction of your wrong answers is subtracted from your right answers—but National Physical Therapy Examination for Physical Therapist Assistants does not penalize you for guessing. The number of questions you answer correctly yields your raw score. So you have nothing to lose and everything to gain by guessing.

The more complicated answer to the question "Should I guess?" depends on you—your personality and your guessing intuition. There are two things you need to know about yourself before you go into the exam:

- Are you a risk taker?
- Are you a good guesser?

You'll have to decide about your risk-taking quotient on your own. To find out if you're a good guesser, complete the worksheet Your Guessing Ability that follows. Frankly, even if you're a play-it-safe person with lousy intuition, you're still safe in guessing every time. The best thing would be if you could overcome your anxieties and go ahead and mark an answer. But you may want to have a sense of how good your intuition is before you go into the exam.

Step 7: Reach Your Peak Performance Zone

Time to complete: Ten minutes to read, weeks to complete!
Activity: Complete the physical preparation checklist.

To get ready for a challenge like a big exam, you have to take control of your physical, as well as your mental, state. Exercise, proper diet, and rest will ensure that your body works with, rather than against, your mind on test day, as well as during your preparation.

Your Guessing Ability

The following are ten really hard questions. You are not supposed to know the answers. Rather, this is an assessment of your ability to guess when you don't have a clue. Read each question carefully, as if you were expected to answer it. If you have any knowledge of the subject, use that knowledge to help you eliminate wrong answer choices.

1. September 7 is Independence Day in
   a. India.
   b. Costa Rica.
   c. Brazil.
   d. Australia.

2. Which of the following is the formula for determining the momentum of an object?
   a. $p = MV$
   b. $F = ma$
   c. $P = IV$
   d. $E = mc^2$

3. Because of the expansion of the universe, the stars and other celestial bodies are all moving away from each other. This phenomenon is known as
   a. Newton's first law.
   b. the big bang.
   c. gravitational collapse.
   d. Hubble flow.

4. American author Gertrude Stein was born in
   a. 1713.
   b. 1830.
   c. 1874.
   d. 1901.

5. Which of the following is NOT one of the Five Classics attributed to Confucius?
   a. the *I Ching*
   b. the *Book of Holiness*
   c. the *Spring and Autumn Annals*
   d. the *Book of History*

6. The religious and philosophical doctrine that holds that the universe is constantly in a struggle between good and evil is known as
   a. Pelagianism.
   b. Manichaeanism.
   c. neo-Hegelianism.
   d. Epicureanism.

7. The third chief justice of the U.S. Supreme Court was
   a. John Blair.
   b. William Cushing.
   c. James Wilson.
   d. John Jay.

8. Which of the following is the poisonous portion of a daffodil?
   a. the bulb
   b. the leaves
   c. the stem
   d. the flowers

9. The winner of the Masters golf tournament in 1953 was
   a. Sam Snead.
   b. Cary Middlecoff.
   c. Arnold Palmer.
   d. Ben Hogan.

10. The state with the highest per capita personal income in 1980 was
    a. Alaska.
    b. Connecticut.
    c. New York.
    d. Texas.

Answers

Check your answers against the following correct answers.

1. c.
2. a.
3. d.
4. c.
5. b.
6. b.
7. b.
8. a.
9. d.
10. a.

How Did You Do?

You may have simply gotten lucky and actually known the answer to one or two questions. In addition, your guessing was probably more successful if you were able to use the process of elimination on any of the questions. Maybe you didn't know who the third chief justice was (question 7), but you knew that John Jay was the first. In that case, you would have eliminated choice **d** and, therefore, improved your odds of guessing right from one in four to one in three.

According to probability, you should get two and a half answers correct, so getting either two or three right would be average. If you got four or more right, you may be a really terrific guesser. If you got one or none right, you may be a really bad guesser.

Keep in mind, though, that this is only a small sample. You should continue to keep track of your guessing ability as you work through the sample questions in this book. Circle the numbers of questions you guess on as you make your guesses; or, if you don't have time while you take the practice tests, go back afterward and try to remember which answers were guesses. Remember, on a test with four answer choices, your chances of getting a right answer is one in four. So keep a separate "guessing score" for each exam. How many questions did you guess on? How many did you get right? If the number you got right is at least one-fourth of the number of questions you guessed on, you are at least an average guesser, maybe better—and you should always go ahead and guess on the real exam. If the number you got right is significantly lower than one-fourth of the number you guessed on, you would, frankly, be safe in guessing anyway. But maybe you'd feel more comfortable if you guessed only selectively, when you could eliminate a wrong answer or at least have a good feeling about one of the answer choices.

Exercise

If you don't already have a regular exercise program going, the time during which you're preparing for an exam is actually an excellent time to start one. And if you're already keeping fit—or trying to get that way—don't let the pressure of preparing for an exam fool you into quitting now. Exercise helps reduce stress by pumping wonderful good-feeling hormones called endorphins into your system. It also increases the oxygen supply throughout your body, including your brain, so you'll be at peak performance on test day.

A half hour of vigorous activity—enough to raise a sweat—every day should be your aim. If you're really pressed for time, every other day is okay. Choose an activity you like and get out there and do it. Jogging with a friend always makes the time go faster, as does jogging with an iPod. But don't overdo it. You don't want to exhaust yourself. Moderation is the key.

Diet

First of all, cut out the junk. Go easy on caffeine and nicotine, and eliminate alcohol and any other drugs from your system at least two weeks before the exam. Promise yourself a binge the night after the exam, if need be.

What your body needs for peak performance is simply a balanced diet. Eat plenty of fruits and vegetables, along with protein and carbohydrates. Foods that are high in lecithin (an amino acid), such as fish and beans, are especially good "brain foods."

The night before the exam, you might "carbo-load" the way athletes do before a contest. Eat a big plate of spaghetti, rice and beans, or whatever your favorite carbohydrate is.

Rest

You probably know how much sleep you need every night to be at your best, even if you don't always get it. Make sure you do get that much sleep, though, for at least a week before the exam. Moderation is important here, too. Extra sleep will just make you groggy.

If you're not a morning person and your exam will be given in the morning, you should reset your internal clock so that your body doesn't think you're taking an exam at 3 A.M. You have to start this process well before the exam. The way it works is to get up half an hour earlier each morning, and then go to bed half an hour earlier that night. Don't try it the other way around; you'll just toss and turn if you go to bed early without having gotten up early. The next morning, get up another half an hour earlier, and so on. How long you will have to do this depends on how late you're used to getting up.

Step 8: Get Your Act Together

Time to complete: Ten minutes to read, time to complete will vary

Activity: Complete Final Preparations worksheet.

You're in control of your mind and body; you're in charge of test anxiety, your preparation, and your test-taking strategies. Now it's time to take charge of external factors, like the testing site and the materials you need to take the exam.

Find Out Where the Test Is and Make a Trial Run

The testing agency or your instructor will notify you when and where your exam is being held. Do you know how to get to the testing site? Do you know how long it will take to get there? If not, make a trial run, preferably on the same day of the week at the same time of day. Make a note, on the Final Preparations worksheet on page 31 of the amount of time it will take you to get to the exam site. Plan on arriving 10–15 minutes early so you can get the lay of the land, use the bathroom, and calm down. Then figure out how early you will have to get up that morning, and make sure you get up that early every day for a week before the exam.

Gather Your Materials

The night before the exam, lay out the clothes you will wear and the materials you have to bring with you to the exam. Plan on dressing in layers; you won't have any control over the temperature of the examination room. Have a sweater or jacket you can take off if it's warm. Also, keep in mind that candidates are not permitted to bring digital watches, cell phones, pagers, or other electronic devices into the test room. In addition, food and beverages are not allowed into the test room. (Lockers are provided so that candidates may store personal items while testing.) Use the checklist on the Final Preparations worksheet on page 31 to help you pull together what you'll need.

Don't Skip Breakfast

Even if you don't usually eat breakfast, do so on exam morning. A cup of coffee doesn't count. Don't do doughnuts or other sweet foods, either. A sugar high will leave you with a sugar low in the middle of the exam. A mix of protein and carbohydrates is best. Cereal with milk and just a little sugar or eggs with toast will do your body a world of good.

Step 9: Do It!

Time to complete: Ten minutes, plus test-taking time
Activity: Ace the physical therapist assistants exam!
Fast-forward to exam day. You're ready. You made a study plan and followed through. You practiced your test-taking strategies while working through this book. You're in control of your physical, mental, and emotional state. You know when and where to show up and what to bring with you. In other words, you're better prepared than most of the other people taking the physical therapist assistant's exam with you. You're psyched.

Just one more thing. When you're done with the exam, you will have earned a reward. Plan a celebration. Call up your friends and plan a party, or have a nice dinner for two—whatever your heart desires. Give yourself something to look forward to.

And then do it. Go into the exam, full of confidence, armed with test-taking strategies you've practiced until they're second nature. You're in control of yourself, your environment, and your performance on the exam. You're ready to succeed. So do it. Go in there and ace the exam. And look forward to your future career as a physical therapist assistant!

Final Preparations

Getting to the Exam Site

Location of exam site: _____

Date: _____

Departure time: _____

Do I know how to get to the exam site?   Yes ___   No ___   (If no, make a trial run.)

Time it will take to get to exam site: _____

Things to Lay Out the Night Before

Clothes I will wear   _____

Sweater/jacket   _____

Watch   _____

Photo ID   _____

No. 2 pencils   _____

_____   _____

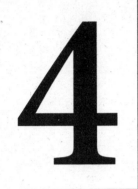

Diagnostic Test

CHAPTER SUMMARY

This Diagnostic Test should be taken before you begin reviewing the topics in Chapters 5 through 8. The practice exam will provide valuable feedback that can be utilized not only to identify your strengths and weaknesses, but also to direct your efforts in preparing for the national exam—the NPTE for PTAs. The variety of academic and clinical application questions are designed to challenge your test-taking skills. You can also refine those skills by slowly reading each question, rereading the question, then reading all possible responses. Strive to develop a test-taking pace of 30–45 seconds per question.

Make a note of the types of questions you miss. Do not neglect any subject area unless you have an almost perfect score in that area. Then develop a study plan, and review the individual topics in Chapters 5 to 8.

Good luck!

Part I

1.	ⓐ	ⓑ	ⓒ	ⓓ
2.	ⓐ	ⓑ	ⓒ	ⓓ
3.	ⓐ	ⓑ	ⓒ	ⓓ
4.	ⓐ	ⓑ	ⓒ	ⓓ
5.	ⓐ	ⓑ	ⓒ	ⓓ
6.	ⓐ	ⓑ	ⓒ	ⓓ
7.	ⓐ	ⓑ	ⓒ	ⓓ
8.	ⓐ	ⓑ	ⓒ	ⓓ
9.	ⓐ	ⓑ	ⓒ	ⓓ
10.	ⓐ	ⓑ	ⓒ	ⓓ
11.	ⓐ	ⓑ	ⓒ	ⓓ
12.	ⓐ	ⓑ	ⓒ	ⓓ
13.	ⓐ	ⓑ	ⓒ	ⓓ
14.	ⓐ	ⓑ	ⓒ	ⓓ
15.	ⓐ	ⓑ	ⓒ	ⓓ
16.	ⓐ	ⓑ	ⓒ	ⓓ
17.	ⓐ	ⓑ	ⓒ	ⓓ
18.	ⓐ	ⓑ	ⓒ	ⓓ
19.	ⓐ	ⓑ	ⓒ	ⓓ
20.	ⓐ	ⓑ	ⓒ	ⓓ
21.	ⓐ	ⓑ	ⓒ	ⓓ
22.	ⓐ	ⓑ	ⓒ	ⓓ
23.	ⓐ	ⓑ	ⓒ	ⓓ
24.	ⓐ	ⓑ	ⓒ	ⓓ
25.	ⓐ	ⓑ	ⓒ	ⓓ
26.	ⓐ	ⓑ	ⓒ	ⓓ
27.	ⓐ	ⓑ	ⓒ	ⓓ
28.	ⓐ	ⓑ	ⓒ	ⓓ
29.	ⓐ	ⓑ	ⓒ	ⓓ
30.	ⓐ	ⓑ	ⓒ	ⓓ
31.	ⓐ	ⓑ	ⓒ	ⓓ
32.	ⓐ	ⓑ	ⓒ	ⓓ
33.	ⓐ	ⓑ	ⓒ	ⓓ
34.	ⓐ	ⓑ	ⓒ	ⓓ
35.	ⓐ	ⓑ	ⓒ	ⓓ
36.	ⓐ	ⓑ	ⓒ	ⓓ
37.	ⓐ	ⓑ	ⓒ	ⓓ
38.	ⓐ	ⓑ	ⓒ	ⓓ
39.	ⓐ	ⓑ	ⓒ	ⓓ
40.	ⓐ	ⓑ	ⓒ	ⓓ
41.	ⓐ	ⓑ	ⓒ	ⓓ
42.	ⓐ	ⓑ	ⓒ	ⓓ
43.	ⓐ	ⓑ	ⓒ	ⓓ
44.	ⓐ	ⓑ	ⓒ	ⓓ
45.	ⓐ	ⓑ	ⓒ	ⓓ
46.	ⓐ	ⓑ	ⓒ	ⓓ
47.	ⓐ	ⓑ	ⓒ	ⓓ
48.	ⓐ	ⓑ	ⓒ	ⓓ
49.	ⓐ	ⓑ	ⓒ	ⓓ
50.	ⓐ	ⓑ	ⓒ	ⓓ

Part II

51.	ⓐ	ⓑ	ⓒ	ⓓ
52.	ⓐ	ⓑ	ⓒ	ⓓ
53.	ⓐ	ⓑ	ⓒ	ⓓ
54.	ⓐ	ⓑ	ⓒ	ⓓ
55.	ⓐ	ⓑ	ⓒ	ⓓ
56.	ⓐ	ⓑ	ⓒ	ⓓ
57.	ⓐ	ⓑ	ⓒ	ⓓ
58.	ⓐ	ⓑ	ⓒ	ⓓ
59.	ⓐ	ⓑ	ⓒ	ⓓ
60.	ⓐ	ⓑ	ⓒ	ⓓ
61.	ⓐ	ⓑ	ⓒ	ⓓ
62.	ⓐ	ⓑ	ⓒ	ⓓ
63.	ⓐ	ⓑ	ⓒ	ⓓ
64.	ⓐ	ⓑ	ⓒ	ⓓ
65.	ⓐ	ⓑ	ⓒ	ⓓ
66.	ⓐ	ⓑ	ⓒ	ⓓ
67.	ⓐ	ⓑ	ⓒ	ⓓ
68.	ⓐ	ⓑ	ⓒ	ⓓ
69.	ⓐ	ⓑ	ⓒ	ⓓ
70.	ⓐ	ⓑ	ⓒ	ⓓ
71.	ⓐ	ⓑ	ⓒ	ⓓ
72.	ⓐ	ⓑ	ⓒ	ⓓ
73.	ⓐ	ⓑ	ⓒ	ⓓ
74.	ⓐ	ⓑ	ⓒ	ⓓ
75.	ⓐ	ⓑ	ⓒ	ⓓ
76.	ⓐ	ⓑ	ⓒ	ⓓ
77.	ⓐ	ⓑ	ⓒ	ⓓ
78.	ⓐ	ⓑ	ⓒ	ⓓ
79.	ⓐ	ⓑ	ⓒ	ⓓ
80.	ⓐ	ⓑ	ⓒ	ⓓ
81.	ⓐ	ⓑ	ⓒ	ⓓ
82.	ⓐ	ⓑ	ⓒ	ⓓ
83.	ⓐ	ⓑ	ⓒ	ⓓ
84.	ⓐ	ⓑ	ⓒ	ⓓ
85.	ⓐ	ⓑ	ⓒ	ⓓ
86.	ⓐ	ⓑ	ⓒ	ⓓ
87.	ⓐ	ⓑ	ⓒ	ⓓ
88.	ⓐ	ⓑ	ⓒ	ⓓ
89.	ⓐ	ⓑ	ⓒ	ⓓ
90.	ⓐ	ⓑ	ⓒ	ⓓ
91.	ⓐ	ⓑ	ⓒ	ⓓ
92.	ⓐ	ⓑ	ⓒ	ⓓ
93.	ⓐ	ⓑ	ⓒ	ⓓ
94.	ⓐ	ⓑ	ⓒ	ⓓ
95.	ⓐ	ⓑ	ⓒ	ⓓ
96.	ⓐ	ⓑ	ⓒ	ⓓ
97.	ⓐ	ⓑ	ⓒ	ⓓ
98.	ⓐ	ⓑ	ⓒ	ⓓ
99.	ⓐ	ⓑ	ⓒ	ⓓ
100.	ⓐ	ⓑ	ⓒ	ⓓ

Part III

101.	ⓐ	ⓑ	ⓒ	ⓓ
102.	ⓐ	ⓑ	ⓒ	ⓓ
103.	ⓐ	ⓑ	ⓒ	ⓓ
104.	ⓐ	ⓑ	ⓒ	ⓓ
105.	ⓐ	ⓑ	ⓒ	ⓓ
106.	ⓐ	ⓑ	ⓒ	ⓓ
107.	ⓐ	ⓑ	ⓒ	ⓓ
108.	ⓐ	ⓑ	ⓒ	ⓓ
109.	ⓐ	ⓑ	ⓒ	ⓓ
110.	ⓐ	ⓑ	ⓒ	ⓓ
111.	ⓐ	ⓑ	ⓒ	ⓓ
112.	ⓐ	ⓑ	ⓒ	ⓓ
113.	ⓐ	ⓑ	ⓒ	ⓓ
114.	ⓐ	ⓑ	ⓒ	ⓓ
115.	ⓐ	ⓑ	ⓒ	ⓓ
116.	ⓐ	ⓑ	ⓒ	ⓓ
117.	ⓐ	ⓑ	ⓒ	ⓓ
118.	ⓐ	ⓑ	ⓒ	ⓓ
119.	ⓐ	ⓑ	ⓒ	ⓓ
120.	ⓐ	ⓑ	ⓒ	ⓓ
121.	ⓐ	ⓑ	ⓒ	ⓓ
122.	ⓐ	ⓑ	ⓒ	ⓓ
123.	ⓐ	ⓑ	ⓒ	ⓓ
124.	ⓐ	ⓑ	ⓒ	ⓓ
125.	ⓐ	ⓑ	ⓒ	ⓓ
126.	ⓐ	ⓑ	ⓒ	ⓓ
127.	ⓐ	ⓑ	ⓒ	ⓓ
128.	ⓐ	ⓑ	ⓒ	ⓓ
129.	ⓐ	ⓑ	ⓒ	ⓓ
130.	ⓐ	ⓑ	ⓒ	ⓓ
131.	ⓐ	ⓑ	ⓒ	ⓓ
132.	ⓐ	ⓑ	ⓒ	ⓓ
133.	ⓐ	ⓑ	ⓒ	ⓓ
134.	ⓐ	ⓑ	ⓒ	ⓓ
135.	ⓐ	ⓑ	ⓒ	ⓓ
136.	ⓐ	ⓑ	ⓒ	ⓓ
137.	ⓐ	ⓑ	ⓒ	ⓓ
138.	ⓐ	ⓑ	ⓒ	ⓓ
139.	ⓐ	ⓑ	ⓒ	ⓓ
140.	ⓐ	ⓑ	ⓒ	ⓓ
141.	ⓐ	ⓑ	ⓒ	ⓓ
142.	ⓐ	ⓑ	ⓒ	ⓓ
143.	ⓐ	ⓑ	ⓒ	ⓓ
144.	ⓐ	ⓑ	ⓒ	ⓓ
145.	ⓐ	ⓑ	ⓒ	ⓓ
146.	ⓐ	ⓑ	ⓒ	ⓓ
147.	ⓐ	ⓑ	ⓒ	ⓓ
148.	ⓐ	ⓑ	ⓒ	ⓓ
149.	ⓐ	ⓑ	ⓒ	ⓓ
150.	ⓐ	ⓑ	ⓒ	ⓓ

Part I

1. A PTA is working with a patient in the early postoperative phase, following a recent reverse (Putti-Platt) posterior shoulder reconstruction. Which of the following movements should be avoided?
   a. abduction and external rotation
   b. abduction and internal rotation
   c. adduction and internal rotation
   d. adduction and external rotation

2. A PTA is reviewing the physical therapist's initial evaluation and a pediatric patient's history. She notes that the patient sustained a traction injury to the lower brachial plexus (Klumpke's or Klumpke-Dejerine paralysis) as an infant during childbirth. What nerve levels does this involve?
   a. C3 and C4
   b. C5 and C6
   c. C8 and T1
   d. C7 and C8

3. A student PTA is preparing for a clinical education rotation on a cardiac rehabilitation unit. What is the normal cardiac index (CI) range?
   a. 2.5 to 3.5 L/min/m^2
   b. 0.5 to 1.5 L/min/m^2
   c. 1.0 to 3.0 L/min/m^2
   d. 1.0 to 4.0 L/min/m^2

4. A PTA is working with a pediatric patient. At what month should sitting alone steadily be present in normal development?
   a. 4–5 months
   b. 8–9 months
   c. 10–11 months
   d. 6–7 months

5. A PTA is working with a pediatric patient. At what month should walking alone be present in normal development?
   a. 5–6 months
   b. 7–8 months
   c. 9–10 months
   d. 11–12 months

6. A patient reports pain at the humeral lateral epicondyle after playing racquet ball. Which resisted motion, when applied by a PTA, would stress the tissue?
   a. wrist extension
   b. wrist flexion
   c. wrist ulnar deviation
   d. wrist radial deviation

7. A PTA is working with a 12-year-old male patient with a diagnosis of Osgood-Schlatter's disease. Where would this patient complain of pain?
   a. tibial tuberosity
   b. ischial tuberosity
   c. lateral malleolus
   d. greater trochanter

8. A PTA is working with a patient with piriformis syndrome. What motion will stretch the piriformis muscle?
   a. external rotation
   b. flexion
   c. internal rotation
   d. extension

9. A PTA is observing a pressure ulcer. She notes full thickness loss with extensive destruction and tissue necrosis with damage to muscle present. Using the pressure ulcer classification system adopted by the National Pressure Ulcer Advisory Panel (NPUAP), what stage is this ulcer as described?
   a. stage I
   b. stage II
   c. stage IV
   d. stage III

10. A PTA desires to strengthen the posterior rotator cuff and maximize supraspinatus muscle activity. What is the best position to achieve this treatment goal?
    a. prone horizontal abduction to eye level with the arm in full external rotation
    b. standing flexion to eye level with the arm in full internal rotation
    c. side lying horizontal abduction to eye level with the arm in full internal rotation
    d. supine adduction to eye level with the arm in full external rotation

11. A patient is performing a straight leg raise (SLR) exercise. A PTA desires to make the exercise the most difficult to perform without increasing the size of the cuff weight. Where should the PTA place the cuff weight?
    a. ankle joint
    b. knee joint
    c. mid-calf
    d. upper thigh

12. A PTA is working with a patient with a postoperative shoulder. Which procedure involves suturing the capsule and labrum back down to the anterior glenoidal rim?
    a. Bankart
    b. Putti-Platt
    c. Magnuson-Stack
    d. Bristow

13. The physical therapist evaluation indicates your patient is on a beta blocker. A normal heart rate reaction in your patient while exercising on a treadmill should be
    a. a slight elevation.
    b. no elevation.
    c. an extreme elevation.
    d. a normal decrease in HR.

14. Knowing that blood pressure (BP) = cardiac output (CO) × total peripheral resistance (TPR), your burn patient presents with an elevated BP and a decrease in blood flow (Q). The PTA then would expect the patient's body to respond by
    a. an increase in HR secondary to a decrease in stroke volume.
    b. BP not related to blood flow.
    c. a decrease in HR secondary to a decrease in stroke volume.
    d. an increase in BP and stroke volume and a decrease in HR.

15. Knowing that blood pressure = cardiac output × total peripheral resistance, what would be a normal response to exercise?
    a. increase in CO and increase in TPR
    b. decrease in CO and increase in TPR
    c. no response or change
    d. increase in cardiac output and decrease in total peripheral resistance

16. Which of the following is correct if normal ejection fraction (EF) values fall between 60%–80%, and a patient's heart fills with 100 mL of blood and pumps out 50 mL?
    a. Patient has 100% EF and is not compromised.
    b. Patient is within normal range.
    c. Patient has 50% ejection fraction and is compromised.
    d. The heart cannot fill with 100 mL of blood.

17. A clinical presentation of an obstructive pulmonary disease includes
   a. dyspnea, wheezing, and broad chest.
   b. normal physical appearance; no abnormality.
   c. dry cough and clubbing of digits.
   d. cyanosis, tachypnea, and stiff lungs.

18. The patient is diagnosed with left ventricle heart failure and presents to the PT department for exercise therapy. The PTA would be aware of
   a. bradycardia.
   b. postural blood pressure changes.
   c. decreased level of exercise tolerance.
   d. pulsation visible above right clavicle.

19. A PTA is performing a home health visit of a patient who sustained a T6 spinal cord injury three months earlier. The patient complains of severe pounding headache, blurred vision, and sweating. The PTA takes his blood pressure and pulse finding hypertension and bradycardia. Which of the following is the most likely cause of these symptoms?
   a. autonomic dysreflexia
   b. pneumonia
   c. swine flu
   d. allergic reaction

20. A PTA is instructing a patient who is in a wheelchair, full-time, due to a spinal cord injury, on the importance of weight shift to prevent pressure ulcers. What time frequency is prescribed?
   a. 20 minutes
   b. 15 minutes
   c. 30 minutes
   d. 45 minutes

21. A PTA is dressing a burn on a patient with a pseudomonas infection. Which topical medication works best to treat this type of infection?
   a. silver sulfidiazine
   b. silver nitrate
   c. bacitracin
   d. collagenase

22. A PTA is working with a patient who is unable to shift weight on her own. What is the maximum amount of time that should elapse before a change of position is required to prevent tissue breakdown?
   a. 1 hour
   b. 1.5 hours
   c. 2 hours
   d. 2.5 hours

23. A PTA is working with a patient after a stroke who exhibits uncontrolled outbursts of crying which quickly change to laughing. What condition is the patient experiencing?
   a. expressive aphasia
   b. seasonal affective disorder
   c. dementia
   d. pseudobulbar effect

24. A PTA is working with a patient after a stroke who is unaware of recent sensory and motor deficits, resulting in significant difficulty when performing a transfer activity safely. What area of the brain is affected?
   a. left hemisphere
   b. frontal lobe
   c. right hemisphere
   d. limbic system

25. A student PTA is performing a clinical education rotation in a rehabilitation center and will be working with patients with spinal cord injuries. What is the most frequent cause of autonomic dysreflexia in this patient population?
    a. bladder distention
    b. pneumonia
    c. bronchitis
    d. allergic reaction

26. A PTA is working bedside on lying-to-sitting bed transfers with a patient with a recent spinal cord injury when the patient reports dizziness at the completion of the transfer. What should the PTA suspect caused the dizziness?
    a. spasticity
    b. respiratory impairment
    c. Raynaud's phenomenon
    d. postural hypotension

27. Which of the following tissue structures is innervated by the vagus nerve?
    a. diaphragm
    b. bronchioles
    c. serratus anterior
    d. rectus abdominus

28. A PTA is preparing for a rotation on the spinal cord injury unit. What is the highest level of injury at which functional expectations for the patient would include skin inspection and pressure relief, bowel and bladder care, self-feeding, and dressing?
    a. C6
    b. C5
    c. C4
    d. C1, C2, C3

29. A PTA is working with a patient after a stroke who presents left-side unilateral neglect and agnosia. Which area of the brain has been injured?
    a. right brain injury
    b. left brain injury
    c. frontal lobe
    d. limbic system

30. A PTA is working with a patient after a stroke who presents difficulty comprehending and following simple commands. Which area of the brain has been injured?
    a. right hemisphere
    b. left hemisphere
    c. posterior lobe
    d. limbic system

31. A PTA is working with a patient following a stroke who comprehends verbal instructions. However, when asked a related question, the patient is unable to respond. What is the problem?
    a. Broca's aphasia
    b. Wernicke's aphasia
    c. agnosia
    d. psyarthria

32. The PTA has completed muscle-length testing on a patient and has identified that she has a positive Thomas test bilaterally. Given this finding, which of the following postural deviations would the PTA also expect to see?
    a. posterior pelvic tilt
    b. anterior pelvic tilt
    c. elevated pelvis
    d. depressed pelvis

33. Which of the following findings is inconsistent with patellofemoral syndrome?
a. Q angle less than ten degrees
b. positive Ober test
c. positive Thomas test with the hip moving into abduction and internal rotation (IR)
d. 3–/5 strength of the vastus medialis oblique (VMO)

34. Which of the following positions should be avoided until late in the rehabilitation process for a patient who sustained a proximal tendon rupture of the long head of the biceps brachii?
a. elbow flexion, shoulder flexion, and forearm supination
b. elbow extension, shoulder extension, and forearm pronation
c. elbow flexion, shoulder extension, and forearm supination
d. elbow extension, shoulder flexion, and forearm pronation

35. Patients with coxa valga are at increased risk for developing which of the following conditions?
a. toe-in posture
b. hip dislocation
c. toe-out posture
d. femoral neck fracture

36. A PTA instructs a patient in the day's treatment plan. The patient correctly repeats the instructions for a sit-to-stand transfer. As the PTA cues the patient to initiate the transfer, the patient asks the PTA what she is supposed to be doing. This patient is demonstrating impairment of
a. immediate memory.
b. short-term memory.
c. remote memory.
d. long-term memory.

37. A PTA is reviewing a physical therapy evaluation for a patient she is about to treat in the ICU. She notes that the patient was rated at a level III on the Ranchos Los Amigos at the time of evaluation. What kind of behavior should the PTA expect from this patient?
a. automatic appropriate
b. confused inappropriate
c. localized response
d. generalized response

38. The PTA observes the physical therapist performing an initial examination of a patient with an open wound on the distal toes. The therapist is palpating a pulse on the dorsum of the foot. Which artery is the therapist assessing?
a. femoral artery
b. popliteal artery
c. dorsalis pedis artery
d. tibial artery

39. The PTA removes a semipermeable foam dressing from a venous wound and notes a large amount of thin, clear, yellow drainage. What is the most important information needed by the PTA to assess whether or not the drainage is normal?
a. whether or not the wound is infected
b. who applied the last dressing
c. the patient's nutritional status
d. when the dressing was applied

40. Read the following descriptions of a pressure ulcer on the ischial tuberosity. Which is most likely to be infected?
   a. stage II; covered 100% with yellow slough; minimal clear yellow drainage; surrounding skin macerated
   b. stage III; 50% yellow slough, 50% pale, dry granulation tissue; moderate thick, tan drainage; surrounding skin inflamed
   c. stage III; covered with brown eschar; no drainage; surrounding skin reddened
   d. stage IV; 75% yellow slough, 25% red granulation tissue; moderate pink drainage; surrounding skin reddened

41. As a result of a stressful test eliciting an individual's fear of falling, the hormone most likely to be secreted is
   a. glucagon.
   b. cortisol.
   c. norepinephrine.
   d. thyroxine.

42. During tests or measures that cause fear, the body may release _____ in preparation for a _____ response.
   a. epinephrine; fight or flight
   b. cortisol; stress
   c. norepinephrine; fight or flight
   d. cortisol; pain

43. A patient receives the majority of the sensory information regarding balance while standing on a firm, level surface from which system?
   a. vestibular—semicircular canals
   b. vestibular—utricle and saccule
   c. visual
   d. somatosensory

44. Which of the following is NOT a neural adaptation associated with strength training?
   a. increased number of motor units firing
   b. increased twitch contraction time
   c. increased rate of firing
   d. increased synchronization of firing

45. A PTA and a patient are discussing the patient's concerns about falling at home. The patient reports that she worries the most about having to walk down the gravel and dirt driveway to the mailbox in the afternoon. The patient reports no other environment or time of day where she feels unstable. Based on the patient's report, what balance system should the PTA expect to be impaired?
   a. vestibular system
   b. visual system
   c. somatosensory system
   d. auditory system

46. A PTA is performing postural stabilization exercises with a patient following surgery to the lower back. Postural muscles are type ___ muscles and respond best to what type of exercise intensity and duration?
   a. I; high intensity, short duration
   b. II; high intensity, long duration
   c. I; low intensity, long duration
   d. II; low intensity, short duration

47. A patient with coronary artery disease is exercising, and the PTA is monitoring the patient's response to increased cardiovascular activity. Which of the following would the PTA expect to see?
  a. a sharp drop in diastolic blood pressure just after stopping exercise
  b. an increase in HR during and just after stopping exercise
  c. a decrease in RR during and just after stopping exercise
  d. a decrease in systolic blood pressure during exercise

48. The PTA walks into the waiting room to let her next patient know that she is ready for the treatment session. The patient stands from the chair and begins to fall forward. Which muscles must strongly contract to prevent a fall?
  a. hip flexors
  b. hip extensors
  c. trunk flexors
  d. trunk extensors

49. The PTA is observing a group of children playing in the waiting room while the PTA awaits the arrival of her next patient. The PTA observes a young girl trying to walk a straight line on the tiled floor. Another child accidentally and lightly bumps the girl walking on the straight line on the side of her shoulder. Which strategy is the girl walking on the straight line most likely to use for balance in this position?
  a. ankle strategy
  b. hip strategy
  c. stepping strategy
  d. jumping strategy

50. A PTA and physical therapist are working with a social worker to make recommendations for long-term care placement for a stroke patient. What is the best assessment tool to assist with this task?
  a. Functional Independence Measure (FIM)
  b. Nagi Model
  c. International Classification of Impairments, Disabilities, and Handicaps
  d. *Guide to Physical Therapist Practice*

Part II

51. The PTA has a patient with right-sided carpal tunnel syndrome and who is complaining of swelling after typing for more than 30 minutes. The PTA would like to take pre- and post-activity measurements to determine the extent of swelling in the patient's hands. Which of the following tools would be the best choice to accomplish this?
  a. circumferential measurements every 5 cm from the radial styloid
  b. figure-eight measurements from the ulnar styloid
  c. volumetrics up to the radial styloid
  d. limb length from capitate to end of distal phalanx of third digit

52. The PTA's patient is a 40-year-old male with sudden onset of lower back pain and radiating symptoms down into his right lateral calf. His patella and achilles reflex are intact, but he cannot heel walk. His MRI most likely shows a herniated disc at what level?
  a. L4
  b. L5
  c. S1
  d. S2

53. The PTA observes a patient ambulating down the hallway. The patient is lifting the right hip and knee high in the air and does not have a true heel strike because his foot slaps the ground. What is the correct term for this gait pattern?
    a. drop foot
    b. steppage
    c. Trendelenburg
    d. compensated Trendelenburg

54. The PTA observes that a patient is using a reverse action of the gastrocnemius to compensate for a specific weakness that impacts gait. What is the most likely reason that the patient is using this compensation?
    a. drop foot
    b. Trendelenburg
    c. quadriceps weakness
    d. gluteus maximus weakness

55. A patient underwent surgery three days ago. The PTA has been asked to take girth measurements of the patient's right and left lower extremities. The measurements are as follows:
    mid patella—R: 44 cm L: 39 cm
    10 cm above—R: 52cm L: 56 cm
    10 cm below—R: 38 cm L: 37 cm
    Which of the following statements is NOT consistent with the other conclusions?
    a. Surgery was on the knee.
    b. Atrophy is present over the quadriceps.
    c. Edema is primarily around the knee.
    d. Atrophy is present over the gastrocnemius.

56. Which test will assess the patient's risk for falls during ambulation in the shortest amount of time?
    a. Tinetti Performance Oriented Mobility Assessment (POMA)
    b. Berg Balance Scale
    c. timed up and go (TUG) test
    d. Dynamic Gait Index (DGI)

57. The patient is performing isokinetic testing at 60, 180, and 300 degrees/second of the quadriceps and hamstring muscle groups. The patient has been asked to work as hard as he can until the test is terminated, when the patient reaches 50% of peak torque. This test is designed to measure which component of muscular performance?
    a. muscle power
    b. muscle endurance
    c. muscle strength
    d. muscle agility

58. A patient sustained a terrible triad injury to his right knee playing football. Which of the following special tests would not be positive given this injury?
    a. Lachman's test
    b. McMurray's test
    c. varus stress test
    d. valgus stress test

59. Based on the following results, which patient would be at the greatest risk for falls?
    a. single-leg stance test—10 seconds
    b. functional reach test—10 inches
    c. Berg Balance Scale—24
    d. Tinetti Performance Oriented Mobility Assessment—24

60. Which of the following positions would be the best to assess the strength of the vastus medialis against gravity?
   a. seated with hips flexed 90 degrees and hip externally rotated and resist knee extension
   b. seated with hips flexed 45 degrees and hip externally rotated and resist knee extension
   c. seated with hips flexed 90 degrees and hip internally rotated and resist knee extension
   d. seated with hips flexed 45 degrees and hip internally rotated and resist knee extension

61. A PTA has been asked to assist with collecting range of motion measurements for a workers compensation patient with mechanical lower back pain. Which tool would be the most beneficial, given this patient's diagnosis and insurance environment?
   a. bubble inclinometer
   b. dual inclinometer
   c. tape measure to the floor
   d. standard goniometry

62. A PTA is preparing to examine an infant's primitive reflexes. When assessing the Babinski reflex, the PTA should expect which of the following responses?
   a. toe curling
   b. forefoot pronation
   c. toe fanning
   d. forefoot supination

63. A PTA is preparing to examine an infant's neck righting reflex. The most appropriate stimulus for this test is
   a. passive cervical flexion.
   b. passive cervical extension.
   c. passive cervical rotation.
   d. passive lateral cervical flexion.

64. A PTA wants to assess a patient's static and dynamic balance during everyday functional activities such as picking objects up off the floor and reaching forward. The best standardized assessment tool to use is
   a. gait subscale of Tinetti Performance Orientated Mobility Assessment.
   b. Berg Balance Scale.
   c. timed up and go test.
   d. multidirectional reach test.

65. A PTA is performing observational gait analysis with a patient who has documented anterior tibialis weakness. The PTA anticipates that this patient will present with what type of gait pattern?
   a. steppage gait
   b. scissoring gait
   c. Trendelenberg gait
   d. dystrophic gait

66. A PTA is assessing passive movement in the lower extremity of a patient who recently experienced a stroke. She notices that when she performs passive movement there is some resistance to the motion, and the faster she moves the limb, the more resistance she feels. This resistance is best described as
   a. dystonia.
   b. hypotonia.
   c. rigidity.
   d. spasticity.

67. The PTA cannot palpate the pulse in the dorsalis pedis artery on a patient with suspected arterial insufficiency. What is another test and measure that would give information about arterial function?
   a. Ankle-Brachial Index
   b. blood pressure
   c. girth measurement
   d. temperature assessment

68. A patient has sustained burns to the anterior aspect of the right hip. Which joint motions would be most important to measure?
a. hip flexion, adduction, and internal rotation
b. hip flexion, abduction, and external rotation
c. hip extension, adduction, and internal rotation
d. hip extension, abduction, and external rotation

69. To ensure patient safety, which motion should the PTA instruct a patient to avoid when the patient is post-op for recurrent anterior shoulder dislocations?
a. internal rotation
b. external rotation
c. extension
d. adduction

70. A patient is being seen one year following burn injuries. Which of the following would describe the best outcome for scar management?
a. slightly raised, pink in color, and moderately pliable
b. moderately raised, red in color, and moderately pliable
c. slighty raised, normal skin tone in color, and very pliable
d. moderately raised, pink in color, and moderately pliable

71. The physical therapy tests and measures that can have the most significant impact on the metabolic and endocrine systems are
a. anthropometric tests.
b. assistive and adaptive devices.
c. aerobic capacity and endurance tests.
d. arousal and attention assessments.

72. A PTA is performing a work reintegration assessment with an individual who is a mail carrier. The most likely endocrine response to this assessment is
a. increased secretion of norepinephrine.
b. decreased uptake of blood glucose.
c. decreased secretion of norepinephrine.
d. increased uptake of blood glucose.

73. What are the three common ways to assess self-care and independence in the community?
a. self-report, observational screen, and direct examination by a PT
b. medical history review, nursing functional screen, and self-report
c. family member report, observational screen, and self-report
d. observational screen, doctor's physical examination, and direct examination by a PT

74. A PTA takes a pulse oximetry level on a patient who completed ten minutes of bicycle riding at moderate resistance and gets a pulse oximetry value of 85%. What does this value represent?
a. inadequate arterial blood oxygen saturation
b. adequate arterial blood oxygen saturation
c. inadequate venous blood oxygen saturation
d. adequate venous blood oxygen saturation

75. A PTA is listening with a stethoscope to a patient's breathing and hears crackles, or a sound that mimics the opening or closing of a cellophane bag. What medical condition is associated with this breathing sound?
a. congestive heart failure
b. airway obstruction
c. narrowing of the trachea
d. foreign object

76. Which of the following is NOT an appropriate recommendation for patients with patellofemoral syndrome?
   a. minimize ascending and descending stairs
   b. sit with your knee extended out rather than flexed
   c. when squatting, make sure your knees go past your toes
   d. avoid kneeling even on padded surfaces

77. A PTA is treating the ankle of a 15-year-old athlete who sprained his ankle last night in a track event. The PTA received a request from the supervising therapist to apply compression wrapping to the involved ankle and foot, elevate the involved foot above the heart with the patient in the supine position, and apply ice for approximately ten minutes. Just before carrying out the treatment, the PTA notices that the ankle is swollen, very bruised, and warm to the touch. What information would NOT be documented in the objective portion of the daily note?
   a. compression wrapping to involved ankle and foot
   b. ankle is swollen, very bruised, and warm to the touch
   c. apply ice for ten minutes
   d. sprained ankle at track event

78. A patient is two weeks s/p subacromial decompression procedure to his right shoulder. Along with this procedure, he had a small rotator cuff tear repaired in his supraspinatus tendon. The PTA's orders are to begin moving this patient within the patient's pain tolerance. With which of the following movements should the PTA begin?
   a. AROM scapula retraction
   b. PROM shoulder abduction
   c. AROM shoulder flexion
   d. PROM of shoulder internal rotation with shoulder adducted to the side

79. Which of the following activities would be the best choice for a patient with osteoarthritis in both ankles and who is trying to improve his aerobic capacity?
   a. BAPS board in sitting clockwise and counterclockwise movements in sitting
   b. stationary bicycling at 60 RPMs
   c. single leg standing on foam for 30 second sets
   d. ladder drills hopping forward to back and side to side

80. The patient is a 40-year-old male tennis player who injured his right dominant shoulder. He desires to work on his overhand cross-body serve. Which PNF pattern would be most helpful to simulate the sequence of the serve?
   a. D1 flexion of the UE
   b. D1 extension of the UE
   c. D2 flexion of the UE
   d. D2 extension of the UE

81. The PTA is working with a 50-year-old female patient who is now three weeks after an arthroscopic left nondominant rotator cuff repair. Based on the surgical protocol, the patient is to progress to AAROM today. When she arrives for her appointment, she is holding her arm close to her body and reports pain on a 7 out of 10. She reports that she has been working hard on her pulleys at home. What should the PTA do first?
   a. Do not treat the patient at all. Have her go home, take her medicine, and call her physician.
   b. Question the patient further about which activities she did at home that are increasing her pain, and review how she should perform the pulley exercises.
   c. Begin the next phase of the protocol because some increase in pain is expected.
   d. Recognize that the patient likely did too much during her most recent appointment, and change the treatment to ice and electrical stimulation to manage the patient's symptoms.

82. The physical therapist assistant is working with a patient who sustained burns over 25% of his body. The patient is concerned about his pain and does not understand the importance of strength training exercises. What would be the most appropriate statement for the PTA to make to this patient in order to motivate him to participate in strength training activities?

a. "After a burn, you lose body weight and muscle mass. Strength training will help you to regain what you have lost."

b. "Strength training is not as important as making sure we prevent contractures. How about we work on wand exercises instead?"

c. "After a burn, there is a chance you can develop peripheral neuropathy. By performing strength training activities, we can prevent that from occurring."

d. "Strength training will help your burns heal faster."

83. A PTA is monitoring a patient during an exercise program. The patient walked on a treadmill for 20 minutes at 70% of his maximum heart rate with no adverse reaction during exercise. The next day, the patient experienced excessive fatigue that limited his daily activities. What is the best way to adapt this exercise during the next treatment session to prevent another negative response?

a. decrease exercise intensity

b. decrease exercise duration

c. change the mode of exercise

d. decrease exercise frequency

84. The PTA is working with a 47-year-old patient with high blood pressure on a new cardio-vascular training program following a total hip replacement. The Borg Rate of Perceived Exertion (RPE) Scale is being used to monitor the response to exercise due to the patient's cardiac medications. What grade on the 15-point Borg scale is an appropriate starting intensity for an aerobic exercise program?

a. 9

b. 10

c. 13

d. 15

85. A PTA is working with a patient on an endurance training program and is monitoring the patient's response to exercise. At initiation of the session, the patient's blood pressure was 134/86, and his resting HR was 64 bpm. After 15 minutes of activity, the patient's blood pressure is 115/65, and his HR is 112 bpm. What is the most appropriate action for the PTA?

a. increase intensity to 80% HR maximum

b. continue exercising

c. begin a five-minute cool down

d. stop exercise immediately

86. The PTA is initiating treatment with a patient who is having trouble relaxing, and the PTA decides to try the use of diaphragmatic breathing to help calm the patient. What is the best way for the PTA to facilitate diaphragmatic breathing?

a. Place a hand over the diaphragm, and "push" the diaphragm into hand while exhaling.

b. Place a hand over the diaphragm, and "push" the diaphragm into hand while inhaling.

c. Place a hand over the sternum, and "push" the chest up into hand while exhaling.

d. Place a hand over the sternum, and "push" the chest up into hand while inhaling.

87. The PTA's plan for today's treatment session with a 37-year-old female patient is lower extremity strengthening following a quadriceps pull of six weeks ago. The PTA is determining the patient's one repetition max for knee flexion, which she determines is 35 pounds. With this information, the PTA calculates the weight to be used during the strength training program. What is the most appropriate weight for knee flexion strength training with this patient?
- **a.** 15 pounds
- **b.** 20 pounds
- **c.** 25 pounds
- **d.** 30 pounds

88. The PTA is working with a patient who experienced a traumatic brain injury, and the PTA has been working on skilled upper extremity movements in quadruped. The PT asks her to progress through the developmental postures with the patient. What is the next posture that the PTA should use for training?
- **a.** kneeling
- **b.** sitting
- **c.** modified plantigrade
- **d.** standing

89. The PTA would like to use percussion to help loosen secretions with a patient during postural drainage. For which patient would this be most appropriate?
- **a.** a patient with a pulmonary embolus
- **b.** a patient on an anticoagulant medication
- **c.** a patient with chronic bronchitis
- **d.** a patient two days s/p thoracotomy

90. Following a CVA, a patient with lower left extremity extensor spasticity is referred to physical therapy for functional training and spasticity management. The PTA working with this patient would most likely use which of the following techniques to assist in this patient's sit-to-stand training?
- **a.** joint approximation of the left knee before standing
- **b.** prolonged stretching of the hip extensors before standing
- **c.** quick stroking to the knee flexors during standing
- **d.** manual contact to the extensors during standing

91. You are working with a patient status post T10 SCI. Which of the following is the first position on the mat which will promote weightbearing through the hips and facilitate initial control of the lower trunk and hips?
- **a.** prone on elbows
- **b.** long sitting without upper extremity support
- **c.** quadruped
- **d.** supine on elbows

92. You are treating a patient with venous insufficiency. The physical therapist has asked you to provide patient education regarding prevention of open areas. Which of the following activities would be most important in preventing an ulcer?
- **a.** keeping skin clean, dry, and moisturized
- **b.** wearing well-fitting footwear
- **c.** wearing compression garments to minimize edema
- **d.** visual inspection of the skin

93. You are treating a patient with a partial thickness arterial ulcer on the lateral malleolus. Which of the following topical dressings would be most appropriate?
    a. calcium alginate
    b. hydrogel
    c. semipermeable foam
    d. semipermeable film

94. Which of the following interventions is most important in facilitating a flat scar formation following a burn?
    a. keeping the skin clean and dry
    b. moisturizing the skin
    c. applying pressure to the scar
    d. applying massage to the scar

95. All of the following factors increase metabolism EXCEPT
    a. application of cold pack to skin.
    b. a stressful situation.
    c. application of moist heat to skin.
    d. increasing muscle to adipose tissue ratio.

96. Exercise affects the body's response to hormones, including those of the pancreas. Which of the following is the best description of the body's response to exercise?
    a. increased glucagon sensitivity
    b. decreased glucagon sensitivity
    c. increased insulin sensitivity
    d. decreased insulin sensitivity

97. In order to improve balance, a PTA is working with an elderly patient with a history of falls. Which of the following medications may increase the chance of falling in the elderly population?
    a. calcium blockers
    b. antacids
    c. antibiotics
    d. analgesics

98. A PTA is working with a 68-year-old patient who is one week post-op on a surgical above-knee amputation secondary to diabetes. What is the best indicator of cardiovascular functional capacity to be considered in preparation for prosthesis gait training?
    a. maximum oxygen uptake (VO2 Max)
    b. Body Mass Index (BMI)
    c. sit and reach test
    d. Trendelenburg test

99. A PTA is performing postural drainage and desires to drain the upper lobe posterior segments. What is the best patient position to achieve this goal?
    a. The patient leans over a folded pillow at a 30 degree angle.
    b. The patient lies on his or her back with a pillow under the knees.
    c. The patient lies on his or her abdomen with two pillows under the hips.
    d. The patient lies on his or her side, head down, with a pillow under the knees.

100. A PTA is working with a patient who has a neuropathic ulcer on the plantar surface of the foot. The treatment goal is to initiate ambulation on the extremity while reducing weight-bearing stress. What is the best method to reduce stress?
    a. total contact cast
    b. cast shoe
    c. post-op shoe
    d. cushioned athletic shoe

Part III

101. The physical therapist assistant is working on transfers with a patient who has an unstable cervical fracture. What type of cervical orthosis does the PTA expect to find the patient wearing?
  a. SOMI (suboccipital mandubular immobilizer)
  b. Phildelphia
  c. Minerva
  d. Halo

102. An 11-year-old female patient is diagnosed with idiopathic scoliosis. She is being considered for a CTLSO to manage her problem. Given this knowledge, what is the most likely location of her scoliosis?
  a. 10 degree right thoracic curve at T12
  b. 55 degree left thoracic curve at T7
  c. 35 degree left thoracic curve at T5
  d. 22 degree right thoracic curve at T10

103. Which of the following is not necessary to check when assessing the fit of a wrist cock-up splint?
  a. distal end of splint ends proximal to the proximal palmar crease
  b. measures 10–15 degrees of wrist extension
  c. able to slip one finger in between the Velcro strap and the brace
  d. red areas on the dorsum of the forearm

104. Which of the following patients would be most appropriate for teaching ambulation with a rolling walker with five inch casters?
  a. 12-year-old with non-displaced fibular fracture
  b. 34-year-old male who just underwent a right arthroscopic menisectomy
  c. 75-year-old female with an uncemented total hip arthroplasty
  d. 68-year-old male with spinal stenosis and bilateral lower extremity weakness

105. You observe a patient ambulating with axillary crutches. The patient moves both crutches forward together, then the left foot even with the crutches, and finally moves the right foot past the left foot. The patient then repeats the process. Choose the correct pattern that would be documented in the patient's chart.
  a. two point swing-through gait
  b. three point step-to gait
  c. two point step-to gait
  d. three point step-through gait

106. You are asked to evaluate the fit of a permanent prosthesis on a patient with a transfemoral amputation. Which of the following would be an area of concern that should be addressed prior to using the prosthesis independently?
  a. redness over the patella tendon
  b. the shrinker and the residual limb fitting into the prosthesis with good contact
  c. when ambulating, the socket pistons approximately one-half inch during the swing phase
  d. when the patient reports that he is a bit achy after being on his feet for one hour

107. A PTA is performing an orthotic assessment with a patient who has recently started wearing an AFO due to dorsiflexion weakness. During gait, the patient demonstrates excessive knee extension during the stance phase of the involved lower extremity. The most likely cause for this gait deviation is
  a. inadequate plantar flexion stop.
  b. excessive dorsiflexion assist.
  c. inadequate heel lift.
  d. inadequate transverse plane alignment.

108. A PTA is assessing the fit of a KAFO with a patient who has never used this type of device before. The most appropriate approach to aligning the ankle joint of the orthotic is
a. aligning the KAFO ankle joint with the proximal tip of the medial malleolus.
b. aligning the KAFO ankle joint with the distal tip of the medial malleolus.
c. aligning the KAFO ankle joint with the anterior tip of the medial malleolus.
d. aligning the KAFO ankle joint with the posterior tip of the medial malleolus.

109. A PTA is working with patient status post-immobility secondary to a fractured left femur. The patient presents with decreased knee extension ROM on the left, and the PTA chooses static stretching to increase ROM. What is the best provision of static stretching for this patient?
a. moist heat to the knee extensors followed by three reps of 15-second knee extension stretches
b. moist heat to the knee flexors followed by three reps of 30-second knee extension stretches
c. three reps of 15-second stretches to the knee flexors followed by moist heat
d. three reps of 30-second hold stretches to the knee extensors followed by moist heat

110. The supervising PT asks the PTA to fit a new patient for a rolling walker. The PTA reads that the patient is 5'5", and he sets the walker for that height. To verify the fit, the PTA has the patient stand in the walker and grasp the handgrips. What should the PTA look for in order to confirm a good fit?
a. less than 5 degrees of elbow flexion when grasping the handgrips
b. 5 to 10 degrees of elbow flexion when grasping the handgrips
c. 20 to 30 degrees of elbow flexion when grasping the handgrips
d. 35 to 40 degrees of elbow flexion when grasping the handgrips

111. The PTA is working with a patient with advanced type II diabetes mellitus. Following gait training with a new knee-ankle-foot orthosis, which of the following should be the primary concern of the PTA?
a. skin condition of the extremity with the orthotic device
b. the patient's ability to don/doff the orthotic device
c. the patient's cardiovascular response to ambulation
d. the patient's comfort level with the look of the orthotic device

112. A patient is presenting with foot slap at heel strike. Which of the following should an ankle-foot orthosis for this patient include?
a. hyperextension stop
b. rotation stop
c. plantarflexion stop
d. dorsiflexion stop

113. A PTA is performing gait training with a patient status post left hip fracture. The patient's orders include weight-bearing as tolerated, and the patient is using a large-based quad cane. Which of the following is the correct use of the quad cane for this patient?
  a. Hold the quad cane on the left, and advance with the left lower extremity.
  b. Hold the quad cane on the right, and advance with the right lower extremity.
  c. Hold the quad cane on the left, and advance with the right lower extremity.
  d. Hold the quad cane on the right, and advance with the left lower extremity.

114. Which of the following is a normal skin response following a 20-minute application of a superficial heating agent?
  a. strong pink skin color
  b. mottled skin color
  c. cyanotic skin color
  d. chalky white skin color

115. A PTA is about to perform ultrasound to a patient with chronic right piriformis muscle inflammation. Which ultrasound settings would be MOST appropriate to effectively treat this area?
  a. 1.0 MHz, 20% duty cycle at 1.5 watts/cm^2
  b. 1.0 MHz, 100% duty cycle at 1.5 watts/cm^2
  c. 3.0 MHz, 20% duty cycle at 1.5 watts/cm^2
  d. 3.0 MHz, 100% duty cycle at 1.5 watts/cm^2

116. If a patient is a candidate for superficial heat and the PTA wishes to combine it with active exercise of the wrist and hand, the modality of choice would probably be
  a. fluidotherapy.
  b. hydrocollator packs.
  c. infrared.
  d. paraffin bath.

117. A PTA is treating a patient with the diagnosis of psoriasis. Which therapeutic modality below would be the most appropriate to treat the patient's condition?
  a. iontophoresis
  b. phonophoresis
  c. transcutaneous electrical nerve stimulation
  d. ultraviolet light

118. A PTA has a patient who has a history of Raynaud's syndrome. Knowing this information, which modality would NOT be appropriate for this patient?
  a. cold immersion bath
  b. hot pack
  c. massage
  d. ultrasound

119. A PTA is treating a patient diagnosed with a left tibia fracture. The patient is nine weeks status post open reduction and internal fixation (ORIF) with a plate and screw. Which modality below is NOT appropriate for this patient?
  a. hot packs
  b. massage
  c. shortwave diathermy
  d. whirlpool

120. A PTA desires to strengthen the teres minor and infraspinatus muscles. What is the best position to maximize this treatment goal?
  a. standing flexion to eye level with the arm in full internal rotation
  b. side-lying horizontal abduction to eye level with the arm in full internal rotation
  c. supine adduction to eye level with the arm in full external rotation
  d. prone, upper arm supported, forearm over the edge of the table, elbow and shoulder at 90 degrees, and the hand placed in external rotation

121. If cardiac output = heart rate × stroke volume (SV) during exercise, and if heart rate rises with exertion of exercise, what would you also expect?
  a. a decrease in stroke volume and overall cardiac output
  b. an overall increase in cardiac output
  c. no change in cardiac output
  d. cardiac output, heart rate, and stroke volume are not associated with exercise

122. A PTA is treating a patient with a diagnosis of a lumbar strain. With palpation, the PTA feels tight spasms in the patient's lumbar paraspinal muscles. The PTA uses the neuromuscular electrical stimulation unit to fatigue the spasm. Which parameters for electrical stimulation would be most appropriate to achieve this goal?
  a. 5 pulses per second, 1:1 on/off ratio
  b. 35 pulses per second, 1:6 on/off ratio
  c. 50–80 pulses per second, 1:1 on/off ratio
  d. 100 pulses per second, continuous

123. A PTA is treating a patient with the diagnosis of herniated nucleus propulsus to the L5–S1 level. The patient reported that since initiating mechanical lumbar traction two weeks ago, he has increased pain in his lower back, decreased pain in the right lower extremity, and decreased numbness in the right lower extremity. The patient's report would indicate that
  a. the treatment made the condition worse.
  b. the treatment was ineffective.
  c. there is decreased compression on the nerve root.
  d. there is increased pressure on the nerve root.

124. A PT and a PTA observe a patient who is exercising in the gym grab his chest and collapse. What is the best course of action for providing CPR to the patient?
  a. One rescuer gives breaths while the second rescuer provides chest compressions.
  b. One rescuer gives compressions and breaths.
  c. One rescuer checks the pulse.
  d. Both rescuers assess the patient and call 911 and wait for professional help.

125. The physical therapist assistant is treating a 76-year-old male patient with mild Alzheimer's disease who underwent a left hip hemiarthroplasty after a fall. The patient is getting ready to go home, and the PTA is reviewing precautions, home exercise programs, and plans for follow-up with home healthcare. Which of the following is the least appropriate educational intervention at this time?
  a. Include the patient's wife in the discussion.
  b. Provide patient with handouts of home exercise program.
  c. Focus on the details of how to perform each exercise.
  d. Have the patient demonstrate the exercise.

126. A PTA is working with a teenage patient and his mother on home exercise instruction. The PTA describes the exercises and asks the patient if he understands. The patient states that he is not sure that he understands the instructions. What is the best way to verify that the patient understands?
  a. Give the patient pictures of the home exercise program.
  b. Have the patient demonstrate the home exercise program.
  c. Explain the home exercise program to the patient's mother.
  d. Describe the exercises again and make sure the patient is listening.

127. Sherri, the secretary at a therapy clinic, receives a cancellation from Mr. Jones, who has a work conflict. She quickly finds Manuel, the PTA, to see if he wants Mrs. Adams scheduled in Mr. Jones's place. While Manuel performs some stretching on his current patient's knee, Sherri says, "Mr. Jones cancelled again today! Can you believe it? You just need to discharge him. Can I call Mrs. Adams to come instead?" Which of the following statements is true?
   a. Sherri is to be commended for her quick thinking to schedule patients in a timely way.
   b. Sherri is violating appropriate supervision laws, as it is up to the PT to schedule patients.
   c. Sherri is doing her job.
   d. Sherri is in violation of HIPAA.

128. The PTA, Manuel, who is in the middle of helping a patient, immediately answers the secretary, "Yes, I know that Mr. Jones is taking up valuable appointment time from patients who really need it. However, schedule Miss Smith, because I have a hard time understanding Mrs. Adams with that thick accent of hers." Which one of the following statements is true?
   a. Manuel's behavior is both legal and ethical.
   b. Manuel's behavior is legal even though it is not ethical.
   c. Manuel's behavior is illegal and unethical.
   d. Manuel is doing his job.

129. Which of the following also describes Manuel's behavior?
   a. He is demonstrating informed consent.
   b. He is demonstrating a lack of cultural awareness.
   c. He is demonstrating cultural competency.
   d. He is demonstrating on-site supervision.

130. The PTA observes that on each of three home health visits, Mrs. Brown is sallow, has body odor, and wears the same worn housecoat and slippers with holes in the toes. When encouraged to practice her walking out of her room, Mrs. Brown becomes visibly shaken and panicky and she quickly refuses. After gentle prodding, Mrs. Brown confides that her family told her that she must stay in her room or, she says, "They'll send me away." The PTA's responsi-bilities include all but which of the following?
   a. discussing this situation with the family, as this may be a misunderstanding
   b. being aware of state/federal regulations affecting the types of patients/clients with which the PTA works
   c. reporting concerns to the supervising PT
   d. reporting suspicions to appropriate authorities in accordance with company policy

131. The issue being described in the previous question is commonly referred to as _____ and is classified as _____.
   a. elder care; informed consent
   b. elder care; required reporting
   c. elder abuse; informed consent
   d. elder abuse; required reporting

132. The patient's or client's right to refuse physical therapy treatment is an example of
   a. confidentiality.
   b. safety.
   c. informed consent.
   d. HIPAA.

133. Forcibly transferring a competent patient from the bed to the chair "max assistance × three" so that the bed can be changed despite the patient's request "to be left alone" is
   a. a required part of acute care physical therapy.
   b. often necessary.
   c. required if the PT puts this in the plan of care.
   d. illegal and unethical.

134. The number one way for a PTA to reduce the risk of cross contamination in the healthcare environment is through
   a. hand washing.
   b. routine inspections.
   c. continued competence.
   d. proper body mechanics.

135. Which of the following purposes is defined as interrupting, establishing barriers to the infection cycle, and/or preventing the transmission of microorganisms?
   a. patient safety considerations
   b. emergency preparedness
   c. using the proper cleaning solutions
   d. personal protective equipment (PPE)

136. Which of the following is NOT an important rule of proper body mechanics?
   a. Pull (don't push) objects when moving them from point A to point B.
   b. Plan the action ahead of time.
   c. Take the time to get help—even if "time is money."
   d. Face the object you will lift or move.

137. In the event of a tornado, the PTA should do what?
   a. Call 911.
   b. Contact the therapist of record immediately.
   c. Competently use emergency management procedures.
   d. Nothing, as this is outside the PTA's scope of work.

138. A recent PTA graduate lands a job at the new outpatient orthopedic clinic in her hometown. She begins to dread going to work whenever the PT owner of the clinic sees patients out in the gym because he frequently makes suggestive comments about her and brushes up against her as though there is not enough room to walk by. Which of the following is true with regard to her employee rights?
   a. The PTA should enact the whistle blowing law.
   b. This unacceptable behavior is punishable by law.
   c. She should contact OSHA to report this behavior.
   d. She needs to play along to keep her job.

139. Which of the following is NOT documented in a patient's medical record?
   a. specifically what occurred while in the presence of the PTA
   b. accurate time and date of all interaction or communication with the patient
   c. incident report
   d. notification or communication with other healthcare team members

140. Which of the following legally determines the specific expectations and limitations of the PTA within the clinical setting?
   a. standards of practice
   b. code of ethics
   c. company policy
   d. practice act

141. Effective delegation strategies that have been widely adopted within the physical therapy profession include a systematic approach based on the process of decision making and delivering the interventions. Who does what with regard to the role and responsibilities of the PT versus the PTA?
   a. PT tasks weigh heavily on the process of decision making.
   b. PTA tasks weigh heavily on the process of decision making.
   c. PT tasks and PTA tasks are virtually equally divided.
   d. PT tasks are essentially "doing" tasks.

142. PTAs may provide services under the direction of which of the following healthcare members?
   a. physical therapists
   b. both physicians and physical therapists
   c. physicians, chiropractors, and physical therapists
   d. depends on the state

143. A direct-access patient enters the clinic and reports having injured his ankle two days prior. He experienced pain at the time of injury followed by mild swelling, local tenderness, and pain with movement. What grade tissue injury should the PTA suspect?
   a. grade I
   b. grade II
   c. grade III
   d. grade IV

144. A patient with an obstructive lung disease presents with
   a. a decreased ability to inhale air.
   b. a decreased ability to expire air.
   c. an increased ability to expire air.
   d. no problem with air exchange.

145. Knowing type I fibers are aerobic and type II are anaerobic, a patient with COPD would most likely have
   a. increased type I fibers.
   b. increased type I and II fibers.
   c. decreased type I fibers.
   d. decreased type II fibers.

146. Maceration of skin may contribute to the development of open wounds. What does this mean?
   a. Pressure over the bony areas is increased.
   b. Excessive moisture can cause skin breakdown.
   c. Friction and shear forces can cause skin breakdown.
   d. Patients with poor sensation are more prone to skin breakdown.

147. A PTA is treating a 76-year-old patient with a kyphotic posture and balance loss. The patient has a timed up and go score of 38 seconds when ambulating with a standard cane. What does this score indicate regarding the patient's safety in the community?
   a. The patient will need assistance to ambulate safely in the community.
   b. The patient will be a safe, independent community ambulator if you give the patient a quad cane.
   c. The patient is a safe community ambulator using a standard cane.
   d. The patient is at low risk for falls.

148. A 45-year-old male presents to the clinic with hip flexion contractures measured at −20 degrees. The contractures are secondary to muscle shortening from sustained sitting posture. Which of the following treatment interventions would be most effective to address the mobility deficits associated with this condition?

  a. theraband activities to strengthen hip flexors

  b. stationary recumbent bicycling for 20 minutes

  c. facilitated agonist contraction techniques to hamstrings

  d. single leg standing on foam with vision unoccluded

149. A patient presents with impingement syndrome of the right dominant shoulder. The PTA is asked to implement a therapeutic exercise program focused on increasing range of motion and on strengthening. The patient is in the acute stage, reporting pain at 5 out of 10 after medication. Which exercise would be the most appropriate to begin treatment?

  a. flexion to 90 degrees performed passively by the physical therapist assistant

  b. walking on a finger ladder from 0 to 140 degrees

  c. resisted abduction with yellow theraband to 90 degrees

  d. isokinetic exercises at 60 degrees per second for internal and external rotation

150. A PTA is providing vibration as part of the chest therapy program to remove lung secretions. When is the appropriate time to apply vibration to ensure patient safety?

  a. only during expiration as patient is deep-breathing

  b. only during inspiration as patient is deep-breathing

  c. during early inspiration and late expiration

  d. prior to postural drainage

Answers and Explanations

1. b. The posterior reconstruction for posterior dislocations such as the Putti-Platt is performed to decrease posterior capsule laxity. The mechanism for dislocation is the motion of internal rotation. The infraspinatus muscle is used, postoperatively; the patient is positioned in neutral or external rotation. Abduction and internal rotation movements are avoided. The posterior deltoid and rotator cuff are strengthened during rehabilitation. (Gould 1990, page 517)

2. c. Klumpke's or Klumpke-Dejerine paralysis involves the lower brachial plexus at the C8 and T1 levels. The distal area of the forearm and hand of the limb would be affected with this level of injury. (Hollinshead 1974, page 189)

3. a. The cardiac index (CI) is the cardiac output in relation to the surface area of the body (BSA) and is calculated $CI = CO/BSA$. The normal cardiac index range is 2.5 to 3.5 L/min/m^2. (O'Sullivan and Schmitz 2007, page 595)

4. d. The average age of accomplishment of sitting alone steadily is 6.6 months, while the range is 5–9 months. (Tecklin 1999, page 9)

5. d. The average age of accomplishment of walking alone is 11.7 months, while the range is 9–17 months. (Tecklin 1999, page 9)

6. a. The musculoskeletal disorder described involves the strain and inflammation of the common extensor tendon at its insertion on the lateral epicondyl, within the tendon or at the musculotendinous junction. Although this is referred to as tennis elbow, many cases do not arise from playing tennis. The condition is aggravated by extension of the wrist, supination of the forearm against resistance, and squeezing or gripping with the hand. (Saunders 1985, page 167)

7. a. Osgood-Schlatter's disease occurs primarily in active boys between ages 10–15 years of age. Observable swelling and tenderness over the tibial tuberosity are the major symptoms. (Saunders 1985, page 165)

8. c. The piriformis muscle externally rotates the femur. Internal rotation of the hip will stretch the piriformis muscle while external rotation of the hip will shorten the piriformis muscle. (Saunders 1985, pages 155–156)

9. c. NPUAP descriptions are as follows: Stage I—intact skin with non-blanchable redness of a localized area usually over a bony prominence; darkly pigmented skin may not have visible blanching; its color may differ from the surrounding area. Stage II—partial-thickness loss of dermis presenting as a shallow open ulcer with a red pink wound bed, without slough; may also present as an intact or open/ruptured serum-filled blister. Stage III—full-thickness tissue loss; subcutaneous fat may be visible, but bone, tendon, or muscle are not exposed; slough may be present but does not obscure the depth of tissue loss; may include undermining and tunneling. Stage IV—full-thickness tissue loss with exposed bone, tendon, or muscle; slough or eschar may be present on some parts of the wound bed; often included under mining and tunneling. (McCulloch, Kloth, and Feedar 1995, page 196)

10. a. Blackburn's (1981) and Jobe and Moynes's (1986) EMG studies determined when a patient is positioned in prone horizontal abduction to eye level with the arm in full external rotation, the action of the supraspinatus muscle is abduction of the shoulder. (Gould 1990, pages 508–509)

11. a. The ankle joint is the most distal position and makes the exercise with resistance the most difficult to perform. This applies the concept of moments of force (torque). The moment of force generated depends on the magnitude of force and the length of the lever arm; moment (m) = force (F) × distance (D). Thus, the greater amount of force or a longer lever arm increases the moment of force. (Gould 1990, pages 75–76)

12. a. The Bankart repair involves suturing the capsule and labrum to the glenoidal rim. Postoperatively, the patient wears an internal rotation sling for two to three weeks and the patient may perform submaximal isometric activation of the muscles that were not cut during surgery. From three to six weeks following surgery, a sling is worn only at night. Activities include active abduction to 90 degrees and external rotation is limited to neutral. More aggressive range of motion can be performed at 7 to 8 weeks, while functional activities can be performed from weeks 8 to 12. (Gould 1990, page 517)

13. a. Beta blockers appear to reduce oxygen consumption resulting in a reduction in heart rate and the force of heart muscle contraction. Exercise increases the demand of oxygen consumption and increases the heart rate allowing for a slight elevation despite ingestion of a beta blocker. (Lippincott 2000, page 593)

14. a. One of the factors controlling the HR is the autonomic nervous system. When the SV falls, the nervous system is stimulated to increase the HR and thereby maintain adequate CO. (Lippincott 2000, page 657)

15. d. Although cardiac output during exercise is high, vasodilation reduces peripheral resistance to maintain a relatively low diastolic blood pressure. Systolic blood pressure will increase in proportion to the workload. (O'Sullivan and Schmitz 2007, page 110)

16. c. With each ejected stroke, 42% (right ventricle) to 50% (left ventricle) or more is ejected by the normal heart. Thus, EF measures myocardial contractibility; the EF decreases

if contractibility is depressed. (Lippincott 2000, page 537)

17. a. Obstructive pulmonary disease includes reduced air flow resulting in excessive accumulation of mucus and secretions which block the airway. This causes impaired gas exchange and destruction of over-distended alveoli walls. The lungs are in a chronic state of hyper-expansion, causing the broad chest. (Lippincott 2000, page 446)

18. c. The decrease in ejected ventricular volume causes the heart rate to increase and the pulse to become weak and thready. Without adequate output, the body cannot respond to increased energy demands, so the patient is easily fatigued and has decreased activity tolerance. Exercise is alternated with periods of rest. (Lippincott 2000, page 665)

19. a. Autonomic dysreflexia (hyperflexia) is a pathological autonomic reflex that generally occurs in lesions above T6. Symptoms include hypertension, bradycardia, headache (often severe and pounding), profuse sweating, increased spacticity, restlessness, vasoconstriction below the level of lesion, vasodilation (flushing) above the level of the lesion, constricted pupils, nasal congestion, piloerection (goose bumps), and blurred vision. (O'Sullivan and Schmitz 2007, page 943)

20. b. Kosiak (1959) determined pressure on the buttocks was 70 mm Hg supine and increased to 300 mm Hg at the ischial tuberosity in the seated position. Chairbound patients who are able to shift their weight should be instructed to shift their weight every 15 minutes. (Clinical Practice Guideline Number 15, Treatment of Pressure Ulcers 1994, page 42)

21. a. Medications and descriptions are as follows: silver sulfadiazine is a commonly used topical antibacterial agent that is effective against pseudomonas infections; silver nitrate is an antiseptic germicide and astringent that will penetrate only 1–2 mm of eschar—it is useful for surface bacteria and stains black; bacitracin is a bland ointment which is effective against gram positive organisms; and collagenase is an enzymatic debriding agent that selectively debrides necrotic tissue with no antibacterial action. (O'Sullivan and Schmitz 2007, page 1,103)

22. a. Kosiak (1959) determined pressure on the buttocks was 70 mm Hg supine and increased to 300 mm Hg at the ischial tuberosity in the seated position. Chairbound patients who are able to shift their weight should be instructed to shift their weight every 15 minutes. Therefore, it is paramount to reposition the patient at least every hour. If an hourly schedule cannot be met or is kept inconsistently with overall treatment goals, the patient should be returned to bed. (Clinical Practice Guideline Number 15, Treatment of Pressure Ulcers 1994, page 42)

23. d. Pseudobulbar affect (PBA), also known as emotional lability or emotional dysregulation syndrome, presents in approximately one out of five stroke patients. The hallmark is emotional outbursts of uncontrolled laughing or crying that occur inconsistently with patient mood. Episodes are uncontrolled and quickly change with little or no stimulation. (O'Sullivan and Schmitz 2007, page 724)

24. c. A patient who sustained right hemisphere damage displays difficulty with comprehension and performance of a spatial-perceptual task. The patient's behavior is often described as quick and impulsive, resulting in an overestimation of abilities and poor judgment. Patient safety is a major concern. Repetition and verbal feedback are required. (O'Sullivan and Schmitz 2007, page 724)

25. a. The most frequent cause of autonomic dysreflexia in spinal cord injury patients is bladder distention (urinary retention). Other causes include rectal distention, pressure sores, urinary stones, bladder infections, noxious cutaneous stimuli, kidney malfunction, urethral or bladder irritation, and environmental temperature changes. Autonomic dysreflexia also has been reported following passive stretching at the hip. (O'Sullivan and Schmitz 2007, page 943)

26. d. Postural hypotension (orthostatic hypotension) is caused by a decrease in blood pressure that occurs in erect or vertical positions, such as during the performance of transfers from lying-to-sitting or sit-to-stand. This condition is caused by the loss of sympathetic vasoconstriction control. Inactivity (such as bed rest) causes a lack of muscle tone, creating peripheral and splenic bed blood pooling. The reduced blood flow and decreased venous return to the heart causes symptoms of lightheadedness, dizziness, or fainting. (O'Sullivan and Schmitz 2007, page 944)

27. b. The vagus nerve (cranial nerve X) enters the thoracic cavity, from which many branches arise to innervate visceral organs of the thorax and abdomen. The diaphragm is innervated by the phrenic nerve C3, 4, 5. Serratus anterior is innervated by the long thoracic nerve C5, 6, 7, 8. Rectus abdominus by the thoracic nerves T5, T6, T7–12, and T12. (Burt 1993, page 377, and Kendall 2005, pages 194, 236, 332)

28. a. The nerve root innervation of muscles at the C6 level include extensor carpi radialis, infraspinatus, latissimus dorsi, pectoralis major, pronator teres, serratus anterior, and teres minor. These muscles allow motions of shoulder flexion, extension, internal rotation, and adduction; scapular abduction and upward rotation; forearm pronation and wrist extension, all of which are required to perform the ADLs in question. (O'Sullivan and Schmitz 2007, page 962)

29. a. Right hemisphere damage results in left-side hemiplegia and paresis. Common visual-perceptual impairments may include a left-side unilateral neglect, agnosia, and visuospatial impairment. (O'Sullivan and Schmitz 2007, page 725)

30. b. Left hemisphere damage may result in speech and language impairments, including nonfluent (Broca's) aphasia, fluent (Wernicke's) aphasia, and global aphasia. (O'Sullivan and Schmitz 2007, page 725)

31. a. Nonfluent aphasia (Broca's expressive aphasia) results from a lesion in the premotor area of the left frontal lobe. Characteristics include slow, labored speech with limited use of vocabulary and impaired syntax (word arrangement in a sentence). Fluent aphasia (Wernicke's/sensory receptive aphasia) results from a lesion in the left lateral temporal lobe which impacts auditory comprehension. (O'Sullivan and Schmitz 2007, page 722)

32. b. A positive Thomas test suggests tight hip flexors. Tight hip flexors can result in an anterior pelvic tilt of the pelvis. (Kisner and Colby 2002, page 395)

33. a. A normal Q angle is between 5 to 15 degrees. Q angles greater than normal are associated with patellofemoral syndrome. Positive Ober test suggests a tight iliotibial band. Positive Thomas test with hip moving into abduction and IR suggests a tight TFL, which is attached to the ITB. Tightness of these structures is associated with PFS. Weak VMO is also associated with patellofemoral syndrome. (Kisner and Colby 2002, page 712–713)

34. b. This position would maximally elongate the biceps and place tension upon it. This tension could disrupt the healing process in the inflammatory and proliferative phases of healing. Maximal stretching would be appropriate in the remodeling and maturation phase. (Kisner and Colby 2002, pages 578, 615)

35. b. Coxa valga is where the angle of inclination of the femoral head is greater than 125 degrees. This puts the patient at increased risk for hip dislocation. Less than 125 degrees is known as coxa vara and puts the patient at increased risk for femoral neck fractures. Femoral anteversion, which is associated with torsion angles greater than 15 degrees, is associated with a toe-in posture, and femoral retroversion is associated with torsion angles less than 12 degrees and a toe-out posture. (Konin 1998, page 134)

36. b. The ability to recall information within minutes or hours is short-term memory. Immediate memory involves recalling information within an interval of a few seconds and long-term, or remote, memory involves intervals of years. (O'Sullivan 2007, page 1,167)

37. c. Level III on the Ranchos Los Amigos Scale is a localized response. Generalized response is level II, confused appropriate is level VI, and automatic appropriate is level VII. (O'Sullivan 2007, page 901)

38. c. The dorsalis pedis artery is palpated on the dorsum of the foot, between the tendons of the extensor hallucis longus and extensor digitorum brevis muscles. (Hoppenfeld 1976, page 214)

39. d. Interpreting the amount of drainage requires that the PTA know when the dressing was applied. A large amount of drainage on a dressing only two hours old indicates a much higher rate of drainage than the same amount on a dressing applied 24 hours ago. While infection can result in increased drainage, it would also tend to create cloudy or discolored exudate. Thin, clear, yellow drainage is normal. (Myers 2004, page 53)

40. b. The stage of the wound does not matter in determining whether or not a wound is infected. Key factors pointing to infection are the pale, dry granulation tissue, the presence of thick, tan drainage, and the inflammation of surrounding skin. The other choices describe wounds that are not necessarily healthy, but do not show hallmark signs of infection. (Myers 2004, pages 52–53)

41. b. The hormone that would most likely be secreted as a result of a stressful test that may elicit an individual's fear of falling is cortisol. Cortisol is the hormone most closely linked to the stress response. (Scanlon 1999, page 225)

42. a. During tests or measures that cause fear, the body may release epinephrine in preparation for a fight or flight response. (Widmaier, 2006, page 375)

43. d. When a patient is standing on a firm, level surface, the patient is receiving the majority of the sensory information regarding balance from the somatosensory system. The vestibular system is designed primarily to detect linear acceleration (utricle and saccule) and angular acceleration (semicircular canals) and is used when there is confusion between the visual and somatosensory systems. The visual system is a secondary system that supports the other two. The primary system working on level surfaces is the somatosensory system, which includes mechanoreceptors and proprioceptors in the joints and skin. (Kisner and Colby 2007, pages 258–260)

44. b. Increased twitch contraction time is not a neural adaptation associated with strength training. Increased twitch contraction time indicates that it will take longer for a muscle contraction to occur when the muscle is stimulated. This is not because the speed of the twitch contraction time decreases or becomes faster. Increased number of motor units firing, increased rate of firing, and increased synchronization of firing are all neural adaptations associated with strength training. (Kisner and Colby 2007, page 158)

45. c. The PTA should expect the somatosensory system to be impaired. Walking on an uneven pebbled driveway during daylight is most challenging to the somatosensory system. If walking on this surface leads to falls, then the patient most likely has an impairment of the somatosensory system for which she is not able to compensate with vision. (O'Sullivan 2007, page 503)

46. c. Postural muscles are type I muscles and respond best to low intensity, long duration exercise because these types of muscle must work at a low intensity throughout the day to maintain posture. (O'Sullivan 2007, page 493)

47. b. The PTA should expect to see an increase in heart rate during and just after stopping exercise. After a period of rest, the heart rate will return to the resting level. For a patient with a cardiovascular history, the heart rate may plateau; however, the PTA should anticipate an increased heart rate during and just after stopping exercise. (O'Sullivan 2007, page 598)

48. b. As part of the hip strategy, the extensor muscles must strongly contract in order to prevent a forward fall. (Umphred 1995, page 807)

49. b. Due to the narrow base of support with tandem walking and the lack of a very forceful perturbation, the child walking on the straight line is most likely to use the hip strategy for balance in this position. (O'Sullivan 2007, page 253)

50. a. The Functional Independence Measure is widely used and has demonstrated reliability, validity, and sensitivity. As a result, it is used extensively in rehabilitation facilities for stroke patients. The assessment examines functional mobility skills that include bed mobility, movement transitions, transfers, locomotion, stairs, basic ADL skills that include feeding, hygiene, and dressing and instrumental ADL skills that include communication and home chores. (O'Sullivan and Schmitz 2007, pages 387, 388, 735)

51. c. Because of the odd shape of the hand, volumetrics is the best choice. Volumetrics looks at water displacement of the entire hand and even small changes can be documented. (O'Sullivan and Schmitz 2007, page 658)

52. b. Lateral calf is the dermatome for L5. Weakness of dorsiflexors could correspond with L4 or L5 but the patella reflex (which is L4) is intact and the achilles reflex is intact (which is S1). This suggests that L5 is the best choice for the level impacted by herniated disc. (Cook and Hegedus, 2008, pages 35–36)

53. b. The patient has a steppage gait. Although dorsiflexors are weak and a drop foot pattern might be possible, what is described is the compensation for a drop foot. The Trendelenburg and compensated Trendelenburg are deviations in the frontal plane and imply a gluteus medius weakness. (Lippert 2006, page 311)

54. c. A reverse action of the gastrocnemius can be used to extend the knee when the quadriceps are weak. (Lippert 2006, page 310)

55. d. Choices **a**, **b**, and **c** are consistent with right knee surgery with quad atrophy and swelling around the right knee. Atrophy of the gastrocnemius is not consistent with the rest of the data. (O'Sullivan and Schmitz, 2007, page 659)

56. c. All four tests will assess fall risk for gait; however, the timed up and go will take the least amount of time to complete. (O'Sullivan and Schmitz 2007, pages 255–258)

57. b. The example given is the definition of a muscular endurance test. For muscle power, the test would be to perform as many maximal reps as possible in a period of time. For muscle strength, we would want to assess peak torque. Agility tests require alternating directions while functionally moving, not in the controlled format of the isokinetic testing

environment. (O'Sullivan and Schmitz 2007, page 183)

58. c. A terrible triad injury to the knee involves the medial collateral ligament, medial meniscus, and the anterior cruciate ligament. The Lachman's test assesses the integrity of the ACL, McMurray's is either the medial or lateral meniscus, a valgus stress test assesses the MCL, and a varus test assesses the integrity of the LCL. The varus test is not needed. (Cook and Hegedus 2008, pages 284, 304, 332, 334)

59. c. The single leg stance and functional reach are in low risk ranges. The Tinetti composite score is out of 28, and scores between 24–28 are considered low risk for fall. The Berg is out of 56; therefore, a score of 24 is in the high-risk-for-fall category. (O'Sullivan and Schmitz, 2007, pages 255–256)

60. a. To test the rectus femoris, the hip must not be in 90 degrees of flexion because that puts it on active shortened insufficiency. Therefore, rectus is typically tested in 45 degrees of flexion. All the vasti are tested in 90 degrees of flexion. To emphasize the vastus lateralis, the hip is internally rotated, and to test the vastus medialis, it is externally rotated. The best answer is **a**. (O'Sullivan and Schmitz 2007, page 1,272)

61. b. Dual inclinometers are the best choice for range of motion for a spinal segment. Although a bubble inclinometer would be a second choice, given the insurance environment, the dual inclinometer measurements can be used to assist the disability rating of the patient. Tape measure to the floor will give you an objective measurement to compare from one session to another, but there are no normative values. Standard goniometry is not effective because it requires several joints to make composite lumbar motion.

(American Medical Association 2007, page 485)

62. c. The normal reaction to Babinski test in an infant is fanning and extension of the toes. (Martin 2007, page 18)

63. c. During the neck righting reflex, the infant tries to align the body with the head. The stimulus is passive cervical rotation, and in response the child will rotate the rest of the body to align with the head. (Umphred 2006, page 47)

64. b. The Berg Balance Scale is the only option that involves everyday functional activities such as picking objects up off the floor and reaching forward. (O'Sullivan 2007, page 257)

65. a. Anterior tibialis weakness affects the control of the eccentric dorsiflexion during foot flat. A lack of the foot lowering to the walking surface results in a foot slap, and the result is a steppage gait pattern. (O'Sullivan 2007, page 328)

66. d. Velocity-dependent resistance to passive movement defines the term spasticity. Rigidity is resistance that is not velocity dependent. Hypotonia does not involve increased resistance to movement, and dystonia is disordered tone. (O'Sullivan 2007, page 233)

67. a. If arterial insufficiency is suspected or lower extremity pulses are not readily palpable, the Ankle-Brachial Index should be calculated. (Myers 2004, page 210)

68. d. With a burn to the anterior aspect of the hip, contractures would tend to limit extension and abduction. Rotation may or may not be involved. (O'Sullivan and Schmitz 2007, page 1,106)

69. b. The mechanism for anterior shoulder dislocation is external rotation. Therefore, the patient should be instructed to avoid functional activities such as throwing, placing the hand behind the head to comb hair, or drying the back with a towel. (Gould 1990, page 500)

70. c. The ideal scar would be the color of the surrounding skin, it would have a high degree of pliability, and it would be flat. (Myers 2004, page 343)

71. c. Aerobic capacity and endurance tests have the potential for the most significant metabolic and endocrine responses due to the high physical demands of this type of testing. (American Physical Therapy Association 2001, page 548)

72. d. The most likely endocrine response to the work reintegration assessment is increased uptake of blood glucose. This is due to the physical demands of a mail carrier's position, which is a position that requires prolonged walking. (Widmaier 2006, page 627)

73. a. Three common methods of assessing self-care and ADL status are self-report, observational screen, and direct examination by a physical therapist. (Lewis 2002, page 29)

74. a. Pulse oximetry provides a measure of arterial blood oxygenation levels with each pulse. Normal oxygen saturation levels range between 96–100%. When oxygen saturation levels fall below 90%, this is considered inadequate and requires additional testing such as arterial blood gas analysis. Supplemental oxygen administration may also be initiated. (O'Sullivan and Schmitz 2007, page 102)

75. a. Crackles or rales are the rattling or bubbling sounds produced as a result of secretions in the air passages of the respiratory tract. The sounds may be detected with the ear but are best heard with a stethoscope. The crackles or rales breathing sounds are commonly apparent in patients with congestive heart failure. (O'Sullivan and Schmitz 2007, pages 106–107 and 1,330)

76. c. Choice **c** is not an appropriate recommendation for patients with patellofemoral syndrome. Extension puts the least amount of pressure on the patellofemoral joint, and the

more flexion of the knee the greater the compressive forces. Allowing the knee to go past
the big toe increases the pressure on the
patellofemoral joint significantly and should
be avoided with all patients, but especially
with patients with patellofemoral syndrome.
(Kisner and Colby 2007, pages 711–712)

77. d. Choice **d** would not appear on the objective
portion of the daily note. The treatment and
clinical observations all belong under objective. The fact that the patient is a 15-year-old
athlete who sustained an injury to his ankle
at a track event belongs under a subjective
portion of the note, since it is history. (Erick-
son and McKnight 2005, pages 24–25)

78. a. The PTA should begin with AROM scapula
retraction. Scapula retraction does not
directly involve the glenohumeral joint and
will be the easiest of the motions to complete.
Typically, range of motion after surgery is
done passively beginning with the easiest
motions (extension and flexion) and pro-
ceeding backward through the capsular pattern IR, abduction, and ER. (Kisner and
Colby 2007, page 509)

79. b. The best choice for this patient with osteoarthritis to both ankles is stationary bicycling at
60 RPMs. Stationary bicycling is both an aerobic activity and appropriate for someone
with osteoarthritis to both ankles. BAPS
board is good for range of motion; single leg
balance on foam is good for proprioception;
and balance and ladder drills are good for
agility and could be used to improve aerobic
capacity, but these would be inappropriate
for osteoarthritis ankles. (Kisner and Colby
2007, pages 239–240)

80. d. D2 extension begins with the shoulder
abducted, flexed, and ER. It ends with the
shoulder moving into extension, adduction,
and IR. This most closely mimics an overhand

cross-body serve used in tennis. (Kisner and
Colby 2007, page 196)

81. b. The PTA should question the patient further
about which activities she did at home that
are increasing her pain and review how she
should perform the pulley exercises. It is
important for the PTA to reassess the area
prior to taking any action. Once the PTA has
questioned the patient further about her
symptoms and gained insight about how the
patient was performing activities, the PTA
will be able to determine whether it is necessary to reinstruct the patient. Ignoring new
symptoms may worsen the change noted.
Having the patient go home, take medication,
and call the physician leaves out the supervising PT and does not address the concern.
Finally, changing the treatment plan scheduled for the day may be appropriate after
assessment has been done, but if this is
necessary it should be done in consultation
with the supervising PT. (Kisner and Colby
2007, page 506)

82. a. The PTA should explain to the patient that
after a burn he or she is likely to lose body
weight and muscle mass. Strength training
will help the patient to regain this lost muscle
mass. Choice **b** does not address the question.
Choice **c** is incorrect because although
peripheral neuropathy may occur after burns,
strength training is not likely to prevent it
from occurring. Choice **d** is incorrect because
there is no evidence that strength training
will help burns heal faster. (O'Sullivan and
Schmitz 2007, page 1,108)

83. a. The best way to adapt this exercise during the
next treatment session to prevent another
negative response is to decrease exercise
intensity. Exercise intensity should be
decreased before other components of the
program. If the exercise is still too much for

the patient, then the duration should be decreased. (Lewis 2002, page 160)

84. c. The grade of 13 is an appropriate starting intensity for an aerobic exercise program for this patient. The grade of 13 corresponds to "somewhat hard" on the Borg RPE Scale, and this is recommended for the initiation of a cardiovascular exercise program. (Strunk 2006, page 16)

85. d. The PTA should stop the exercise immediately due to the significant drop in blood pressure during exercise. A drop in blood pressure during exercise is not a normal response to exercise. (O'Sullivan 2007, page 600–601)

86. b. The best way for the PTA to facilitate diaphragmatic breathing is to place a hand over the patient's diaphragm and "push" the diaphragm into his or her hand while inhaling. (Martin 2007, page 293)

87. d. The most appropriate weight for knee flexion strength training with this patient is 30 pounds. The recommended percentage of one repetition max for strength training is a minimum of 80%. Therefore, a weight of 30 pounds is the closest weight to 80% of the one repetition max for this patient. (Nyland 2006, page 175)

88. b. The next posture that the PTA should use for training is sitting, because it is the next posture in the developmental progression. Once skilled movements and balance are gained in the quadruped position, the next position to work in would be sitting. (O'Sullivan 2007, page 482)

89. c. Chronic bronchitis is an indication for postural drainage with percussion. The other conditions are relative contraindications for percussion. (Kisner and Colby, 2007, page 870–871)

90. b. The PTA working with this patient would most likely use prolonged stretching to assist in this patient's sit-to-stand training. Prolonged stretching is an inhibitory technique that can be used to decrease spasticity in preparation for mobility. The hip extensors would be the muscles to which the PTA should apply the technique. Prolonged stretching before the movement will allow for more normal movement and retraining. (O'Sullivan 2007, page 744)

91. c. The first position on the mat that will promote weight bearing through the hips and facilitate initial control of the lower trunk and hips is quadruped. Quadruped is the only choice that will allow weight-bearing through the hips while working on control of the trunk and hips. (O'Sullivan 2007, page 972)

92. c. The most important therapeutic measure for prevention of venous leg ulcers is compression therapy. Increased pressure in the lower extremity veins starts a cascade of events leading to skin breakdown. (O'Sullivan and Schmitz 2007, pages 652–653)

93. b. Arterial ulcers are dry and require moisture to be added to them. Hydrogel can add moisture; the other dressings listed absorb it. (Myers 2004, pages 128, 220)

94. c. Pressure is most effective in preventing excessive scar tissue formation, which would increase the height of the scar. The other choices contribute more to keeping the skin pliable. (O'Sullivan and Schmitz 2007, pages 1,110–1,111)

95. c. The application of moist heat to the skin would decrease metabolism. Cold, stress, and increasing muscle mass all increase metabolism. (Scanlon 1999, page 397)

96. c. Exercise results in increased insulin sensitivity of the cells of the body, resulting in decreased blood sugar. (Widmaier 2006, page 629)

97. a. Research by Sullivan and Markos (1982) reported that patients taking cardiac medications (digitalis and calcium blockers) may be at greater risk for falling. (Guccione 2000, page 299)

98. **a.** Research by Sanders, Colin, and Burgess (1992) reported healthy adults in the sixth decade of life use 41% of their maximum aerobic capacity during ambulation. Aerobic energy costs using a prosthesis increase significantly during ambulation, ranging from 40 to 60% with a unilateral transtibial amputation and 90 to 120% with unilateral transfemoral amputation. Measurement of maximum oxygen uptake (VO2 max) provides a good indication of cardiovascular functional capacity. (Guccione 2000, page 329)

99. **a.** Postural drainage places the patient in the best position to permit the bronchus of the involved lung segment perpendicular to the ground. This allows gravity to assist the process. The following segments are drained in the subsequent patient positions:

Upper lobes, posterior segments—patient leans over folded pillow at 300° angle.
Upper lobes, anterior segments—patient lies on back with pillow under knees.
Lower lobes, superior segments—patient lies on abdomen with two pillows under hips.
Lower lobes, anterior basal segments—patient lies on side, head down, with pillow under knees. (O'Sullivan and Schmitz 2007, page 580)

100. **a.** Once infection and edema are controlled, the application of a total contact cast is an effective method to achieve reduction of weight-bearing stress on the foot for a healing ulcer. The technique utilizes plaster padding and rubber inserts. It is worn for seven to ten days. The limitation is the lack of visibility of the ulcer when the cast is intact. A cast shoe and post-op shoe are the same thing and offer a temporary but lesser degree of wound off-loading. (O'Sullivan and Schmitz 2007, page 685)

101. **d.** A Halo device is designed for unstable cervical fractures. The other devices are examples of cervical orthoses for patients with soft tissue or stable fractures. (O'Sullivan and Schmitz 2007, page 1,233)

102. **c.** Curves between 30–45 degrees are considered for orthotic management. Choices **a** and **d** would be monitored, and choice **b** is a surgical candidate. (Highsmith, "Demonstration Project on Prosthetics and Orthotics," http://oandp.health.usf.edu/orth/orthotics _ov/orthotics_ov.html, slide # 47)

103. **d.** Cock-up splints are usually positioned over the palmar or volar aspect of the forearm. Although checking for red areas is an appropriate item to assess, it is unlikely with the type of splint described. (Highsmith, "Demonstration Project on Prosthetics and Orthotics," http://oandp.health.usf.edu/orth/orthotics_ ov/orthotics_ov.html, slide # 24)

104. **c.** The walker will give her stability while still allowing her to perform activities in an energy-efficient manner. Choice **a** is likely to use axillary crutches, **b** will also use axillary crutches or a cane, and choice **d** axillary or Loftstrand crutches. (Pierson and Fairchild 2008, page 219–220)

105. **d.** The gait described is a three-point gait because there are three points of contact made separately. It is a step-through gait because the uninjured leg moves past the injured leg. With a two point swing-through gait, the crutches would be advanced and then the patient would swing through landing on the uninjured leg. A step-to gait implies that the uninjured leg moves to the same level as the injured leg. (Pierson and Fairchild 2008, pages 232–233)

106. c. All the other answers are consistent with normal checkout except choice **c.** Pistoning should not occur more than one-quarter inch. (Cerny 1995, page 682)

107. a. Inadequate plantar flexion stop would result in excessive plantar flexion during the stance phase of gait. With the ankle in a position of plantar flexion, the knee hyperextends as a result. (Seymour 2002, page 394)

108. b. The ankle joint of a lower extremity orthotic is most appropriately aligned with the distal tip of the medial malleolus. (Seymour 2002, page 394)

109. b. The best provision of static stretching for this patient is moist heat to the knee flexors followed by three reps of 30-second knee extension stretches. Moist heat applied to the area prior to stretching can enhance the static stretching technique, and static stretches should be held for a minimum of 30 seconds. The knee flexors are the muscles that are tight if a patient has decreased knee extension ROM. (O'Sullivan 2007, page 495)

110. c. The PTA should look for 20 to 30 degrees of elbow flexion when grasping the handgrips in order to confirm a good fit for the walker. This measurement allows the patient enough leverage to put weight through the upper extremities to take weight off the lower extremities. (O'Sullivan 2007, page 552)

111. a. Following gait training with a new knee-ankle-foot orthotic, the primary concern of the PTA should be the condition of the skin for the extremity on which the orthotic device is worn. This is because the PTA must be sure that the patient is not experiencing any friction or pain from the device. (Seymour 2002, page 380)

112. c. An ankle-foot orthotic for this patient should include a plantar flexion stop, which will prevent the foot from slapping at heel strike. (O'Sullivan 2007, page 1,218)

113. d. The correct use of the quad cane for a patient status post left hip fracture is for the patient to hold the quad cane on the right and advance with the left lower extremity. Canes are placed on the opposite side of the involved extremity and are advanced with the involved extremity. Therefore, in this example, the cane is placed on the right and advanced with the left lower extremity. (O'Sullivan 2007, page 545)

114. a. Strong pink skin color is a normal skin response following a 20-minute application of a superficial heating agent. This strong pink appearance is due to vasodilation of the blood vessels in the dermis. Mottling is an indication of overheating. Cyanosis and a chalky white appearance occur after cold applications. (Behrens and Michlovitz 2006, pages 24–25)

115. b. A 1.0 MHz sound head penetrates deeper than the 3.0 MHz. Additionally, because the condition is chronic, it is most appropriate to treat the piriformis with a 100% duty cycle. (Behrens and Michlovitz 2006, page 64)

116. a. While all four choices are superficial heat modalities, only with fluidotherapy is a patient encouraged to move during treatment. The other three require the patient to minimize movement during the treatment session. (Behrens and Michlovitz 2006, page 45)

117. d. Ultraviolet is the only modality stated in which psoriasis is a specific contraindication. (Hayes 2000, pages 44–45)

118. a. Individuals with Raynauds syndrome do not tolerate cold well. Hot packs, massage, and ultrasound are indicated. (Behrens and Michlovitz 2006, page 51)

119. c. Metal implants are a contraindication with diathermy. Hot packs, massage, and whirlpools are indicated. (Behrens and Michlovitz 2006, page 48)

120. d. Blackburn's (1981) and Jobe and Moynes's (1986) EMG studies determined when a patient is positioned prone, upper arm supported, forearm over the edge of the table, elbow and shoulder at 90 degrees, and the hand is placed in external rotation, the action of the teres minor and infraspinatus muscles is external rotation of the shoulder. (Gould 1990, pages 508–509)

121. b. Cardiac output is responsive to changes in the metabolic demands of the tissues. During exercise, the cardiac output may increase fourfold. This increase is accomplished by doubling the heart rate and stroke volume, thus increasing the cardiac output. (Lippincott 2000, pages 536–537)

122. c. The pulse rate for choice **a** is too low. It will not allow a tetanic contraction. For choice **b**, the off time for the on/off ratio will not likely cause muscle fatigue. The pulse rate and continuous mode would not be comfortable for the patient and could actually cause muscle cramping. The higher pulse rate and equal on/off ratio are appropriate, and choice **c** is the best choice to produce muscle fatigue. (Behrens and Michlovitz 2006, pages 177–178)

123. c. Increased centralized pain, decreased peripheral pain, and radicular symptoms indicate that the condition is resolving and the treatment is effective in decreasing pressure on the involved nerve root. (Hayes 1993, page 80)

124. a. To effectively apply two-rescuer CPR, one rescuer provides the breaths while the second rescuer gives chest compressions. Rescuers should alternate performing compressions after every five cycles (approximately two minutes) to reduce fatigue. (American Heart Association, Basic Life Support for Healthcare Providers 2006, pages 25–26)

125. c. Given the fact that the patient has had a hemiarthroplasty and has mild Alzheimer's disease, education should be focused on safety, ensuring correct follow-up with the next healthcare provider, and a home exercise program. Although all of these recommendations are appropriate in general, a patient with Alzheimer's disease may have difficulty remembering detail. However, including the patient's spouse in the discussion, providing written information on the exercise, and actually having the patient demonstrate the exercise will help the patient and the spouse to maintain activities until a home health therapist can begin to work with the patient. (O'Sullivan and Schmitz 2007, page 1,157)

126. b. The best way to verify a patient's understanding of exercise instructions is to have the patient demonstrate them. This allows the PTA to see the positioning and movement of the patient during the exercises to determine whether or not the patient understands all aspects of the instructions. (Dreeben 2010, page 29)

127. d. Sherri is in violation of HIPAA because she is speaking with Manuel about confidential information in front of another patient. The Health Insurance Portability and Accountability Act of 1996 is a federal law, administered through the U.S. Department of Health and Human Services, which regulates the use and disclosure of individuals' health information. Any information that can identify a patient is protected, including the patient's name, address, telephone number, date of birth, or Social Security number. Violations for disclosing personal identifying information—even if the disclosure was accidental—can result in heavy fines. Knowingly releasing identifying information without proper authorization can lead to infractions against the healthcare provider and the institution. (Hosley and Molle 2006, page 196; Nicholson 2008, page 233)

128. c. Manuel's behavior is illegal and unethical, because he is talking about confidential information in front of another patient, and this compromises patient privacy and confidentiality. Healthcare professionals have a clear legal and moral obligation to protect the privacy of those entrusted to their care. Confidentiality deals with private affairs that are not available to those not needing to know. The Standards of Ethical Conduct for the Physical Therapist Assistant provides a foundation of conduct expected by all physical therapist assistants. These standards require that the PTA both keep patient information confidential and report others who violate confidentiality. Many states' physical therapy practice acts include language requiring physical therapist assistants to maintain confidentiality and to report licensed colleagues who commit any infraction to the practice act and code or standards of ethical conduct. (APTA Standards of Ethical Conduct for the PTA 2010, Standards 2D and 4C)

129. b. Manuel is demonstrating a lack of cultural awareness by not wanting to treat a patient who has an accent. Cultural awareness describes a set of skills, knowledge, and attitudes that demonstrates awareness of and acceptance of difference, awareness of one's own cultural values, development of cultural knowledge, and commitment to seek approaches to service delivery that appreciates the uniqueness of every person. The Continuum of Cultural Proficiency describes skills or behaviors ranging from awareness through culturally sensitive proficiency in healthcare delivery. The physical therapist assistant is expected to recognize patients' individual and cultural differences and adapt accordingly. The PTA is also expected to display sensitivity when interacting with patients or clients, their caregivers, and other members of the healthcare team by treating patients regardless of differences in race, ethnicity, religion, gender, age, national origin, sexual orientation, disability, or health status. (Curtis and Newman 2005, pages 185–190)

130. a. The PTA does not have to discuss this situation with the family. This is a situation in which the PTA has been told of possible abuse. In many states, a PTA who is made aware of abuse has a responsibility to report the situation to the PT and to the proper authorities. The PTA should be aware of state and federal regulations affecting the types of patients or clients with which the PTA works. Abuse can be physical, psychological, medical, or financial, and can include neglect. At times, it may be difficult to identify abuse because the cause of the injury, behavior, or situation can often be attributed to causes other than abuse. Seniors may be hesitant to report abuse due to fear of retaliation. Each state has a division responsible for receiving and investigating suspected or confirmed cases of child or elder abuse or neglect. (Hosley and Molle 2006, page 193; Pozgar 2010, pages 380–382)

131. d. Required reporting is defined as follows: Abuse may occur in an institution, as well as in a person's home. Each state has a division responsible for receiving and investigating suspected or confirmed cases of child or elder abuse/neglect. Most states protect healthcare workers reporting with a good-faith belief that the facts being reported are true. The criminal and civil risks for healthcare workers lie in failing to report suspected incidents of elder and/or child abuse, not in good-faith reporting. (Pozgar 2010, pages 380–382)

132. c. The patient or client's right to refuse physical therapy treatment is an example of informed consent. Informed consent is voluntary agreement by a person with the mental capacity to make an intelligent choice to allow a treatment or procedure suggested by another person to be performed on him or her. Courts in the United States have emphasized and upheld that a competent adult has the right to decline any and all forms of medical intervention including lifesaving or life-prolonging choices. (Pozgar 2010, page 352)

133. d. Forcibly transferring a competent patient from the bed to the chair despite the fact that the patient has asked to be left alone is illegal and unethical because the person is being treated without his or her consent. Consent is voluntary agreement by a person with the mental capacity to make an intelligent choice to allow a treatment or procedure by another person to be performed on him or her. Courts in the United States have emphasized and upheld that a competent adult has the right to decline any and all forms of medical intervention including lifesaving or life-prolonging choices. (Pozgar 2010, page 352; APTA 2010, Standards of Ethical Conduct)

134. a. The number one way for a PTA to reduce the risk of cross contamination in the healthcare environment is through hand washing. The PTA should wash his or her hands both before and after providing patient care in order to reduce the risk of the spread of infection from one person to another. (Pierson and Fairchild 2007, page 9)

135. d. Personal protective equipment (PPE) serves as a barrier to prevent contamination between human beings. The purpose of the PPE (including proper removal and disposal) is to interrupt or establish barriers to the infection cycle. (Myers 2004, page 110)

136. a. Pull (don't push) objects when moving them from point A to point B is not a rule of proper body mechanics. (The rule is push, don't pull.) Adherence to proper body

mechanics reduces stress and strain and prevents PTAs from injury. It also helps PTAs care for the patient or client safely. Important considerations in body mechanics include:

- Plan activity/actions ahead of time.
- Face object you will lift—do not twist.
- Lift with leg muscles and stabilize your core or trunk muscles.
- Ensure your base of support is wide enough to enhance your balance.
- Position yourself close to the object.
- Push don't pull.
- Get adequate help—invest the time for your and your patient's safety. (Pierson 2007, page 109)

137. c. The PTA should competently use emergency management procedures. Effectively responding to a patient or client and to environmental emergencies in one's practice setting is a competency expectation for a PTA. Effective emergency preparedness includes competent use of emergency management procedures to protect and save patients or clients and others from fire, tornado, hurricane, or other disasters; using disaster evacuation measures; or using seizure precautions. (APTA Normative Model PTA Education 2009)

138. b. This unacceptable behavior is punishable by law. A variety of federal and state laws have been enacted to protect employees from unfair treatment at work. The Equal Employment Opportunity Commission (EEOC) enforces this and other laws related to fair employment practices. Employee rights include the right to be free from sexual harassment and intimidation; the right to be treated with dignity and respect; and employment at will and fair treatment practices. (Pozgar 2010, page 348)

139. c. An incident report provides a place to document the circumstances depicting an event and an opportunity for an internal investigation. This investigation surrounds the what, how, and why and details what can be done to reduce the risk of it happening again. Incident reports are often documents created in anticipation of litigation and are typically not required to be submitted to the other party or documented in the patient's medical record. (Pozgar 2010, page 232)

140. d. The specific limitations and expectations of the physical therapist assistant within the clinical setting are dictated by the practice act of that particular state. (Umphred and Carlson 2006, page 4)

141. a. The physical therapist's tasks weigh heavily with the process of decision making. Effective delegation strategies were proposed as a taxonomy by Nancy Watts in a landmark article in 1971. Within this systematic approach for the division of responsibility, tasks are analyzed in terms of the process of decision making ("deciding" behaviors) versus delivering an intervention ("doing" behaviors) required in the practice of physical therapy. (Watts 1971, pages 23–25)

142. a. PTAs provide physical therapy services only under the direction and supervision of physical therapists. (Curtis and Newman 2005, page 4; Umphred and Carlson 2006, page 4)

143. a. Severity of tissue injury: Grade I (first degree)—mild pain at the time of injury or within the first 24 hours; mild swelling and local tenderness occur when the tissue is stressed. Grade II (second degree)—moderate pain that requires stopping the activity; stress and palpation of the tissue greatly increase the pain; ligaments injuries with torn fibers increase joint mobility. Grade III (third degree)—near-complete or complete tear or avulsion of the tissue (tendon or ligament) with severe pain; stress to the tissue is usually painless; palpation may reveal the defect;

increased ligament fiber tears result in instability of the joint. (Kisner and Colby 2007, page 297)

144. b. Obstructive lung disorders are characterized by an increase in airway resistance and a resultant decrease in airflow during expiration. (Moffat and Frownfelter 2000, page 87)

145. c. Type I fibers need oxygen to make ATP used for muscle activity. 95% of ATP comes from aerobic respiration. When the lungs are compromised by chronic lung disease, this activity is altered. (Pearson, Benjamine, and Cummings 2007, page 302)

146. b. Maceration is skin damage due to excessive moisture. (Myers 2004, page 26)

147. a. Timed up and go scores are categorized as follows: Normal range is 7–10 seconds. If the patient takes longer than 20 seconds, the patient will have mild to moderate mobility problems resulting in the need for assistance when ambulating in the community. The presented scenario indicates a patient with high risk of falls without physical assistance despite the use of an assistive device. Treatment goals must be realistic and age appropriate. The treatment plan should strive to achieve normal quality and velocity of ambulation as well as patient safety during ambulation. (Guccione 2000, pages 309–310)

148. c. Facilitated agonist contraction techniques to hamstrings would be most effective to address the mobility deficits associated with hip flexion contractures measured at −20 degrees. Agonist contraction technique is a facilitated stretching technique designed to stretch the hip flexors. This would be most appropriate to address loss of mobility. Strengthening the hip flexors will generally make them tighter. Recumbent bicycling positions the hip in more than 25 degrees of hip flexion, which would not address the flexibility at the hip. Balance on foam would also not address mobility at the hip. (Kisner and Colby 2007, page 86)

149. a. The most appropriate exercise to begin treatment for a patient with impingement syndrome of the right dominant shoulder is flexion to 90 degrees performed passively by the physical therapist assistant. Passive range of motion is the only intervention listed that is appropriate in the acute stage of rehab. While the other activities may be appropriate later on—such as the finger ladder or, when in subacute, resisted thera-band activities and isokinetic activities—they are not appropriate during the acute stage of rehabilitation. (Kisner and Colby 2007, page 506)

150. a. Vibration is a manual technique used after postural draining to help move secretions to larger airways. Vibration is safely applied only during the expiratory phase as the patient is deep-breathing. Strict adherence to this sequence reduces the chance of secretions remaining in smaller airways. (Kisner and Colby 2007, page 871)

Clinical Application of Physical Therapy Principles and Foundational Sciences

CHAPTER SUMMARY

The material in this chapter is intended to allow the student to review the anatomy and physiology of the major body systems with which physical therapy is involved. These are the cardiovascular and pulmonary systems, the musculoskeletal system, the neuromuscular system, the integumentary system, and the endocrine and metabolic systems. A solid understanding of normal anatomy and physiology is integral to understanding the pathologies reviewed in this chapter and also serves as the basis for applying the data-collection techniques covered in Chapter 6 and the interventions discussed in Chapter 7. The overall goal of this chapter is to help the student understand how problems in each system affect, and are affected by, physical therapy treatment.

Cardiac, Vascular, and Pulmonary Systems

This section covers anatomy and function of the heart as well as the vascular, lymphatic, and pulmonary systems. It also covers common pathologies of the cardiac, vascular, lymphatic, and pulmonary systems. This foundational information provides the understanding necessary for the safe and effective treatment of patients in the physical therapy setting.

Normal Anatomy and Function of the Heart

Blood flow can be traced through the heart beginning at the right atrium. Blood flows from there through the right atrioventricular, or tricuspid, valve into the right ventricle. Blood leaves the right ventricle, flowing through the pulmonary semilunar valve into the pulmonary artery. After the gas exchange occurs in the lungs, the blood passes through the pulmonary vein and into the left atrium. The pulmonary artery is the only artery in the body that carries relatively deoxygenated blood, and is the only vein that carries oxygenated blood. From the left atrium, the blood moves through the left atrioventricular, or mitral, valve into the left ventricle and then to the aorta. At the very beginning of the aorta and just behind the aortic semilunar valve, the left and right coronary arteries branch off to supply blood to the myocardium. Many Americans suffer and die from coronary disease each year, so knowledge of the distribution pattern of these arteries is important. The highest percentage of blood supply moves to the left ventricle in accordance with the amount of work done in this area. Each atrium receives blood from the corresponding coronary artery, while the ventricles receive their blood supply from branches of both the right and left coronary arteries.

Heart Rate and Contractility

The heart rate is normally controlled by impulses from the sinoatrial (SA) node. The primary modifier of this rate is the ratio of impulses from the sympathetic (stimulatory) and parasympathetic (inhibitory) nervous systems. The parasympathetic impulses reach the SA node via the vagus nerve, which is cranial nerve X. The sympathetic impulses are carried by chemicals such as epinephrine and norepinephrine, and reach the SA node via the bloodstream. Other factors such as hormones, exercise, pain, body temperature, and emotions can play an important role in influencing heart rate.

Cardiac Conduction

The cardiac conduction system is made up of four bundles of highly specialized cardiac tissue. Impulses initiate from the sinoatrial node causing the atria to contract. The impulse passes quickly to the atrioventricular node (AV) where it slows down to allow complete contraction of the atria before the ventricles are stimulated. After passing through the AV node, the impulse passes quickly through the bundle of His (or atrioventricular bundle) into the ventricles. The terminal point for the impulse is the Purkinje fibers which relay the electrical impulse to the heart muscle cells causing ventricular contraction.

Electrocardiogram

The electrocardiogram (EKG or ECG) assesses heart rate, rhythm, coronary perfusion, and conduction delays. An EKG is a record of the electrical activity (action potentials) leading up to the contractions of the chambers of the heart. The action potentials are represented by a sequence of waves designated by the letters P, QRS complex, and T. The individual letters contain no significance and do not represent other words. Instead, meaning is centered on their sequential patterns. The P wave indicates depolarization of the atria. The QRS complex gives a clear picture of ventricular depolarization. The T wave shows ventricular repolarization. Measurement of these interval wavelengths provides valuable information on heart rate, heart rhythm, and on the rate of conduction of the action potential as it passes through the system. Measurement of the intervals' height can be used to interpret the degree of contractility of the heart and coronary perfusion.

Common Pathologies

In the role of physical therapist assistant, many pathologies of the cardiac system may be encountered. It is important to understand these pathologies by definition as well as by signs and symptoms. This section also includes common medical management.

Angina Pectoris

Angina pectoris is a transient ischemia that occurs when the coronary arteries are unable to supply the heart muscle with adequate oxygen. Coronary artery disease (CAD) accounts for almost all (90%) of angina. Causative factors are usually physical activity or stress. Signs and symptoms include sudden onset of temporary pain that usually lasts one to five minutes. The pain may originate in the chest but can also radiate into the neck, jaw, or arms. This condition is usually treated with rest and nitroglycerin. It can be confused with an acute myocardial infarction (MI). If rest and medication do not relieve symptoms, emergency medical intervention is required.

Cardiomyopathy

Cardiomyopathy is a term used to describe a group of diseases affecting the myocardium or muscular layer of the heart. The three disease categories are dilated, hypertrophic, and restrictive. All types hinder the heart's ability to contract and relax, thus decreasing its ability to pump blood effectively. Symptoms include neck vein distension, fatigue or weakness, possible chest pain, and exercise intolerance. There is no cure for cardiomyopathy, and the only lasting treatment is a heart transplant.

Congestive Heart Failure

Congestive heart failure is the end result of several conditions—including coronary artery disease—and is essentially pump failure. Back pressure from stagnant blood causes congestion in other organs and extremities because of this pump failure. Clinical signs include fluid retention in the extremities, pulmonary edema, orthopnea, elevated resting heart rate, and nonproductive cough. Treatments include reversing or enhancing the underlying problem through medications such as digitalis, ACE inhibitors, or beta-blockers or utilizing lifestyle changes, such as a salt-restricted diet to prevent fluid retention. Surgical interventions that may be effective in treating this condition include heart transplant, left ventricular assist device (LVAD)—a temporary device used to bolster a failing heart—or pacemaker.

Coronary Artery Disease

Coronary artery disease is the result of atherosclerosis (fatty buildup inside vessel walls) in the coronary arteries. This condition results from cumulative buildup over many years and results in narrowing or blockage of the coronary vessels. This condition could result in ischemia or necrosis of heart tissue. Contributing factors include genetics, smoking, obesity, and hypertension. Signs and symptoms may vary, from being asymptomatic to angina. Symptoms usually occur after approximately 75% blockage has occurred. If the condition goes untreated, an MI or sudden death may occur. The most common treatment is insertion of a stint to open the vessel and prevent further occlusion. Medications may be utilized based on physiological need such as alpha-adrenergic blocking agents to dilate arterioles and veins and decrease blood pressure. (Examples would be Cardura® and Minipress®.) Calcium channel blockers will decrease the heart's demand for oxygen by reducing the flow of calcium, thus allowing increased peripheral vasodilation. (Examples would be Procardia® and Norvasc®.) Other medications including nitrates and diuretics may be prescribed. Surgical intervention would include a coronary artery bypass.

Endocarditis

Endocarditis is an inflammatory infection of the inner lining of the heart. Bacteria and fungi are the most common causes. The most commonly damaged structure is the mitral valve, but endocarditis can also damage the aortic and tricuspid valves. It can occur after an invasive medical or dental procedure. Symptoms may occur suddenly or may take months to appear and include fever, chest pain, valvular murmurs, congestive heart failure, and myalgia. The potential for damage to the involved valves is high, and they may require replacement with artificial ones. Bacterial and fungal infections can be treated with medications.

People who are at risk for endocarditis may be advised to use antibiotics prophylactically.

Myocardial Infarction

Myocardial infarction is a sequence of events that leads to irreversible heart tissue damage. Several conditions including atherosclerotic occlusion, poor coronary perfusion, or occlusion of a major artery could lead to prolonged ischemia of an area of the heart. Symptoms include sudden crushing pain or pressure in the chest; radiation of pain into the neck, jaw, upper back or arms; shortness of breath; profuse sweating; and fatigue. If a large portion of the heart is involved, an arrhythmia may occur. If the situation goes untreated, death will occur within minutes. Treatment consists of restoring cardiac rhythm via CPR or electrical defibrillation. Tissue damage cannot be repaired, but patients who recover from the infarct may undergo coronary bypass to open blocked vessels and restore circulation. Some patients may require a heart transplant.

Pericarditis

Pericarditis is inflammation of the pericardial sac. It usually occurs in conjunction with other infections of the heart and is most often caused by bacteria or viruses. It may also develop as a result of cardiac surgery or malignant disease. The inflammation causes fluid to collect in the sac, which can become very painful. Symptoms may include chest pain, diffuse ST segment elevation, cough or hoarseness, joint pain, fever, and weakness. Treatment could include managing the underlying condition, controlling pain, and drainage of fluid through a chest tube.

Rheumatic Heart Disease

Rheumatic heart disease (RHD) is a multisystem condition that also affects joints, subcutaneous connective tissue, and less frequently the brain. A common cause of RHD is streptococcal infections of the throat and upper respiratory system. It may involve all layers of the heart tissue (presenting as endo-, myo-, or pericarditis) and frequently causes valve damage. Symptoms would be chest pain, acute onset of polyarthritis, palpitations, fever, joint pain, and weakness. There is no treatment, as most lesions that occur from this disease are irreversible. Surgical intervention may be used to replace damaged valves.

Normal Anatomy and Function of Vascular System

The vascular system is made up of arteries, veins, and capillaries. Arteries carry blood away from the heart. Except for the pulmonary artery, all arteries carry oxygenated blood. Small arteries are called arterioles.

Veins carry blood toward the heart and, with the exception of the pulmonary vein, carry deoxygenated blood. Small veins are called venules.

Capillaries—the smallest of vessels—connect these two parts of the vascular system and provide an avenue for distribution of oxygen and nutrients to the cells of the body.

Location of Major Veins and Arteries

The superior and inferior vena cava carry blood from the body to the heart. The brachiocephalic vein receives blood from the head and upper extremities, while the common iliac vein receives blood from the lower extremities. The pulmonary artery takes blood from the heart to the lungs, and the pulmonary vein brings blood back to the heart from the lungs. The aorta is the main artery carrying blood away from the heart to the rest of the body.

The vertebral and carotid arteries supply the head, the axillary artery supplies the upper extremities, and the femoral artery supplies the lower extremities.

Structure of Arteries and Veins

Although veins and arteries carry the same substance—blood—they are made up of very different types of tissue. The arteries are under higher pressure from the force of the ventricular contraction and must therefore have slightly thicker walls. The veins have an additional structure arising from the endothelium in the form of valves that assure one-way movement of the blood toward the heart. As blood vessels decrease in size, so does their relative thickness. The smallest of vessels, the capillaries, are also the thinnest. This is an important attribute because the capillary walls must allow for efficient exchange of gases and other materials between the blood and interstitial fluid.

Common Pathologies of the Vascular System

Conditions in the peripheral vascular system can lead to impairments, such as pain, weakness, sensory changes, and open wounds. These conditions will benefit from effective interventions.

Chronic Arterial Insufficiency

Chronic arterial insufficiency is one form of peripheral vascular disease (PVD). It refers to a lack of blood flow to an area of the body. The areas primarily involved are the lower extremities. Several disorders such as arteriosclerosis, atherosclerosis, and Reynaud's disease can contribute to the development of chronic arterial insufficiency by narrowing the diameter of the arteries. The most common symptom of this disorder is cramping or aching in the calves during exertion. This pain is caused by intermittent claudication as the muscles are not receiving the blood perfusion required for the exertion level. An important test administered to examine the function of the arterial system is the Ankle-Brachial Pressure Index. The single most important intervention for PVD is smoking cessation. Other helpful treatments include keeping body weight down and managing hypertension.

Chronic Venous Insufficiency

Chronic venous insufficiency is the most common type of PVD that refers to inadequate drainage of the venous system of a body part. This typically affects the lower extremities and is the primary cause of leg ulcers. Aging, obesity, prolonged standing, and genetics may predispose a person to this disorder. Edema is often the first sign, while varicosities and ulceration may follow. Treatment usually consists of compression and elevation to aid blood flow.

Deep Vein Thrombosis (DVT)

Deep vein thrombosis is a disorder involving one of the deep veins of the body, most often the iliac or femoral vein. A thrombus forms, occluding blood flow through the vessel. This is a potentially life-threatening condition. For example, an embolus from this thrombus could lodge in the lungs or heart and result in death. Although patients could be asymptomatic, most will complain of pain or heat in the affected area. They may also have skin redness and swelling. Doppler ultrasound is the most often used test to diagnose a DVT, though an MRI can also detect presence of thrombi. Treatment options include anticoagulant and thrombolytic drug therapy to prevent the clot from growing larger or from forming an embolus that could move to a more dangerous location. Patients who form repeated clots, or who cannot take anticoagulants, may have a filter placed in the inferior vena cava to prevent emboli from reaching the heart and lungs.

Normal Anatomy and Function of the Lymphatic System

The two main functions of the lymphatic system are to maintain fluid balance and to fight infection. As plasma from the circulatory system filters through the tissues, some is absorbed into the tissue cells, some is reabsorbed by the blood, and a small percentage remains in the interstitial spaces. This interstitial fluid could accumulate, causing massive edema and resultant tissue destruction or death, if not for the presence of the lymphatic drainage system. This drainage system parallels the venous system. The fluids collected here are eventually returned to the circulatory system after passing through the lymph nodes. The lymph nodes help the body fight infection by filtering out dead cells and bacteria and by creating antibodies.

Other structures associated with this system include the thymus gland, tonsils, and spleen.

Pathology of the Lymphatic System

Lymphedema, an important pathological condition of the lymphatic system, can occur for different reasons in a variety of patients. Patients with lymphedema may benefit from effective interventions.

Lymphedema

Lymphedema is a condition that arises from an accumulation of lymph fluid in the tissue. It can be caused by an inflammation, an obstruction, or by removal of the lymph channels. It can occur in any part of the body but is most common in the lower extremities. Another common site is the upper extremity of a person who has undergone a radical mastectomy with lymph node removal. There are two types of lymphedema—primary lymphedema and secondary lymphedema.

Primary lymphedema is the least common type and arises from a congenital or hereditary condition. Secondary lymphedema is the most prevalent and is usually triggered by damage to the lymph system due to surgery or radiation treatment, although it can also be the result of paralysis or trauma to regional lymph nodes. Symptoms are numerous and include swelling in tissues near the area of lymph impairment that is not relieved by elevation; pitting edema; fatigue; numbness or tingling; increased susceptibility to infection; loss of mobility and ROM; and impaired wound healing. In most cases, special testing is not necessary to arrive at a diagnosis of lymphedema. Patient history and physical presentation are usually adequate for accurate diagnosis. There is no cure for the condition, but treatment can work to improve lymph drainage from the extremity and should include elevation, compression, and moderate exercise. Light massage, diuretics, and avoidance of spicy or salty foods may also be beneficial. Therapeutic intervention for a patient with lymphedema is most effective if begun early and best performed by someone trained in the specialty. This training is not provided by entry-level professional programs.

Normal Anatomy and Function of Pulmonary System

The respiratory system functions as both an air distributor and a gas exchanger. It works in conjunction with the circulatory system to accomplish the gas exchange necessary for optimal functioning of the body's cells. The respiratory system is divided into the upper and lower tracts. The upper respiratory tract includes the nose, nasopharynx, oropharynx, laryngopharynx, and larynx. The lower respiratory tract is composed of the trachea, all segments of the bronchial tree, and the lungs. At the lower end of the trachea, the two branches of the bronchus divide to send air into each of the two lungs. An interesting anatomical fact is that the right bronchus is slightly larger and more vertical than the left which explains why, when aspiration occurs, the object is more frequently lodged in the right bronchus. The bronchi branches are divided into smaller tubes called bronchioles which eventually terminate in the alveolar sacs. It is at the point of the alveoli that the gaseous exchange with the blood occurs. The right lung is divided into three lobes, while the left lung has only two. Each lobe is divided into segments named for their location, such as apical, anterior, lateral, etc.

The air distribution portion of the lung function is performed by the bronchial tree. The gas exchange portion of the lung function is performed by the alveolar sacs in conjunction with the capillaries that envelop them. Breath sounds can be broken into categories.

Normal Breath Sounds

Normal tracheal and bronchial sounds are high-pitched, loud, and tubular and can be heard during inspiration and expiration with a pause between the two. Sounds can be heard in the more distal airways primarily during inspiration and are noted as soft and low pitched. These are called vesicular breath sounds and are also normal sounds.

Abnormal Breath Sounds

Abnormal sounds, called adventitious breath sounds, include sounds that are heard outside of the normal phase of breathing or location. The sounds are heard through a stethoscope. They include: wheeze, which is a continuous, high-pitched sound that generally indicates airway obstruction; rhonchi are continuous, adventitious breath sounds occurring with both inspiration and expiration and are low in pitch. They indicate obstruction in the larger airways; stridor is also a continuous adventitious breath sound heard on both inspiration and expiration and contains a high-pitched wheeze. It can indicate an upper airway obstruction. If this is heard without a stethoscope it can signal a medical emergency; crackles (previously termed rales) are the pops and bubble sounds that usually represent movement of fluid (wet sounds) or opening and closing of airways (dry sounds); decreased or diminished breath sounds are less audible sounds that usually indicate extreme congestion, advanced emphysema, or other conditions resulting in hypoventilation; absent breath sounds may indicate severe compromise to the system, such as atelectasis or pneumothorax.

Lung Volumes and Capacities

The amount of air moving in and out of the lungs can be quantified in a number of ways. Residual volume is the amount of air left in the lungs after maximal expiration. Tidal volume is the amount of air moved during a relaxed inspiration and relaxed expiration. The total lung capacity is the amount of air in the lungs after a maximal inspiration. The vital capacity is the amount of air moved during a maximal inspiration and a maximal expiration.

Common Pathologies

The following are common pathologies of the pulmonary system.

Chronic Obstructive Pulmonary Disease

This is a category of diseases marked by increased resistance to the passage of air either in or out of the lungs due to narrowing of the bronchial tree. Several diseases fall in this category: asthma, bronchiectasis, chronic bronchitis, and emphysema.

Asthma

Asthma is a condition where the respiratory system is characterized by bronchospasm and increased mucous production. Triggers include exercise, stress, and allergens such as mold, pollen, or animal dander. Asthma attacks may range from mild to life-threatening. Symptoms include increased respiration rate, increased utilization of accessory muscles, dyspnea, wheezing, prolonged expiration, and nonproductive cough. Medical intervention may be warranted and patients may use a bronchodilator.

Bronchiectasis

Bronchiectasis is a progressive obstructive disorder that manifests itself by abnormal dilation of a bronchus. This

Determining Pulmonary Volume

Inspiration reserve volume + tidal volume + expiratory reserve volume + residual volume	= total lung capacity	5,700–6,200 mL
Inspiratory reserve volume + tidal volume + expiratory reserve volume	= vital capacity	4,000–5,000 mL
Tidal volume + inspiratory reserve volume	= inspiratory capacity	3,000–4,000 mL
Expiratory reserve volume + residual volume	= functional residual capacity	2,200–2,400 mL

Values for pulmonary volume can be determined using these equations.

condition is irreversible and is usually associated with other chronic conditions, such as infection, cystic fibrosis, or aspiration. Symptoms include crackles, wheezes, loud breath sounds, chronic productive cough, and hemoptysis.

Chronic Bronchitis

Chronic bronchitis is diagnosed if a productive cough is present for three months during two consecutive years. This results in increased mucous secretions as well as structural changes to the bronchi. Symptoms include dyspnea, cyanosis, systemic edema, persistent cough, wheezing, increased pulmonary artery pressure, and thick sputum.

Emphysema

Emphysema is the last of the COPD conditions and results from chronic irritation of the pulmonary tissue. It is often associated with smoking. The air spaces within the alveolar sacs become permanently distended making expiration difficult and causing dead air space to increase. Symptoms include dyspnea, chronic cough, barrel chest, increased respiratory rate, and orthopnea.

Cystic Fibrosis

Cystic fibrosis (CF) is an autosomal-recessive disorder that causes excessive secretion by the exocrine glands of the body. The glands most affected are found in the lungs, pancreas, and sweat glands. In the lungs, the most difficulty comes from the excessive, thick mucus that fills the lumen of the bronchial tree causing difficulty with breathing. Symptoms include chronic cough, frequent foul-smelling stools, and persistent upper respiratory infections. There is no cure for CF and treatment focuses on dislodging secretions using techniques such as postural drainage, breathing exercises, and antibiotics prophylactically to prevent infection. Heart-lung and double-lung transplants have been successful in treating CF.

Pulmonary Embolus

A pulmonary embolus is the blockage of a pulmonary artery by fat, air, or a part of a blood clot that arises from a peripheral vein. Predisposing factors can include stagnation of blood due to immobility after procedures such as childbirth or surgery, damage to blood vessels walls, or excessive coagulation. It can be difficult to distinguish from a myocardial infarction, as the symptoms are very similar and include dyspnea, anxiety, cyanosis, and sudden chest pain. Diagnostic tests used to detect a pulmonary emboli include chest X-ray and pulmonary angiography. The majority of patients with pulmonary emboli die within a few hours. Treatment beyond that time could include an embolectomy and use of anticoagulants to prevent further clot formation. Introduction of ambulation, exercise, and modalities to increase lower extremity circulation can be used prophylactically.

Restrictive Pulmonary Disease

Restrictive pulmonary disease is a disorder characterized by diminished lung volumes and capacities due to lung expansion or chest wall restrictions. This condition can be caused by weak respiratory muscles, thoracic deformities such as scoliosis, or diseases such as tuberculosis and pneumonia. It may also occur following a thoracotomy. Symptoms include shortness of breath, ineffective cough, and increased respiratory rate.

Tuberculosis

Tuberculosis (TB) is a bacterial infection that is transmitted via droplets in the air. TB can affect several structures in the body besides the lungs. Symptoms include fatigue, loss of weight, dyspnea, anorexia, productive cough, and low-grade fever. Diagnosis can be made by X-ray. This condition can be treated with drug therapy and can be prevented by childhood immunization.

Practice 1

1. Which of the following statements best explains chronic bronchitis?
   a. A condition characterized by thickened pulmonary secretions that obstruct the airway.
   b. A condition characterized by limited airflow as a result of airway inflammation.
   c. Episodic periods of airway narrowing secondary to bronchospasm of the airways.
   d. A condition in which lung volume is reduced with decreased lung expansion.

2. A PTA assesses a patient two days post THR, and the patient complains of sudden chest pain and difficulty breathing. The PTA notes cyanosis of the nail beds. Which of the following is the most likely cause of this patient's distress?
   a. myocardial infarction
   b. bronchitis
   c. pulmonary embolus
   d. pneumonia

3. Which of the following diagnostic tests would give the least information regarding patient status with regard to a patient suffering from a pulmonary embolism?
   a. blood gas analysis
   b. chest X-ray
   c. lung scan
   d. EKG

4. What is the equation used to determine inspiratory capacity?
   a. tidal volume and inspiratory reserve volume
   b. tidal volume and expiratory reserve volume
   c. residual volume and expiratory reserve volume
   d. residual volume and inspiratory reserve volume

5. The PT is working with a pulmonary patient, and you notice an equation in the patient's chart that reads "inspiratory reserve volume + tidal volume + expiratory reserve volume + residual volume." From this information, you know that the therapist was looking for which of the following values?
   a. inspiratory capacity
   b. vital capacity
   c. functional residual capacity
   d. total lung capacity

6. A PTA is providing treatment for a pediatric patient. The patient's mother is concerned that the child may have aspirated a small toy while lying on the mat table waiting for the session to begin. You know that if lung aspiration has occurred the toy will probably show up in the right lung. Which of the following is the correct justification for this rational?
   a. The right bronchus is slightly smaller and more horizontal.
   b. The left bronchus is larger and more vertical.
   c. The right bronchus is larger and more vertical.
   d. The position of the child when the object disappeared.

7. Blood enters the heart from the vena cava and travels through the atrium into the ventricle via which of the following valves?
a. right atrioventricular (tricuspid) valve
b. left atrioventricular (mitral) valve
c. semilunar valve
d. bicuspid valve

8. A PTA reads a patient chart in preparation for treatment. Which of the following values will give the most complete picture of the patient's cardiac condition?
a. stroke volume
b. cardiac index
c. cardiac output
d. blood volume

9. Which of the following statements is true regarding an electrocardiogram?
a. It can be used to assess the amount of air exchanged in the lungs.
b. It can be used to assess heart rate and the electrical conduction system of the heart.
c. It can be used to identify the amount of blood flowing through the heart.
d. It can be used to assess vascular insufficiency in the extremities.

10. A PTA is monitoring an exercise program when the patient complains of chest pain and shortness of breath. The patient has a diagnosis of angina. The PTA suspends the exercise and places the patient supine and the patient self-administers nitro-glycerin. After the prescribed dosage and time has elapsed, the patient still complains of symp-toms but wants to continue the exercise routine. Which of the following is the most appropriate course of action for the PTA?
a. end session and activate emergency procedures
b. end session and advise the patient to see his or her physician
c. allow patient to resume exercise
d. allow patient to resume exercise, decrease resistance and repetitions, and monitor closely

11. When viewing an ECG or EKG, the QRS complex is assessing which of the following?
a. atrial depolarization
b. atrial repolarization
c. ventricular depolarization
d. ventricular repolarization

12. Which of the following is a true statement regarding the Ankle-Brachial Pressure Index?
    a. It can be used to assess the amount of air exchanged in the lungs.
    b. It can be used to assess heart rate and the electrical conduction system of the heart.
    c. It can be used to identify the amount of blood flowing through the heart.
    d. It can be used to assess arterial insufficiency in the extremities.

13. The lymphatic system is made up of vessels and nodes. All of the following are accessory structures to this system EXCEPT
    a. the thymus.
    b. the spleen.
    c. the pancreas.
    d. the tonsils.

14. Lymphedema is a condition that arises from an accumulation of lymph fluid in the tissue. The most common form of lymphedema is which of the following?
    a. primary lymphedema
    b. secondary lymphedema
    c. acute lymphedema
    d. chronic lymphedema

15. A patient presents with symptoms that include swelling that isn't relieved by elevation alone, pitting edema, fatigue, and numbness or tingling in the right lower extremity. Upon review of the patient chart, which of the following would be most likely noted as the patient diagnosis?
    a. chronic arterial insufficiency
    b. DVT
    c. lymphedema
    d. chronic venous insufficiency

16. A patient has a complaint of calf pain brought on by intermittent claudication. This is most commonly seen in which of the following diagnoses?
    a. chronic arterial insufficiency
    b. chronic venous insufficiency
    c. DVT
    d. pulmonary embolus

17. Which of the following is the abbreviation for the diagnosis defined most simply as "pump failure"?
    a. COPD
    b. MI
    c. CHF
    d. CAD

Practice 1 Answers

1. b. Additionally, chronic bronchitis has a strong connection with smoking and involves increased mucus production due to inflamed pulmonary tissue.

2. c. This patient has just undergone a lower extremity surgical procedure, so embolus is mostly likely. The cyanotic nail beds would also indicate an oxygenation problem and often aren't seen in MIs until later in the process.

3. d. While an EKG may be performed, it will not give information on the status of the pulmonary vessel function, location of the embolus, or blood oxygen levels, all of which are vital to sustaining the patient's life.

4. a. See chart titled Determining Pulmonary Volume on page 81.

5. d. See chart titled Determining Pulmonary Volume on page 81.

6. c. The larger, more vertical position of the right bronchus leads to aspirants, in this case a toy, moving in that direction.

7. a. Blood enters the right atrium from the vena cava and passes through the right atrioventricular, or tricuspid, valve into the right ventricle.

8. b. Cardiac index provides a more complete assessment of a patient's cardiac output by looking at the amount of blood being pumped from the heart per minute per square meter of body mass. Normal CI range is 2.5 to 3.5 L/min/m^2.

9. b. The electrocardiogram (EKG or ECG) assesses heart rate, rhythm, coronary perfusion, and conduction delays.

10. a. This condition is usually treated with rest and nitroglycerin. It can be confused with an acute MI. If rest and medication do not relieve symptoms, emergency medical intervention is required.

11. c. The QRS complex gives a clear picture of ventricular depolarization.

12. d. An important test administered to examine the function of the arterial system is the Ankle-Brachial Pressure Index.

13. c. This drainage system parallels the venous system and in fact the fluids collected here are eventually returned to the circulatory system after passing through filtering tissues called lymph nodes. Other structures associated with this system include the thymus gland, tonsils, and spleen.

14. b. Secondary lymphedema is the most prevalent and is usually triggered by damage to the lymph system due to surgery or radiation treatment, although it can also be the result of paralysis or trauma to regional lymph nodes.

15. c. Symptoms of lymphedema are numerous and include swelling in tissues distal or adjacent to the area of lymph impairment that is not relieved by elevation, pitting edema, fatigue, numbness or tingling, increased susceptibility to infection, loss of mobility and ROM, and impaired wound healing.

16. a. Patients with chronic arterial insufficiency often have calf pain caused by intermittent claudication, as the muscles are not receiving the blood perfusion required for the exertion level.

17. c. Congestive heart failure is the end result of several conditions, including coronary artery disease, and is essentially defined as pump failure.

Musculoskeletal System

The musculoskeletal system is an integral part of physical therapy practice throughout all clinical settings impacting patients across the lifespan continuum. This section will cover the anatomy and associated physiology of the musculoskeletal system as well as the kinesiology by major joint complex. It will also discuss diseases and conditions that impact the system along with the appropriate medical management.

The musculoskeletal system is necessary to achieve voluntary movement that accomplishes our daily activities. In an adult, 206 bones form the structural framework of the body divided into the axial and appendicular skeleton. The skeleton is then connected via a series of joints, the most mobile of which are synovial joints. The amount of movement or stability of a joint is dependent on the shape of the articular interfaces and the associated ligaments and capsule. The striated or voluntary muscles are anchored to the skeletal system through tendons and create movement around the joint through electrochemical signals initiated by the nervous system and sent along specific nerve pathways.

Normal Anatomy and Kinesiology by Joint Complex

Understanding the normal anatomy and kinesiology of each of the major joints is a foundational element necessary to treat patients with musculoskeletal disorders. Each joint's unique features endow it with specific characteristics that provide mobility or stability to a given area and work in concert with other joints to produce functional movement. Loss of function is often a result of abnormal joint formation or movement. With greater understanding of normal joints and joint accessory movements, physical therapist assistants can help patients resume normal mobility, strength, and function.

Shoulder Complex

The highly mobile shoulder complex is actually comprised of four joints:

- glenohumeral joint
- scapulothoracic joint
- acromioclavicular joint
- sternoclavicular joint

The glenohumeral joint consists of the glenoid fossa of the scapula articulating with the head of the humerus. This ball and socket joint, or spheroidal synovial joint, is the most mobile of all our joints. Two-thirds of the movement of the shoulder joint into elevation (flexion, abduction, or scaption) comes from the glenohumeral joint. The arthrokinematics in an open-chained environment where the distal segment or humerus is free to move—the convex shaped humeral head moves on the concave glenoid fossa. This results in the joint play motion at the glenohumeral joint to be in the opposite direction of the observed movement.

TAKE NOTE

There is a two to one relationship between motions from the glenohumeral joint to the scapulothoracic joint. For every 90 degrees of shoulder joint motion, 60 degrees comes from the glenohumeral joint and 30 degrees from the scapulothoracic joint.

The stability of the glenohumeral joint is dependent on the functioning of a strong rotator cuff or SITS group. The supraspinatus, infraspinatus, teres minor, and subscapularis help to hold the head of the humerus into the smaller glenoid fossa. The glenoid fossa is surrounded by the glenoid labrum, which helps to deepen the cup for the humeral head. The superior, middle, and inferior glenohumeral ligaments are present anteriorly and the coracohumeral ligament is superior and slightly posterior. These ligaments are weak and are ineffective in maintaining joint stability on their own without the help of the rotator cuff. Surrounding the glenohumeral joint is the joint capsule. It is redundant inferiorly to allow for 180 degrees of shoulder complex elevation.

INFORMATION IN ACTION

Patients who have pain in their glenohumeral joint after surgery or injury or are fearful of movement often hold the arm closely adducted and internally rotated toward their body. Prolonged immobility may result in the redundant capsule adhering to itself, resulting in adhesive capsulitis.

Above the glenohumeral joint is a unique ligament called the coracoacromial arch. This ligament attaches two landmarks on the scapula. Rather than stabilize a joint, it forms the roof of the glenohumeral joint where the tendons of the rotator cuff, the long head of the biceps brachii, and the subacromial or subdeltoid bursa pass through. Anteriorly, the subscapular bursa facilitates the movement of the subscapularis tendon.

The scapulothoracic joint is a functional joint rather than a true synovial joint. The scapula and its associated musculature slide over the rib cage and make up one-third of the available movement of the shoulder complex. Maximum mobility of the shoulder girdle complex is achieved through a force couple of the upper and lower trapezius and the serratus anterior. These muscles act together to produce upward rotation which when coupled with glenohumeral elevation allow for full mobility of the shoulder joint.

The acromioclavicular joint is a synovial plane or gliding joint with limited movement in three planes of movement. Its stability is reinforced by the acromioclavicular ligament as well as the coracoclavicular ligaments, the conoid, and trapezoid. Motion at the acromioclavicular joint is primarily at end range of elevation. Despite the limited movement at this joint,

it helps to stabilize the clavicle, achieving greater strength and power at the glenohumeral joint.

The sternoclavicular joint is a saddle, or sellar, joint. There is an articular disc, centrally located to absorb shock that is translated through the upper extremity. In addition to the articular disc, there is a sternoclavicular ligament as well as an interclavicular ligament which spans between the two clavicles over the manubrium of the sternum and the costoclavicular ligament which stabilizes the clavicle to the first rib. This joint along with the acromioclavicular joint helps to stabilize the clavicle. Instability in the clavicle may diminish the functional strength of the shoulder complex by as much as 50%.

Elbow and Forearm

The deceptively simple elbow joint is actually composed of three joints within the capsule. These are:

- humeroulnar joint
- radiocapitular joint
- proximal and distal radioulnar joint

The humeroulnar joint is a ginglymus, or hinge, joint and moves in a single plane allowing for flexion and extension. The trochlea, which is the hourglass-shaped condyle on the medial side of the humerus, articulates with the trochlear fossa of the ulna. In an open-chained environment, the concave trochlear notch moves over the convex trochlea producing arthrokinematic joint play in the same direction. The humeroulnar joint is a very stable joint and achieves this through the bony articulation as well as by the strong medial (ulnar) collateral and lateral (radial) collateral ligaments. These ligaments are tight in full extension, and with the bony shape of the articulation you can lock out your arms to become a long, straight, and stable unit. The tendons of the triceps brachii distally attach to the olecranon which is on the posterior side of the ulna. Between the olecranon and the triceps brachii there is an olecranon bursa to help cushion direct trauma to the elbow and facilitate sliding of the tendons.

The capitulo-radial, or humeroradial, joint is a modified ball and socket joint that allows the radius to roll over the ulnar during pronation and supination as well as participate in the flexion and extension of the elbow. Like the humeroulnar joint, the concave head of the radius articulates with the convex capitulum allowing for arthrokinematic joint play in the same direction.

Pronation and supination of the forearm occurs simultaneously through the proximal and distal radioulnar joints, as well as the syndesmosis (interosseous membrane) which connects the radius and ulna. The proximal and distal radioulnar joints are both pivot, or trochlear, joints which allow for the radius to move over the ulna. The head of the radius is held in place by the annular ligament.

INFORMATION IN ACTION

A parent is walking along a path with her four-year-old, holding his hand. Suddenly, she hears a bicyclist behind her on the path and quickly pulls up on her son's arm to move him out of the path of the bicyclist. A loud pop is heard and the little boy is crying that his arm hurts. Children under the age of six are at increased risk for dislocating the radial head with quick extension and distraction of the elbow because the annular ligament is not yet mature and stable. When picking up children, ensure that their elbows are flexed as you lift from the hands or better yet, lift them up under their arms.

When your arm hangs at your side, your forearm and hands are positioned slightly away from the body. The carrying angle is normally 5 to 15 degrees and allows for your arms to swing and carry objects without interference or contacting your body. Women generally will have a larger carrying angle than men, but this predisposes them to increased valgus stress on the medial (ulnar) collateral ligament and also puts the ulnar nerve under increased stress. This may increase risk of injury to these structures.

TAKE NOTE

The carrying angle at the elbow is 5 to 15 degrees as is the Q-angle, or Quadriceps angle, at the knee.

Wrist and Hand

The wrist is actually made of three joints. The radiocarpal joint, a condyloid joint, provides the majority of the movement we associate with the wrist. It moves in two planes to allow for flexion and extension as well as abduction and adduction, or radial and ulnar deviation, respectively.

TAKE NOTE

The combination of all four motions—flexion, extension, radial, and ulnar deviation—produce circumduction. There is no rotation at the radiocarpal joint.

The convex-shaped carpal bones move on the concave-shaped distal radius which results in accessory motions that are in the opposite direction to that of the joint motion.

The midcarpal or intercarpal joints located between the first and second row of carpal bones are irregular in shape and are classified as plane or gliding joints. The motion at the radiocarpal joint plus the midcarpal joint is added together for total wrist motion.

On the medial side of the wrist, the ulna styloid does not extend distally enough to articulate with the triquetrum and lunate. The transverse fibrocartilage complex (TFCC) fills in the space between the distal ulna and the carpal bones and acts as a shock absorber.

There are a series of small ligaments referred to generally as intrinsic ligaments that help the wrist to function as a single unit instead of eight separate bones. The major support to the wrist is provided by the radial collateral and ulnar collateral ligaments (which limit ulnar and radial deviation, respectively) and the palmer and dorsal radiocarpal ligaments. The dorsal radiocarpal ligament limits excessive flexion of the wrist, while the thick and fibrous palmer radiocarpal ligament limits extension. Above the long extrinsic tendons that travel into the wrist is the flexor retinaculum. It is made up of the palmar ligament and the transverse carpal ligament which forms the roof of the carpal tunnel. Finally, the palmar fascia covers the palm of the hand and helps to protect its structures.

INFORMATION IN ACTION

Carpal tunnel syndrome is compression of the median nerve between the transverse carpal ligament and the nine tendons that pass through the carpal tunnel. It can be brought on by repetitive activity, such as keying, direct trauma, or swelling that results from pregnancy.

Although there is a carpo metacarpal (CMC) joint for each of the digits, the joint for digits 2–5 is more for stability of the arch than mobility. The only one that truly is functional is the first CMC of the thumb. The first metacarpal joint articulates with the trapezium in a saddle, or sellar, joint. Both surfaces are convex and concave and, depending on the movement in question, the accessory motions will be in the same or opposite direction of the joint motion. The metacarpal phalangeal (MCP) joints are condyloid joints and allow for both flexion and extension and abduction and adduction. There are two interphalangeal joints, a proximal (PIP) and distal (DIP) for digits 2–5, and one interphalangeal (IP) joint for the thumb. These

are simple hinge, or ginglymus, joints and only allow for flexion and extension.

TAKE NOTE

If you remember that the proximal end of the phalanx is called the base and the distal end is the head, you will know that at both the MCP and IP joints the distal segment is concave and the proximal segment is convex. This means that the accessory motion for all of these joints is in the same direction as the joint motion.

On the palmar aspect of the metacarpophalangeal and interphalangeal joints is a palmar plate. This fibrocartilage plate helps to support the fingers in extension and allows you to point without using a lot of muscle energy. On the dorsum of each digit is an extensor mechanism. This structure provides an attachment for the extensor digitorum muscles as well as for the lumbricles and interossei. There are lateral bands that run on the medial and lateral side of each digit that help to anchor the extensor mechanism and, together with the palmar plates, require little muscular energy to support the finger in full extension.

Hip and Pelvis

The pelvic girdle is a critical pivot point in the human body and serves several important functions in the body. First, the pelvis supports the weight of the trunk and upper body and transmits the axial load to each of the lower extremities. Conversely, it transmits the ground reaction forces that are transmitted up the lower extremities to the rest of the body. Finally, the pelvic girdle transmits forces horizontally, vertically, and laterally to allow for smooth transition during gait. The pelvic girdle is made up of two innominate bones and the sacrum, joined together at the two sacroiliac joints and the pubic symphysis. The innominate is the fusion of the ilium, the ischium, and the pubis bones. The sacroiliac joint is a plane, or gliding, joint, however, the joint surfaces are very irregular to help hold them in place. The pelvis moves on the sacrum in three planes producing anterior and posterior pelvic tilt in the sagittal plane, elevation and depression in the frontal plane, and left and right rotation in the transverse plane. In addition, the sacrum moves on the innominate for nutation and counternutation. Nutation occurs when the base of the sacrum (superiorly) moves anteriorly and inferiorly—sometimes referred to as sacral flexion. Counternutation is just the opposite, where the base of the sacrum moves posteriorly and superiorly and is referred to as sacral extension. The pubic symphysis is a cartilaginous joint that has very little independent movement. These joints are held firmly in place by a series of sacrotuberous and sacrospinous ligaments posteriorly and the iliolumbar, lumbosacral, and anterior sacroiliac ligaments anteriorly.

INFORMATION IN ACTION

During pregnancy, the hormone relaxin allows for laxity in the ligaments to allow for expansion and mobility of the pelvis to accommodate the growing fetus. Some 69 % of pregnant women complain of back pain during their pregnancy, and one source of this pain is the increased hypermobility of the pelvis. Although modalities are usually contraindicated, gentle stabilization and muscle energy techniques can be helpful in managing this discomfort.

The coxo femoral joint, or hip joint, is a spheroidal, or ball and socket, joint. The head of the femur articulates with the acetabulum which is on the posterior lateral aspect of the innominate. All three of the innominate bones—ilium, ischium, and pubis—join together in the acetabulum, ensuring the greatest amount of strength. Unlike the shoulder, the coxo femoral joint gains a great deal of stability from the bony shape of the joint. However, what the joint gains in stability it loses in mobility. Adding to the stability of the coxo femoral joint is the acetabular labrum and three ligaments. The iliofemoral ligament, or Y-ligament, is located anteriorly along with the pubofemoral ligament. The ischiofemoral ligaments lie posteriorly. It is important to note that all of these ligaments are tight in full extension, which allows for maximum stability of the hip joint during push-off with gait. Like the glenohumeral joint, the convex femoral head moves on the concave acetabulum to produce joint accessory motions in the opposite direction.

TAKE NOTE

Remember that with lower extremity joints—such as the hip, knee, and ankle—many of the activities are performed in a closed-chain environment. Arthrokinematics of the joint in a closed-chain environment will be opposite of the accessory motions produced in an open-chain environment.

Knee

The knee is the largest joint in the body and is classified as a modified hinge, or ginglymus, joint. It is different than the humeroulnar joint (which is a true hinge joint) in that, in addition to flexion and extension, there is a rotational component necessary for locking and unlocking the knee. The convex-shaped distal femur is larger on the medial side than it is on the lateral side. When it articulates with the concave-shaped tibia, it must rotate in order to stay congruent with the tibial surfaces. In an open-chain environment, the concave tibia moves on the convex femur producing accessory motions in the same direction. During the last 20 degrees of extension, the tibia also externally rotates to accommodate for the large surface area of the medial condyle. This additional rotation component locks the knee and is known as the "screw-home" mechanism. This rotation is primarily as a result of concentric contraction of the vastus lateralis and is controlled eccentrically by the tendons of the pes anserine (goose foot) which are the sartorius, gracilis, and semitendinosus. Conversely, in the first 20 degrees of flexion, the popliteus unlocks the knee and facilitates a medial rotation force. In a closed-chain environment, with the femur moving on the tibia, the motions are opposite.

Superimposed on the tibiofemoral joint are the patellofemoral joint motions. This is commonly referred to as patella tracking. The patella, which is actually the distal attachment of the quadriceps femoris group, attaches into the tibial tuberosity via the patella ligament. The patellofemoral joint is a gliding, or plane, joint which articulates between the medial and lateral femoral condyles. The patella glides superiorly because the quadriceps femoris group is contracting during the last 20 degrees of extension. Simultaneously, the "screw-home" mechanism is occurring at the tibiofemoral joint. The external rotation of the tibia is supported primarily by the vastus lateralis. Because the vastus lateralis is pulling strongly, the patella will tend to move superiorly and laterally. In order for the patella to stay in line with the femoral condyles at terminal knee extension, the vastus medialis (specifically the vastus medialis oblique (VMO)) must pull the patella superiorly and medially.

The Q-angle, or quadriceps angle, reflects the pull angle of the quadriceps femoris group as a whole. It is measured from the anterior superior iliac spine (ASIS), to the middle of the patella, and then to the tibial tuberosity. The normal Q-angle is 5 to 15 degrees. Men tend to have smaller Q-angles—from 5 to 10 degrees—while women tend to have large ones—from 10 to 18 degrees. Higher Q-angles give the vastus lateralis a mechanical advantage while simultaneously putting the vastus medialis, and especially the VMO, at a disadvantage.

INFORMATION IN ACTION

Patellofemoral syndrome or chondromalacia patella is a common knee complaint that is often seen in young women. Tightness in the iliotibial band and vastus lateralis, a Q-angle greater than 15 to 18 degrees, and weakness of the VMO are all common findings with this population. Physical therapy interventions such as stretching tight lateral structures, strengthening the quadriceps femoris group (especially the VMO), and cross friction massage to the distal iliotibial band are all effective tools to help manage this problem. Education on proper footgear and the impact of flat feet (pes planus) or high arches (pes cavus) is also helpful.

The knee joint is most stable in full extension. The two intrinsic ligaments—the anterior and posterior cruciate as well as the collateral ligaments, the medial and lateral collateral—are all tight in full extension. In addition, the lateral side of the knee is further reinforced by the iliotibial band, and the medial side is supported by the tendons of the pes anserine which include the sartorius, gracilis, and semintendinosus. These are easily remembered with the abbreviation SGT (T is for tendinosus) or the phrase "Say Grace before Tea." There are also two menisci—a C-shaped medial meniscus and an O-shaped lateral meniscus. These structures not only help to better support the femoral condyles, but they also provide shock absorption and add to the stability of the knee structure in full extension. There are more than 13 bursa in the knee. These are designed to facilitate the gliding of tendons between bony prominences. There is a prepatella bursa, suprapatella bursa, and infrapatella bursa, which are named based on their location in relation to the patella. In addition to the infrapatella bursa, there is also an infrapatella fat pad. This acts as a shock absorber when you are kneeling or fall onto your knees. The other bursa are posterior bursa. Oftentimes, when there is trauma to the knee because of surgery or injury, a Baker's cyst will develop. A Baker's cyst is a general name for inflammation of the posterior patella bursa. These are common and the swelling often results in limiting range of motion.

Foot and Ankle

The foot and ankle are usually the body's first contact with the ground during ambulation. The ground reaction forces are as much as three to five times your body weight with walking and more than ten times your body weight with running and jumping. For a 200-lb. man going out for a jog, as much as one ton (2,000 lb.) of force is impacting the body, every time he takes a step. In the time it takes you to transfer from one foot to another while walking, your body must change from a flexible shock absorber to a rigid lever. The ability to transition so quickly from one function to another makes the foot and ankle a fascinating area of study.

The talocrural joint is made up of the tibia, fibula, and the talus. The tibia and fibula are joined together by the interosseous membrane and the distal tibiofibular joint so that they function essentially as a single unit. The tibia and fibula surround the superior aspect of the talus the way a carpenter's mortise fits to form a solid connection. The talocrural joint is also called the mortise joint for that reason. The convex talus articulates with the concave opening in the tibia and fibula to create a hinge, or ginglymus, joint that moves in one plane of motion allowing for dorsiflexion and plantarflexion. The accessory motions are in the opposite direction in an open-chain environment. The deltoid ligament stabilizes the medial aspect of the talocrural joint while laterally the anterior talofibular, calcaneofibular, and posterior talofibular ligament support the lateral side.

INFORMATION IN ACTION

The much more stable deltoid ligament on the medial side of the ankle is so strong that it is more common to sustain for an avulsion fracture of the medial malleolus than a sprain to this ligament. Conversely, the anterior talofibular ligament is the most common ligament sprained with an inversion ankle sprain.

The subtalar joint is difficult to separate from the midtarsal joint. Together these joints function to accommodate rotational forces without allowing for significant joint erosion. The subtalar joint has three facets on the inferior surface of the talus which articulate with three corresponding facets on the calcaneus. The midtarsal joints include the calcaneocuboid which is saddle, or sellar, in shape while the talonavicular has a modified ball and socket shape. The ability for the foot and ankle to convert between a rigid lever to a mobile adapter and shock absorber happens here through pronation and supination. Pronation, which is associated with shock absorption and adaptation to the ground surface, is a combination of dorsiflexion, eversion, and abduction. Supination, which is associated with a rigid or locked foot, helps the joint surfaces to come close together and helps ligamentous structures lock the foot into plantarflexion, inversion, and adduction. Adding to the stability of the foot is the windlass mechanism formed through the positioning of the plantar fascia. The plantar fascia is a tough, fibrous band which runs from the calcaneous to the base of the proximal phalanges of the toes. When the foot is in toe off, the head of the metatarsal traps the plantar fascia. As the foot plantar flexes over the extended toes, the fascia becomes tight and pulls the bony surfaces closer together, forming a rigid foot which is easy to push off. It also increases the height of the medial longitudinal arch, acting to store kinetic energy to spring forward. In addition to the plantar fascia, the medial arch is also supported by the spring, or calcaneonavicular, ligament; the bifurcate ligament; the long and short plantar ligaments; and the tendons of the fibularis (peroneus) longus, tibialis posterior, flexor digitorum longus, and flexor hallucis longus.

TAKE NOTE

The tibialis posterior, flexor digitorum longus, and flexor hallucis longus are known collectively as "Tom, Dick, and Harry." They are named because they cross behind the medial malleolus in this order. "Pop" (the popliteus) and his three sons "Tom, Dick, and Harry" all live in the deep posterior compartment of the leg. "Pop" stays behind to unlock the door (knee) when "Tom, Dick, and Harry" go out.

The metatarsophalangeal (MTP) joints and the interphalangeal (DIP, PIP) joints are similarly aligned as in the hand. It is important to note however that 50% of the body weight is carried over the base of the first metatarsal, while the other 50% is divided equally between digits two through five.

The Spine

The spine is made up of a total of 24 individual vertebrae, the sacrum, and the coccyx. There are seven cervical vertebrae, twelve thoracic vertebrae, and five lumbar vertebrae which form the individual vertebrae; five fused sacral vertebrae which form the sacrum; and three to four coccyx bones. Each vertebra has a pair of superior and inferior articulating facets. The superior facets articulate with the vertebra above and the inferior, articulating facets connect the vertebra below, forming pairs of gliding or plane joints. Each joint can only provide a small amount of movement yet cumulatively demonstrate significant mobility and flexibility in multiple planes. The plane in which the facets are oriented dictates the degree of mobility in a particular plane of movement.

Between each vertebral body is the intervertebral disc which is a cartilaginous synchondrosis. Although there is significantly less mobility than with the gliding joints, these intervertebral discs absorb shock and help the body adapt to the many combinations of motions that the spine can configure. The intervertebral disc is made up of the tough, fibrous rings of the annulus fibrosus. These concentric rings create a stable and strong support for the much softer and liquid nucleus pulposus. The jellylike center moves opposite to the movement of the vertebrae to absorb shock and to equalize pressure. The disc is firmly attached to the vertebra above and below through the vertebral endplate. Although patients will mention their "slipped disc," discs do not in fact slip.

The seven cervical vertebrae are identified because they are small in size, they each have a large central vertebral foramen, a transverse foramen for vertebral arteries to pass through, and often will have bifid spinous processes to allow for many muscular attachments. Anteriorly, there are joints of Luschka which provide some additional anterior stability of the cervical spine. The cervical vertebrae are quite mobile and, with the exception of the atlas (C1) and axis (C2), the articulating facets are not oriented in any one plane but cross several to allow for good overall mobility. Atlas, or C1, articulates with the occipital condyles. Capital flexion and extension occurs here, as a small nod similar to indicating yes. Atlas also articulates with axis (C2). Axis has a large, superior projection called the dens, or odontoid, process that functions as an axis. Some 50% of the rotation movement of our head and neck comes from this pivot joint, which allows us to shake our head and say no.

Thoracic vertebrae have a much larger vertebral body and a smaller vertebral foramen. There are two costal facets for ribs two to eight—one on the body and one on the transverse process—which allow the 12 pairs of ribs to articulate with the thoracic spine.

The transverse processes are both lateral and posterior and the spinous process is quite long and moves inferiorly. The orientation of the articulating facets is in the frontal or coronal plane, which promotes lateral bending. Were it not for the ribs, we would have significantly greater mobility to the right and to the left. The orientation of the spinous process limits extension. There is significantly greater ability to perform flexion than extension in the thoracic spine.

TAKE NOTE

When performing palpation in the thoracic spine, it is important to remember the length of the spinous process. When palpating, the spinous process of the seventh thoracic vertebra (if you move laterally) you will be palpating the transverse process of the eighth thoracic vertebra. They are not at the same level. Make sure you remember to go up one and over to find the correct transverse process.

The lumbar vertebrae have the largest vertebral bodies and the smallest vertebral foramen. The transverse processes are oriented more in the frontal plane, and the spinous process is short and stubby. The articulating facets are oriented in the sagittal plane promoting flexion and extension of the trunk and limiting rotation.

The sacrum, specifically the sacroiliac joint, was discussed with the pelvis and hip. The lumbosacral joint is the transition point between the lumbar spine and the sacrum. Because the sacrum is formed of five fused bones, there is often a significant amount of stress at the lumbosacral joint, and it is a frequent location for injury. The small coccyx bones do not have functional articulations and are usually only problematic after a traumatic fall, which might cause malpositioning.

The stability of the spine comes from several sources. The ligamentous structures such as the anterior and posterior longitudinal ligaments provide strong, anterior stability to the spine as they support anteriorly and posteriorly around the vertebral body. The posterior ligaments are not as stable because there is more mobility on the posterior aspect of the spine. The ligamentum flavum is located within the vertebral foramen anterior to the spinous process. The interspinal and intertransversarii ligaments are as their name implies between each spinous process and between each transverse process. Most superficial are the supraspinous ligaments, which connect the spinous processes in a long line. A thickening of this ligament in the cervical spine is called the ligamentum nuchae. Trunk stability is dependent on core strength or dynamic spinal stability from abdominals and spinal extensor muscles. The ability to support the lumbar spine in its natural position with cervical and lumbar lordosis and thoracic kyphosis requires muscular support. It is important to differentiate dynamic muscle support from a valsalva maneuver which will provide some temporary stability. Physical therapists and physical therapist assistants can assist patients in differentiating these two methods of trunk support and educate patients on more desirable techniques that will allow long-term support of the trunk and no increase in blood pressure.

Practice 2

1. Using standard goniometric measurements, you measure 90 degrees of active shoulder flexion on your patient with adhesive capsulitis. How much of that motion, in degrees, comes from the glenohumeral joint?
   a. 90 degrees
   b. 70 degrees
   c. 60 degrees
   d. 30 degrees

2. Your patient sustained a Colles fracture and has just come out of a cast. After the initial evaluation, the supervising physical therapist discusses the plan of care and wants to focus on improving wrist flexion. You know that in order to improve wrist flexion, joint accessory motion will need to be applied in which direction?
   a. posterior to anterior
   b. anterior to posterior
   c. lateral to medial
   d. medial to lateral

3. During the first 20 degrees of knee flexion, the popliteus facilitates the joint accessory motions to move as follows:
   a. Femur moves posteriorly and medially rotates on the tibia.
   b. Tibia moves anteriorly and externally rotates on the femur.
   c. Femur moves anteriorly and externally rotates on the tibia.
   d. Tibia moves posteriorly on the femur and externally rotates on the tibia.

4. Which of the following functions of the foot is best represented at the end of the stance phase?
   a. mobile adapter
   b. base of support
   c. rigid lever
   d. shock absorber

5. All of the following are negative results of a forward head rounded shoulder posture EXCEPT
   a. loss of glenohumeral joint elevation.
   b. limited thoracic chest expansion.
   c. TMJ dysfunction.
   d. loss of lower cervical (C5–C8) joint mobility.

6. You are assessing a patient who demonstrates signs of inflammation in the right knee. Which of the following is not a cardinal sign of inflammation?
   a. pallor
   b. rubor
   c. tumor
   d. calor

7. Which type of lower extremity amputation is most likely to develop an equinus deformity of the foot?
   a. fourth and fifth ray amputation
   b. symes
   c. chopart
   d. transmetatarsal

8. Which of the following features is not consistent with rheumatoid arthritis?
   a. flares and remission
   b. impacts women more than men
   c. multijoint involvement
   d. stiffness late in the day

9. Which of the following activities would not be encouraged for a patient after a right posterior lateral total hip replacement with precautions?
   a. backing up with a walker to sit on the toilet
   b. turning to the right when ambulating with a rolling walker
   c. bridging up in bed
   d. standing up from a wheelchair using a walker with right knee flexed

10. Tenderness to the common wrist extensor tendon, pain with resisted supination, and strong gripping is consistent with which of the following conditions?
    a. medial epicondylitis
    b. lateral epicondylitis
    c. golfer's elbow
    d. little league elbow

11. Which of the following is NOT consistent with the proliferative phase of healing?
    a. parallel collagen formation
    b. controlled motion
    c. increased vascularization
    d. wound contraction

12. Which of the following substances is associated with the formation of damaging crystals which can destroy a joint with gout?
    a. calcium
    b. sodium
    c. uric acid
    d. lactic acid

13. Which type of fracture will necessitate the most conservative weight-bearing status initially?
    a. transverse
    b. spiral
    c. greenstick
    d. fissure

14. A 15-year-old basketball player enters the clinic for a sports medicine evaluation following a twisted ankle in practice yesterday. Evaluation reveals that the lateral ankle is swollen with limited range of motion. However, good ligament stability is present. The ligament most commonly injured in an ankle sprain is which of the following?
    a. anterior tibiofibular ligament
    b. deltoid ligament
    c. anterior talofibular ligament
    d. calcaneonavicular ligament

15. All of the following tendons will glide over the pes anserine bursa with one exception. Which muscle will not glide over that bursa?
    a. semimembranosus
    b. semitendinosus
    c. sartorius
    d. gracilis

Practice 2 Answers

1. c. There is a 2 to 1 ratio between glenohumeral and scapulothoracic movement. For every 2 degrees of glenohumeral movement, 1 degree comes from the scapulothoracic. So for 90 degrees of total shoulder motion, 60 degrees comes from the glenohumeral joint and 30 comes from the scapulothoracic joint.

2. b. Since in an open-chain environment the radiocarpal joint accessory motions are in the opposite direction of the joint motion, to facilitate flexion you would need to move opposite of flexion, which would be anterior to posterior. Answer **a** would be correct for extension, **c** would be correct for radial deviation, and **d** is correct for ulnar deviation.

3. c. The two answers beginning with the tibia imply it is an open-chain movement because the tibia is moving on the femur. The arthrokinematics are in the same direction as the movement. Since we are talking about flexion, posterior is correct. However, flexion is associated with medial rotation, not lateral rotation. For the two answers beginning with the femur, it's implied that this is a closed-chain activity. Here the arthrokinematics are in the opposite direction of the joint motion. So for flexion, the femur must move anteriorly and externally rotate to unlock the knee.

4. c. At the end of the stance phase, the foot is in heel off to toe off. The foot is plantar flexed and ready to push off. The foot and ankle become supinated, and the windlass mechanism also helps complete this process. The foot must be rigid in order to translate muscular force to push off the ground. Both feet act as your limits of the base of support at all times. During the early part of stance phase heel strike (foot flat to midstance), the foot and ankle are pronated and the foot is working as a shock absorber and mobile adapter to the ground.

5. d. All of these answers are associated with a forward head rounded shoulder posture except **d**.

There is an increase in lower cervical mobility resulting in degenerative changes and a loss in upper cervical mobility.

6. a. The signs of inflammation are rubor—redness; calor—heat; dolar—pain and tumor; swelling. Pallor or paleness of the skin is not a sign of inflammation.

7. c. Both the Chopart and Lisfranc are often associated with equinus deformities of the foot.

8. d. Rheumatoid arthritis is associated with all of the features described as well as early morning stiffness.

9. d. Hip precautions after a posterior lateral hip replacement include no hip flexion > 90 degrees, no trunk flexion > 90 degrees, no adduction and no IR. All of the mentioned activities do not include one of these components except standing up from a wheelchair using a rolling walker keeping the right knee flexed. Likely you will need to keep hip flexed > 90 degrees. Knee should be extended.

10. b. Medial epicondylitis and golfer's elbow are the same condition. Little league elbow is an injury to the medial collateral ligament of the elbow. Lateral epicondylitis is correct. It involves inflammation of the common wrist extensor tendon and difficulty with wrist extension, gripping, and supination.

11. a. All of these are consistent with the proliferative phase of healing except parallel collagen formation. This does not occur until the remodeling stage.

12. c. Uric acid crystals are associated with gout.

13. b. Spiral fractures have a twist within them that encourages the bony segments to pull apart. This would likely have the most restricted weight-bearing status because too early weight bearing may result in the fracture splitting apart.

14. c. Anterior talofibular ligament is the most common ligament sprained with an inversion sprain.

15. a. Use the mneumonic "Say Grace before Tea" for the sartorius, gracilis, semitendinosus muscles.

Neuromuscular System

The neuromuscular system is an integral part of the functioning human being. Without proper development and maturation, the human body cannot perform movement in a synchronized, coordinated manner. The nervous system is divided into the central and peripheral nervous systems. The central nervous system includes the brain and spinal cord, while the peripheral nervous system includes the cranial nerves, the spinal nerves, and the autonomic nervous system. The autonomic nervous system is further subdivided into the sympathetic and parasympathetic systems. The ability to produce normal motor and sensory responses is dependent on the ability of each section of the nervous system to communicate with the others.

Normal Development of the Nervous System

Embryological development of the nervous system begins at 21 days of gestation with the development of the neural tube from flattened neural tissue. From this point on, the central nervous system develops and common pathologies such as neural tube defects (spina bifida) can occur.

Development of the neuromuscular system occurs in a cephalocaudal (head to toe), proximal-distal (near the joint to away from the joint), gross-fine (large motor skills to small, finite motor skills) pattern and is dependent on repetition through links between the sensorimotor systems.

The Brain

The brain enables us to perceive, communicate, remember, and understand. It also helps us to appreciate, understand, and initiate motor movements associated with more involved levels of consciousness. The major sections of the brain include the cerebrum, the cerebellum, and the midbrain.

Cerebrum

The human body is made up of the central nervous system (CNS)—the brain and spinal cord—and the peripheral nervous system (PNS), which includes everything outside of the CNS. The cerebrum is the main part of the functioning CNS that helps control motor and sensory responses.

The brain has two cerebral hemispheres. In most individuals, the left hemisphere of the brain controls concrete functions such as speech, writing, language, and calculation. The right hemisphere of the brain controls imaginative functions such as spatial abilities, knowledge of music, and intuition. The thin outer layer of the cerebral hemispheres, which is composed of gray matter (mostly non-myelinated nervous tissue), is called the cerebral cortex. The basal ganglia lie at the base of the cerebral cortex. The inner white matter (mostly myelinated nervous tissue) of the cerebrum is composed of those nerve fibers and their axons.

Cerebral Cortex

The cerebral cortex initiates movement and thought processes and is responsible for voluntary motor responses and conscious awareness of sensory stimuli. It is divided into the frontal lobe, the parietal lobe, the temporal lobe, and the occipital lobe.

1. **Frontal lobe.** The frontal lobe initiates voluntary muscle movement and contains the principle motor areas. The areas of the body controlled by the motor cortex are illustrated by the motor homunculus. A cortical homunculus is a pictorial representation of the anatomical divisions of the motor and somatosensory cortex. It represents that portion of the brain directly responsible for the movement and exchange of sense and motor information for the rest of the body.

   The frontal lobe also contains Broca's area, which controls the motor portion of speech.

Other functions of the frontal area include reasoning, problem solving, memory, personality, concentration, and behavior control.

> ## TAKE NOTE
>
> Damage to the frontal lobe can result in personality changes, memory loss, and impulsivity, as well as motor control impairments. At times, the behavioral changes can create more rehabilitation challenges than the motor control issues.

2. **Temporal lobe.** The temporal lobe provides information for communication and is the primary auditory area. It includes Wernicke's area, which controls the understanding or receptive portion of speech, language, singing, and hearing. The hippocampus is located in the temporal lobe and is responsible for memory.

3. **Parietal lobe.** The parietal lobe of the brain is responsible for sensation and perception in addition to integration of sensory input. The areas of the body that send information to the sensory cortex are illustrated by the somatosensory homunculus.

   The parietal lobe also works with the visual system in the occipital lobe for spatial coordination.

4. **Occipital lobe.** The occipital lobe is the center of the visual perceptual system and works with the parietal lobe to enable a person to see the world around them. The visual cortex responds to the shape, color, size, location, and movement of objects. Damage to this lobe can cause a type of blindness known as cortical visual impairment (CVI) and, if in concert with damage to the parietal lobe, causes word blindness.

Basal Ganglia

The basal ganglia are so named because they are a group of nerve cell bodies (ganglia) located at the base of the cerebral cortex. They are responsible for the regulation of posture and muscle tone and play a role in the control of voluntary and automatic movement. This area also controls motor activity by modifying or altering instructions from the motor cortex that call for voluntary movement. Damage to the basal ganglia leads to abnormalities in movement such as chorea, athetosis, and rigidity. Disorders include extrapyramidal cerebral palsy, Parkinson's disease, Huntington's disease, and torsion dystonia.

The Cerebellum

The cerebellum rests just below the cerebral hemispheres. The cerebellum is responsible for control of equilibrium, muscle tone, and motor coordination. It controls these parameters by regulating the rate, force, range, and rhythm of muscle activity. Damage to this area causes ataxia, nystagmus, poor balance, and low muscle tone.

Other Important Structures in the Brain

There are many other structures in the brain that contribute to the successful completion of skilled, voluntary movement.

1. **Thalamus.** The thalamus is part of the diencephalon. It is considered the inner room of the brain. The thalamus evaluates sensory signals from the spinal cord tracts and send that information to the pre-motor cortex for processing of an appropriate motor response. Problems with the thalamus can result in tremors or decreased coordinated movements. Pain syndrome surfaces with CVA damage in this area of the thalamus.

2. **Hypothalamus.** The hypothalamus is one of the master glands of the brain, which helps maintain homeostasis in many organ systems.

It participates in the regulation of blood pressure, heart rate (HR), body temperature, wake cycles, and endocrine function.

3. **Pituitary gland.** The pituitary gland is a small, oval endocrine gland that lies at the base of the brain. It is sometimes called the master gland of the body because all of the other endocrine glands depend on its secretion for stimulation.

4. **The reticular activating system (RAS).** The reticular activating system is located in the medulla, pons, and midbrain. Its functions are to help maintain arousal, filter many inputs, and regulate visceral functions.

5. **The hippocampus.** The hippocampus is located in the temporal lobe and is responsible for memory.

Cerebral Spinal Fluid (CSF) and Meninges

The nervous tissue is delicate and sensitive to pressure changes and has the consistency of pudding. The barrier of the cerebral spinal fluid and blood helps preserve its safe status. The brain and spinal cord are enclosed by membranes called the meninges. Meninges are a tough connective tissue that cover and protect the brain tissue physically. Meninges contain the CSF and form partitions within the tissue consisting of layers. These layers include the dura (tough outer layer), arachnoid (spiderlike) middle layer, and the pia (inner soft) covering. Meningitis occurs when there is inflammation from a virus or bacteria that enters the brain tissue.

The CSF provides a liquid cushion for the brain and unweights it by 97%. The CSF physically protects the brain from trauma and nourishes it. It is similar to plasma but has different ion concentrations. It circulates in the ventricles and the spinal canal. Hydrocephalus is a compression or blockage of the CSF within the system of ventricles (the laterals, the third and fourth ventricles) and canals.

Cerebral Vascular Supply

The brain receives most of its arterial supply through the anterior, middle, and posterior cerebral arteries with help from the anterior and posterior communicating branches. The anterior portion of the brain's arterial supply comes from the internal carotid artery, while the posterior portion is supplied by the vertebral arteries. Extracranial blood supply to the brain is provided by the right and left internal carotid arteries and by the right and left vertebral arteries. The anterior communicating artery communicates with the anterior cerebral arteries of both sides. The vertebral artery is either one of two arteries that branches off the subclavian artery. It then travels through the foramina of the transverse processes of the upper six cervical vertebrae to the foramen magnum and into the brain, where it unites with the vertebral artery from the other side to form the basilar artery. The cerebellum is supplied by the vertebral-basilar system. Posterior communicating arteries connect the posterior cerebral arteries with the internal carotid arteries and complete the circle of Willis (at the base of the brain).

The main arteries that supply the cerebral hemispheres and subcortical structures include the anterior (ACA), middle (MCA), and posterior (PCA) cerebral arteries. Cerebral blood flow varies with the size of the vessels. The MCA is the most common area for a cerebral vascular accident to occur. As in coronary heart disease, symptomatic changes generally result from a restriction of flow greater than 80%.

The Brain Stem

The brain stem lies between the cerebral hemispheres and the spinal cord and contains the medulla, pons, midbrain, and all of the cranial nerves with the exception of the olfactory and optic nerves. It controls breathing, swallowing, seeing, hearing, facial expressions, eye and tongue movement, and salivation through the 12 cranial nerves. Damage to this area causes sucking or swallowing problems, strabismus, and excessive salivation and speech disorders. The brain stem (part of the mesencephalon) is programmed to maintain automatic functions for survival. It houses the cranial nerves and contains the crossing point (decussation) for the corticospinal tracts. It controls many involuntary functions such as heart rate, blood pressure, respiration rate, and digestion.

The Spinal Cord

The spinal cord lies below the brain and extends from the brain stem to the lower back and ends at L2 in the conus medullaris. The cervical and lumbar regions are enlarged to house the anterior horn cells, which send messages to the peripheral nerve fibers of the arms and legs. The spinal cord transmits motor and sensory messages. Damage to this area can cause paralysis and sensory loss in the trunk and extremities.

The Peripheral Nervous System (PNS)

The peripheral nervous system involves the autonomic nervous system (ANS), the cranial nerves, and the spinal nerves. Two major types of nerve fibers are contained in peripheral nerves: motor (efferent) and sensory (afferent) fibers. Sensory impulses are afferent and send messages toward the cerebral hemispheres from the peripheral parts of the body. For example, when someone touches your hand to get your attention, a sensory impulse travels from your hand toward the cerebral hemispheres of your brain. You sense the touch by your body afferently, sending the touch impulse from the peripheral part of the body (your hand) up to the spinal cord and then to your brain for interpretation. Motor impulses are efferent and send messages toward the body from the cerebral hemisphere. Your brain interprets what type of sensory information it receives and from where the sensory information originates. Your brain receives this sensory message in the cerebrum and sends a motor impulse or efferent impulse back down to the muscle to let you respond to the sensory impulse, if need be. Will you withdraw your hand if you touch something painful? Will you squeeze the hand when someone places theirs in yours? These are examples of motor impulses.

The Autonomic Nervous System

The autonomic nervous system controls all involuntary activities, such as cardiovascular, respiratory, digestive, endocrine, urinary, and reproductive systems. In addition, it controls systems such as the fight or flight response in the sympathetic system and the digestive responses, for example, of the parasympathetic system. Control centers for the ANS are found in the brain stem and hypothalamus. Motor neurons are located within spinal nerves that innervate smooth muscle, cardiac muscle, and glands.

The Somatic Nervous System (SNS)

The somatic nervous system involves 12 pairs of cranial nerves located in the brain stem and can be sensory, motor, or mixed in function. The cranial nerves are designated by both name and roman numeral, according to the order in which they appear on the inferior surface of the brain. One-third of the nerves have both sensory and motor components. Three of the nerves are associated with the special senses of smell, vision, hearing, and equilibrium and have only sensory fibers. Five other nerves are primarily motor in function, but do have some sensory fibers for proprioception. The remaining four nerves consist of significant amounts of both sensory and motor fibers.

Cranial Nerves

1. Olfactory—sensory (smell)
2. Optic—sensory (sight)
3. Oculomotor—motor (eye movements)
4. Trochlear—motor (eye movements)
5. Trigeminal—mixed (sensation to face and chewing)
6. Abducens—motor (eye movements)
7. Facial—mixed (taste and facial expressions)
8. Vestibulocochlear (acoustic)—sensory (hearing and equilibrium)
9. Glossopharyngeal—mixed (sensory to tongue and swallowing)

10. Vagus—mixed (sensory to larynx, trachea, heart, and other thoracic and abdominal organs and movements of organs)
11. Spinal accessory—motor (movement to muscles of the pharynx and soft palate, shoulder, and neck)
12. Hypoglossal—motor (tongue movements)

Spinal Nerves

Spinal nerves consist of both a sensory and motor component and exit the intervertebral foramen. The cervical, brachial, and lumbosacral plexuses are also a part of the peripheral nervous system. The plexuses are composed of nerves that innervate the cervical, brachial (upper extremity), pelvis, and lower extremity.

Spinal Nerves

1. Cervical—8 nerves
2. Thoracic—12 nerves
3. Lumbar—5 nerves
4. Sacral—5 nerves
5. Coccygeal—1 nerve

Nerve Cell Function

A nerve contains a bundle of nerve fibers, either axons or dendrites, surrounded by connective tissue. These fibers can carry sensory or motor signals depending on their position within the CNS. Each nerve is made up of several layers that help contribute to its function. The first outer layer of a nerve is made up of connective tissue called the epineurium. Within each nerve is a bundle of nerve fibers called a fasciculus. Each fasciculus is surrounded by a layer of connective tissue called the perineurium. Within each fasciculus, the individual nerve fiber with its myelin and neurilemma is surrounded by connective tissue called the endoneurium. The neuron or nerve cell is the basic unit of the nervous system and consists of a cell body with a long fiber called an axon extending from the cell body and shorter, jutting tendrils called dendrites running into the cell.

Neurons do not multiply or cannot regenerate unless the axon is intact. Neurons exhibit longevity, are non-replaceable if damaged, and work at a high metabolic rate, which means that they need a lot of energy. Dendrites can collaterally sprout, are not myelinated, and receive impulses. Axons send impulses from the cell body and may be myelinated.

Action Potential

Nerve impulses are propagated along the axon as a result of an action potential. The action potential occurs when positive ions flow into the neuron. The resting potential, or differences between the inside and the outside of the neuron at rest, is between −60mV and −90mV. When enough positive ions flow into the neuron to raise this value to −55mV, an action potential occurs, sending an impulse along the nerve. An action potential along an afferent nerve will carry sensory information from the periphery to the central nervous system. An action potential along an efferen nerve will carry a motor impulse from the brain and spinal cord to a muscle, resulting in a muscle contraction.

Common Pathologies

Common pathologies related to the neuromuscular system include cerebral vascular accidents (CVA), traumatic brain injuries (TBI), spinal cord injuries (SCI), and upper motor neuron (UMN) and lower motor neuron (LMN) lesions.

Cerebral Vascular Accidents (CVAs)

Cerebral vascular accidents occur due to an occlusion or hemorrhage in an artery within the brain causing death to neurons within specific areas. Causes can include hypertension (HTN), elevated cholesterol levels, diabetes, smoking, valvular heart disease, and arteriosclerosis. In addition, contributing factors can include age, ethnicity, and lifestyle choices. Diagnosis is imperative and a CAT scan is used to determine whether the CVA is from an occlusion or a hemorrhage. Occlusions can be treated with "clot busting" medications if done so within several hours of onset. Clinical signs and symptoms can include impairments in motor, sensory, mental, perceptual, and language functions. They can also include paralysis (hemiplegia) or weakness (hemiparesis). CVAs or strokes range from slight to severe, and the symptoms can be temporary or permanent.

Traumatic Brain Injury (TBI)

Head injuries most often result from traumatic brain injuries related to motor vehicle accidents, diving accidents, or incidences of violence and cause damage to a local or diffuse area of the brain. Damage is caused by bleeding and destruction of cranial tissue within the closed cranial cavity or due to fractures of the skull opening up the head to infection and subsequent neural damage. Head injuries can be minor or profound and irreversible. Damage from a head injury can include brain stem involvement, contusions, diffuse matter lesions, blood vessel damage, and cranial damage. Clinical signs and symptoms can include loss of consciousness or impairments in motor, sensory, mental, perceptual, and language functions. Signs can also include paralysis (hemiplegia) or weakness (hemiparesis) similar to those seen with a CVA. Injuries can be closed or open in nature, and the severity of the injury depends on the type of insult, response to commands, and return of function.

Spinal Cord Injuries (SCI)

Spinal cord injuries are divided into traumatic and nontraumatic, with the majority of injuries occurring traumatically and caused by motor vehicle accidents. Diagnosis is determined though assessment of sensory and motor function and loss. The level of SCI and the determination regarding complete versus incomplete must also be made. Causes of SCI include damage to the vertebral column with resulting damage to the soft spinal cord and surrounding tissue. Damage to the spinal cord is generally irreversible. Treatment in the emergency room can include the use of corticosteroids to reduce the amount of swelling within the spinal canal and resulting damage to the tissue. Determination regarding the level of the injury must be made and the patient must be evaluated for tetraplegia (also called quadriplegia) or paraplegia.

Upper Motor Neuron (UMN) Lesions

Lesions that involve the upper motor neurons (within the brain and spinal cord) are caused from damage from chemical changes or disease. These types of changes are not related to CVAs or TBIs and include such diseases as:

1. **Parkinson's disease (PD).** Parkinson's disease is a degenerative disorder of the basal ganglia, with the substantia nigra most often affected. Parkinson's disease is a degeneration of nerve cells and the neurotransmitting chemical dopamine. This decrease in the production of dopamine produces a disorder of body movement that is progressive in nature. Signs and symptoms include postural instability, decreased balance reactions, decreased trunk rotation, damage to automatic functions and coordinated movements, slowed movements (bradykinesia), muscle rigidity (cogwheel or lead pipe), masklike face, resting tremors ("pill rolling"), festinating gait (short, running steps), restlessness, difficulty initiating movement (akinesia), muscle cramps, depression, and drooling. Common medications include monoamine oxidase (MAO) inhibitors, L-dopa, and Carbidopa (Sinemet®).

2. **Alzheimer's disease.** Alzheimer's is a progressive disorder characterized by "premature, severe, diffuse cerebral atrophy, particularly of the frontal lobes." It is the most common form of dementia, affecting approximately 5.2 million people in the United States. The clinical picture varies with Alzheimer's disease, however intellectual loss always occurs before motor loss. Posture, stance, and gait are preserved until mental deterioration is extensive. Common medications utilized to treat Alzheimer's can include, but are not limited to, Aricept®, Razadyne®, Exelon®, Cognex®, and Namenda®.

3. **Poliomyelitis.** Polio, or poliomyelitis, is a contagious viral infection affecting the central nervous system. It produces no symptoms in about 95% of cases. Most commonly, the polio virus attacks the anterior horn cells mimicking a lower motor neuron pathology, when, in fact, it may also strike the upper motor neuron (UMN). For that reason, polio is considered a UMN lesion. Abortive polio is manifested by mild flu-like symptoms, such as a mild upper respiratory infection, diarrhea, fever, sore throat, and general feeling of malaise. Nonparalytic polio is associated with aseptic meningitis and neurological symptoms such as sensitivity to light and neck stiffness. Paralytic polio produces severe, debilitating problems, such as atrophy, muscle weakness, flaccidity, and inability to ambulate without supportive orthotics.

4. **Post-polio syndrome (PPS).** Approximately 50% of patients with polio experience an abrupt onset of disorders ten or more years after the initial bout with polio. These new disorders may include pain of an orthopedic nature, fatigue, muscle weakness of either a previously affected or unaffected muscle or group of muscles, muscle atrophy, fasciculations, breathing difficulty, cold intolerance, or a change in functional status. These problems are collectively referred to as post-polio syndrome. The pain arises from the chronic stress placed on joints and tendons due to muscle weakness and abnormal movement mechanics. The progressive weakness is thought to arise from the ongoing degeneration of motor units. Over time, this progressive degeneration leads to further complications and loss of function. The specific underlying cause of PPS is unknown.

5. **Multiple sclerosis (MS).** Multiple sclerosis (MS) is a slowly progressive disease characterized by disseminated patches of demyelination in the brain and spinal cord, resulting in multiple and varied neurological symptoms and signs, usually with remissions and exacerbations. Patients present with changes in vision, balance, and strength that may be transient and difficult to pinpoint. Symptoms may be mild, such as numbness in the limbs, or severe, such as paralysis or loss of vision. As the disease progresses, increased weakness, fatigue, and paralysis worsen, and the patient can be confined to a wheelchair. It is important to work with patients with MS in the early morning to combat fatigue. Other symptoms can include walking, balance, and coordination problems; bladder dysfunction; dizziness and vertigo; sexual dysfunction; pain; cognitive deficits; emotional changes; depression; and spasticity.

6. **Amyotrophic lateral sclerosis (ALS).** ALS is often referred to as Lou Gehrig's disease, after the famous baseball player who was diagnosed with the disease in the 1930s. It is a rapidly progressing, fatal neurodegenerative disease that damages the anterior horn cells (gray matter) in the spinal cord and destroys the pyramidal tracts (motor pathways), resulting in muscle atrophy. Unlike multiple sclerosis, no sensory, cognitive, visual, or hearing changes occur with ALS. Symptoms of ALS can include muscle weakness and atrophy in the hands, arms, or legs; muscle weakness and atrophy in the muscles of speech, swallowing, or breathing; twitching (fasciculation) and cramping of muscles, especially those in the hands and feet; impaired use of the arms and legs; thick speech and difficulty in projecting the voice; shortness of breath; difficulty in breathing and swallowing; and hyperactive deep tendon reflexes (DTR) initially progressing to hypoactive with disease progression.

7. **Acute transverse myelitis.** Acute transverse myelitis is a neurological syndrome caused by inflammation of the spinal cord. The deficit is usually severe, resulting in global sensorimotor paraplegia below the level of the lesion, urinary retention, and loss of bowel control. The thoracic area is most often involved so that abdominal paralysis also occurs. Eventual improvement is only slight, except in cases caused by viral encephalomyelitis or an acute inflammatory edema.

Lower Motor Neuron (LMN) Lesions

Lower motor neuron lesions affect the peripheral nervous system. Damage can be due to injury, disease, or other metabolic causes and can be reversible if addressed in a timely manner. LMN lesions include some of the following:

1. **Peripheral nerve dysfunction.** The peripheral nervous system (PNS) is composed of all the neurons that are not in the central nervous system. A neuropathy is the term used to describe an injury affecting the peripheral nerve due to infection, a toxin, or a metabolic disorder. A polyneuropathy refers to widespread, bilateral insults to the peripheral nerve. Polyneuropathies are common and are due to toxins, metabolic disorders, or hereditary disorders. The axon continues to die back as long as the toxin or metabolic problem remains and then the axon regenerates. Symptoms include muscle atrophy, glove/stocking sensory and motor loss, tingling in toes and fingers, decreased forearm and ankle reflexes, and decreased nerve conduction velocity (NCV). Regeneration occurs at the rate of approximately 1 to 2 mm per day if the axon hillock is still intact.

2. **Metabolic neuropathies (e.g., diabetes).** Metabolic neuropathies are those nerve deficits that develop secondary to systemic disease with a metabolic origin. Common diseases can include, but are not limited to, diabetes mellitus (most common cause), hypoglycemia, uremia (second most common cause), hypothyroidism, hepatic failure, polycythemia, amyloidosis, acromegaly, porphyria, disorders of lipid or glycolipid metabolism, nutritional or vitamin deficiencies, mitochondrial disorders, and any disorder that alters the function of the myelin and axons through the metabolic pathways.

3. **Traumatic lesions (e.g., severing nerves or stretching nerves).** Traumatic lesions can be mild to very severe depending on the type of injury and the amount of tissue damage resulting from the trauma. These types of injuries are classified in three ways:

   - **Class 1**—mild to moderate compression of nerve; recovery takes three months.
   - **Class 2**—caused by closed-crush or percussion injuries; recovery takes several months to years (proximal to distal).
   - **Class 3**—caused by stab wounds, bullet wounds, or severe stretch injury (brachial plexus).

These types of lesions involve total motor, sensory, and autonomic dysfunction (often caused by MVA or forcible downward displacement of the shoulder or traction of head during delivery or breech presentation, causing damage to or severing of the brachial plexus). Symptoms can include motor weakness, sensory loss, muscle atrophy (after one month), and areflexia below the level of the lesion.

4. **Other types of nerve injuries (e.g., brachial plexus injury, ulnar, median, and radial nerve injury).** Nerve injuries can occur in any area of the body and for multiple reasons. Common types include brachial plexus, ulnar, median,

radial, femoral, tibial, and common peroneal injuries. Symptoms include loss of motor and/or sensory function, tingling, shooting pains, discoloration, and loss of circulation.

5. **Carpal tunnel syndrome.** Carpal tunnel syndrome (CTS) is an example of a compression syndrome. It is the entrapment of the median nerve at the wrist beneath the flexor retinaculum. Carpal tunnel syndrome causes multiple signs and symptoms. If the resulting entrapment cannot be resolved, surgical intervention will be necessary. Carpal tunnel syndrome is known to occur during pregnancy due to the changes in fluid dynamics but generally resolves following delivery. Signs and symptoms of carpal tunnel syndrome can include numbness, tingling, and burning in the hands and fingers; radiating pain to the forearm, elbow, shoulder or neck; night pain; loss of sensation of the first three and a half fingers; and the feeling that the hand is asleep in the morning. Diagnosis of carpal tunnel syndrome is usually confirmed with an NCV test. A positive Tinel (a tingling sensation) over the wrist or aggravation of symptoms by wrists extension may also be present. Treatment includes steroid injection, splinting, or surgery.

6. **Charcot-Marie-Tooth disease.** Charcot-Marie-Tooth (CMT) disease is a hereditary neuropathy (autosomal dominant) with onset in the 20s or 30s. It affects 1 in 2,500 people in the United States. It is also known as a hereditary motor sensory neuropathy (HMSN) or peroneal muscular atrophy. It leads to weakness in the muscles of the feet and lower legs resulting in foot drop and a high-stepped gait pattern. As the disease progresses, it can affect the muscles of the hands leading to difficulty performing fine motor tasks. Symptoms include loss of function of the muscles of the lower leg and feet and degeneration of the muscles of the lower leg and feet and resulting weakness.

7. **Guillain-Barré syndrome.** Guillain-Barré syndrome is a post-infectious polyneuritis or acute idiopathic polyneuropathy of unknown etiology. It is theorized that Guillain-Barré is an inflammatory disorder caused by an allergic or hypersensitive reaction or an autoimmune response of the body. However, some individuals believe Guillain-Barré results from a virus. Symptoms include abrupt onset, autonomic dysfunction, sensory changes (pain or cramping in the muscles), parasthesias (tingling or numbness), and muscle weakness. The muscle weakness is symmetrical and usually begins in the distal lower extremities; it appears as a flaccid, ascending weakness evolving from hours up to ten days and causes decreased DTRs. Neuropathies related to Guillain-Barré syndrome almost always resolve completely.

Pediatric Pathologies

There are three neurologically based pediatric pathologies that occur commonly and require physical therapy intervention.

Spina Bifida

Spina bifida is a congenital defect in the spinal column with incomplete closure of the vertebral canal due to failure of fusion of vertebral arches. This is the most common congenital anomaly and occurs in 1 or 2 in every 1,000 live births.

Spina bifida is further categorized into three main types:

1. **Spina bifida occulta.** The vertebral arches remain unfused, but there is no herniation or displacement of the meninges.

2. **Spina bifida cystica meningocele.** The vertebral arches are unfused, there is no herniation

of the meninges, part of the cord or nerve may be in a sac, and function is mildly involved or normal.

3. **Spina bifida cystica myelomeningocele.** This is the most common type and usually occurs in the lumbosacral region. The vertebral arches are unfused, and herniation is usually present. There is displacement of or disruption of the nerve/cord with the presence of neurological signs and abnormal development of the spinal cord. Hydrocephalus is present in 80% of these cases and requires placement of a shunt because flow of cerebral-spinal fluid is obstructed from the fourth ventricle to the cerebral sub-arachnoid space.

Cerebral Palsy (Little's Disease)

Cerebral palsy is a diagnosis based on a definite motor deficit and classification according to type of motor abnormality. It is caused by damage to an immature central nervous system and can cause mental retardation, seizures, hearing deficits, speech impairment, and visual-motor perception deficits.

Children who are diagnosed with cerebral palsy typically have neurological and developmental issues in the areas of vision, hearing, sensation, language, mobility, and manual competence. Causes of the impairment include anoxia, hemorrhage, infection, trauma, prematurity, breech delivery, compromised umbilical cord, forceful delivery, drug exposure, diseases, and meconium aspiration.

Cerebral palsy can be divided into specific types and subtypes:

- Types of cerebral palsy
  - spastic—increased tone
  - hypotonic—decreased tone
  - athetoid—mixed tone
  - ataxic—decreased tone
  - opisthotonos—increased tone, fluctuating tone

- Subtypes of cerebral palsy
  - monoplegic—involvement of one extremity
  - quadriplegic—involvement of all four extremities
  - diplegic—involvement of either upper or lower extremities
  - hemiplegic—involvement of one side
  - triplegic—involvement of three extremities

Down Syndrome

Down syndrome is diagnosed due to specific physical features and presence of an extra chromosome on number 21. On average, it occurs in 1 in 600 live births.

The risk factor that predisposes a mother to have a baby with Down syndrome increases with age:

- maternal age 20–24, 1 in 2,500 births
- maternal age 25–29, 1 in 1,500 births
- maternal age 30–34, 1 in 750 births
- maternal age 35–39, 1 in 280 births
- maternal age 40–44, 1 in 100 births
- maternal age over 45, 1 in 35–50 births

Common health problems and physical features related to Down syndrome include:

- instability of the atlantoaxial joint
- Abnormal muscle tone
- congenital heart defects
- mental/physical retardation
- slanted eyes and spaced wide apart
- flat bridge of nose, low set ears, short neck
- small mouth with large tongue
- moderate to severe joint laxity
- hand/foot crease is complete across palm with space between big toe and next toe

Practice 3

1. The peripheral nervous system consists of nerves leading to and from the CNS. The PNS involves the _____ and _____ nervous systems.
   a. somatic; sensory
   b. somatic; autonomic
   c. autonomic; automatic
   d. autonomic; motor

2. Which one of the choices below describes the types of losses caused by damage to the frontal lobe of the brain?
   a. Loss of visual input and the ability to understand what someone tells you.
   b. Loss of voluntary movement and the ability to express oneself with speech.
   c. Loss of the ability to communicate expressively and the ability for voluntary sensation.
   d. Loss of pain and temperature sensations.

3. For most people, the _____ side of the brain contains the language center.
   a. right
   b. left
   c. posterior
   d. anterior

4. Which specific part of the brain is responsible for our ability to coordinate and produce the appropriate force, rate, and rhythm of our motor functions?
   a. cerebrum
   b. thalamus
   c. hippocampus
   d. cerebellum

5. Which type of TBI causes no fracture of the skull but can lead to minor or profound damage to the brain?
   a. local brain injury
   b. open head injury
   c. closed head injury
   d. amnesia

6. A patient has symptoms of ascending paralysis from the feet upward following a respiratory infection two weeks ago. What pathology or disease should the PTA think this patient has developed?
   a. ALS
   b. MS
   c. Guillain-Barré syndrome
   d. Bell's palsy

7. Carpal tunnel syndrome causes entrapment of which specific nerve?
   a. ulnar nerve
   b. radial nerve
   c. axillary nerve
   d. median nerve

8. What is Charcot-Marie-Tooth disease caused by?
   a. genetic transmission
   b. metabolic disease
   c. crush injury
   d. stretch injury

9. Development occurs in a specific order dependent on the nervous system. Identify the correct order from the following:
   a. cephalocaudal, distal-proximal, fine-gross
   b. caudal-cepahlo, proximal-distal, gross-fine
   c. cephalocaudal, proximal-distal, gross-fine
   d. caudal-cephalo, distal-proximal, fine-gross

10. The temporal lobe of the brain is responsible for the function of which specific type of speech?
a. expressive
b. receptive
c. global
d. aphasia

11. Damage to the cerebellum can lead to which specific clinical signs?
a. spasticity, loss of voluntary motor control
b. flaccidity, athetoid movements
c. nystagmus and ataxia
d. sensory deficits and flaccidity

12. At what level does the spinal cord end?
a. T1
b. T2
c. L2
d. L5

13. Identify the number and functions of the facial nerve.
a. one; motor
b. three; sensory and motor
c. five; sensory
d. seven; sensory and motor

14. Identify the function of the hippocampus.
a. memory
b. vision
c. sensation
d. coordination

15. What is the most common site for a CVA to occur?
a. ACA
b. MCA
c. PCA
d. DCA

16. Damage to the basal ganglia leads to specific types of abnormalities in movement. Identify an abnormality from the following that you might see with damage to this area.
a. flaccidity
b. athetosis
c. hemiparesis
d. clonus

17. The functions of which area of the brain includes maintaining arousal, regulating visceral functions, and filtering input?
a. hippocampus
b. thalamus
c. reticular activating system
d. basal ganglia

18. Identify the correct cranial nerve responsible for sensory responses to the larynx, trachea, heart, and other thoracic and abdominal organs and movements of those organs.
a. trochlear
b. optic
c. abducens
d. vagus

19. Identify the pathologies considered upper motor neuron lesions.
a. PD and MS
b. MS and Erb's palsy
c. Guillain-Barré and PD
d. diabetes mellitus and MS

20. Identify the upper motor neuron lesion that initially presents with hyperactive deep tendon reflexes and then progresses to hypoactive deep tendon reflexes.
a. Guillain-Barré
b. ALS
c. PD
d. MS

21. What are some common lower motor neuron lesions?
a. CP and PD
b. MS and Guillain-Barré
c. PPS and ALS
d. brachial plexus injury and CIS

22. We can identify traumatic LMN lesions using a classification system. If an injury is caused by a closed-crush or percussion injury and recovery takes several months to years, the injury is classified as
a. Class 1.
b. Class 2.
c. Class 3.
d. Class 4.

23. Injury to the _____ nerve results in a drop foot.
a. ulnar
b. sciatic
c. peroneal
d. radial

24. Charcot-Marie-Tooth disease is commonly referred to as
a. femoral nerve atrophy.
b. tibial nerve atrophy.
c. ulnar nerve atrophy.
d. peroneal nerve atrophy.

25. Most individuals can completely recover from the following disorder:
a. multiple sclerosis
b. Guillain-Barré
c. diabetes mellitus
d. Parkinson's disease

Practice 3 Answers

1. b. The peripheral nervous system is comprised of the somatic (voluntary) and the autonomic (involuntary) systems.

2. b. Loss of voluntary movement and the ability to express oneself with speech are the types of losses caused by damage to the frontal lobe of the brain. The frontal lobe is responsible for expressive speech (Broca's area) and voluntary motor movements. It also controls our emotional state and our ability to determine socially appropriate behaviors.

3. b. For most people, the left side of the brain contains the language center. The left side of the brain is responsible for the majority of our expressive (Broca's area) and receptive (Wernicke's area) knowledge of speech.

4. d. The cerebellum is responsible for coordination of voluntary motor movements through the control of rate, rhythm, and force.

5. c. A closed head injury—with or without a skull fracture—can result in varying amounts of damage to the brain—from little to profound damage.

6. c. A patient with symptoms of ascending paralysis from the feet upward, following a respiratory infection two weeks ago, has developed symptoms consistent with Guillain-Barré syndrome. This syndrome is thought to occur following a respiratory infection and causes ascending paralysis to major portions of the body. It can also involve the respiratory system, which may result in a patient that needs ventilator support. Most patients recover from this pathology.

7. d. Carpal tunnel syndrome is an entrapment pathology that occurs in the carpal tunnel within the wrist and results in compression of the median nerve.

8. a. Charcot-Marie-Tooth disease is caused by transmission of an autosomal dominant gene. The disease develops when the person is 20–30 years old.

9. c. Development occurs in a cephalocaudal, proximal-distal, gross-fine pattern.

10. b. The temporal lobe of the brain houses the speech center called Wernicke's area and is responsible for receptive speech.

11. c. The lesions in the cerebellum can cause nystagmus and ataxia.

12. c. The spinal cord ends at the L2 level called the conus medullaris.

13. d. The facial nerve is the seventh cranial nerve and is responsible for both sensory and motor control.

14. a. The hippocampus is responsible for memory.

15. b. The MCA is the most common area for CVAs to occur.

16. b. Athetosis is a common result because of damage to the basal ganglia.

17. c. The reticular activating system is responsible for these functions.

18. d. The functions of the vagus cranial nerve include both motor and sensory functions.

19. a. Parkinson's disease, post-polio syndrome and multiple sclerosis are types of upper motor neuron lesions.

20. b. Amoytrophic lateral sclerosis (ALS) begins with hyperactive deep tendon reflexes and progresses to hypoactive DTRs.

21. d. The brachial plexus and the median nerve (involved in CTS) are in the peripheral nervous system.

22. b. Class 2 traumatic lesions recover over several months to years.

23. c. The peroneal nerve innervates the ankle dorsiflexors.

24. d. Charcot-Marie-Tooth disease is often called a peroneal nerve atrophy because symptoms are first manifested in this area with a foot drop.

25. b. Most individuals that contract Guillain-Barré recover fully from the symptoms.

Integumentary System

This section will cover the anatomy and physiology of the integumentary system. It will also discuss diseases and conditions of the system, as well as their medical management. This information serves as the foundation for understanding integumentary system involvement in the treatment of patients across the lifespan.

Anatomy and Physiology

The integumentary system, or skin, is the largest organ system in the body. It accounts for 7% of total body weight in the average adult, and receives roughly one-third of resting cardiac output. The three layers of the skin are the epidermis, the dermis, and the subcutaneous tissue layer, or hypodermis. Also contained in the system are appendages such as the nails, sweat glands, sebaceous (oil) glands, hair follicles, and hair.

The integumentary system varies in thickness from 1.5 mm to 5 mm and functions as a barrier against ultraviolet radiation, bacteria, and water-soluble substances. It maintains body temperature, prevents loss of bodily fluids, manufactures vitamin D, serves as a reservoir for blood, and functions as a sensory organ. Finally, it is an integral component of one's personal identity.

The Epidermis

The epidermis ranges in thickness from .06 mm to 0.6 mm, and is composed of five different layers. The innermost layer is attached to the dermis and serves as the launching site for new skin cells. Cells are produced and slowly migrate upwards, becoming longer and drier. By the time the cells travel up and form the outermost layer, over the course of 14 to 21 days, they are dead and flattened, creating a tough, waterproof barrier. These dead cells rub off constantly, resulting in a new epidermis every one to two months. The epidermis contains cells that produce fibrous protein, fight infection, produce pigment, and detect light touch. There is no blood supply in the epidermis, so it relies on oxygen and nutrients to diffuse into it from the dermis.

The Dermis

The dermis ranges in thickness from two to four millimeters and is composed of two layers. The thin upper layer contains loose connective tissue and helps anchor the dermis to the epidermis. The deeper layer contains dense connective tissue and provides increased structural support to the skin. The dermis is rich in blood supply, lymphatic capillaries, and nerve innervations. It contains epidermal appendages, or structures that go from the dermis to the epidermis. These include hair follicles, sweat glands, and oil glands. Epidermal cells can migrate along these structures from the dermis up to the epidermis if the epidermis is damaged.

Subcutaneous Tissue

The hypodermis, or subcutaneous tissue, ranges greatly in thickness, increasing with weight gain, and thinning with weight loss. It contains adipose tissue, loose connective tissue, and lymphatic vessels. It functions to adhere the skin to underlying structures, such as muscle. It cushions and insulates the body and is a source of energy.

Functions of the Skin

Protection
Sensory organ
Vitamin D production
Thermoregulation
Cosmesis

The integumentary system, or skin, is the largest organ system in the body.

Common Pathologies

Lesions of the skin can occur as a result of trauma, pressure, an infectious process, or a disease. This section will discuss pathologies of the integumentary system commonly encountered in physical therapy.

Shingles

Herpes zoster, or shingles, is a painful skin eruption caused by the varicella (chicken pox) virus. It most often affects people between the ages of 50 and 70 who have a compromised immune system. Shingles occurs due to a reactivation of the virus, which is stored in the dorsal root ganglion of cranial and spinal nerves during its dormant period. The virus spreads down the nerve, causing painful blisters to erupt along the associated dermatome. In rare cases, the infection can spread in the central nervous system, causing muscle weakness and atrophy. Persons with shingles are infectious two to three days before symptoms occur until the lesions have dried. Persons at risk are those who have never had chicken pox and pregnant women. Steroids, antiviral medications, and pain medications are used to diminish symptoms. A vaccine is available to prevent infection in those who have not had chicken pox.

TAKE NOTE

When treating a patient with shingles, the therapist should wear gloves and make sure the open sores are covered.

Skin Cancer

Skin cancer is the most rapidly increasing cancer in the United States. There are three main types. Basal cell carcinoma is slow growing and rarely metastasizes. It is seen most often in Caucasians with prolonged sun exposure. It is diagnosed with a biopsy and treated by surgical excision. Squamous cell carcinoma is also most common in fair-skinned Caucasians. It grows more rapidly than basal cell carcinoma and can metastasize. It is associated with prolonged sun exposure and exposure to carcinogens such as arsenic, tar, or oil. It is diagnosed with a biopsy and treated by excision. Malignant melanoma can occur anywhere that pigment exists. It is associated with periods of intense sun exposure, such as a beach vacation or a tanning bed. Lesions deeper than .75 mm are at risk for metastasis. Over 85% of patients with metastasis to the brain, lungs, bones, or liver die within one year. Early clinical assessment of suspicious lesions using the ABCDE method is encouraged. A biopsy confirms the diagnosis. Treatment is surgical excision and immunotherapy.

Clinical Assessment for Malignant Melanoma

A: Asymmetry—The shape of the lesion is irregular.
B: Border—The border of the lesion is irregular, or poorly defined.
C: Color—The lesion contains many colors, including black, brown, tan, red, or blue.
D: Diameter—The lesion is larger than 6 mm in diameter (size of a pencil eraser).
E: Elevation—The lesion is above the surface of the skin.

The ABCDE method is used for clinical assessment of suspicious skin lesions.

TAKE NOTE

Make sure the physical therapist is aware of any unusual or suspicious skin lesions that you notice on a patient, and include a description in your documentation.

Open Wounds

The physical therapist assistant often assists the physical therapist in caring for patients with open areas that occur as a result of pressure, arterial insufficiency, venous insufficiency, or diabetes.

A pressure ulcer occurs because an external force compresses the blood supply to a region, resulting in ischemia and tissue death. This most often occurs over bony prominences of the lower extremity. Factors that increase the risk of a pressure ulcer include the application of shear forces and friction to the body part, excessive moisture causing skin maceration, impaired mobility, impaired sensation, poor nutrition, advanced age (over 70), and a previous pressure ulcer. The depth and severity of a pressure ulcer is described by a staging system.

INFORMATION IN ACTION

You are treating an elderly woman following surgical repair of a hip fracture. In slipping her shoes off, you notice that the eschar that covers a pressure wound on her heel has partially loosened. You are able to glimpse red granulation tissue and the yellow fat pad that is superficial to the calcaneus. You inform the physical therapist of the change in the condition of the patient's wound, adding that it appears to be a stage III pressure ulcer.

The characteristics of open areas are described using the 5 PT system: **p**ain, **p**osition, **p**resentation, **p**eri-wound condition, **p**ulses, and **t**emperature.

Ulcers due to arterial insufficiency are caused by tissue ischemia.

TAKE NOTE

Proper positioning and good skin care are critical to prevention of pressure ulcers.

Staging of Pressure Ulcers

STAGE	APPEARANCE	TISSUES INVOLVED
I	Skin is intact but red; does not blanch; feels firm or "boggy"; painful or itchy	Epidermis; or early indication of deeper tissue involvement
II	Blister; shallow crater; "rug burn"	Epidermis and part of dermis
III	Crater; eschar; distinct margins; undermining; exposed subcutaneous tissue	Epidermis; dermis; and subcutaneous tissue
IV	Deep crater; eschar; distinct margins; undermining; tunneling; exposed muscle, tendon, or bone	Epidermis; dermis; subcutaneous tissue; and muscle/tendon/bone

Characteristics of Open Wounds

POINT	PRESSURE	ARTERIAL	VENOUS	DIABETIC
Pain	Only with intact sensation—calcaneus; greater trochanter; sacrum; ischial tuberosity; lateral malleolus	Severe—lateral malleolus; tibial crest; dorsum of foot; toes	Dull, achy pain; fatigue; heaviness—medial aspect of lower leg; tibial crest; medial malleolus	Little or none—plantar aspect of foot; any bony prominences of foot
Position	See previous table	Round, symmetrical; pale wound bed; black or yellow eschar; dry	Irregular; lots of drainage; red wound bed; thin, stringy yellow	Round, "punched out"; rim of callus; little drainage
Presentation	Red; inflamed; mottled; thickened	Thin, shiny; loss of hair; cyanotic	Red; dermatitis; cellulitis; brown staining; firm	Dry, cracked skin with callus buildup
Periwound	Normal	Decreased or absent	Normal	Variable
Pulses	Red-warm	Cool	Warm	Warm
Temperature	Eschar-cool			

The 5 PTs describe key characteristics of open wounds.

Risk factors contributing to open wounds in patients with arterial insufficiency include high blood fat and cholesterol levels, smoking, diabetes, high blood pressure, trauma, and advanced age. The severity of an arterial ulcer is described by the depth of tissue involvement. Superficial wounds involve the epidermis. Partial-thickness wounds involve the epidermis and part of the dermis. Full-thickness wounds involve the epidermis, dermis, and subcutaneous tissues. The deepest wounds are those extending below the subcutaneous tissue into the muscle, tendon, or bone.

Ulcers associated with venous insufficiency most likely result from local hypoxia caused by tissue congestion.

Risk factors contributing to open wounds in patients with venous insufficiency include venous hypertension, edema, trauma, diabetes, advanced age,

and previous venous ulcer. The depth of venous ulcers usually involves only the epidermis and dermis.

INFORMATION IN ACTION

A physical therapist was asked to consult on a patient with open wounds on the medial aspect of the left lower leg. The wounds were shallow, irregular in shape, and had a large amount of drainage. The patient's legs were both very edematous, and the skin around the open areas was dark brown in color (the patient was Caucasian). Based on these clinical signs, the therapist was able to confirm that the patient's history of venous insufficiency was the cause of these wounds.

Diabetic, or neuropathic, ulcers result primarily from the impact of sensory, motor, and autonomic neuropathy.

Motor neuropathy leads to wasting of the intrinsic muscles of the foot, which alters biomechanics and increases pressure and shear forces on the foot. Autonomic neuropathy results in dry, inelastic skin, which is more prone to breakdown, and increased callus formation, resulting in areas of increased pressure. Sensory neuropathy diminishes the ability of the patient to sense pressure areas and pain on the foot and allows skin breakdown to progress. Risk factors contributing to the development and poor healing of diabetic ulcers include decreased immune response, vascular disease, poor vision, poor footwear, poor glycemic control, and/or a previous ulcer or amputation. The severity of a neuropathic ulcer may be described in the same manner as an arterial ulcer.

TAKE NOTE

Over 20% of patients with type II diabetes will experience foot or toe ulcers and/or amputation.

Phases of Wound Healing

An open wound normally progresses through three phases of wound healing—the inflammatory, the proliferative, and the maturation/remodeling phases. The goals of the inflammatory phase are to control bleeding, clean the wound, and bring in cells to start the rebuilding process. Clinical signs of the inflammatory phase are redness, warmth, edema, and tenderness. The goals of the proliferative phase are building new blood vessels and granulation tissue, wound contraction, and formation of new skin (re-epithelialization). Clinical signs of this phase are tiny red dots of tissue in the wound as blood vessels are formed, a beefy red appearance as granulation tissue is produced, a tightened appearance around the wound as it contracts, and thin, pink skin as the wound is resurfaced. The goals of the remodeling/maturation phase are to strengthen and properly orient the newly developed tissue. A healed wound early in this phase will appear thin and pink, and a wound that is fully remodeled will be pale, or similar in color to the surrounding skin.

Factors Affecting Wound Healing

Elements of the wound itself, the area around the wound, and the patient's condition all affect wound healing. Delayed healing is associated with wounds that are larger, deeper, dried out, infected, or located in the lower extremities or over bony prominences. These may be referred to as chronic wounds. Poor circulation, poor sensation, and mechanical stresses will delay wound healing. The overall health of the patient is critical. Those with diseases that impair circulation, oxygenation, or the immune system will experience slower healing. Medications such as steroids and chemotherapy interfere with the healing process. Poor nutrition, nicotine, and alcohol are also detrimental to healing. Finally, the elderly will heal more slowly than those who are younger.

TAKE NOTE

The best wound care available will not be effective if a patient has inadequate nutrition or unstable medical issues.

Medical Management of Open Wounds

Wounds that are infected may be treated with systemic antibiotics. Wounds with extensive necrosis may be debrided surgically and left open to heal or covered with a graft of skin and/or muscle. Amputation may be necessary in the case of complete necrosis of a digit or intractable infection (sepsis).

Burns

Burns may be caused by excessive heat, chemicals, electricity, or radiation. The exposure to heat may be caused by contact with flames, hot liquids, hot surfaces, or steam. Short exposures to temperatures over 111°F will result in tissue damage. Chemicals used in industrial settings, such as cleaning compounds or asphalt, can cause damage depending upon the type of chemical, its amount, and the duration of skin exposure. Low-voltage electrical burns can be caused by placing a metal object into an electrical socket. High-voltage electrical burns are usually caused by power lines or lightening. Tissue damage is usually deep and may be unpredictable with an electrical burn. Radiation burns are uncommon but may occur due to industrial exposure or as a result of radiation treatment for cancer.

Burn Description

The severity of a burn is described by the percentage of the body that is burned and by the depth of tissue involved. The most common method of quickly determining the extent of a burn is the rule of nines, which allows you to estimate the body surface area on a body that has been burned by using multiples of nine. When a body has been burned, the percent of the entire body involved can be calculated as follows:

Head = 9%
Chest (front) = 9%
Abdomen (front) = 9%
Upper/mid/low back and buttocks = 18%
Each arm = 9%
Each palm = 1%
Groin = 1%
Each leg = 18% total (front = 9%, back = 9%)

Therefore, if both legs (18% × 2 = 36%), the groin (1%), and the front chest (9%) were burned, this would involve 46% of the body.

A superficial burn involves only the epidermis. The skin will appear red, possibly with mild edema. The skin will blanch when pressed and will be tender to the touch. Bumping one's finger against a hot iron

or sun exposure can also cause superficial burns. A superficial partial-thickness burn involves the epidermis and the upper layer of the dermis. Skin with superficial burns will appear red, moist, weeping, or blistered, with mild to moderate edema. The skin will blanch when pressed and be very sensitive to touch or even to air exposure. Severe sunburn, flash burns, or scalds can result in superficial partial-thickness burns.

A deep partial-thickness burn involves the epidermis and the second layer of the dermis. The skin will appear a mottled red or a waxy white color. The deeper into the dermis the burn extends, the whiter the skin will be since the capillaries will be destroyed. The red skin will blanch when pressed, but the return of the red color will be slow. Extensive edema is characteristic. The burn may be painful, but as the depth of the burn increases, sensation will decrease since more sensory receptors are destroyed. Contact with hot objects, liquids, or chemicals, may cause a deep partial-thickness burn.

A full-thickness burn destroys the epidermis and dermis and extends down into the subcutaneous tissue. The skin is destroyed and the remaining tissue is hard eschar that may be red, black, or a grayish white. Edema may be forming under the eschar, but it will not be evident because the eschar is rigid and does not expand due to the pressure of the fluid. There is no blanching to pressure since the capillaries are destroyed and no pain or other sensation since the sensory receptors are destroyed. Immersion in scalding liquid, contact with chemicals, or electrical currents may cause a full-thickness burn.

A subdermal burn reaches below subcutaneous tissue to muscle, tendon, and/or bone. The tissue will appear charred and dry, without edema. As with the full-thickness burn, there is no intact sensation. Prolonged exposure to hot objects, strong chemicals, or electrical currents, to mention a few, may cause a subdermal burn.

Characteristics of Burn Injuries

BURN DEPTH	APPEARANCE	SENSATION
Superficial	Red; dry; mild edema	Tender to touch
Superficial partial-thickness	Red; moist; blistered; mild to moderate	Very painful
Deep partial-thickness	Mottled red; waxy white	Painful, with decreasing sensation
Full-thickness	Red, gray, white; dry; hard; no edema	Asensate
Subdermal	Charred; dry; no edema	

The appearance and sensory status of a burn is associated with the depth of tissue injury.

Prognosis for Healing

Not surprisingly, the speed and quality of healing of a burn is directly associated with the depth of tissue involved. A superficial burn may peel after a few days, but the skin will still maintain its abilities to serve as a barrier to bacteria and to prevent excessive fluid loss. This will diminish complications that delay healing. The superficial burn will heal without any intervention within three to five days without any scarring, assuming no other health complications or comorbidities exist. The superficial partial-thickness burn is more susceptible to an infection since the dermis is damaged and there is a lot of moisture present. However, it will still heal without surgery because epithelial cells can be produced from the remaining dermis, or can migrate in from the edges of the burn. Healing takes one to two weeks, and the new skin may be slightly lighter in color due to damage to melanocytes.

A deep partial-thickness (DPT) burn will contain some epithelial cells, clinging to what is left of structures such as the hair follicles. A small DPT burn can heal without surgical intervention in three to five weeks. The skin will be thin and light in color and may be dry and itchy due to the lack of oil production from sebaceous glands. This compromised skin can be easily injured and is prone to hypertrophic scarring. More extensive DPT burns will be covered by skin grafting. A deep partial-thickness burn is at risk for converting to a full-thickness burn due to a tenuous blood supply or as a consequence of an infection. Full-thickness and subdermal burns require surgical intervention for healing.

Prognosis for Burn Healing

BURN DEPTH	SURGERY REQUIRED	HEALING TIME
Superficial	No	3 to 5 days
Superficial partial-thickness	No	1 to 2 weeks
Deep partial-thickness	Maybe	3 to 5 weeks
Full-thickness	Yes	Depends on surgery
Subdermal	Yes	Depends on surgery

More superficial burns generally do not require surgery and may heal in a few days to a few weeks time.

Complications of Burns

The loss of extensive skin surface area that occurs with serious burns causes many systemic complications. Other injuries, such as fractures or smoke inhalation, may occur in conjunction with the burn. Finally, the patient's age and health influence the effect of the burn. The following are specific complications related to burns.

Cardiovascular Complications of Burns

After a burn, fluid leaks out of capillaries due to vessel damage and vasodilation. This fluid evaporates quickly from the burned areas due to the loss of the protective barrier of the skin, resulting in a low circulating blood volume and decreased cardiac output. This condition is termed hypovolemic shock, or burn shock. The delivery of oxygen and nutrients to the body is diminished, possibly resulting in tissue destruction, organ dysfunction, or death. Heart rate will increase to compensate for the diminished cardiac output, which will make the patient less able to tolerate activity. Fluid replacement is accomplished through intravenous (IV) placement and by encouraging the patient to drink water frequently.

Another consequence of fluid leakage from vessels is edema. Edema over joints will limit range of motion. It creates compression on tissues and blood vessels, especially in burned areas that cannot expand. This increased pressure can cause blood clots and nerve injury and may need to be relieved surgically.

Arrhythmias caused by an electrical burn are another potential cardiovascular complication of burns.

Pulmonary Complications of Burns

Inhalation of toxic gases or smoke may cause direct damage to the lungs. Fluid leakage from blood vessels can cause pulmonary edema. Burns around the torso may impair chest expansion. All these factors will impair ventilation and may lead to hypoxia or death. Patients with burns are often intubated to maintain pulmonary function.

Metabolic Complications of Burns

A patient's metabolic rate increases substantially following a burn injury. This increases the core body temperature as much as 2.5°F. The patient's room should be kept around 85°F to minimize stress on the patient. The increased metabolic rate also causes an accelerated breakdown of the body's proteins. Patients may exhibit weakness due to loss of muscle mass. Careful nutritional supplementation is critical.

Immunologic Complications of Burns

There are many reasons for impaired immune system function following a burn. The most obvious reason is that the skin, which is the major barrier protecting the body from pathogens, has been compromised. In addition, the damaged tissues create an environment that is very conducive to bacteria growth. Damaged blood vessels limit delivery of cells that clean up dead tissue and fight infection. Finally, the physiological stress on the body from the burn injury diminishes the function of the immune system. Topical antibiotics, aggressive wound debridement, early skin closure, and use of sterile techniques are important in preventing infection.

Psychological Complications of Burns

Sleep disorders, depression, and anxiety are common reactions to the physical pain, prolonged recovery time, and altered personal appearance associated with a burn injury. As with any patient, explanations of the rationale behind treatment activities, a consistent approach, and including the patient in goal setting and decision making will enhance rapport and trust and decrease anxiety.

Complications of Burns

BODY SYSTEM	COMPLICATIONS
Cardiovascular	Hypotension; low cardiac output; arrythmias; edema
Pulmonary	Hypoxia
Metabolic	Increased metabolic rate; increased core temperature; protein breakdown
Immune	Infection
Psychological	Anxiety; depression
Multisystem	Neuropathy; kidney failure; gastrointestinal ulcers

Burn injuries have a serious negative impact on many of the body's systems.

Medical Management of Patients with Burns

Because comprehensive management of a patient with burns requires an integrated team approach, it is important that the PTA understand aspects of medical management and how physical therapy management intersects with medical management.

Acute Medical Intervention

Patients with burn injuries require extensive medical management in the acute phase due to the systemic challenges that were discussed previously. Aggressive fluid management with intravenous fluids is necessary to replace vital fluids and electrolytes. An airway must be established and maintained to prevent respiratory distress and to ensure adequate tissue oxygenation. Cardiac rhythm abnormalities must be monitored and managed. The percent of total body surface area (TBSA) burned is estimated and the burns are classified. Clothing is removed and initial debridement and dressing of wounds are performed.

Medications

The two main areas of focus for medical management are prevention and management of infection and pain. With the large amount of necrotic tissue, the presence of foreign matter, and the impairment of the immune system, the risk of an infection developing in a burn is great. Topical antibiotics are routinely applied to the burns and intravenous antibiotics may also be used. Pain is a constant factor for a patient with burns. There is pain due to the tissue damage itself and pain due to the interventions, such as wound care or stretching exercises.

Ideally, patients should report pain at no more than four on a ten centimeter visual analogue scale. Pain is controlled with intravenous narcotics, oral narcotics, non-narcotic pain relievers, and nonsteroidal anti-inflammatory medications (NSAIDs).

Medications may also be used to control anxiety, to manage cardiac arrhythmias, to improve kidney function, or to address any other medical issue that arises during the care of the patient with burns.

Surgical Management

The goals of surgical management are to reduce pressure on intact tissues, to remove devitalized tissue and eschar, and to provide coverage for deep or extensive burns to promote healing.

Escharotomy

An escharotomy is an incision made into hard eschar to relieve the pressure on underlying, intact tissues. When systemic edema develops, unburned, elastic skin will expand, resulting in a swollen appearance.

The hard eschar that covers deeper burns cannot expand and the tissue underneath will be subjected to high pressure. The pressure can occlude blood vessels, causing death of the tissues they supply. Pressures are monitored, and an escharotomy is performed as needed to prevent tissue damage.

Surgical Debridement

Patients with full thickness and subdermal burns usually have the burns debrided surgically. This allows most of the eschar to be removed at one time, instead of during multiple debridement sessions. This is typically less painful for the patient, diminishes the chance of infection, and promotes earlier wound closure.

Skin Grafting

Skin grafts are applied to deep partial-thickness and full-thickness burns. The graft allows strong, rapid closure of the burn with less scarring.

An autograft is one taken from the patient's body and provides permanent coverage of the burn. If there is not enough tissue area available from which to harvest the graft, temporary coverage can be obtained with a graft from a cadaver, from an animal, or from a synthetic material. Typical autograft donor sites are the thighs, buttocks, and back.

Harvesting a split-thickness graft requires removing the epidermis and part of the dermis. The graft can be applied as a sheet, or it can be made into a mesh by running it through a press that cuts little diamonds into it. This allows the graft to cover more area, but it heals with a rougher texture than the sheet graft. A split-thickness donor site heals quickly, allowing another graft to be taken from it in 10 to 14 days.

Harvesting a full-thickness graft requires removing the epidermis and dermis. It is applied in sheet form only and provides a better cosmetic result than a split-thickness graft. However, the disadvantage is that the donor site requires a long healing period and is generally not available for further grafting.

Stress cannot be placed on the grafts for at least three to five days while new blood vessels grow into the grafted tissue. A graft may fail to adhere to the underlying tissue due to infection, the presence of necrotic tissue on the wound bed, too much movement after graft placement, or edema collecting under the graft.

Practice 4

1. A stage II pressure ulcer on a patient's greater trochanter has a beefy-red wound bed and a puckered look around the edges. The pressure ulcer is in which stage of healing?
   a. inflammatory stage
   b. proliferative stage
   c. regressive stage
   d. remodeling/maturation stage

2. A patient has a flame burn on the forearm. It is waxy white in appearance with moderate edema present. The patient reports diminished sensation. What is the classification of this burn injury?
   a. superficial partial-thickness
   b. deep partial-thickness
   c. full-thickness
   d. subdermal

3. A patient presents with a wound on the plantar aspect of the third metatarsal head. It is round, dry, and painless and has a buildup of callus surrounding it. What is the etiology of this wound?
   a. pressure
   b. arterial insufficiency
   c. venous insufficiency
   d. diabetes

4. Of the epidermis, dermis, and hypodermis, which of the following are found only in the dermis?
   a. a top layer of dead, flattened cells
   b. sensory receptors
   c. adipose tissue
   d. sebaceous (oil) glands

5. Which of the following statements is true concerning herpes zoster (shingles)?
   a. It is caused by a strain of resistant bacteria.
   b. It is most common in infants and children.
   c. It can be spread by contact with the open sores.
   d. There is no way to immunize against herpes zoster.

6. Which of the following is the most fatal form of skin cancer?
   a. malignant melanoma
   b. meningioma
   c. basal cell carcinoma
   d. squamous cell carcinoma

7. You are practicing bed mobility activities with a patient while assisting nursing staff to change the patient's soiled brief. You notice an area on the sacrum that appears like a "rug burn" abrasion. In what stage is this ulcer?
   a. stage I
   b. stage II
   c. stage III
   d. stage IV

8. You are treating a patient who presents with a series of small, irregular open areas just proximal to the medial malleolus. There is a moderate amount of drainage from the wounds. The surrounding skin is edematous and it is a mottled brown color. What is the etiology of this wound?
   a. arterial insufficiency
   b. venous insufficiency
   c. diabetic
   d. pressure

9. Which of the following risk factors is most applicable for development of a venous ulcer?
   a. smoking
   b. hypertension
   c. lower extremity edema
   d. poor glycemic control

10. Which of the following types of burns causes the most unpredictable amount of tissue damage?
   a. flame burns
   b. scalding burns
   c. electrical burns
   d. chemical burns

11. One of the most serious complications following a burn is the loss of fluids. What is the term describing this condition?
   a. immunological compromise
   b. hypovolemic shock
   c. inhalation injury
   d. metabolic alteration

Practice 4 Answers

1. b. The ulcer is most likely to be in the proliferative stage of healing. In the proliferative phase of wound healing, granulation tissue forms that is beefy red in color. The wound starts to close by contraction, giving rise to a puckered look around the edge.

2. b. The most likely classification of this burn injury is deep partial-thickness. A deep partial-thickness burn is characterized by a mixed red or waxy white color, marked edema, and diminished light touch sensation.

3. d. The most likely etiology of this wound is diabetes. Characteristics common to both arterial and diabetic ulcers include round shape and dry wound bed. The lack of pain and presence of callus distinguish this wound from an arterial wound.

4. d. Oil glands are found only in the dermis. They serve to lubricate the epidermis and keep it supple. The top layer of the epidermis is a layer of dead, flattened cells. The dermis and epidermis both contain sensory receptors. Adipose tissue is located in the hypodermis.

5. c. Herpes zoster is caused by the virus that causes chicken pox (varicella). It is most common in adults aged 50 to 70 years old. People are contagious from a few days before sores are evident up until the sores dry. A vaccine is available for prevention.

6. a. Malignant melanoma is often fatal within a year if it has metastasized. Basal cell carcinoma is very slow growing and rarely metastasizes. Squamous cell carcinoma grows a little faster and can metastasize. Meningioma is a form of brain tumor.

7. b. Stage II ulcers involve the epidermis and dermis and appear as blisters or abrasions. In stage I, the epidermis is not broken. In stage III, the subcutaneous tissue would be evident, and in stage IV, muscle, tendon, or bone would be visible.

8. b. The characteristics described are classic for ulcers caused by venous insufficiency.

9. c. Edema control is critical to prevent ulcers due to venous insufficiency. Smoking and hypertension are risk factors for arterial ulcers. Poor glycemic control is a risk factor for development of a diabetic ulcer.

10. c. Electrical burns are the most unpredictable because the electricity travels deep in the body, following the path of least resistance. The internal damage caused by electrical burns may not be readily apparent from the surface.

11. b. Hypovolemic shock describes the low blood pressure and low cardiac output that results from the sudden fluid shift that occurs following a burn injury.

Normal Anatomy and Physiology of the Endocrine and Metabolic Systems

There are a variety of chemical and physical actions of the human body required for normal growth, normal development, and maintenance of normal body function. The metabolic and endocrine systems regulate many of these actions with the goal of maintaining a balanced state of homeostasis.

Metabolic System

The process of metabolism creates energy for the cells of the body through biochemical processes that convert food and nutrients to energy. There are two primary metabolic processes carried out in the body. Catabolism is a type of metabolism involving the breakdown of organic compounds to provide heat and energy. Cell respiration is made up of catabolic reactions to break down food molecules. Anabolism is a metabolic process that involves the building of complex compounds by the bonding together of smaller compounds. The synthesis of glycogen (by liver cells) and of fat (for storage) are examples of anabolism. Enzymes are catalysts for both of these metabolic processes and facilitate metabolism processes that would not occur on their own. The body has many enzymes and each relates to a specific reaction of metabolism.

The body's metabolic rate refers to the amount of heat that the body is producing. There are many processes in the body that create energy which produce heat. Therefore, the metabolic rate is an indirect measure of energy. The energy required for a body at rest is known as the basal metabolic rate. Beyond the basal metabolic rate, all activities have specific energy expenditure. Factors such as exercise, age, body composition, stress, food intake, and climate can affect the body's metabolism. Factors such as exercise and cold climates increase metabolic rate due to increased energy expenditure to create more heat. Factors such as increased age and prolonged decreased food intake lower metabolic rate in order to conserve the energy sources that are available to the body.

TAKE NOTE

Metabolic rate is high in children due to the energy requirements of their growing bodies. When the body is no longer growing, metabolic rate slows approximately 2% per decade. An inactive body has a decreased metabolic rate of approximately 5% per decade. As a PTA, it is very important to promote physical activity in clients of all ages—especially those of increasing age—in order to maintain metabolic rate, as well as function and independence.

Endocrine System

The endocrine system is made up of glands that produce, store, and secrete hormones. Hormones are molecules carried by the circulatory system to distant sites in the body, such as organs. These molecules act as chemical messengers, sending information throughout the body from cell to cell in order for the body to perform vital functions. Cells that receive information through hormones contain sites called receptor sites, which allow hormones to bind to the cells and transmit information. Hormones influence sites throughout the body, regulating processes such as metabolism, stress response, sexual reproduction, regulation of blood pressure, and balance of electrolytes.

The endocrine system uses a feedback mechanism to control the stimulation and release of hormones. A feedback system involves a multiple-step process to maintain the correct amount of hormones in circulation. A signal is sent from a master gland by way of a releasing hormone that stimulates the receiving gland to secrete a stimulating hormone. The stimulating hormone is released into the bloodstream and binds to the target gland. The target gland then releases its hormone because it has just been stimulated by the stimulating hormone messenger. The level of this hormone then increases in the bloodstream. The level of hormone is sensed by the body, and the master gland reacts when the level becomes too high. The master gland stops sending the hormone, which results in no additional stimulating hormone being released. Without the stimulating signal, the target gland will no longer release hormones. This system is continuously working to ensure a steady level of hormones in the bloodstream.

Abnormalities or pathologies of the primary gland responsible for a particular hormone can lead to endocrine system dysfunction. In addition, circulation problems or abnormalities of the target organ can result in dysfunction of the endocrine system. If a gland secretes an excessive amount of a hormone, it is overactive; if it does not secrete enough of a hormone, it is hypoactive. Dysfunctions of the endocrine system are described as hypofunction or hyperfunction.

Glands of the Endocrine System

The hypothalamus indirectly regulates many of the glands of the body by direct regulation of the pituitary gland. The pituitary gland is responsible for sending the stimulating message to many of the glands of the endocrine system.

The hypothalamus is important in directly regulating metabolism and body temperature. In addition, the hypothalamus secretes hormones that stimulate the pituitary gland to secrete hormones. One non-stimulating hormone released by the hypothalamus is a hormone that stops the release of the growth hormone.

The pituitary gland is a small gland that plays a very large role in the endocrine system by controlling the function of many of the endocrine glands. There is an anterior and posterior lobe of the pituitary, each secreting different hormones. The anterior lobe is known as the adenohypophysis, and the posterior lobe is known as the neurohypophysis. The pituitary gland is regulated by the hypothalamus.

The thyroid gland produces thyroid hormones that contain iodine. The thyroid's hormone, thyroxine, controls cellular oxygen consumption and assures that the body produces enough heat to maintain normal body temperature. The thyroid gland is stimulated by the anterior pituitary gland that releases the thyroid stimulating hormone (TSH). As a result of secretion of TSH, the thyroid releases thyroxine into

Glands of the Endocrine System

GLAND	LOCATION
Hypothalamus	Lower central brain
Pituitary	Base of the brain beneath the hypothalamus
Thyroid	Lower front neck
Parathyroid	Embedded in the surface and on either side of the thyroid gland
Adrenal	On top of each kidney
Pineal body	Middle of the brain
Pancreas	Back of the abdomen behind the stomach
Ovaries	Both sides of the uterus
Testes	Scrotum

All glands of the endocrine system are "ductless," meaning there are no pathways to guide the hormones to a specific location in the body. All hormones of the endocrine system are released into the bloodstream.

circulation. When the level of thyroxine circulating in the blood is high, the anterior pituitary is inhibited and stops the release of TSH. This is known as a negative feedback loop. Overall, the hormones of the thyroid regulate metabolism, bone growth, and development of brain and nervous tissue in children, as well as the maintenance of blood pressure, heart rate, digestion, muscle tone, and reproduction.

The parathyroid glands are located on the surface of the thyroid gland and are important in regulating the level of calcium and phosphate in the circulatory system. There is a continuous exchange of calcium and phosphate between the bone and blood. During bone breakdown and bone buildup activity of the osteoblasts and osteoclasts, calcium and phosphate are released into the bloodstream. The balance of calcium and phosphate is controlled by the parathyroid glands. When blood calcium decreases, parathormone is secreted; when the body detects increased levels of blood calcium, parathormone is inhibited.

The adrenal glands sit on top of each kidney and regulate body metabolism, the balance of salt and water, the immune system, and sexual function. The adrenal glands also release a hormone that helps the body cope with physical and emotional stress through regulation of the heart rate and blood pressure. Each adrenal gland consists of two main parts: an outer adrenal cortex and an inner adrenal medulla. The adrenal cortex secretes steroid hormones—primarily mineralocorticoids, glucocorticoids, and sex hormones. Mineralocorticoids regulate the salt balance in the body; the primary mineralocorticoid is aldosterone. Glucocorticoids regulate carbohydrate, lipid, and protein metabolism; the primary glucocorticoid is cortisol. Sex hormones secreted by the adrenal glands include the male hormone androgen and the female hormone estrogen. The adrenal medulla secretes epinephrine and norepinephrine, which are secreted in situations of stress. Epinephrine causes vasodilation as well as increased heart rate, blood pressure, and respiratory rate, which are all needed in a stressful situation requiring fight or flight. Norepinephrine causes

general vasoconstriction and reduces the overall effects of epinephrine.

The pineal gland secretes melatonin. It regulates sleep-wake cycles. The pineal gland is positioned deep in the brain and is about the size of a grain of rice.

The primary role of the pancreas is regulating blood sugar. The secondary functions of the pancreas include digestive and hormonal functions. The pancreas produces, stores, and secretes two hormones—insulin and glucagon. Insulin is secreted by beta cells of the pancreas, and glucagon is secreted by alpha cells. Insulin decreases the level of the blood glucose, and glucagon increases the level of blood glucose. When blood glucose rises, insulin is secreted, facilitating the entry of glucose into the cells, resulting in decreased glucose in the bloodstream. When blood glucose falls below normal, glucagon is released, stimulating the release of glucose from storage so that it can enter the bloodstream.

TAKE NOTE

It is important to keep track and monitor the blood sugar of patients with the diagnosis of diabetes, as well as monitor for signs of abnormal blood sugar in patients who do not have a diagnosis of diabetes. Exercise and physical activity facilitate the body's use of glucose and therefore decrease blood sugar levels. For patients with diabetes, it is important to monitor blood sugar before, during, and after activity in order to maintain normal levels even during the physical activity required in therapy sessions. Patients without the diagnosis of diabetes may also present with signs of low blood sugar during exercise due to the body's increased use of glucose during activity.

The pancreas is an endocrine gland as well as an exocrine gland. The exocrine function of the pancreas is digestion. The primary endocrine role of the pancreas is the regulation of blood sugar.

Hormones of the Endocrine System

GLAND	HORMONES	FUNCTION
Thyroid	Thyroxine	Regulates metabolism and bone growth; maintains blood pressure, heart rate, digestion, muscle tone, and reproduction.
Parathyroid	Parathormone	Regulates calcium-phosphate balance.
Adrenal	Steroid hormones	Regulates metabolism, response to stress, salt balance, and sexual reproduction.
Pineal	Melatonin	Regulates the sleep-wake cycle.
Pancreas	Insulin; glucagon	Regulates blood sugar.
Ovaries	Estrogen; progesterone	Regulates the development of sexual characteristics.
Testes	Androgens; testosterone	Regulates the development of sexual characteristics.

Each hormone of the endocrine system has specific functions and specific target organs.

The ovaries and testes secrete sex hormones directly into the bloodstream. The ovaries produce estrogen and progesterone, which control the development of female physical characteristics and reproductive function (such as pregnancy and the menstrual cycle). The testes secrete androgens such as testosterone, which affect male physical characteristics and sperm production. Hormones of the ovaries and testes, which are secreted directly into the bloodstream, can have effects on both the male and female body.

The pituitary gland, or master gland, serves many functions and specific target organs.

Hormones of the Anterior Pituitary

HORMONE	FUNCTION
Growth hormone (somatotropin)	Increases protein synthesis; facilitates growth of bone and tissue.
Thyroid stimulating hormone (TSH)	Stimulates production and release of thyroid hormone.
Adrenocorticotropic hormone (ACTH)	Stimulates production of corticosteroids; increases metabolism; responsible for skin and nail color.
Follicle stimulating hormone (FSH)	In females—stimulates growth of ovarian follicles and secretion of estradiol; in males—stimulates epithelium of seminiferous tubules and spermatogenesis.
Luteinizing hormone (LH)	In females—stimulates progesterone production; in males—stimulates testosterone.

The pituitary gland, also known as the hypophysis, with the adenohypophysis, or anterior pituitary lobe

Hormones of the Posterior Pituitary

HORMONE	FUNCTION
Vasopression (antidiuretic hormone, or ADH)	Constricts blood vessels; increases blood pressure; stimulates reabsorption of water by kidneys.
Oxytocin	Stimulates contraction of uterus; stimulates secretion of milk by mammary glands.

The pituitary gland, also known as the hypophysis, with the posterior pituitary lobe, or neurohypophysis.

The process of metabolism, a vital function of the body, is carried out by all reactions of the body. In addition, the endocrine system regulates many processes of the metabolic system and is a very important system to the overall function of the body. As a physical therapist, it is important to understand the function of metabolism and the role of the endocrine system in order to recognize the effects of PT intervention on these systems.

Practice 5

1. Catabolism is a process involved in the body's metabolism. Catabolism is best described as the
   a. building of complex compounds using heat and energy.
   b. building of complex compounds from smaller compounds.
   c. breakdown of complex compounds into smaller compounds.
   d. breakdown of complex compounds to produce heat and energy.

2. Which of the following is the "master" gland that is involved in direct control of the functions of other endocrine glands?
   a. hypothalamus
   b. pituitary gland
   c. thyroid gland
   d. parathyroid gland

3. Which of the following is the endocrine system's primary mechanism to control the release of hormones?
   a. feedback mechanism
   b. feed-forward mechanism
   c. negative stimulation mechanism
   d. positive stimulation mechanism

4. Most glands of the endocrine system only have endocrine functions. Which gland of the endocrine system has both endocrine and exocrine functions, controlling digestion and blood sugar?
   a. pituitary gland
   b. parathyroid gland
   c. pineal gland
   d. pancreas

5. Which of the following glands secrete a hormone which contains iodine, with the primary function of regulating metabolism?
   a. pineal gland
   b. thyroid gland
   c. parathyroid gland
   d. adrenal gland

6. The parathyroid glands are important in which of the following functions?
   a. regulation of blood calcium levels
   b. regulation of blood sugar levels
   c. regulation of blood nitrogen levels
   d. regulation of blood iodine levels

7. When the body is placed in a stressful situation, which gland can facilitate the fight-or-flight response?
   a. thyroid gland
   b. pineal gland
   c. adrenal gland
   d. pancreas

8. What is the primary role of the pancreas?
   a. regulation of blood calcium levels
   b. regulation of blood sugar levels
   c. regulation of blood nitrogen levels
   d. regulation of blood iodine levels

9. Melatonin is the hormone of the _____ gland and helps to regulate the
   a. pineal; sleep-wake cycle.
   b. pineal; response to stress.
   c. parathyroid; sleep-wake cycle.
   d. parathyroid; response to stress.

10. Which of the following hormones regulates the development of sexual characteristics?
    a. parathormone
    b. androgen
    c. melatonin
    d. thyroxine

11. Which of the following hormones is secreted by the anterior pituitary gland and is responsible for increased protein synthesis?
    a. adrenocorticotropic
    b. luteinizing
    c. growth
    d. follicle stimulating

12. Which of the following hormones is most responsible for the fight-or-flight response to stress?
    a. norepinephrine
    b. epinephrine
    c. aldosterone
    d. progesterone

Practice 5 Answers

1. d. Catabolism involves the breakdown of organic compounds to provide heat and energy. Anabolism involves the building of complex compounds by bonding together smaller compounds.

2. b. The pituitary gland is commonly known as the "master" gland because of the influence it has over the majority of the glands of the endocrine system.

3. a. The production or release of a hormone into the bloodstream is controlled by the amount of effect the hormone has on the body. For example, insulin causes blood sugar levels to fall. As the levels fall, less insulin will be released. As the blood sugar levels rise, more insulin will be released. The pancreas gets feedback about blood sugar levels and either allows or inhibits the release of insulin.

4. d. The pancreas has an endocrine function that regulates blood sugar through the secretion of insulin and glucagons; it has an exocrine function that is involved in digestion.

5. b. Thyroxine, the hormone of the thyroid, contains iodine. The thyroid is a vital hormone in the body's metabolism.

6. a. The parathyroid glands maintain the balance of blood calcium and phosphate.

7. c. The adrenal glands—specifically the adrenal medulla—secretes epinephrine, which is the hormone that prepares the body for fight or flight.

8. b. The primary role of the pancreas is to maintain blood sugar.

9. a. The pineal gland regulates the sleep-wake cycle through the secretion of melatonin.

10. b. Androgens are hormones secreted by the testes, and they play a role in the development of sexual characteristics.

11. c. The anterior pituitary gland secretes the growth hormone, which plays a role in increasing protein synthesis.

12. b. Epinephrine causes vasodilation and increase in heart rate, blood pressure, and respiration rate, which are needed for the fight-or-flight response in stressful situations.

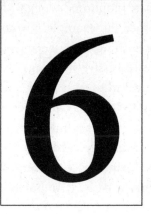

TESTS AND MEASURES REVIEW

CHAPTER SUMMARY

This chapter will review the types and applications of tests and measures used to collect data regarding the cardiovascular and pulmonary circulatory systems, the musculoskeletal system, the neuromuscular system, and the integumentary system. Normal values and the significance of abnormal findings will be reviewed. Changes in metabolism and blood sugar due to various tests and measures will be discussed. Finally, data collection regarding self-care and home management; barriers in home, work, and community; and the ability to assume or resume work, community, and leisure activities will be covered. Performing tests and measures establishes the baseline status of the patient and serves to demonstrate changes in status following physical therapy intervention.

Cardiac, Vascular, and Pulmonary Systems

The ability to collect information accurately and reliably about the cardiac, vascular, and pulmonary systems is a necessary skill for every physical therapist assistant. Whereas pulse rate, respiratory rate, and blood pressure must be measured on *every* patient (regardless of the patient's presenting diagnosis) to determine baseline status and assess the individual's response to activity and exercise, other tests and measures are appropriate only for patients with involvement of the cardiac, vascular, or pulmonary systems. For example, the Ankle-Brachial Index is used to assess circulation in patients with arterial insufficiency.

Many patients have a history of cardiac, pulmonary, or vascular problems even though they may be engaged in physical therapy for another reason. Therefore, every PTA—regardless of the setting of his or her practice—must be knowledgeable about the tests and measures for these systems.

Tests and Measures of the Cardiac System

Data regarding the cardiac system may be taken before, during, and/or after exercise. Data collected prior to the start of exercise may help determine the patient's aerobic capacity. Measurements taken during exercise assess the patient's response to the activity. Information collected after the completion of exercise or activity measures the patient's tolerance to activity.

Aerobic Capacity or Endurance Assessment

Measurement of aerobic capacity or endurance assesses the body's ability to take in, deliver, and utilize oxygen in order to perform an activity over a period of time. This is quantified by determining the volume of oxygen consumed per minute, or VO_2. Assessing aerobic capacity allows the PT and PTA to plan appropriate interventions and assess the effectiveness of those interventions over time.

Standardized Exercise Test Protocols

Exercise test protocols are also referred to as exercise tolerance tests, or stress tests. They can be administered as noted above to plan or assess exercise interventions. They may also be administered to determine a diagnosis of cardiac disease. If stress testing is done in a cardiac lab, extensive patient monitoring will be done. An electrocardiogram (EKG) will assess the heart rate and rhythm, the status of the conduction system through the heart, and the oxygen perfusion into the heart muscle. Nuclear imaging may also be done to assess cardiac perfusion. An echocardiogram can assess cardiac wall motion and left ventricular function. Pulse oximetry may be used to assess the amount of oxygen in the blood. Heart rate, respiratory rate, and blood pressure are monitored, along with the patient's clinical appearance. For example, it would be noted if the patient were flushing, experiencing pallor, or exhibiting diaphoresis (excessive sweating).

The patient will be asked to assess how difficult the activity is by using a standardized rate of perceived exertion scale. If the stress test is administered in a physical therapy clinical setting, typical data collection would include the pulse oximetry, vital signs, RPE, and clinical appearance of the patient. Ambulation on a treadmill, stepping activities, and ergometry (stationary biking) are typical aerobic activities utilized during testing.

Borg Rate of Perceived Exertion Scale

6	
7	Very, very light
8	
9	Very light
10	
11	Fairly light
12	
13	Somewhat hard
14	
15	Hard
16	
17	Very hard
18	
19	Very, very hard

The PTA can use the Borg Rate of Perceived Exertion Scale during activity to monitor the intensity of the activity from the perspective of the patient.

Principles of Stress Testing

Regardless of the setting in which the stress testing is done or the specific aerobic activity that is performed, the principles of stress testing are the same. The test must progress through several levels of workload. The first workload level should be easy (that is, well below the individual's anticipated aerobic capacity). Each workload is maintained for two to six minutes and then progressed by increasing speed, resistance, or elevation. The test is terminated when oxygen uptake does not increase with further increases in workload, when the patient is exhausted, or when the patient demonstrates abnormal vital or clinical signs.

All stress testing procedures begin at a low level or workload and progressively get more difficult. An exercise stress test is terminated if the patient exhibits abnormal vital signs, EKG, or clinical signs. Indications for the termination of the stress test include:

- heart rate greater than 190 bpm
- irregular heart rhythm
- drop in or excessively high blood pressure
- labored respiration
- extreme pallor
- excessive fatigue
- nausea
- dizziness
- altered balance or coordination.

Treadmill Tests

Treadmill stress tests are common, and they have many standardized protocols. A commonly used stress test protocol is the Bruce Protocol. It begins with the patient walking on a 10% incline at 1.7 miles per hour (mph). This corresponds with a metabolic equivalent, or MET level, of 5. Every three minutes the workload is increased. At the highest workload (MET level 22), the treadmill is at a 22% grade and a speed of 6 mph.

Ergometry Tests

Ergometry tests can be performed using a standard stationary bicycle, an upper extremity bike, or even a wheelchair ergometer, which is a device for stationary wheelchair propulsion for those unable to use their lower extremities. Protocols for ergometry tests are often designed to stop short of maximal performance. Equations are used to predict maximal aerobic capacity. As such, they are easily applied in a clinical setting.

Step Tests

Step tests are also frequently applied in a clinical setting. All versions include the patient moving up and down stairs at a prescribed cadence. The height of the step may be constant or progress from 6 to 18 inches in height. There is even a version that allows the person being tested to sit and touch each foot (alternating) onto a stool in front of them. This test is appropriate for a more fragile patient population because the workloads range from only 2.3 to 3.9 METs.

Level Walking Tests

Timed walking can also be used to predict aerobic capacity and endurance. No special training or equipment is required, and walking is an activity familiar to nearly all patients. In the six-minute walk test, the time is kept fixed and the distance assessed. In the one-mile walk test, distance is fixed and the time is assessed.

One-Mile Walk Tests

The patient walks for one mile as quickly as he or she can. In addition to the time taken to complete the distance, the person's age, gender, weight, ending heart rate, and ending RPE are placed into an equation to estimate this individual's VO_2 max.

Six-Minute Walk Tests

Patients with significant cardiac disease or other pathologies may not be able to walk a mile. The six-minute walk test has been used in many different patient populations, including in those with chronic heart failure. For this test, the distance walked is plugged into an equation, along with the patient's age, weight, height, ending heart rate, and ending systolic blood pressure to predict his or her maximal aerobic capacity.

INFORMATION IN ACTION

The patient is a 73-year-old man with end stage chronic heart failure. He is 5'9" and weighs 165 pounds. The physical therapist has asked the PTA to perform a six-minute walk test with the patient to determine his capacity for activity. The patient walks 750 feet in six minutes, with an ending heart rate of 132 beats per minute (bpm) and systolic blood pressure of 92 mm Hg. Plugging these results into a spreadsheet, the patient's VO_2max is estimated at 6.8 mLO_2/kg/min, which is about two METs. Activities consistent with the patient's current aerobic capacity would include using a computer or playing cards. The PTA shares this information with the PT, and the PT is then able to use the information to develop an appropriate exercise program.

TAKE NOTE

The units for the volume of oxygen consumed per minute, or VO_2, are mLO_2/kg/min. One MET equals approximately 3.5 mLO_2/kg/min.

MET Level Assessment

MET is an indication of the oxygen cost of an activity. One MET represents the amount of oxygen required to carry out basic metabolic activities while the person is sitting and awake. When sitting and awake, a person burns roughly 3.5 milliliters of oxygen per kilogram of body weight every minute to supply his or her body's needs. Because the MET level of many daily activities has been calculated, an estimate of aerobic capacity can be made by assessing the types of activities a patient is able to tolerate. The MET level is then multiplied by 3.5 to estimate the patient's VO_2. Normal VO_2max varies by sex and age. Generally, for adult men, VO_2max should be over 30 mLO_2/kg/min. For women, it should be over 26 mLO_2/kg/min.

MET Levels for Various Activities

MET LEVEL	ACTIVITIES
2 to 3	Desk work; dusting; standing; walking 1 to 2 mph; bowling; light woodworking
3 to 4	Cleaning windows; mopping floors; golfing; badminton
4 to 5	Ballroom dancing; painting; raking leaves; hoeing; walking 3.5 mph
5 to 6	Digging in garden; shoveling; swimming
7 to 8	Sawing wood; walking 5 mph; biking 12 mph; canoeing
8 to 9	Running 5.5 mph; handball; rope skipping; basketball
10+	Running 6 mph; swimming 40 yds/min; biking 15 mph

MET levels can be used to estimate VO_2max or to guide people toward activities that are appropriate for their endurance level.

Assessment of Response to Activity

The various standardized exercise tolerance tests are excellent tools to determine baseline aerobic capacity and measure the effectiveness of an exercise program after a course of therapy. However, it is also necessary to measure how a patient is handling the activity while he or she is actually doing it. PTAs must be able to assess heart rate, blood pressure, and RPE and compare the results to normal or expected values.

Heart Rate, Rhythm, Volume

The rate, rhythm, and volume of the heart are assessed by palpating arterial pulses. Common locations for measurement during and immediately following activity are the radial and external carotid arteries. Pressure applied with the second and third digits should be firm enough to create turbulence in the vessel without occluding it. Heart rate is measured in beats per minute and can be measured for a full minute or for a shorter period of time and then multiplied by the correct factor. For example, pulse can be counted for 15 seconds and then multiplied by four for the rate per minute. The longer the pulse is assessed, the more accurate the measurement will be. This is particularly important for patients with an irregular pulse. In addition to rate, for those with an irregular pulse, rhythm and volume are assessed. The rhythm is noted as regular or irregular. The volume is noted as normal, as weak or thready, or as strong or bounding.

Normal Values

Normal values for heart rate vary by age. Normal values range from 60 to 85 bpm for adults, from 80 to 100 bpm for children, and over 100 bpm for infants. In addition to activity level and tolerance, many factors may affect pulse. These include cardiac pathologies, infection, fever, emotional stress, sex, and medication. For example, beta blockers, a class of medications typically used to treat heart failure and high blood pressure, will prevent a normal increase in heart rate, even during exertion. It is critical that the PTA understand all factors that may affect heart rate to avoid drawing erroneous conclusions when assessing it.

Heart Rate and Exercise

Heart rate should increase proportionally in response to exercise. It should plateau during steady-state exercise and decline back to resting values within a few minutes after the exercise ends.

TAKE NOTE

If the PTA has trouble finding a patient's radial pulse, he or she would try the brachial artery. Proximal arteries usually have a stronger pulse. It may feel less invasive to the patient to have his or her pulse taken using the brachial artery than it would to have it taken using the external carotid artery.

Blood Pressure

Blood pressure assesses the force of the blood against the walls of the arteries during systole and diastole. It is assessed at the brachial artery using a sphygmomanometer and a stethoscope. Care should be taken not to inflate the cuff more than 20 mm Hg above the systolic pressure to avoid compressing the artery.

Normal Values for Blood Pressure

Normal systolic blood pressure for adults ranges from 90 to 140 mm Hg. Normal diastolic pressure for adults ranges from 60 to 90 mm Hg. However, optimal pressure is considered to be below 120/80 mm Hg. Many factors, in addition to physical activity, may influence blood pressure, including age, emotional status, vascular pathology, blood volume, and medications. Postural hypotension is a side effect of many medications.

Response to Exercise

It is ideal to take blood pressure during exercise to assess the patient's response, but this may be technically difficult or impossible. If blood pressure is taken after exercise, it should be done with the patient in the same position as during the activity. Systolic blood pressure increases in proportion to the intensity of the exercise. Diastolic blood pressure may increase or decrease slightly. A cool-down period after exercise should be utilized to prevent a sudden drop in blood pressure.

Borg Rate of Perceived Exertion

The Borg Rate of Perceived Exertion Scale is a standardized way for the patient to measure how hard he or she is working. It is a valuable adjunct to vital sign measurement and an important indicator of tolerance when heart rate and/or blood pressure are not reliable.

Electrocardiogram

In some settings, patients may be hooked directly through EKG leads to a monitor. Patients may also be monitored through telemetry. When a patient is monitored through telemetry, a small portable device carried by the patient sends radio signals to a centrally located monitor. Abnormal rate or rhythm changes can be assessed by the physical therapist or other medical staff. It is not the responsibility of the PTA to interpret EKG readings.

Clinical Signs

In addition to taking quantifiable measurements, the PTA should be continually observing the patient's appearance for signs of exercise intolerance. These may include shortness of breath; cyanosis of the nail beds, lips, or earlobes; and complaints of dizziness or excessive fatigue. Increased edema in the distal lower extremities may indicate a worsening of chronic heart failure in patients with that condition.

INFORMATION IN ACTION

A PTA is conducting a treatment session at a skilled nursing facility (SNF) with an 82-year-old woman whom the PTA knows well. The patient has a complicated medical history, which includes congestive heart failure (CHF). The patient had a recent decline in function and was referred for physical therapy to improve her transfer and ambulation status. The PTA notices that the patient is complaining of increased fatigue today and is more short of breath than usual following a walk. Because the patient takes a beta blocker, the PTA asks the patient to rate how hard she feels she is working using the RPE scale, instead of taking her pulse or blood pressure. The rating is higher than normal. The PTA also notices that the patient's feet and ankles are more swollen than normal. The PTA suspects that the patient is having an exacerbation of her CHF. The PTA ends the therapy session early and shares the clinical signs observed with the PT and with the nursing staff.

Assessment of Cardiac Risk

Using standardized assessment tools, patients without cardiac disease should be assessed for their risk of disease. During testing, some factors cannot be modified, such as a person's age, family history, or past medical history. Other factors can be modified, such as smoking, diet, activity level, and weight. Percentage of body fat and Body Mass Index (BMI) are measurements that contribute to an understanding of a person's risk factors for cardiac disease.

Percent Body Fat Measurement

The most reliable way to assess percentage of body fat is with hydrostatic, or underwater, weighing. However, this requires equipment not found in a physical therapy setting. Electrical impedance and ultrasound can also be used to estimate body fat. A more reliable and more accessible method in the clinic is the use of a caliper to assess skin fold measurements. Skin fold measurements are usually taken from three areas on the body. Common areas are behind the triceps, above the anterior superior iliac spine, and below the inferior angle of the scapula. The measurements are summed. A chart is then used to find the person's percent body fat. Normal body fat percentage is 5% to 20% for men and 12% to 25% for women. The greater the increase over normal body fat percentage, the greater the risk for cardiac disease.

Body Mass Index

BMI is an indirect measure of body composition which compares weight to height.

A BMI over 25 is considered overweight. Cardiac risk increases as BMI increases over this value.

TAKE NOTE

Body fat that is concentrated in the abdominal area has been found to increase risk for cardiac disease more than it would if the fat were distributed in other areas of the body.

Body Mass Index Table

	Normal						Overweight					Obese										Extreme Obesity														
BMI	19	20	21	22	23	24	25	26	27	28	29	30	31	32	33	34	35	36	37	38	39	40	41	42	43	44	45	46	47	48	49	50	51	52	53	54
Height (Inches)															Body Weight (pounds)																					
58	91	96	100	105	110	115	119	124	129	134	138	143	148	153	158	162	167	172	177	181	186	191	196	201	205	210	215	220	224	229	234	239	244	248	253	258
59	94	99	104	109	114	119	124	128	133	138	143	148	153	158	163	168	173	178	183	188	193	198	203	208	212	217	222	227	232	237	242	247	252	257	262	267
60	97	102	107	112	118	123	128	133	138	143	148	153	158	163	168	174	179	184	189	194	199	204	209	215	220	225	230	235	240	245	250	255	261	266	271	276
61	100	106	111	116	122	127	132	137	143	148	153	158	164	169	174	180	185	190	195	201	206	211	217	222	227	232	238	243	248	254	259	264	269	275	280	285
62	104	109	115	120	126	131	136	142	147	153	158	164	169	175	180	186	191	196	202	207	213	218	224	229	235	240	246	251	256	262	267	273	278	284	289	295
63	107	113	118	124	130	135	141	146	152	158	163	169	175	180	186	191	197	203	208	214	220	225	231	237	242	248	254	259	265	270	278	282	287	293	299	304
64	110	116	122	128	134	140	145	151	157	163	169	174	180	186	192	197	204	209	215	221	227	232	238	244	250	256	262	267	273	279	285	291	296	302	308	314
65	114	120	126	132	138	144	150	156	162	168	174	180	186	192	198	204	210	216	222	228	234	240	246	252	258	264	270	276	282	288	294	300	306	312	318	324
66	118	124	130	136	142	148	155	161	167	173	179	186	192	198	204	210	216	223	229	235	241	247	253	260	266	272	278	284	291	297	303	309	315	322	328	334
67	121	127	134	140	146	153	159	166	172	178	185	191	198	204	211	217	223	230	236	242	249	255	261	268	274	280	287	293	299	306	312	319	325	331	338	344
68	125	131	138	144	151	158	164	171	177	184	190	197	203	210	216	223	230	236	243	249	256	262	269	276	282	289	295	302	308	315	322	328	335	341	348	354
69	128	135	142	149	155	162	169	176	182	189	196	203	209	216	223	230	236	243	250	257	263	270	277	284	291	297	304	311	318	324	331	338	345	351	358	365
70	132	139	146	153	160	167	174	181	188	195	202	209	216	222	229	236	243	250	257	264	271	278	285	292	299	306	313	320	327	334	341	348	355	362	369	376
71	136	143	150	157	165	172	179	186	193	200	208	215	222	229	236	243	250	257	265	272	279	286	293	301	308	315	322	329	338	343	351	358	365	372	379	386
72	140	147	154	162	169	177	184	191	199	206	213	221	228	235	242	250	258	265	272	279	287	294	302	309	316	324	331	338	346	353	361	368	375	383	390	397
73	144	151	159	166	174	182	189	197	204	212	219	227	235	242	250	257	265	272	280	288	295	302	310	318	325	333	340	348	355	363	371	378	386	393	401	408
74	148	155	163	171	179	186	194	202	210	218	225	233	241	249	256	264	272	280	287	295	303	311	319	326	334	342	350	358	365	373	381	389	396	404	412	420
75	152	160	168	176	184	192	200	208	216	224	232	240	248	256	264	272	279	287	295	303	311	319	327	335	343	351	359	367	375	383	391	399	407	415	423	431
76	156	164	172	180	189	197	205	213	221	230	238	246	254	263	271	279	287	295	304	312	320	328	336	344	353	361	369	377	385	394	402	410	418	426	435	443

$$BMI = \frac{weight\ (kg)}{height\ (m)^2}$$

INFORMATION IN ACTION

A 62-year-old man is attending physical therapy at an outpatient clinic following a left total knee replacement. He is nearing the end of his therapy and has expressed to the PTA with whom he is working a desire to lose weight. The patient states that he knows that weight loss will help his joints as well as his heart. The PTA shares this information with the supervising PT, and the PT instructs the PTA to assess the patient's BMI during that session. During the next session, the PT conducts a submaximal ergometry stress test. Based on the results of these tests, the PT designs an aerobic exercise routine for this patient and has the PTA instruct the patient in it.

Tests and Measures of the Pulmonary System

Some patients with pulmonary pathologies will need a detailed examination of their respiratory status, including an assessment of their breathing pattern, pulmonary volumes, cough, thoracic cage mobility, and posture. Other patients may just need an assessment of their respiratory rate or pulse oximetry to determine their readiness for and response to exercise. The PTA must be knowledgeable about the full range of tests and measures applied to the pulmonary system.

Posture

Patients with chronic lung problems typically exhibit an increased thoracic kyphosis and a forward head, with scapular protraction. In a sitting position, the person tends to lean forward on the arms for stability in order to use accessory muscles of respiration. This places the trunk in a flexed position. When the person looks up from this position, it places the head in a forward head posture. The PT or PTA must determine if this is a postural fault or a fixed deformity. The anterior/posterior diameter of the thorax enlarges due to loss of elastic recoil, giving rise to the typical barrel-chest appearance.

Range of Motion

During inspiration, the rib cage expands in all directions. An increase in anterior/posterior (A/P) diameter requires movement at the sternocostal joints and thoracic spine extension. This is referred to as "pump handle" motion, with the sternum visualized as the handle of a water pump pulling the thoracic cage up and forward. An increase in medial/lateral (M/L) diameter requires motion at the sternocostal and costovertebral joints. This is referred to as "bucket handle" motion, with the ribs visualized as the handle of a bucket moving up and out.

The ribs must be observed during inspiration to ensure that they are moving appropriately. The PT can assess the joint play of the sternocostal and costovertebral joints. Spinal extension can be assessed with a tape measure or inclinometer.

TAKE NOTE

The PTA can quickly assess rib cage movement by placing his or her hands on the sides of the patient's rib cage and asking the patient to take a deep breath. The patient's ribs should move up and out symmetrically.

Muscle Length

Muscle length assessment of the pectoralis major, pectoralis minor, and sternocleidomastoid muscles should be assessed. These are muscles that are shortened with the postural deformities mentioned previously.

Ventilation and Respiration

When assessing respiration, the PTA should take note of rate, rhythm, depth, and character. Normal respiratory rate is 30 to 50 breaths per minute for infants, 15 to 35 breaths per minute for children, and 12 to 18 breaths per minute for adults. In addition to exercise, respiratory rate can be affected by altitude, air quality, emotional status, disease, and medications. The rhythm of breathing is either regular or irregular. The depth of breathing is normal, shallow, or deep. Character of breathing refers to any sounds during respiration. Normal respiration observed without a stethoscope should not make any noise. Other factors related to ventilation and respiration must be assessed.

Breathing Pattern

People normally demonstrate a diaphragmatic breathing pattern at rest. With contraction of the diaphragm during inspiration, the abdomen rises. Although accessory muscle use may occur normally after exertion, it also may be seen during quiet respiration in those with pulmonary pathology. The accessory muscles include the sternocleidomastoid, the scalenes, and pectoralis major and minor. These muscles pull upward on the clavicle and ribs to increase the inferior/superior diameter of the rib cage and improve inspiration. If the PTA notes use of accessory muscles at rest, that is an indication of an abnormal breathing pattern. The ratio of inspiration to expiration should be 1 to 2 at rest and 1 to 1 during exertion. Normal expiration occurs passively through relaxation of the muscles. The PTA may notice that some patients with obstructive lung disorders do a forced expiration through pursed lips in order to improve this phase of breathing.

Cough

An effective cough is critical to good pulmonary health. A cough protects the airway from aspiration and clears secretions that have accumulated. Patients with chest wall pain, weak abdominal muscles, or the inability to take a deep breath may demonstrate a weak and ineffective cough.

Pulse Oximetry

A pulse oximeter attaches to a patient's finger or earlobe and measures the amount of oxygen in the blood at those points. Normal values range from 95% to 100%. Patients with chronic lung pathologies may normally run in the low 90s. Oxygen saturation below 88% is considered an indication for supplemental oxygen. Oxygen saturation should be monitored before, during, and after exertion in patients with pulmonary pathologies. Exercise should be tailored to keep the patient's saturation level above that determined by the PT. Again, 88% is a value typically used.

Clinical Signs

Signs the PTA may observe which indicate acute or chronic pulmonary distress include shortness of breath and cyanosis of fingertips, lips, or earlobes. Patients with chronic pulmonary problems may have clubbing of the digits.

INFORMATION IN ACTION

A PTA is seeing a 43-year-old man four days after a thoracotomy for removal of a cancerous lung tumor. The PTA observes that the man takes shallow breaths and has a weak cough. When placing her hands on the sides of the man's rib cage, the PTA notes little lateral expansion during inspiration. The PTA instructs the patient in diaphragmatic breathing and an effective cough and does segmental breathing to improve lateral costal expansion. She then reassesses the patient's breathing pattern, coughing, and lateral expansion following the treatment session.

INFORMATION IN ACTION

A PTA is treating a 67-year-old woman with chronic obstructive pulmonary disease. Prior to the session, the PTA notices the patient sitting hunched forward with her arms on the armrests of her chair. The PTA observes the patient's use of accessory muscles during inspiration and pursed lip breathing upon expiration. Her oxygen saturation is 92% at rest and 86% after ambulating 120' with a wheeled walker. The PTA times her recovery to baseline saturation and notes that it takes 3.5 minutes.

Tests and Measures of the Peripheral Vascular System

The peripheral vascular system includes the arterial, venous, and lymphatic circulation. A primary symptom of venous and lymphatic disorders is edema, so data collection focuses on its measurement. Data collection for arterial disorders assesses the delivery of oxygenated blood to the periphery.

Girth Measurement

Edema can be measured by assessing the girth of an extremity. A tape measure is placed firmly around the circumference of the limb, and the girth is noted in centimeters. The distance from adjacent bony landmarks is also recorded in order to reproduce the measurement location accurately. For example, edema of the lower leg may be measured at the level of the tibial tubercle, 10 cm below the tibial tubercle, and 5 cm proximal to the lateral malleolus.

Limb Volume Measurement

Edema can also be measured by assessing the volume of the limb. It requires more equipment and is more time-consuming than a girth measurement, but it accommodates for variations in limb size more accurately. The distal portion of the limb is placed into a container filled to the brim with water. The volume of water displaced is measured and recorded.

Pulse Palpation

Detection of a pulse is an indication of good arterial blood flow. Pulses are assessed proximally to distally in patients suspected of arterial insufficiency. For example, the patient's pulse would be palpated first at the femoral artery, next at the popliteal artery, and then at either the dorsalis pedis or posterior tibial artery.

The PTA should take note primarily of the volume of the pulse; rate and rhythm are not the main concern at this time.

Ankle-Brachial Index

When a pulse cannot be detected manually, measurement of the Ankle-Brachial Index can give more accurate information about the quality of arterial circulation. The ABI is the ratio between the systolic blood pressure taken at the brachial artery and the systolic blood pressure taken at the posterior tibial artery. Instead of a stethoscope, a Doppler ultrasound is used to identify the pulse. The blood pressure is measured in both upper extremities, and the higher of the two is recorded. The blood pressure is then measured in the involved lower extremity and divided by the upper extremity pressure. Normal ABI is .95 to 1.2. A value above or below this range would indicate arterial disease.

Pain

Lack of oxygenated blood flow to tissues results in ischemia and pain. Patients with arterial insufficiency often experience lower extremity pain after ambulation, a condition known as intermittent claudication. The PTA should assess the intensity of the patient's pain on a rating scale and the time or distance at which the patient experiences the pain. Patients with severe arterial insufficiency may experience pain at rest, indicating that their arteries are not able to supply enough oxygen for even resting metabolism. Patients with venous and lymphatic disorders may report aching, but they do not have the sharp pain associated with ischemia.

Trophic Changes

Lack of oxygenated blood flow impairs the health of the structures in the skin. Patients with chronic arterial insufficiency will exhibit loss of hair, dry skin, shiny skin, and thickened nails.

Skin Color

The PTA can observe changes in skin color that may indicate the presence of peripheral vascular disorders. With arterial insufficiency, the limb will appear pale when elevated and red when dependent (dependent rubor). The nail beds may appear cyanotic. Capillary refill time may also give information about the quality of the arterial circulation. The PTA presses on the nail bed to create blanching and then releases and times how long it takes for the color to return. Normal capillary refill time is less than three seconds. The skin on the lower legs of patients with chronic venous insufficiency may be brown and blotchy. Known as hemosiderin staining, this is due to leakage of red blood cells from the veins into the surrounding tissue spaces.

Across the lifespan, accurate and reliable data collection of cardiovascular and pulmonary parameters is important for patients with problems in any practice pattern. Accurate measurement of these parameters can serve as the basis for goal setting, intervention planning, and outcome assessment.

Practice 1

1. How many METs does it require for a person to be awake and sitting?
   a. one
   b. two
   c. five
   d. ten

2. A healthy person is undergoing a treadmill stress test as part of a physical examination. Which of the following symptoms would indicate that the exam should be terminated?
   a. heart rate of 120 bpm
   b. systolic blood pressure dropping 20 mm Hg
   c. respiratory rate of 22 breaths per minute
   d. patient stating that he or she is getting tired

3. Which of the following activities has the highest MET level?
   a. walking 3 mph
   b. painting
   c. biking 13 mph
   d. water skiing

4. What is the amount of oxygen used when at rest?
   a. 1 mLO_2/kg/min
   b. 2.5 mLO_2/kg/min
   c. 3.5 mLO_2/kg/min
   d. 5 mLO_2/kg/min

5. What is the most reliable way to measure exercise tolerance in a patient who is taking a beta blocker?
   a. heart rate
   b. respiratory rate
   c. blood pressure
   d. rate of perceived exertion

6. Which of the following postural faults would most likely be noted in a patient with COPD?
   a. loss of cervical lordosis
   b. loss of thoracic kyphosis
   c. increased thoracic kyphosis
   d. scoliosis

7. A patient presents with a history of COPD. Results from which of the following muscle length assessments should the PTA expect to see on the initial examination?
   a. pectoralis major
   b. levator scapula
   c. back extensors
   d. hamstrings

8. The PT asks the PTA if a patient with COPD is using accessory muscle for respiration at rest. Which of the following muscles would the PTA be looking for?
   a. diaphragm
   b. internal intercostals
   c. external intercostals
   d. sternocleidomastoid

9. The PTA observes a patient sitting quietly in the gym prior to his therapy session. Which of the following clinical signs could indicate a chronic pulmonary problem?
   a. diaphragmatic breathing pattern
   b. pink nail beds
   c. clubbing of the digits
   d. 1:2 ratio of inspiration to expiration

10. Which of the following tests and measures would be most appropriate for a patient with arterial insufficiency?
   a. limb girth measurement
   b. limb volume measurement
   c. ankle range of motion
   d. distance walked until intermittent claudication occurs

11. Which of the following tests and measures would be most appropriate for a patient with venous insufficiency?
   a. limb girth measurement
   b. Ankle-Brachial Index
   c. time walked until intermittent claudication occurs
   d. pulse assessment in the foot

12. The PTA reads the following information from the PT's initial examination of the patient: "The skin on the lower legs and feet is dry and shiny. Dorsalis pedis pulses are absent bilaterally. Nail beds are cyanotic." What pathology does this suggest to the PTA?
   a. deep vein thrombosis
   b. arterial insufficiency
   c. primary lymphedema
   d. congestive heart failure

Practice 1 Answers

1. a. It requires one MET, or metabolic equivalent, for a person to be awake and sitting. One MET represents the basic systemic oxygen requirements at rest.

2. b. If systolic blood pressure drops 20 mm Hg, then the exam should be terminated. Systolic blood pressure should increase as exercise intensity increases. A drop of over 10 mm Hg would be an indication to terminate a stress test.

3. c. Walking 3 mph requires 3 to 4 METs. Painting requires 4 to 5 METs. Water skiing requires 6 to 7 METs. Biking 13 mph requires 8 to 9 METs.

4. c. The basic systemic oxygen requirement for a person at rest is roughly 3.5 mLO$_2$/kg/min.

5. d. Rate of perceived exertion gives the best indicator of a patient's exercise tolerance for a patient taking beta blockers. Beta blockers blunt the rise in heart rate and blood pressure with exercise. Respiratory rate is not precise enough to indicate exercise tolerance.

6. c. Patients with COPD develop an increased thoracic kyphosis and an increase in the A/P diameter of the thorax.

7. a. Common postural faults in patients with COPD include an increased thoracic kyphosis and a forward head. The pectoralis major would become tight with these postural faults and should be routinely assessed in this patient population.

8. d. Accessory muscles of respiration are those which can elevate the rib cage and which are not normally used during quiet breathing. The sternocleidomastoid pulls up on the clavicle to increase the inferior/superior diameter of the rib cage. The diaphragm and intercostals are normal muscles of respiration.

9. c. Clubbing of the digits is an indicator of chronic hypoxia and could be due to a chronic pulmonary problem. All other clinical observations listed are normal.

10. d. Intermittent claudication is the most common complaint in patients with chronic arterial insufficiency. Limb girth and limb volume measurements are assessments of edema, which is a symptom of venous and lymphatic system problems.

11. a. Edema is the major symptom of venous insufficiency. Limb girth measurement assesses edema. All other measures listed assess the arterial system.

12. b. These are signs of trophic changes and decreased oxygen supply and are characteristic of arterial insufficiency.

Musculoskeletal System

Tests and measures provide objective data that is critical to ensure reimbursement; establish clear communication to other healthcare providers, insurance professionals, and employers regarding changes in functional mobility; and also demonstrate outcomes and effectiveness of therapists' interventions. This section will outline many of the tests and measures used by physical therapists and physical therapist assistants to assess the status of patients with musculoskeletal disorders.

Anthropometric Characteristics

Anthropometric (or body) measurements vary considerably among human beings. By measuring length, width, circumference, and volume of extremities, we can assess edema and limb length. By measuring subcutaneous tissue thickness, we can assess body composition. One way in which this information may be applied is in ensuring the correct fit of adaptive equipment, orthotics, and prosthetics.

Body Composition

Health risks associated with obesity, such as hypertension, diabetes mellitus type II, cardiovascular disease, respiratory dysfunction, elevated cholesterol, and increased stress to joints, are all well documented. However, fat within the body is also essential for maintaining body temperature and as an important fuel source for energy expenditure.

Lean body mass is made of essential structures such as water, muscle, bone, and internal organs. Fat is broken into three categories to include: essential fat, storage fat, and nonessential fat. Understanding the body's fat composition versus lean muscle mass is essential in order to safely advise patients on how to reduce fat content within the body.

The minimum recommended body fat for a male is 5% and 12% for a female. The average percentage of body fat for a healthy male will range between 15% to 18% and for a female between 22% to 25%. Overweight is defined as a fat percentage greater than 25% to 35% for a male and 30% to 40% for a female. Obesity is defined as a fat percentage greater than 35% for a male and 40% for a female.

Methods for Measuring Body Fat

There are a variety of methods to determine body fat. Hydrostatic weighing uses Archimedes's principle of displacement, which assumes that lean muscle mass weighs more than water and that fat tissue weighs less than water, so a fatter person will weigh less underwater. Hydrostatic weighing is currently the gold standard for determining Body Mass Index; however, newer and more sophisticated measurement systems may make this obsolete in the future.

Skin fold measurements require the use of a caliper (which is a tool to determine the thickness of fat in various body regions) to determine overall percentage of body fat. According to the American College of Sports Medicine, the measurements are 98% accurate compared to hydrostatic weighing, which is the gold standard for measuring body fat percentage. There are several sites that may be used to collect measurements. These include the triceps, pectorals, subscapula, midaxillary, abdomen, suprailiac, and quadriceps areas. Measurements are typically taken at three or four locations and added together. This total value is then located on a chart or plugged into a formula to calculate body fat percentage.

Another tool for measuring body fat is bioelectrical impedance analysis, or body fat analysis. Although not generally considered as accurate as the methods listed above, it is simple and quick. A safe, low-level electrical current is sent through a specific area of the body. Body fat is determined based on a calculation that examines the amount of lean tissue versus fat, as the electrical current travels at different speeds through the various types of tissues. Many digital scales have incorporated this feature.

The Body Mass Index is another simple tool that looks at height and weight to estimate the percent of body fat. It is not considered as accurate as some of the other methods previously discussed, but it is a simple measurement that can be used to track an individual's progress in a weight loss program. The BMI is determined by dividing the individual's weight in pounds by his or her height in inches squared, and then multiplying that number by 703. BMI = weight/(height)^2 × 703. BMI between 18 and 24.9 is considered normal, 25 to 29.9 is overweight, and over 30 is considered obese.

Body Dimensions

Length, width, circumference, or girth can be determined by using a tape measure. It is important to use bony landmarks as references for consistency. Some PTAs prefer to use a grease pencil to mark a small dot on the patient—but you must be careful when measuring wounds or fragile skin, as the pen may cause a skin reaction.

When measuring a wound that is being treated by secondary intention, it is important to take measurements from 12 o'clock to 6 o'clock, and then from 3 o'clock to 9 o'clock. You may also refer to length and width, but the standard orientation uses a clock, positioned based on the orientation of the limb, with a superior or proximal orientation being characterized as 12 o'clock and a more distal or inferior location as 6 o'clock. A location of 90 degrees from this plane is either a 3 o'clock or a 9 o'clock orientation.

You must also use consistent tension on the tape measure. If tension is too loose or too tight, you may decrease the reliability of the measurement. Some tape measures have a spring so that when you pull on the tape measure a line or dot appears. You should pull until you see that dot or line each time, to ensure the same tension on the tape measure.

Although standard American measurement units are used in the United States, many length, width, and circumferential measurements are measured in metric units. These have smaller increments and are easier to divide into decimal equivalents.

To measure residual limb length, the PTA should begin from either the middle of the patella or the anterior superior iliac spine (ASIS) and measure down to the end of the tibia or femur, respectively. If you are using a caliper instead of a tape measure, it is important to keep the caliper parallel to the long axis of the residual limb. Circumferential measurements must be positioned perpendicular to the long axis of the residual limb. It is also important to read either the top edge or the bottom edge of the tape measure consistently. Even small inconsistencies can significantly impact the accuracy of measurements.

Edema Measurement

Girth measurements are appropriate for determining the amount of edema or atrophy present in a local area. Measurements are made from a known landmark using a tape measure. Although measurements may be made using standard American or metric units, metric units are used more commonly. The centimeter, which lends itself to decimal increments, can easily be broken down into ten millimeter components, while the inch must be broken into fractional components, such as $\frac{1}{4}$, $\frac{1}{8}$, or $\frac{1}{16}$, which are more difficult to compare.

Circumferential girth measurements are measured from a nearby bony landmark, and if necessary, additional measurements can be made above and below the landmark at 10–15 cm intervals. A left-right comparison is necessary, as there is no normative data for comparison. If a left-right comparison is not possible, then the measurements can be compared over time; however, the initial measurements do not have any relative value except as comparison numbers. Measurements can be used to identify both edema and evidence of atrophy.

TAKE NOTE

Usually type IIb muscle fibers, or fast twitch fibers, will atrophy more quickly than type I or type IIa fibers. Powerful muscles, such as the quadriceps femoris group, the gastrocnemius, and the biceps brachii, will atrophy more quickly than other surrounding muscles.

Figure-Eight Measurements

The hand and the foot are often more challenging when it comes to collecting circumferential measurements. A figure-eight measurement can be performed to gain a single measurement to determine swelling around the wrist or the ankle.

The figure-eight measurement for the wrist begins at the ulnar styloid process. It moves across the palm to the proximal palmar crease at the base of the first metacarpal, then to the dorsum of the hand along the metacarpal-phalangeal joint. Next it moves to the palmar surface underneath the fifth metacarpal, across to the thenar eminence, and then on the dorsum of the hand at the wrist.

The figure-eight measurement for the ankle begins at the lateral malleolus. It moves over the dorsum of the foot to the middle of the medial longitudinal arch, then laterally under the base of the fifth metatarsal, up over the dorsum of the foot to the medial malleolus, and then on the posterior side of the leg to the lateral malleolus. These measurements are useful if you need a single gross measurement of swelling to either the ankle or the wrist.

Volumetrics

Should you need more specific measurements involving the foot or the hand, volumetrics is the most accurate. In this method, a clear plastic container is filled with water. There is a shunt off of the container, and next to it is a graduated cylinder which measures the displaced water in millimeters. The hand or the foot is placed into the container up to styloid processes or malleoli, respectively. Water is displaced into the graduated cylinder. The amount of water displaced represents the volume of the hand or foot. These can be done as a pre- and post-activity measurements, or a left-right comparison. Changes of more than 10% are considered significant.

Ergonomics and Body Mechanics

Ergonomics is the study of the interaction between the human body and tools or equipment. This includes aspects of engineering, psychology, and kinesiology. Physical therapists and physical therapist assistants use the principles of ergonomics to assist patients to safely return to work. The Americans with Disabilities Act of 1992 cited physical and occupational therapists as experts in determining reasonable accommodations for injured workers. This requires using skills to analyze work performance and technique and to identify modifications to reduce stress to injured body areas. Body mechanics focuses more on the techniques used by the individual to perform activities in the safest and most energy-efficient manner while putting the least amount of stress on the body.

Functional Capacity Evaluation

The American Physical Therapy Association has developed occupational health guidelines that include guidance for performing Functional Capacity Evaluations (FCE). An FCE is a detailed examination and evaluation that objectively measures the patient's current level of function, primarily within the context of the demands of competitive employment, activities of daily living, or leisure activities. Measurements of function from an FCE are used to make return-to-work/activity decisions, disability determinations, or to design rehabilitation plans.

An FCE measures the ability of an individual to perform functional or work-related tasks and predicts the potential to sustain these tasks over a defined time frame. This supports tertiary prevention by preventing needless disability or activity restrictions (according to the APTA Occupational Guidelines on Functional

Physical Demand Characteristics

PHYSICAL DEMAND LEVEL	OCCASIONAL: 0–33% OF THE DAY	FREQUENT: 34–66% OF THE WORKDAY	CONSTANT: 67–100% OF THE WORKDAY
Sedentary	1–10 lb.	Negligible	Negligible
Light	11–25 lb.	1–10 lb.	Negligible
Medium	21–50 lb.	11–25 lb.	1–10 lb.
Heavy	51–100 lb.	26–50 lb.	11–20 lb.
Very Heavy	Over 100 lb.	Over 50 lb.	Over 20 lb.

According to the U.S. Department of Labor, work is characterized into five categories based on material handling (lifting) abilities.

Capacity Evaluations 3.2). Functional Capacity Evaluations are further divided into General Purpose FCEs (which identify a physical demand category of work) and a job-specific FCE. The latter is designed to match an injured employee with the physical demands of a specific job. FCEs were developed during the 1980s as a response to the workers' compensation insurance industry's need to quantify an injured employee's ability to return to work. This necessitated an understanding of the U.S. Department of Labor's occupational work guidelines and how work was characterized into five categories based on material handling (lifting) abilities.

The evaluations may take three to six hours for a one-day exam or five to eight hours for a two-day exam. There is no single standardized methodology for performing Functional Capacity Evaluations. There are various models that require advance training and or specialization prior to being able to perform them using a specific methodology. They may be manually performed or computer-assisted. Computer-assisted formats do not interpret data; however, they usually speed up the documentation process. Some of the more common formats include ErgoScience, Isernhagen Work Systems, Matheson Work System, Blankenship System, ERGOS, BTE ER, and Key Systems. As there are many more types of Functional Capacity Evaluation models, this is not intended to be an exhaustive list but simply to identify some of the more commonly used models.

Functional Job Analysis

When performing a job-specific Functional Capacity Evaluation, it is necessary to also have a Functional Job Analysis. This is different than the typical job description that the human resource department might provide, as it has the physical demands of the job as well as the essential functions necessary to perform the job. This can then be used later to compare functional abilities to this job description or determine how a position might be modified. This also has other applications in that a functional job analysis could be used to identify ergonomic design or work process changes and can also be used to develop a pre-placement or post-offer screen for new employees.

Characteristics of Work

When describing work tasks, it is important that there is a common understanding of what the work requires. The Department of Labor has defined characteristics of work so that we have a common language to describe work tasks. Material handling tasks, which include activities such as lifting, pushing, pulling, and carrying, are divided in five categories: sedentary, light, medium, heavy, and very heavy. These are classified by the weight of the loads lifted as well as the frequency with which they are handled.

Occasional, frequent, and constant describe how often these activities occur within an eight-hour day. Occasional implies up to 33% of the workday; frequent is up to 67% of the workday; and constant implies more than 67% of the workday.

Nonmaterial handling activities are activities that do not require force,and are positional- or movement-related. Examples of nonmaterial handling activities include: walking, sitting, standing, reaching, handling, fingering, stooping, kneeling, crawling, crouching, and climbing. These also can be described by the terms occasional, frequent, and constant.

Functional job analyses are most accurate when a qualified individual goes out and observes and measures one or more individuals performing the job. Through interviews with employees, supervisors, and management, evaluators can reach a consensus about what is required for a job. Title I of the Americans with Disabilities Act (ADA) ensures that the hiring, firing, transfers, and benefits of employees are equitable. It requires employers to identify essential functions of the job. An essential function is defined as the reason a job exists, a job that can only be performed with the skills or certifications of a specific individual, or a job which has no one else available to perform this task. Although physical and occupational therapists and assistants can assist employers in identifying essential functions, the ultimate determination is up to the employer. Qualified individuals with disabilities are eligible for reasonable accommodations. Based on information provided by the Equal Employment Opportunity Commission (EEOC), which enforces Title I of the ADA, the majority of reasonable accommodations cost less than $500. There are provisions that if it poses undue hardship, employers are not required to implement the accommodations.

Assessment of Body Mechanics during ADLs and IADLs, Work, and Recreational Activities

Body mechanics is the use of the correct sequence of muscles and muscle actions to produce an efficient and safe movement, without undue strain on muscles and joints. Physical therapists and physical therapist assistants are frequently called on as experts to assist other healthcare providers, caregivers, and employers to identify and instruct in good body mechanics.

Principles of Good Body Mechanics

Depending on a patient's diagnosis and the activity in question, a wide variety of recommendations might be made. Preventing joint deformities in the hand of a patient with rheumatoid arthritis, for example, has little in common with preventing a back injury for a construction worker. However, the principles involved are remarkably similar. Using the larger joints of the body, such as the hips and knees or shoulders and elbows (rather than the smaller joints of the spine or fingers), can help to place stress on joints that are better able to handle it. Keeping loads close to the body while maintaining a wide base of support and low center of gravity can help an individual remain stable and still allow larger muscles to perform the task. The following is a list of principles to keep in mind:

- Use larger joints.
- Keep center of gravity low.
- Maintain the normal lordosis in your spine.
- Keep objects close to your body.
- Avoid twisting or pivoting through your feet.
- Use a ladder to get to hard to reach places.
- Ask for help when something is beyond your capabilities.
- Push or pull rather than lift or carry.
- Avoid using momentum to initiate movements.
- Loads are easier to manage in the center of your body between knuckle and chest height rather than overhead or from the floor.
- Pivot from the hip rather than flex the trunk.
- Keep your body flexible and strong so you can handle these day-to-day stresses.
- Change positions often throughout the day.
- Breathe—don't hold your breath (avoid Valsalva maneuver).

Although this is a general list of principles to keep in mind, it is important to look at each individual activity and how it impacts a patient's diagnosis and his or her functional abilities. An individual with a knee problem who has difficulty with crouching may be shown techniques different from those shown to a person with a back injury. Whenever possible, activities that are very difficult might be reduced or eliminated. Moving items in low or high cabinets to an area that is easy to reach might eliminate a problematic activity completely. Creativity and flexibility are necessary to provide the most optimal outcomes for your patients. Remember to share your ideas and network with other professionals. Sharing an idea learned from someone else is much easier than starting from scratch each and every time.

Gait, Locomotion, and Balance

Safely moving patients from one location to another and teaching them to do the same independently or with caregiver assistance is a focal point of the profession. Ensuring the safety of the patient through the use of safety devices and correct guarding techniques is vital to building the trust and rapport that therapists seek with patients. Watching patients progress from needing maximum assistance to complete independence will fill you with a sense of accomplishment that you have made a difference in a person's life.

Assessment of Level of Assistance Required for Gait

When gait training, an assessment of the level of assistance a patient may require begins with a review of the medical record. Gaining insight into the patient's premorbid functional abilities, need for ambulation aids, and the environment into which he or she is likely to return all set the stage for your intervention. Then an assessment of the patient's strength, mobility, and balance, as well as tolerance for sustained upright postures, will be necessary prior to choosing an assistive device. Finally, the patient's diagnosis (and specifically weight-bearing status, as well as any other functional limitations) will be used to determine the level of assistance necessary for gait training.

Monitoring vital signs and being alert to unexpected circumstances will ensure that any fluctuations in balance can be accommodated. Ensure that the patient is wearing the proper footgear, including a nonslip sole and closed-back shoe, prior to standing in order to begin ambulation.

Non-weight-bearing (NWB) and toe-touch weight-bearing (TTWB) are the most restrictive weight-bearing statuses. Essentially, no weight can be accepted by the injured extremity, and balance must be achieved through the remaining limb and the upper extremities. Partial weight-bearing (PWB) and weight-bearing as tolerated (WBAT) allow for some weight-bearing through the injured extremity and are therefore more stable.

Assistive Devices

The most stable assistive device is walking within parallel bars. However, for independent ambulation, a walker gives the greatest amount of stability. A standard walker is very stable, especially if a NWB or TTWB status is observed. A rolling walker requires less energy expenditure for the patient, but it may be slightly unsteady with fewer casters than a standard walker. A rolling walker may have only two of the four casters, and they may be two inches to five inches in diameter. Usually, the fewer the casters (two versus four) and the larger the casters (five inches versus two inches), the more stable the walker is.

Axillary crutches or Canadian or Lofstrand crutches provide more stability than a cane but less than a walker. Because of the narrow base of support, significant upper extremity strength is required. Axillary or Lofstrand crutches provide the least amount of support with which a NWB or TTWB gait can be performed. Progressing further to less stability is a four- or three-point cane, called a quad- or tri-cane. A hemi walker is another tool that has unilateral support;

however, it is typically used with patients with hemiparesis or hemiplegia from a neurological insult. Finally, the least amount of support is provided by a straight cane.

Types of Gait Patterns

In addition to the assistive device, the type of gait pattern will also contribute to the need for assistance during gait training. A four-point reciprocal gait is a very slow gait that is performed with axillary or Lofstrand crutches or two canes. It necessitates that only one point moves at a time. Depending on the side of injury, it may be right crutch, left foot, left crutch, and right foot. This pattern is very stable. The progression of this pattern is a two-point reciprocal gait which moves two points, the crutch and opposite leg, together. This is also a stable pattern and especially appropriate for someone with bilateral lower extremity weakness. With a unilateral problem, a three-point step-to pattern achieves both stability and speed. It can be done with all of the assistive devices and with all weight-bearing statuses. A step-through pattern is considered a progression to a more functional gait while still maintaining stability. A two-point, step-to, or step-through pattern is the least stable of the patterns prior to ambulating without an assistive device.

Guarding

Guarding assistance varies depending on the stability of the patient with the assistive device. Assistance with guarding ranges between minimum, moderate, and maximal assistance. Maximal assistance of one or more clinicians requires that the clinician provides 50% to 75% assistance in positioning the assistive device, weight shifting, and advancing limbs. Moderate and minimal assistance require that clinicians provide up to 50% or 25%, respectively. Contact guarding is usually performed with the physical therapist assistant's standing to the side and slightly behind the patient, on the side that he or she is most likely to lose balance. One hand is placed on the pelvis on the gait belt, and the second is placed on the

front of the shoulder. It is important not to grip clothing or grasp under the patient's axilla, as it is likely to cause damage and not provide adequate stability should a loss of balance occur.

Close guarding requires the PTA to be positioned close to—but not touching—the patient. The PTA is close enough that should a loss of balance occur, contact can be made to stabilize balance quickly. Similar to this is stand-by guarding, or supervision. In this, the patient receives primarily verbal cues, yet the clinician is close by should assistance be necessary. These require very little support and are for patients that are familiar with the assistive device and are close to achieving independence with its use. With advance planning and review of medical record information, safe and effective gait training can be accomplished with the appropriate assistive device.

Assessment of Level of Assistance Required for Locomotion

Moving a patient from one surface to another requires a significant amount of planning. Begin by understanding the patient's mental and physical capabilities to perform the transfer, including the patient's weight-bearing status. Then ensure that the patient is dressed appropriately for the transfer, which includes footwear that is nonslip and will not easily slide off of his or her foot. As you determine which surface you are transferring to (for example, a wheelchair or a bed), ensure whenever possible that you transfer leading with the patient's strong side and that obstacles are removed from your path. Once you have determined all of these factors, you are ready to determine the level of assistance necessary for the transfer.

Levels of Assistance

Independent. The patient does not require any physical assistance or supervision to consistently perform an activity safely and in an acceptable amount of time.

Supervision (stand-by) assistance. The patient requires verbal or tactile cues, directions, or instructions from the PTA, who is positioned close to the patient (but is not touching the patient). The PTA is close enough to provide assistance should the patient's safety be threatened.

Close guarding. The PTA is positioned close to, but not touching the patient (no contact). The patient may be offered verbal or tactile cues, such as directions or instructions similar to supervisory assistance described previously. The primary difference between close guarding and the other levels of assistance is that with close guarding, the PTA is much closer to the patient because there is a higher risk that contact guarding or assistance may need to be offered, even if it is momentary assistance.

Minimal assistance. Minimal assistance is necessary when the patient can perform more than 75% of the transfer on his or her own and needs only up to 25% assistance from the PTA. Contact guarding is maintained throughout the transfer.

Moderate assistance. Moderate assistance is necessary when the patient can perform 50% to 75% of the transfer and needs only 25% to 50% assistance from the PTA. Contact guarding is maintained throughout the transfer.

Maximal assistance. Maximal assistance is necessary when the patient can perform 25% to 50% of the transfer and requires 50% to 75% assistance from the PTA. Contact guarding is maintained throughout the transfer.

Dependent. Dependent transfers are necessary when the patient is able to perform less than 25% of the transfer and requires 75% to 100% assistance from two or more clinicians. Additionally, a patient who requires the use of mechanized equipment is considered dependent.

Identification of Gait Deviations

Pain, weakness, and loss of range of motion are all common problems that may result in a gait deviation. Understand that, depending on the diagnosis, one or more of these deviations may be present simultaneously—and the patient may have multiple methods of compensating for the gait deviation. Although gait deviations are common with many diagnoses, this section limits discussion to those with musculoskeletal dysfunctions.

Prior to beginning your assessment of the gait deviation, review the patient's subjective complaints and past medical history. Then observe the patient, when it is appropriate, walking without an assistive device. It is important to observe from the front, the side, and the back to see all the planes of movement that the gait deviation may impact. It is also helpful to check the wear pattern on shoes and even the calluses on the feet, as this may indicate a long-term pattern.

Common Gait Deviations

Antalgia: An antalgic gait is associated with pain when weight-bearing results in a limp or a shortened step length on the affected side and a shortened stance time.

Hammer toes: Hammer toes impact the pre-swing phase of gait the most. It is difficult for the patient to achieve a smooth toe-off, so the patient moves from heel-off abruptly into swing. This typically results in a shortened step length, shortened stance on the affected side, and diminished balance.

Hallux valgus: With a hallux valgus, or bunion, weight shift over the first metatarsal is difficult. Weight tends to stay more on the back side, and there is a late heel rise. Toe-off is over the side of the foot or avoided all together. This diminishes the balance on the affected side.

Drop foot: Drop foot results from weakness to one or more of the dorsiflexors of the foot, or muscles that cause flexion in a backward direction. This typically results from damage to the deep fibular nerve, which stimulates the anterior compartment. Together, all of the muscles perform dorsiflexion. Drop foot impacts the swing phase of gait, in that the patient is unable to clear the foot on the affected side secondary to weakness. It also impacts the heel strike (the point at which the foot first makes contact with a surface) to the flat part of the foot because there is no ability to control dorsiflexion. This results in a foot slap, where the patient strikes with the foot flat (or toe to heel) first. When compensating for this gait, a steppage gait is seen.

Steppage gait. This kind of gait compensates for drop foot by increasing hip and knee flexion so the foot can clear during swing. When the leg is moving into stance, the foot can strike flat foot or a toe heel pattern.

Trendelenburg gait. A Trendelenburg gait is a result of weakness to the gluteus medius and minimus along the pelvis. This impacts the midstance phase of gait on the stance side. Damage to the superior gluteal nerve may result in this problem, as well as many other conditions that can lead to progressive weakness over time. During midstance, the gluteus medius is to use a reverse action to depress the pelvis so that the contralateral side swings through without contacting the foot. When it is weak, the contralateral side appears to drop.

Compensated Trendelenburg gait. In this variation, the patient laterally flexes to the weak side (or compensates) to avoid the discomfort of the Trendelenburg gait. This effectively depresses the stance side and raises the swing side, allowing the limb to clear.

TAKE NOTE

When observing a patient with a Trendelenburg gait, the most obvious indication is the dropping of the pelvis on the swing side. Remember, the weakness is on the other side, not the side on which you observe the drop. Take care to avoid making this common error.

Circumducted gait. A circumducted gait may be observed when the limb on the affected side is lengthened, possibly because of a cast or brace or to compensate for weakness in areas such as the gluteus medius or hip flexors. The patient swings the affected side in a half-circle rather than keeping it in the saggital plane.

Weak quadriceps. Weakness in the quadriceps femoris group (lower leg muscles) impacts the ability of the affected limb to move into extension during stance. This may be the result of trauma from surgery, injury, or weakness in the femoral nerve. Weakness may result in buckling or falling to the ground from initial contact through midstance. It is especially a problem when moving into loading response, because of the eccentric control required to perform this movement. This may result in a jarring or a slight foot slap. The compensation for this is to lock the knee through alternative means. For example, the gastrocnemius (calf) may extend the knee as a reverse action. Unfortunately, this often results in hyperextension of the knee. A knee-ankle-foot orthosis, or KAFO, may be necessary to minimize the damage from hyperextension.

Weak plantar flexors. Weak plantar flexors may be a result of trauma such as surgery, an Achilles tendon rupture, or damage to the tibial nerve. Plantar flexors primarily affect the foot and ankle during heel- and toe-off. Weak plantar flexors will limit the patient's ability to propel the body forward. Significant weakness may result in knee flexion to lift the foot into swing. This will result in a short step length, stance time, and diminished balance.

Inadequate knee flexion. Inadequate knee flexion is often the result of injury to the knee, resulting in either loss of motion or bracing which will limit knee flexion. This condition may be compensated in a variety of ways. Circumduction (circular movement of a limb) is one possibility and has already been discussed. Another possibility is vaulting which is observed during the swing phase on the affected side. As the limb is longer because of the limited knee flexion, the patient quickly moves to early heel-off on the opposite side to help clear the affected side. Other compensations may include increased hip flexion or trunk movement to clear the limb during the swing phase.

Gluteus maximus weakness. The gluteus maximus is a hip extensor that works primarily during deceleration of the swing phase to slow the limb moving into hip flexion and to prepare for initial contact. In addition, the gluteus maximus helps to achieve extension of the hip during midstance and is important for balance and stability. Weakness to the inferior gluteal nerve or direct trauma to the gluteus maximus may result in injury that could cause this gait deviation. This will be observed primarily during the stance phase, when the patient's shoulders will be retracted and the trunk will be extended to position the hip in its close-packed position (abduction, extension, and external rotation). This will allow the ligaments to stabilize the hip, as they are all taut and extended.

Weak hip flexors. Weak hip flexors may be a result of surgery to the front of the hip or knee or from excessive tightness, which has adaptively shortened the muscle and made it weak. The primary function of the hip flexors is to initiate the swing phase of gait. Weak hip flexors will result in a shortened step length and a longer time in stance, because the swing phase will also be shortened. The patient may easily compensate for this by externally rotating the hip so that the hip adductors act as hip flexors to initiate the swing. Circumduction is another strategy that may be used.

Functional Assessments of Gait

The gait deviations described in the previous section are important to identify, as they often help direct the focus of the PTA's therapeutic exercise interventions to the weak muscles or limited ranges of movement. A functional assessment of gait looks at the overall quality of the gait pattern with or without an assistive device. This is vital to assess a patient's risk for future falls or his or her ability to walk safely. In a functional assessment of gait, the therapist considers time as well as quality of movement while also assessing control of movement during transitions from one position to another.

Timed up and go test. The timed up and go test is a quick test used to assess functional walking speed, stopping, starting, and turning. The test begins with the person's sitting back in a chair with arms resting on the armrest. The person wears his or her usual footwear and may use an assistive device if necessary. The individual then is asked to rise from the chair and walk a distance of approximately 10 feet (three meters), turn around and walk back to the chair, and then sit down again. Next, the individual is asked to walk quickly and safely. The test is timed from the moment the individual begins to rise from the chair until he or she is seated again. The average time to complete the test is between 7–10 seconds. Those who require more than 20 seconds are at increased risk for falls. This is an excellent gross, or general, screening test that is not only fast but also easy to administer.

Tinetti Performance Oriented Mobility Assessment. The Tinetti test is divided into two sections. One part examines stationary balance, and one examines gait. All test items are graded on a three-point scale ranging from 0 to 2. The balance test assesses the ability to rise from a chair without using arms as support, stand still, maintain balance (with vision obstructed), and turn in a small circle. There is a total of 16 possible points in this portion of the test. The second part of the test assesses gait on a 12-point scale. The patient is asked to rise from a seated position, walk approximately 15 feet, turn, and return to the starting point. A composite score is used to determine the patient's fall risk. Patients who score less than 19 points have a high fall risk, patients who score between 19 and 24 have a medium fall risk, and patients who score between 25 and 28 have a low fall risk.

Dynamic Gait Index. The Dynamic Gait Index assesses eight qualities of gait on a 24-point scale. In this test, the patient is asked to walk 20 feet, to increase and decrease speed, to change head positions both horizontally and vertically, to move over and around obstacles, to turn, and to go up and down stairs. Patients with scores of less than 19 points have been shown to have an increased risk of falling. This is a comprehensive analysis of gait and is appropriate for community ambulators. These are patients who need to ambulate in community settings, such as through parking lots, over curbs, and through stores or restaurants.

Standardized Balance Assessments

Similar to the functional gait assessments, standardized balance assessments help to rate the patient's ability to balance in situations that are likely to require adjustment. The better patients are able to cope with a variety of changes, the more successful they are likely to be in managing activities of daily living (ADLs) and instrumental activities of daily living (IADLs) in the community setting. Conversely, the more difficulty patients have with moving outside the center of gravity and with changes in speed, body, and head position, the greater the risk that the patient will fall.

Berg Balance Scale. The Berg Balance Scale is a series of 14 activities to assess balance for community ambulators. Each test is scored on a 0 to 4 scale, with a maximum of 56 points. The scores that identify a person who is likely to fall range from 45–49. The tests begin with the patient's simply maintaining sitting balance. Other activities include rising out of a chair, maintaining standing balance, and moving to and from another surface. The tests become progressively more difficult: performing tasks with eyes open and closed, narrowing the base of support, turning in a small circle, extending forward by reaching outside of the base of support, turning and looking behind, and retrieving an object from the floor. Finally, the patient is tested on the most challenging activities: shifting weight, touching the top of a step with alternating feet, tandem stance, and standing in a single-leg stance.

As you may recall from the previous section, the balance component of the Tinetti assessment is similar in structure to the first few parts of the Berg balance test. The Berg balance test has higher time-based goals, however, and is more appropriate for community ambulators. The Tinetti test is appropriate for use in a home health setting—or perhaps in a skilled nursing facility or assisted living location.

Functional reach test. The functional reach test is technically a component of the Berg balance test but can be done as an individual test as well. The patient is positioned standing with feet shoulder width apart. The shoulder of the reaching arm is positioned at 90 degrees (relative to the flexion). A yardstick is parallel to the long axis of the arm, extending past the arm. The patient is asked to pivot at the hips, and PTA measures the difference between the standing position and the reached position. If the patient steps to regain balance, the trial is not valid. The patient is considered to have a low fall risk if he or she is able to reach further than ten inches, a moderate fall risk if he or she reaches from six to ten inches, and a high fall risk if his or her reach is less than six inches.

Multidirectional reach test. The multidirectional reach test is similar to the functional reach test: The shoulder is positioned at 90 degrees; the yard stick is positioned in line with the long axis of the arm; and the measurement is the difference between the starting position and the reached position, with both feet remaining firmly on the ground. Although both tests measure a patient's forward reach, the multidirectional reach test also measures backward reach, as well as left and right reach. The multidirectional reach test defines the limits of stability in four directions. Note that patients who describe a fear of falling usually have a low backward reach score.

Single-leg stance test. The single-leg stance test is a simple test in which the patient stands and maintains balance on a single leg for as long as he or she can, without touching down or propping the other leg on the stance leg. Ideally, this is performed with shoes off and arms crossed in front of the chest. A patient who can do this for ten seconds or longer is considered a low fall risk. According to a 2006 article in *Physiotherapy Research International*, approximately 90% of community ambulators can maintain the single-leg stance for ten seconds or longer, while residents of skilled nursing facilities are able to do so less than 50% of the time.

Joint Integrity and Mobility (Appendicular Skeleton)

Special testing designed to assess the integrity of joint structures is often performed as part of the diagnostic process. Although these are typically performed by a physician or physical therapist, understand that these tests provide vital information for the physical therapist assistant. As many of these tests are provocative in nature (in that they produce pain associated with the original injury), it is also beneficial to know what positions can avoid or minimize re-injury—as well as to educate the patient on potentially problematic positions. Finally, therapeutic interventions that involve range of motion, mobilization techniques, and stretching all require an understanding of normal versus abnormal end feels. This requires ongoing reassessment of the activity being performed to ensure it is being performed safely and within patients' tolerance levels.

Ligament Stress Testing

Ligaments limit excessive joint mobility and are frequently examined to determine the extent of ligamentous sprain or to determine ligament stability after a repair. A grade I sprain results in micro-tearing of the ligament but continues to have a solid end point with ligament testing. A grade II sprain also has a solid end point. However, it allows for greater movement than normal on the contralateral side. A grade III sprain is a complete ligament disruption (or tear) and usually requires surgery to repair.

Varus and valgus stress tests are performed at the elbow, knee, and the ankle. The tests are usually performed with the elbow or the knee slightly flexed and with the ankle in neutral position. This allows the ligaments to be slightly lax. The testing can also be performed when the elbow and knee are in full extension. However, because there is bony stability in this position, usually only significant grade II or grade III sprains will be identified in these positions.

Varus testing places a stress on the lateral side of the joint in an attempt to move the distal bone medially.

Ligaments tested with a varus stress include the radial collateral ligament of the elbow, the lateral collateral ligament of the knee, the calcaneofibular ligament of the ankle, and the anterior and posterior talofibular ligaments of the ankle. Valgus testing places a stress on the medial aspect of the joint in an attempt to move the distal bone laterally. Ligaments tested with a valgus stress include the ulnar collateral ligament of the elbow, the medial collateral ligament of the knee, and the deltoid ligament of the ankle.

The knee also contains cruciate ligaments, which limit anterior and posterior mobility. The Lachman test is done to test the integrity of the anterior cruciate ligament. Similar to the varus and valgus testing, the Lachman test is generally performed with the knee flexed to about 25 degrees. An anterior force is placed on the tibia while the femur is stabilized.

Apprehension Tests

Apprehension tests are provocative tests in which the patient perceives that his or her shoulder or patella is likely to dislocate and is apprehensive about this posture. In an attempt to protect the joint, the patient often moves away from the position of apprehension and either holds or protects the body.

Ninety to 98% of shoulder dislocations occur anteriorly (in the front of the shoulder). In this kind of injury, the shoulder is abducted and externally rotated. An extension force is applied to the shoulder, resulting in the anterior dislocation. In the shoulder apprehension test, the PT will position the patient's shoulder in abduction and external rotation and then slowly move the shoulder into extension. A positive result will occur if the patient moves quickly into adduction, flexion, and internal rotation or if he or she has a look of concern or apprehension. This occurs because the patient will feel that the test position mimics the position of the shoulder in the past when dislocation has occurred.

A patella dislocation is commonly seen in young females with patellofemoral syndrome. Frequent signs of patellofemoral syndrome include: tight iliotibial band, strong vastus lateralis, and weak vastus medialis, as well as a large Q-angle. Even under these conditions (which would tend to pull the patella laterally), the patella does not often dislocate unless there is a depressed lateral femoral condyle which allows the patella to move off the femur. Pushing the patella laterally reproduces this sensation; and it is considered a positive test for those who are apprehensive with the lateral movement.

Drawer Tests

Drawer tests are similar to varus and valgus tests, in that they move the joint to its end limits—much like a drawer is pulled out or pushed in. Drawer tests can be performed at the shoulder, the knee, and the ankle. In a drawer test, the PTA should stabilize the proximal segment and then move the distal segment anteriorly (forward) or posteriorly (backward). In the shoulder or the knee, the PTA can assess both anterior and posterior instability. At the ankle, the PTA primarily assesses anterior instability. It is important to note that these are general tests of instability. For example, at the knee, a positive test may result if the patient has undergone a meniscectomy or had other surgery where the capsule has been compromised. Although primarily considered a ligamentous test, the drawer test is less specific and can assess generalized capsular instability.

Impingement Tests

Impingement syndrome is a generic term applied to the glenohumeral joint, which contains many structures that could possibly be pinched or compressed. Impingement tests are designed to help differentiate which structures specifically are being compressed. Poor posture, especially forward head and rounded shoulder posture, closes the interval between the acromion and the head of the humerus. The subdeltoid or subacromial bursa may become impinged as well as the biceps brachii long head tendon or the tendons of the rotator cuff, specifically the supraspinatus, infraspinatus, and teres minor.

In a general impingement test, the affected shoulder is positioned at 90 degrees of flexion and then horizontally adducted with the elbow flexed. When end range (or close to end range) of horizontal adduction occurs, pain will be reported at the level of the acromion.

There are several tests which might be used to identify impingement. The first is a Neer test, which brings the shoulder into flexion and, with controlled force, moves it into full flexion. Pain is a positive sign in this test.

The Kennedy-Hawkins impingement test requires the patient to move to 90 degrees of flexion, beginning with the elbow flexed and the forearm pointed to the ceiling. Once again, with a quick and controlled force, the PTA moves the shoulder into internal rotation. Pain is considered a positive sign.

Also specific to the biceps brachii's long head is Speed's test. The arm is flexed to 60 degrees, with the elbow extended. Force is placed on the distal forearm to produce an isometric contraction. While resistance is being given, palpation of the biceps brachii long head tendon will be painful.

Yergason's test is performed with the shoulder flexed to 90 degrees and the forearm pronated. Supination is resisted, and this will be painful over the biceps brachii at the shoulder, if positive. Variations on this test include the Lippman and DeAnquin tests. In the Lippman test, the forearm remains pronated and the evaluator palpates the biceps tendon and shifts it medially and/or laterally. The DeAnquin test allows for palpation of the biceps brachii long head tendon but moves the shoulder into internal and external rotation rather than moving the tendon.

Aside from the biceps brachii, the rotator cuff tendons (which attach to the greater tubercle) are also at risk for impingement. The supraspinatus is the most commonly injured rotater cuff tendon according to Kisner and Colby's *Therapeutic Exercise: Foundations and Techniques*. The two most common tests are the drop arm test and the empty can test. The drop arm test has the patient abduct to 180 degrees (or as high as he or she can) and slowly, eccentrically lower the arm. If the patient is unable to sustain a smooth eccentric contraction, the test is positive.

The empty can test positions the patient in abduction to 90 degrees and then horizontal adduction to 30 degrees. The elbow is extended, the shoulder is internally rotated, and the forearm is pronated with the thumb pointing down. Resistance is applied proximal to the shoulder. If pain is elicited or the arm drops, this suggests injury to the supraspinatus.

End Feel

The end feel is defined as the quality of movement that the therapist or therapist assistant feels when pressure is applied at the end range of available motion. There are normal and abnormal end feels. Normal end feels vary based on both the soft tissue surrounding the joint and the bony formation of a joint. A hard or bony end feel is an abrupt stop to movement when bone contacts bone. This is observed when the trochlear notch locks into the trochlea. A soft end feel occurs when the soft tissue of two body segments come together—such as when the knee is flexed and the thigh meets the hamstring. A firm end feel is a firm or slightly springy sensation associated with muscle, fascia, or ligament stretch. The last type of normal end feel is a capsular stretch. This is slightly different than a soft end feel in that the end feel is more leathery. Passive shoulder external rotation results in this end feel.

Abnormal end feels may have similar qualities to normal end feels. However, they can occur before the normal end of motion, which makes them pathological. For example, a hard or bony end feel, which ends well in advance of normal range, would likely be related to degenerative joint disease or loose bodies within the joint. A pathological soft end feel has some flexibility, which feels similar to using a squeegee on your windshield. This would represent synovitis, or soft tissue swelling. An abnormal firm end feel is often a result of a soft tissue contracture. An empty end feel occurs when pain is so severe that the patient requests that you stop before you reach the end range of the joint.

Motor Function

While the function of each individual muscle or group is important, the coordinated sequence of moving several muscles and muscle groups together comprises motor function. Performing tasks in a smooth, coordinated fashion requires a highly evolved communication between the sensory system and the motor system, facilitated through neuromuscular control. Motor function is generally broken down into gross (or large muscle) function and fine (or small muscle) function. It is this neuromuscular control that makes coordinated work, sports, leisure, and functional tasks possible.

END FEEL	NORMAL	ABNORMAL
Hard	Bone limits motion	Fracture, loose body, severe OA limits motion
Firm	Tension in muscle, tendon, ligament, joint capsule limits motion	Same, but before full motion is obtained
Soft	Soft tissue approximation	Edema in joint capsule
Empty	N/A	Pain limits motion prior to any tissue limits are reached

Normal and abnormal end feels describe the tissues that limit joint motion.

Assessment of Dexterity, Coordination, and Agility

Dexterity is the skill and coordination of performing fine motor tasks. Dexterity is required at various levels to perform a wide variety of tasks. Fine motor coordination is necessary to type on a keyboard, use the keypad on your cell phone to send a text message, or embroider with a counted cross-stitch. Gross motor coordination is necessary for handling balls in various sports, juggling, or manipulating knobs and levers to operate equipment and machinery. In many manufacturing employment environments, payment for a job task is incentive-based: the more pieces completed in an hour or a day, the greater the rate of pay. The ability to assess functional dexterity is generally done with standardized tests and compared to normative values for age and gender. Although a wide number of tests are commercially available, the two most common are the Purdue pegboard test for fine motor function and the Minnesota manual dexterity test for gross motor function. The Purdue pegboard uses a board and a series of small straight pins, washers, and collars. The patient performs several timed trials, either unilaterally with dominant or nondominant hands, or bilaterally with a bimanual (two-handed) assembly task. Each of these tests is then compared to normative data for assessment. The Minnesota manual dexterity test uses a wide rectangular board with circles cut out. The patient is asked to retrieve and position small round disks into the cutouts as quickly as possible. This could be done unilaterally, bimanually, or bimanually with a turning component. As with the Purdue test, data is then compared to normative data figures.

Coordination and agility tests are done usually in the later, or chronic, phase of rehab or as part of athletic or job screening. A physical agility test specifically tests the physical capabilities of a potential employee to ensure that he or she is able to perform the job. These tests came about as a result of the Americans with Disabilities Act. Physical therapist assistants may perform these tests, as they are performed on well individuals.

PTAs are not providing physical therapy services but rather prevention services, which are paid for directly by the employer.

> ### TAKE NOTE
>
> Differentiate a physical agility test from a preplacement screen. Both are discussed in the Americans with Disabilities Act, but each has a different role. The preplacement screen is a medical screen—but it is only appropriate to perform this screening after an offer for employment has been given. Information learned in this process can't be used to fire an employee, unless it can be shown that they are a direct threat. A physical agility test is a functional qualifications exam. It can be done prior to employment, and if the candidate does not pass, it means that they are not qualified to do the job. This test is based on the essential tasks that the candidate would encounter on the job. All employees in that job category must take this type of physical agility test.

Agility and coordination training is often performed later in the rehabilitation process, when the patient is getting ready to return to activities like sports, leisure, or work. These activities improve the patient's ability to perform a series of sudden power movements in rapid succession in opposing directions. There are a wide variety of activities to choose from, and you can even design your own agility drills based on the activity to which the patient desires to return. Laying a pattern that looks like a ladder on the floor with tape can be used to have the patient quickly hop in and out of the "ladder" while moving forward. Carioca drills, which involve lateral movements while performing a grapevine or braiding pattern of the lower extremity, are good for activities that require cutting movements. Patients with knee or ankle stability issues benefit from these type of drills prior to going back to activities like soccer or tennis because the drills mimic the aspects of the activity that might be most challenging for the patient.

Muscle Performance

Muscle performance, which is composed of muscle strength, endurance, and power, is frequently assessed and addressed in therapeutic exercise interventions to improve the patient's functionality and reduce disability. There is a wide variety of factors which influence strength, including age, gender, muscle size, type of contraction, speed of contraction, and the effects of training. The following sections will review the various aspects of muscle performance and the tools that can be used to assess muscle performance.

Manual Muscle Testing

Manual muscle testing was first described by Lovett in 1912 and has been used as the standard physical therapy methodology for measuring muscle strength. Manual muscle testing is a convenient, versatile, and inexpensive tool used to determine strength of either a muscle group or specific muscles and to document progress. For the most reliable and valid testing, it is important that the physical therapist assistant keeps in mind that consistency of testing procedures (including positioning and stabilization) needs to be maintained, that a standardized grading system is used, and that substitution patterns are eliminated. Unfortunately, manual muscle testing inter-rater reliability is estimated at 50–60%. While it may not be the best tool, it is the standard of the profession, and therefore efforts should be made to keep testing as consistent as possible. Pain will invalidate the testing, so you will not be able to compare between individuals; however, testing can still be used to assess the progress of a single patient. Other factors which may impact testing include fatigue, the strength of the assessor, and the environment. Therefore, whenever possible, the testing should be performed by the same individual, at the same time of day, in the same environment. The

use of handheld dynamometers is becoming more prevalent, as the devices allow the assessor to better quantify the force of the contraction. There are limitations to these devices as well—and care and significant practice should be undertaken before they're used with patients.

When performing manual muscle testing, you may choose to perform a break test or a make test. A break test uses an isometric hold of the muscle while the assessor is attempting to "break" the muscle contraction. The advantage of this type of testing is that it is an isometric muscle contraction and easy to reproduce. The disadvantage is that it only measures strength at one point in the range and may not accurately reflect the area of complaint. The make test, on the other hand, is a concentric contraction that is performed throughout the available range of motion and ends with an isometric contraction. Or if the patient can not sustain an isometric contraction, an eccentric contraction results. The advantage to this type of testing is that you have an understanding of the limitations throughout the entire range. The disadvantage is that it requires significant control on the part of the assessor to accurately balance and meet the patient's strength consistently.

Daniels and Worthingham's *Muscle Testing: Techniques of Manual Examination* describes a system of muscle grading that incorporates the impact of gravity and resistance on the muscle testing. This system rates strength on a scale from 0–5. Pluses and minuses have been added to the scale to address more subtle changes within that range. Kendall and McCreary's *Muscles, Testing and Function* describes percentages of normal strength associated with each grade. Daniels and Worthingham advocated gross testing of muscle groups (e.g., elbow flexors), while Kendall and McCreary advocated testing of specific muscles (e.g., biceps, brachioradialis, brachialis). Because both methods are taught in schools throughout the United States, both are provided here as a reference. The following is a table which describes the grades and the definition associated with each:

Manual Muscle Testing

NUMERICAL GRADE	PERCENTAGE	LETTER GRADE	DESCRIPTION
5	100%	N (Normal)	Able to move throughout entire available range of motion against gravity and against maximal resistance
4+		G (Good plus)	Able to move throughout entire available range of motion against gravity and moderate to maximal resistance (break occurs)
4	80%	G (Good)	Able to move throughout entire available range of motion against gravity and moderate resistance
4–		G– (Good minus)	Able to move throughout entire available range of motion against gravity and minimal to moderate resistance
3+		F+ (Fair plus)	Able to move throughout entire available range of motion against gravity with minimal resistance
3	50%	F (Fair)	Able to move throughout entire available range of motion against gravity
3–		F– (Fair minus)	Able to move more than half the available range of motion against gravity
2+		P+ (Poor plus)	Able to move less than half the available range against gravity
2	20%	P (Poor)	Able to move the full available range of motion in a gravity eliminated position
2–		P– (Poor minus)	Able to move through greater than one-half of the available motion in a gravity eliminated position
1+		T+ (Trace plus)	Able to move through less than one-half of the available motion in a gravity eliminated position
1	5%	T (Trace)	None of the available range of motion in a gravity eliminated position and a palpable or observable flicker of a muscle contraction
0	0%	0 (Zero)	None of the available range of motion in a gravity eliminated position and no palpable or observable muscle contraction

Dynamometry

A dynamometer is an instrument that measures force. Dynamometers are used for assessment purposes to measure grip strength, pinch strength, or force associated with manual muscle testing. Grip and pinch dynamometers are common pieces of equipment found in physical therapy clinics. The dynamometer has five positions, ranging in size from approximately 1.5 inches to 3.5 inches wide. Normal values based on age, gender, and hand dominance are available for hand grip, two-point pinches, three-jaw-chuck pinches, and lateral (or key) pinches. Handheld dynamometers are also used when performing manual muscle testing. The handheld dynamometer is placed in the tester's hand between the patient and the therapist assistant. As force is produced by both the patient and the therapist assistant, the device measures the force produced. Intra-rater reliability requires a significant amount of practice to get repeatedly accurate measurements.

Drop-Arm Test

The drop-arm test is done to assess the integrity of the supraspinatus tendon. The therapist or therapist assistant will raise the patient's arm to 180 degrees of abduction or as high as it can go. Then the patient will slowly lower the arm, performing an eccentric muscle contraction of the deltoid and supraspinatus. If the patient loses control of the eccentric contraction and the arm drops, that is considered a positive drop-arm test. Also, if the patient is able to complete one test, a second trial may be attempted—but at 90 degrees of abduction, lightly tap the distal end of the arm. A positive test may result with the light tap. This test is frequently used to diagnose rotator cuff tears.

Trendelenburg Test

The Trendelenburg test is a functional test to measure the strength of the gluteus medius and minimus muscles. During midstance in the gait cycle, the gluteus medius and minimus function primarily to depress the pelvis on the stance side, to allow it to elevate on the swing side so that the extremity clears the floor. A Trendelenburg test has the patient stand with weight evenly distributed on both legs. If necessary, the patient may lightly hold onto a table or walker, as needed, for balance. The patient will then lift one leg off the floor. If there is a positive Trendelenburg test result, the leg that is lifted off the floor will drop, suggesting weakness on the contralateral side. A negative test will result in the pelvis remaining level throughout.

Assessment of Muscle Power

Power is the muscles' ability to contract explosively over a short period of time. If work is force multiplied by distance, power is work divided by time. Although power is often considered an important aspect of many sports activities, it is also vital for many basic functional activities, such as getting up out of a chair.

Isokinetic Testing

Isokinetic testing is performed using a piece of equipment that is designed to vary the resistance to the muscle as the speed of the arc of movement remains constant. Isokinetic testing is typically performed in the chronic phase of rehab, when the patient has a full or partial range of motion, pain-free. Speeds ranging from 30 degrees/second to 300 degrees/second are used in isokinetic testing. Torque production, work, and power can be assessed.

INFORMATION IN ACTION

Isokinetic testing involving the quadriceps femoris group and the hamstrings after anterior cruciate ligament (ACL) surgery is often a critical assessment used to determine when the patient is ready to resume functional activities, such as sports. The hamstrings should be able to produce approximately $\frac{2}{3}$ of the torque of the quadriceps for optimal knee stability.

Timed Activity Tests

Timed activity tests are a great way to determine power of a specific muscle group. A patient is asked to perform an activity for a specific period of time—such as one minute—and the greater the number of repetitions performed over that time, the greater the power produced. Many people take these timed activity tests, such as the president's physical fitness test in school or the military version of a physical training test. In each of these scenarios, a person would be asked to perform as many push-ups, sit-ups, pull-ups, etc., that he or she could perform in a specific time frame. The greater the number of repetitions performed, the greater the ability of that person to perform a repeated, powerful contraction over a specific period of time.

Electromyography (EMG)/Biofeedback

Power can also be assessed through the use of electromyography. The reference electrode can be set to a specific threshold of muscle activation. The patient is then asked to contract the muscle to that threshold as many times as he or she can in a finite period of time. As with the timed activity tests described above, goals can be set to encourage more repetitions over a shorter period of time to generate greater power.

Electromyography and biofeedback can also be used to assess muscular endurance. There are two methods to assess muscular endurance. The first identifies the peak threshold where the muscle can successfully activate the biofeedback device. Then this setting is reduced by half. The patient is then expected to repeatedly contract for as long a time as he or she can or until he or she cannot achieve the new lower threshold. This addresses repetitive contraction for muscular endurance. An alternative method for identifying the muscles' ability to sustain a contraction would be to identify the peak threshold again. This setting is again reduced by half. However, rather than repeatedly contracting, the patient sustains a single contraction until they no longer can meet the threshold. This time is the sustained muscular endurance of this muscle. Depending on how the muscle or group functions, it will determine the best way to assess muscular endurance with EMG.

Assessment of Muscle Endurance

Muscle endurance is the ability of a specific muscle, or muscle group, to sustain repeated contractions against resistance for an extended period of time. Postural muscles and muscles used to provide stability at joints require muscle endurance to perform their roles in the body. Physical therapists and physical therapist assistants often work with patients to improve muscle endurance so that the muscle may play an expanded role as a stabilizer if a ligament or other joint structure has been damaged.

Isokinetic Testing

Isokinetic testing can also be configured to assess muscular endurance. Once you have identified the peak torque of a muscle or muscle group, you can ask the patient to continue as long as he or she is able until the torque drops below 50% of the peak torque measured. This time represents the muscular endurance of the muscle.

Timed Activity Testing

Timed activity testing can also be used to determine muscular endurance. A patient is asked to perform a repetitive activity such as a squat. You should initially note the quality and speed of movement. There should be no evidence of substitution patterns or accessory muscle recruitment. When performing timed activity testing for endurance, you should ask the patient to perform the activity for as long as the patient is comfortable with the repetitive activity or until the quality, speed, accessory muscle contraction, or substitutions become evident. This is the point of fatigue, which can then be noted and quantified with a goal of increasing the amount of time this activity could be performed under the same conditions in the future.

Orthotic, Protective, and Supportive Devices

An orthosis is any externally applied device designed to protect or stabilize a body part, prevent deformity, protect against injury, or assist with function. Orthotic devices may be used temporarily during the acute phase of healing or may be used to compensate for a permanent loss. There are four primary goals accomplished with orthotic devices: protection against physical injury, relief of weight-bearing to distal segments, alignment of body segments, and resistance or assistance to joint motion. Orthoses are named for the body part or joint that they cross to perform their actions. A hip-knee-ankle-foot orthosis (HKAFO) crosses at the hip, knee, ankle, and foot. Orthoses may be custom made to fit a specific individual or purchased off-the-shelf (general sizes are from extra-small to extra-extra-large).

Foot orthosis (FO). Foot orthoses are designed to help the foot achieve a neutral position, controlling either excessive pronation or supination of the foot during the gait cycle. Devices may fill in the gap between the foot's fixed position and may be neutral or corrective in nature where the device helps the foot to achieve neutral position.

Ankle-foot orthosis (AFO). An AFO is the most common type of orthotic device used today. It may be articulating or nonarticulating and will either allow or not allow free dorsiflexion or plantar flexion. Total contact AFOs are made of thermoplast and are light and easy to apply. This type of device is often used to accommodate for a foot drop. Immobilizing AFOs such as Cam Walkers or Carcot Restraint Orthotic Walkers (CROWs) are used to support tibia, fibula, and foot bone fractures or Achilles tendon ruptures or repairs. Less restrictive than an AFO is a supramalleolar orthosis (SMO). An SMO is commonly used to support an athlete after an inversion ankle sprain or to otherwise stabilize an ankle.

Knee orthosis (KO). Knee orthoses are frequently used to accommodate misalignment from genu varum or genu valgum and recurvatum. This type of device may be corrective in nature or used to prevent a deformity from developing or worsening. Athletic knee orthoses are frequently used to help prevent re-injury with sports. They are controversial because, despite the short lever arms used, significant forces can still be placed on the knee. It is believed that knee orthoses do help with proprioception, which may also help with prevention. Nonarticulating knee orthoses (frequently called knee immobilizers) are used to limit motion at the knee during the acute phase of rehabilitation. They make transfers more challenging because of the long lever arm.

Knee-ankle-foot orthosis (KAFO). This device is typically chosen when neither an AFO nor KO can sufficiently address the biomechanical issue. KAFOs may be used to address fracture management as well as significant quadriceps weakness, where the gastrocnemius contracts with a reverse action to hyperextend the knee. Since the gastrocnemius crosses both the knee and the ankle, control is needed at both locations. Depending on the needs and control of the patient, there may be multiple devices used to lock or unlock the knee, block hyperextension, or assist with extension.

Hip orthosis (HO). Hip orthoses are most commonly used after a total hip replacement (or hemiarthroplasty) to prevent the hip from dislocating. This hip orthosis is positioned in abduction and is referred to as a hip abduction orthosis. If necessary, a knee-ankle-foot orthosis component can be added, but these are quite cumbersome and labor intensive during gait. Children are often observed in hip orthosis after dislocation, slipped capital femoral epiphysis, or Legg-Calvé-Perthes disease. A Scottish Rite orthosis or a standing, walking and sitting hip (SWASH) orthosis will allow children with these conditions to perform ADLs.

Wrist-hand orthosis (WHO): Rheumatoid arthritis patients may use a wrist-hand orthosis as a resting splint during a flare-up. This is designed to keep the wrist and hand in a neutral and functional position without allowing active movement so that the tendons and joints may rest. A cock-up splint is commonly used for patients with wrist tendinitis and carpal tunnel syndrome. It positions the hand in slight wrist extension (10–15 degrees) and should not be positioned on the hand past the first palmar crease—so that function of the fingers can be maintained without excessive stress. A thumb spica splint may be used for patients with De Quervain's tenosynovitis to limit the motion of the thumb. Wrist-hand orthoses may also be used to support the wrist and hand after fractures, either as transitional devices after a cast or as the primary means of immobilization.

Elbow orthosis (EO). A lateral or medial epicondylitis strap is designed to diminish the force on either the lateral or medial epicondyle, which is the common attachment site for the wrist extensors or wrist flexors, respectively. By positioning the strap slightly distal to the landmark, it acts similar to a guitar fret in that the force is now applied at the new location, allowing the common attachment point to rest. Other elbow orthoses may be designed to prevent contractures, limit elbow hyperextension, or assist with fracture management.

Shoulder orthosis (SO). The most common shoulder orthosis is a sling, or shoulder immobilizer, designed to rest the glenohumeral joint after surgery or injury. Another type of shoulder immobilizer, referred to as an airplane splint, is designed to maintain the shoulder in an abducted position.

Cervical orthosis (CO). A soft collar is an example of a cervical orthosis designed to provide proprioceptive feedback to keep the cervical spine in a neutral position after soft tissue injuries like whiplash. A more rigid type of cervical orthosis might be used after a patient has undergone a cervical fusion. Examples of cervical orthotic devices include Aspen, Philadelphia, and Malibu. More rigid types of cervical orthoses often extend past the cervical spine to the thoracic spine to more fully limit cervical range of motion. For stable fractures, the most common types are Denison, Guilford, Sternal Occipital Mandibular Immobilizer

(SOMI), or Minerva. For unstable fractures, a halo ring, vest, or crown may be used. It is called a halo because it is screwed directly into the skull and surrounds the head like a halo.

Scoliosis orthosis. An orthotic device may be used to treat scoliosis when the curve is between 30–45 degrees. Patients with scoliotic curves of less than 30 degrees will be monitored closely, and curves greater than 45 degrees are considered for surgical correction. The device needs to bridge across the entire area where scoliosis is identified. A cervical-thoracic-lumbar-sacral orthosis (CTLSO) covers the most area, or the orthosis may be limited to a thoracic-lumbosacral orthosis (TLSO). Regardless of the levels of spine the orthosis crosses, it uses a rigid frame design with three points of contact to give kinesthetic reminders and is worn 23 hours per day. There are some softer designs that can be used for sleeping.

Thoracic-lumbosacral orthosis. TLSOs are designed to assist with the management of a variety of conditions, including thoracic compression fractures, osteoporosis, herniated nucleus pulposus, degenerative disc disease, postsurgical fusion, and soft tissue injuries. A body jacket or clam shell is semi-rigid and interlocks two custom-molded pieces together with Velcro to give maximum support. Depending on the rigidity of the brace and the weight that can be tolerated by the patient, various TLSOs limit trunk flexion and include the Taylor or Taylor Knight, CASH, Jewett, and Mother's Hug.

Lumbosacral orthosis (LSO). The lumbosacral orthoses are commonly off-the-shelf braces that are used to increase intra-abdominal pressure and provide soft tissue support. These are frequently used as management after a herniated nucleus pulposus and have also been used to prevent injuries—with mixed results. Concern exists when the LSO is used as a prevention aid, in that the individual wears the brace and learns to depend on it. This may result in muscles atrophying over time and an individual's inability to stabilize the spine without the brace. It is recommended that the brace be used as a prevention tool only to tighten the belt when a patient is lifting—rather than wearing it tight all the time. The Knight brace is an example of a more rigid and usually custom-molded LSO. This may be used postsurgically or to stabilize a spondylolisthesis.

Assessment of Alignment and Fit of Equipment

An orthosis is designed for constant wear, up to 23 hours a day. It may be temporary until a fracture is healed or the acute flare-up of symptoms has resolved, but proper fit of an orthotic device is critical to prevent secondary problems from developing. These problems may range from skin lesions to compensatory movement patterns. It is important to recognize that there is a period of adjustment for a new orthosis. Ideally, a new orthotic should be checked for fit immediately, and then again a short time later (from a few days up to two weeks). Patients who need to use an orthotic throughout the day for 12–16 hours per day should gradually increase the use of the device. Begin with four hours a day and gradually increase the time spent in the orthosis (or decrease the time spent out of the orthosis) until the patient is wearing it as long as necessary. Periodically checking the fit and alignment of the orthotic device will increase the patient's compliance with its use.

Contact. The first area to check is the skin under the device. Look for areas that are reddened or abraded. If the brace has been worn for several minutes up to several hours, also check to see if there is any unusual swelling distally or any reports of numbness or tingling. With off-the-shelf orthoses, too small a size may limit blood flow to the heart when the limb is held dependently, and it may also cause marks or imprints on the skin. Tightness or pinching of the fabric or material may not be evident until after the patient has worn the orthosis for several hours. For orthoses that are designed for the lower extremities (and weight-bearing is expected), there may be uniform redness—but there should not be any specific areas that are tender or red. The patient should be able to move the

joints above and below the orthosis freely, without the orthosis rubbing or chafing nearby areas. For patients who perspire excessively, cornstarch or cotton clothing may be an appropriate barrier to absorb perspiration. Excessive perspiration may increase the friction for an otherwise correctly fitting orthosis and result in problems later on. It is also important to check for odor. Foul odor may indicate an infection. Diminished circulation because of the device may also make this patient more prone to pressure or venous stasis ulcers. Also check that if an orthosis has moving parts, the parts themselves do not rub as it is moving.

Alignment. Examine the patient's posture. The orthosis should facilitate (and not detract) from achieving postural alignment. A wrist cock-up splint should come no farther than the proximal palmar crease so that the fingers can move comfortably and the patient can do more than simply grasp with a lumbrical grip. A Cam boot that increases the patient's leg length should be compensated by a higher heel on the contralateral side. By proactively identifying how the posture may be impacted, compensations can be made, and secondary pain and discomfort can be avoided. The device itself, especially if it was designed to reduce a deformity, should do just that. If the client demonstrates a forward flexed posture of the thoracic spine, the brace should reduce that deformity. A genu valgum or varum deformity should also be reduced with correct application of the device.

Stability. When the device is worn properly, it should stabilize the appropriate structures. Especially in joints that bear weight during gait, the brace should not encourage buckling of the knee or asymmetrical loading of the joint. As the patient begins to move, the device should securely support the area required and not slip or shift. The device should not piston (move up and down) while wearing it.

Function. The patient should be able to independently put on and take off the device. In a case when it is the caregiver's responsibility to do so, this person should be independent of the performance. It is not unusual to find a patient who has a correctly fitting orthosis but who, because it can not be put on or taken off properly, experiences pain and difficulty with the device. As the patient begins to move, have him or her perform movements that should be accommodated by the orthosis. Remember, some movements may need to be avoided, as they are contraindicated. Look to ensure that the orthosis does not snag on clothing. Some orthoses are designed to be worn under clothing, and some above the clothing. Make sure you assess the patient when they are dressed correctly, as the fit may be hampered by a layer of socks or a pant leg. Finally, ensure that the patient can move freely to ambulate and perform simple ADLs.

Workmanship. The workmanship of an orthosis can help to ensure that it will last a long time. If there are moving parts, make sure that they are not noisy and that they do not fall off. Ensure that the Velcro holds securely—and any extra Velcro that is not needed is cut off to an appropriate length so that it does not become a tripping hazard or get snagged on equipment or clothing.

Taking the time to ensure that the patient's orthosis fits properly and will serve its desired purpose will facilitate the patient's rehabilitation and prevent any complications from the use of the device.

Assessment of Effectiveness of Equipment

The fit of the orthosis is the foundation for determining whether it is effective, and it must fit properly to be effective. Once you have determined that the fit is correct, then it is time to determine if the orthosis is successful in meeting the intended goal. As stated previously, there are four main goals associated with the use of orthoses: protection, relief of distal weight-bearing forces, alignment, and facilitation or reduction of motion. Each of these goals will be explained further to address the effectiveness of the orthosis.

Protection. Orthoses called immobilizers or braces have the function of protection. This may be to protect the area from contact during normal ADLs or to stabilize a fracture. The patient will be the primary resource to determine if the orthosis is effective because if it is not, he or she will experience increased pain. The orthosis should limit shifting of the body segment and limit joint motion in the area. The orthosis should be comfortable and padded appropriately so that it can cushion any impact from functional tasks. If an assistive device is used in addition to the orthosis, the assistive device should not bump or otherwise connect with the orthosis. By allowing the patient to simulate a variety of activities, including walking, dressing, bathing, eating, and using the toilet, you will be able to identify if there are limitations of the orthosis and determine if the patient requires some additional education on alternate methods for performing tasks.

Relief of distal weight-bearing. Spinal orthoses are designed to relieve the pressure on the spine by increasing the intra-abdominal pressure and relieving pressure to the spinal segments. This relieves back pain and also allows the patient to be upright for longer periods of time before becoming fatigued. In addition, fracture management orthoses also stabilize the fracture segments adequately to keep them from shifting. Just as with the protection goal, the patient will be able to provide feedback as to how well the orthosis is working because pain will be significantly reduced (if not eliminated) with the orthosis.

Alignment. When the orthosis is designed to aid in alignment, note that perfect alignment may not be possible. Also, too much correction at any one time may result in increased pain and discomfort for the patient. Foot orthoses can overcorrect and result in discomfort higher up the kinetic chain. Poor alignment may also result in a new gait deviation (if it is a lower extremity orthosis), and subtle compensations with functional activities. This can sometimes be challenging to assess, as some improvement in gait or functional activities is generally expected. Overcorrection, reports of stress in new areas after a few hours or a few days, or new gait deviations are all indications that the orthotic device may not be correctly aligned.

Facilitation or reduction of motion. When an orthosis is designed to limit motion, there is an expectation set by how much that motion is limited. For example, with a KAFO, the knee recurvatum should be limited to zero degrees of extension. Functional observation of gait, as well as range of motion measurements while the patient is in the orthosis, will accomplish this. Usually the limitation in the motion will also improve the quality of the gait or other functional activities as intended. In cases where the range of motion is designed to facilitate motion, it will best be observed during functional activities. The loss of motion that necessitates the orthosis likely results in a compensation or gait deviation. By wearing the orthosis, that compensation or gait deviation should diminish. For example, a patient with a drop foot that is compensating with a steppage gait should reduce or eliminate the steppage gait once a properly fitting AFO has been applied.

Overall, there are three areas that will help to determine if the orthosis is effective. The first indication is the patient's report, especially after the performance of normal functional tasks. The second indication would be the reduction or elimination of the original compensation (or gait deviation), or just overall improvement in the quality of the functional activity. Finally, goniometric measurements and postural alignment should improve with the addition of the orthosis. In some cases, gradual correction over time may be necessary to reduce compensatory muscle, capsular, or joint irritation associated with making corrections too quickly or with too large an amplitude.

Pain

Pain is more than simply the activation of a nociceptor to recognize a noxious stimulus. Pain is both physiological in nature and a learned behavior. No two individuals experience pain in the same manner, yet it is the most common complaint for which patients come to physical therapy, with the expectation that it will be addressed. Pain is a warning signal from the body that there is something wrong. Ignoring pain is just as problematic as always giving in to pain. It is vital that physical therapist assistants teach patients to differentiate between hurt (discomfort) and harm (something that will cause greater damage). Because pain is partly a learned behavior, our interaction with the patient will influence how this individual responds to pain in the future. Encouraging patients to listen to their pain and then take appropriate action to reduce or manage symptoms is vital for successful rehabilitation. The commonly repeated phrase "no pain, no gain" is not the best advice for patients. Teaching patients to respond to pain appropriately requires that we have tools to assess and quantify what is essentially a subjective report. The following are some of the more commonly used tools to assist you with quantifying pain.

Ten-Centimeter Visual Analogue Scale

The Visual Analogue Scale is a ten-centimeter line (either horizontal or vertical). At one end of the scale, usually the far left or the bottom (depending on orientation), the scale is marked "no pain at all." At the other end of the scale, usually the far right or the top, the scale is marked "pain as bad as it could be." The patient is then asked to look at the scale and mark, based on the two qualifiers given, where the patient's pain is located. The physical therapist assistant would then take a ten-centimeter ruler and measure the line with the zero point at the bottom or far left and measure to the mark where the patient indicated he or she had pain. The number is then assessed similar to the traditional numeric scale, with 1–3 indicating mild pain, 4–6 moderate pain, 7–9 severe pain, and 10 excruciating pain. Patients with pain levels reported at 7 or above would be expected to demonstrate objective signs like facial grimacing, decline in the quality and speed of functional activities, and substitution patterns.

Faces Pain Scale

The Faces Pain Scale is a series of six images of a face, ranging from smiling to crying. Each image is designed to represent an image that corresponds to the traditional numeric pain scale. The advantage of the Faces Pain Scale is that it correlates to children ages 4–16, as well as to adults for whom English is a second language (or who do not speak English at all). The patient is asked to choose the face that best corresponds with how he or she is feeling. The images correspond to zero and the even numbers on the numeric scale. The resulting number is based on the scale described above.

The McGill Pain Questionnaire

The McGill Pain Questionnaire is a series of 20 groups of words which describe pain. Each group of words, which may contain anywhere from three to five adjectives, describes a quality of pain. Patients are asked to choose words that best describe how they are feeling. They do not need to pick a word from each category—but for each of the groups they choose, only one word in that group should be chosen. Categories 1 through 10 describe the sensory qualities of pain, while 11 through 15 describe emotional (affective) qualities. Category 16 describes the overall intensity of the total pain experience, and categories 17–20 are miscellaneous. Scoring can be done using one of two methods. The first is to describe how many words are chosen in each category. These will be either sensory (groups 1–10), affective (11–15), evaluative (16), or miscellaneous (17–20). The second method is to assign a value to each of the words within a word group. The first word in the group is considered the lowest intensity, and the last is the highest. The words are numbered consecutively 1, 2, 3, etc., until all the words in the word group are numbered. The score is based on adding the number value assigned for all the words chosen. There is no specific criterion to compare this number to—however, you can do a pre- and post-intervention assessment. The higher the number is, one can infer that the greater

pain is a factor in this patient's rehabilitation and ultimate recovery.

Oswestry Low Back Pain Disability Questionnaire

The Oswestry Low Back Pain Disability Questionnaire examines the patient's perception of the disability or functional limitation that is a result of his or her lower back pain. There are ten questions, each with a series of six answers. Each of the answers implies progressively more difficulty with a task or limitations in performance. The patient chooses the best answer of the six for each question. Once the questionnaire is completed, the physical therapist assistant scores the test by assigning a score to the answer. The first answer in each category is rated as a zero, and then successively numbered 1 through 5. The minimum score is a zero and maximum raw score is 50. Once the raw score is determined, it is multiplied by two so that a percentage can be given. Scores that go from 0–20% suggest the patient perceives minimal disability; 20–40% moderate disability; 40–60% severe disability; 60–80% crippling disability; and 80–100% disability that either renders the patient bed-bound or suggests he or she is displaying exaggerated behavior compared to functional performance. There is also an Oswestry questionnaire for the cervical spine as well.

Western Ontario and McMaster Universities Index of Osteoarthritis (WOMAC)

The WOMAC is used to assess patients with osteoarthritis involving the hip or knee. In it, 24 functional activities are assessed. The patient is asked to rate the difficulty he or she is having with the performance of the activity on a scale of 0–4. The 24 activities address pain, stiffness, and physical function. Scores may range from 0–96 for the entire test, with the following subsections: 0–20 for pain, 0–8 for stiffness, and 0–68 for physical function. The higher the score, the greater the difficulty the patient is having with this aspect of osteoarthritis.

Assessment of Nonverbal Indicators of Pain

Pain is an individual experience, and it is difficult to compare one person's interpretation of pain to another's. Because pain is both physiological as well as learned, each response may be influenced by a variety of factors. Some patients are very stoic about their pain and tend to ignore symptoms until they can no longer do so. Some patients may be prone to exaggerate their symptoms for a secondary gain. Secondary gain implies that remaining in the sick role provides benefits that may not be known to the clinician—and in many cases, the patient may not be aware of this behavior. For this reason, it is important to recognize objective behaviors that either correlate or do not correlate with subjective reports by the patient.

The patient may demonstrate facial grimacing, which includes wincing, squinting, or other facial expressions which indicate discomfort. These are often associated with corresponding sounds that indicate discomfort. Facial grimacing can be feigned, so it should not be the only observation made. The patient may also have flushed skin, which is consistent with vasodilation and increased demand on the cardiovascular system. Perspiration is another objective sign that is difficult to feign. Finally, with strong isometric contractions, you may observe white knuckles, which suggest a strong muscle contraction.

Typically, as patients report increases in pain, the quality and speed of movement decline. Evidence of breakdown in body mechanics, the use of substitution patterns, and recruitment of accessory muscles are all signs that are consistent with these findings. A physical therapist assistant may also observe tremors and a decrease in the range of motion necessary for an activity.

Many people believe that heart rate should increase with onset of pain. While this is true with acute pain, studies have not shown this same correlation with chronic pain. Heart rate increases 20–30 beats per minute with static or isometric activities. Chronic pain has been associated with an increase in the resting heart rate, possibly because of deconditioning.

Observing the patient when he or she is aware or unaware of direct observation can be helpful. A patient who demonstrates limited trunk flexion when under direct observation, but who is able to flex forward without difficulty to reach the water fountain, is inconsistent. Because the patient is not aware how various activities have similar components, these can be used as cross-comparison measures to look at consistency as well. The ways that most physical therapist assistants determine that an exercise is too hard or too easy for a patient are the same ways that are used to decide whether or not the patient's subjective reports are consistent with demonstrated functional abilities.

Posture

A systematic approach to assessing posture ensures that you view the patient from various directions and determine alignment via consistent bony landmarks. Identifying postural deviations assists the physical therapist and physical therapist assistant in correctly identifying muscles that are short and tight versus muscles that are overly stretched. It also helps the clinician determine which structures are most likely under stress and may impact functional activities. When performing an assessment, the patient should have minimal clothing on so that relationships between body segments can be identified and bony landmarks can be easily seen and palpated. A two-piece bathing suit for women and shorts for men are ideal. The patient should stand in a comfortable and relaxed posture. If the patient uses an assistive device or wears an orthosis, the patient should be assessed both with and without these devices so that you can determine the effectiveness of the device on the patient's posture. Hand dominance often accounts for asymmetries in postural alignment. Even people that have no musculoskeletal complaints are likely to have evidence of postural asymmetry that can be detected through postural analysis.

Assessment of Posture from Anterior-Posterior and Lateral Views Using Plumb Bob or Grid

Postural examination is most commonly performed by assessing the body's alignment from an anterior, lateral, and posterior view. A plumb line (also known as a plumb bob), which is simply a piece of string suspended from the ceiling with a small weight attached to the bottom, is an excellent reference point as a straight line. With a mirror and the plumb line, the clinician can assess postural alignment in reference to the line. As an alternative, grid lines may be referenced on the wall, and the grid line can be used in place of the plumb line.

Lateral View

The clinician should examine the patient in a comfortable, relaxed posture. It is important to look at the patient from both sides in case there is an asymmetrical postural deviation that can only be detected on one side. The plumb line should fall through the following landmarks:

- external auditory meatus
- acromion
- chest (symmetrically)
- abdomen and back (midway between)
- sacroiliac joint (slightly anterior)
- hip joint (posterior)
- greater trochanter
- knee (slightly anterior to the midline)
- lateral malleolus (slightly anterior)

Some of the most common postural deformities that can be seen from a lateral observation point are the following:

- **Forward head.** Head anterior to plumb line, typically from tight cervical extensors and stretched cervical flexors
- **Flattened cervical lordotic curve.** Stretched posterior cervical ligaments or tight cervical flexors

- **Excessive cervical lordotic curve.** Tightness of posterior cervical ligaments and neck extensors
- **Forward or rounded shoulders.** Tightness of pectoralis minor and major, or weakness of middle trapezius and rhomboids
- **Increased thoracic kyphosis.** Compression of anterior vertebral bodies, tightness of anterior chest muscles, or stretched posterior thoracic extensors
- **Barrel chest.** Tightness of scapula adductor muscles or overuse of accessory muscles of respiration
- **Decreased lumbar lordosis.** Tightness of hamstrings, weakness of hip flexors, tightness of abdominals
- **Posterior pelvic tilt.** Tightness of hamstring and abdominal muscles
- **Increased lumbar lordosis.** Thoracic kyphosis, stretched anterior hip ligaments, stretched posterior longitudinal ligaments, back extensors, and hip flexors
- **Anterior pelvic tilt.** Tightness of hip flexors and back extensors, stretched abdominals
- **Genu recurvatum.** Hyperextension of the knee, tightness of quadriceps femoris or gastrocnemius
- **Flexed knee.** Tightness of popliteus and hamstrings at the knee, stretched gastrocnemius or quadriceps femoris group
- **Forward lean posture.** Increased dorsiflexion secondary to tight dorsiflexors or stretched plantar flexors

Posterior View

When examining the body from either the anterior or posterior view, it should be with a mind for symmetry. Here, hand dominance may play a role, as it is the most common reason for asymmetry. Although the dominant side is commonly afflicted with asymmetry, the nondominant side may be the source if it is used as a holder or stabilizer (as it is often used in the upper extremity). From a posterior perspective, the plumb line should appear as follows:

- midway through the head through the external occipital protuberance
- midway between the shoulders
- bisecting the spinous processes of the thoracic and lumbar vertebrae
- bisecting and creating symmetry at the spine of the scapula and inferior angle
- bisecting the gluteal cleft
- bisecting the posterior superior iliac spine
- bisecting and creating symmetry at the level of the iliac crest, gluteal folds, and greater trochanters
- bisecting the midpoint between the knees
- bisecting the midpoint between the medial malleoli
- medially from the medial malleolus to the head of the first metatarsal and the navicular tuberosity

Some of the more common postural deformities that can be observed from the posterior view include the following:

- **Head tilt.** Lateral tilt of the head to right or left as a result of asymmetrical tightness of lateral neck flexors
- **Head rotation.** Rotation of neck to right or left as a result of asymmetrical tightness of ipsilateral or contralateral neck rotators
- **Dropped shoulder.** Dominant shoulder is lower, or tightness of rhomboids or latissimus dorsi muscles
- **Shoulder elevated.** Tightness in upper trapezius and levator scapula on one side, or scoliosis
- **Shoulder lateral rotation.** Tightness of external rotators
- **Shoulder medial rotation.** Tightness of internal rotators
- **Abducted scapula.** Tightness of serratus anterior muscle or lengthened rhomboids and middle trapezius
- **Winging scapula.** Medial border of the scapula lifts away from the rib cage because of weakness to serratus anterior.

- **Scoliosis.** Asymmetrical lengthening and shortening of intrinsic back muscles, leg length discrepancy; usually there is a primary and secondary curve if permanent.
- **Lateral pelvic tilt.** Shortening of the contralateral quadrates lumborum, or scoliosis
- **Pelvic rotation.** Tightness of medial rotator and hip flexor muscles on rotated side, or ipsilateral lumbar rotation
- **Hip abducted.** Greater trochanter is higher on affected side because of tightness of hip abductor muscles or contralateral tightness of hip adductor muscles.
- **Genu varum.** Tibia moves toward the midline, creating a bow-legged appearance because of compression of medial joint structures or elongated hip lateral rotators.
- **Genu valgum.** Tibia moves away from the midline, creating a knock-kneed appearance because of a tight iliotibial band, pronation of the foot, and compression of lateral knee joint.
- **Pes planus.** Flat foot, pronated because of shortened fibularis (peroneal) muscles and stretched spring ligament
- **Pes cavus.** High arch, supinated because of shortened posterior and anterior tibial muscles and stretched fibularis (peroneal) muscles

Anterior View

When examining the body from an anterior view, many of the same landmarks as the posterior view can be observed. It is still important to look at them from another perspective, as the orientation of the problem may be more three-dimensional than two-dimensional. From an anterior observation point, the plumb line should appear as follows:

- bisecting the head
- vertically bisecting the sternum, xiphoid process, umbilicus, and pubis
- midway between the lower extremities

Some of the more common postural deformities that can be viewed from the anterior perspective include the following: (Please note that entries that can be observed from both a posterior and anterior perspective are discussed under the posterior observation section.)

- **Lateral tilt**
- **Head rotation**
- **Mandibular asymmetry.** The upper and lower teeth are not aligned secondary to asymmetry in one or more of the muscles of mastication or dentition issues.
- **Shoulder dropped**
- **Shoulder elevated**
- **Clavicle and joint asymmetry.** Previous trauma may result in asymmetry of clavicle, AC joint, or subluxations of sternoclavicular or acromio-clavicular joints secondary to trauma.
- **Cubitus valgus.** The forearm deviates laterally away from the body 5–15 degrees to what is referred to as the carrying angle. Carrying angles which exceed 15 degrees are referred to as cubitus valgus and may be due to a stretched ulnar collateral ligament or elbow hyperextension.
- **Cubitus varus.** The forearm deviates medially at an angle that is less than the standard 5–15 degree carrying angle. This might be related to a stretched radial collateral ligament or a previous fracture at or around the elbow.
- **Swan neck deformity.** A swan neck deformity is described as hyperextension at the proximal interphalangeal joint and flexion at the distal interphalangeal joint. This is commonly seen in patients with rheumatoid arthritis. It can also be caused by trauma.
- **Boutonniere deformity.** A boutonniere deformity is characterized by flexion of the proximal interphalangeal (PIP) joint, with hyperextension of the distal interphalangeal (DIP) joint. It is usually the result of direct trauma to the extensor tendon of the finger over the PIP joint but is also associated with rheumatoid arthritis.

- **Femoral anteversion.** The torsion angle of the femur is normally 12–15 degrees in an adult. This torsion angle develops as a child begins to bear weight through the lower extremity. Children that have excessive anteversion, based on a torsion angle greater than 15 degrees, demonstrate a toe-in posture and are comfortable W-sitting. Strengthening of the hip external rotators is often beneficial. Measurement of the torsion angle is best performed using Craig's test. The patient is positioned prone, with the knee flexed to 90 degrees. The examiner then palpates the greater trochanter and moves the hip into rotation until the most prominent aspect of the greater trochanter is horizontal. The angle between the tibial shaft, midline of the patella, and a vertical line is the torsion angle.
- **Femoral retroversion.** Femoral retroversion results from a femoral torsion angle of less than 12 degrees. Patients present with a toe-out posture and prefer to sit on the floor cross-legged. The femoral torsion angle can be measured with the Craig's test as described above.
- **Coxa vara.** Coxa vara is most commonly a congenital deformity where the angle of inclination between the head and neck of the femur and the shaft of the femur is less than 120 degrees. Because this angle is diminished, it puts the patient at increased risk for the development of femoral neck fractures. Some other bone conditions, such as osteogenesis imperfecta, Paget's disease, and Legg-Calvé-Perthes disease, can also result in the formation of this condition. This is usually compensated at the knee with genu valgum, and the patient may present with a Trendelenburg or compensated Trendelenburg gait.
- **Coxa valga.** Coxa valga occurs when the angle of inclination between the head and neck of the femur and the shaft of the femur is greater than 130 degrees. Because this angle is increased, it puts the patient at increased risk for hip dislocation. This is commonly caused by a slipped capital

femoral epiphysis, which is often observed in overweight adolescent males; or it may also be congenital. This is usually compensated at the knee with genu varum.

- **Hip lateral rotation.** This is most easily observed at the patella, which is turned out. This may be a result of tight hip external rotators or gluteus maximus, femoral retroversion, or internal tibial torsion.

- **Hip medial rotation.** This is most easily observed at the patella, which is turned in. This may be a result of tight hip internal rotation and iliotibial band, weakness of the lateral rotators, femoral anteversion, or external tibial torsion.

- **External tibial torsion.** Twenty-five degrees of external rotation is normal in a mature adult. More than 25 degrees is considered excessive and may be related to tightness in the iliotibial band, femoral retroversion, or a cruciate ligament tear.

- **Internal tibial torsion.** Angles of less than 25 degrees result in the feet pointing straight ahead (without slight toeing out) or medially. This may be a result of tight medial hamstrings and gracilis muscles, femoral anteversion, foot pronation, or genu valgum.

- **Hallux valgus.** More commonly called a bunion, this is a lateral deviation of the proximal phalanx at the metatarsophalangeal joint. It may result from a tight adductor hallucis, short extensor hallucis longus, or joint dislocation.

- **Claw toe.** This is hyperextension of the metatarsophalangeal joint and flexion of the proximal interphalangeal joints and is usually associated with pes cavus. This is typically due to shortened toe flexors and shortened toe extensor muscles.

- **Hammer toe.** This is differentiated from claw toes, in that the metatarsophalangeal joint is hyperextended along with the distal interphalangeal joint, and the proximal interphalangeal joint is flexed. This is due to tightness to toe extensors and stretched lumbricals.

Prosthetic Requirements of the Patient with a Lower Extremity Amputation

According to the Amputee Coalition of America, more the 1.7 million Americans (or approximately 1 in every 200 people) have had a limb amputated, whole or in part. Amputations may be a result of trauma, cancer, a congenital problem, or poor circulation. For the lower extremity amputee, 97% are related to dysvascular conditions, such as peripheral vascular disease and diabetes. Since most lower extremity amputees have preexisting vascular problems, ensuring proper fit and function of the prosthesis is necessary to prevent skin breakdown, maximize stability, reduce discomfort associated with prolonged wear, and manage fatigue.

Assessment of Alignment and Fit of the Prosthesis

The alignment and fit of a prosthesis is a dynamic process. The patient should be examined putting on and taking off the device independently, sitting, standing, and walking on level surfaces and inclines in order to adequately determine if the device is functioning as prescribed. Whether it is a transfemoral, above-knee (AK), transtibial, or below-knee (BK) prosthesis, the assessment is essentially the same.

Before applying the prosthesis, ask:

- *Is the prosthesis as ordered?* Are the components, suspension, and supporting garments all present?

- *Does the patient know how to properly don and doff the prosthesis independently?* Differentiate between a patient education problem and a fit issue.

When the patient is standing, ask:

- *Can the patient stand comfortably, bearing weight approximately equally on both sides, with heels no more than six inches apart?*

- *Does the prosthetic knee or the patient's own knee feel stable?* The knee should not feel like it is going to buckle or be forced into hyperextension (anterior-posterior alignment).

- *Is the shoe resting flat on the floor with no uncomfortable pressure medially or laterally in the socket?* Check the wear of the patient's shoes to see if it is even.
- *Is the prosthesis the correct length?* Palpate the iliac crest height, the anterior superior iliac spines (ASIS), and the posterior superior iliac spines (PSIS) to ensure there is symmetry.
- *Is the piston action minimal during swing phase?* Ensure that the residual limb does not slide up and down during the swing phase of gait and cause rubbing or instability.
- *Are the anterior, medial, lateral, and posterior walls of the prosthesis of adequate height?*
- *Is the patient bearing weight as expected, based on the type of prosthesis?* A patient with a transtibial amputation will use a patellar tendon–bearing prosthesis. Weight is born on the patellar tendon and medial, lateral, and posterior aspects of the limb. A patient with a transfemoral amputation will have either a quadrilateral socket or an ischial containment socket. In the quadrilateral socket, weight is born on the ischial tuberosity and adductor longus tendon. In the ischial containment socket, weight is born primarily on the ischial tuberosity.
- *Does the suspension adequately support the limb?* If there is supracondylar suspension, ensure that the prosthesis goes over the medial epicondyle. If there is a strap or belt, ensure that it is comfortably snug and no tissue is getting trapped underneath.

When the patient is sitting, ask:

- *Can the patient sit comfortably without having tissue bunch?* With transtibial amputation, examine the popliteal space for this problem. The patient should be comfortable, with no excessive discomfort over the hamstring tendons, pressure from sidebars, or a socket that comes up too high.

- *Is the patient walking on level surfaces satisfactorily?* Focus specifically on heel strike, midstance, and heel-off when analyzing gait to identify gait deviations. Those with a BK amputation will usually have fewer gait abnormalities, but the expected functional outcomes are higher. Patients with an AK amputation may have more noticeable gait deviations.
- *Can the patient safely negotiate stairs, inclines, and declines?* Check to see if there is pistoning within the socket when the limb is lifted up to clear the other step. Knee stability and toe clearance will be more significant factors with these changes.
- *Can the patient kneel?* Although this may not be an activity all patients will perform, it is a reasonable goal for many with a BK amputation. It is important to keep in mind the supracondylar suspension may make this more painful and more challenging.

When the prosthesis is off (after being worn for a period of time while the patient performed functional activities), ask:

- *Is there any noise coming from the prosthesis?*
- *Is the size, contour, and color of the prosthesis similar to that of the other limb?*
- *Is the patient's residual limb free from abrasion, discoloration and excessive perspiration immediately after prosthesis is removed?* Focus especially on areas of discomfort for the patient.
- *Is pressure being born on the weight-bearing areas for the prosthesis?*
- *Do the suspension straps have adequate slack for adjustments to be made?*

Assessment of the Effectiveness of the Prosthesis

A lower extremity prosthesis is designed primarily for mobility. Therefore, the assessment for effectiveness is based on functional tasks. Once you have assessed the patient's movement on level surfaces, challenge the patient with more difficult tasks. An incline or decline and stairs are common obstacles that the patient will encounter. Pay close attention as to whether or not the patient drags the foot or pistons excessively during swing. Look at balance when the patient walks on foam or grassy surfaces or transitions from hard floors to carpet. An obstacle course where the patient moves in and out and over obstacles is a great challenge. In addition to gait, determine the length of time the patient can sit before he or she needs to get up again. Is it enough time to watch a movie or only enough time to watch a sitcom on TV? Also, determine whether the patient has to reach overhead, move to retrieve something off the floor, or kneel. Observe whether the patient can get in and out of these postures independently, and document what kind of assistance is necessary.

Assessment of Safe Use of Prosthesis

The patient should be aware of how to clean the prosthesis safely, as well as how to care for the suspension items. Depending on the materials, different cleaning methods may be suggested. This should be part of the patient's education, and part of your assessment should include having the patient verbally explain the procedure to you. In addition, the patient should know how to apply an elastic wrap to the residual limb or to use a shrinker, which is an elastic stocking. If a shrinker or socks are used, the patient should also be familiar with the ply of the socks so that an adequate sock count can be maintained. The patient should be given a schedule for wearing the prosthesis, with instructions for how to gradually progress to wearing the prosthesis all day. In addition, the patient would benefit from awareness that fluid management is very important, and even small gains and losses in weight may impact the fit of the prosthesis.

Assessment of Residual Limb

Over a period of time, the residual limb will undergo changes in shape and size. Physical therapists and PTAs must be able to document changes that are noted.

Strength

Gross muscle testing will be performed as closely as possible to standardize testing, taking into account that there is likely a significantly shorter lever arm which will impact grading. Avoid direct pressure over the distal end of the tibia or femur, as that may cause the patient to self-limit because of pain. Remember that although the prosthetic limb weighs significantly less than the patient's original limb, it is dead weight. The patient must move this load, which extends the lever arm of their leg by the same muscles that now have a shortened lever arm. It is important that the patient understand how important regaining the strength of the muscles is to maximize functional abilities. At a minimum, strength should include knee flexion and extension (when available), as well as hip flexion, abduction, extension, and adduction.

Range of Motion

Patients with amputations are prone to contractures because a significant amount of time is spent sitting and because the amputated limb is more comfortable in flexion. Hip and knee flexors are common contracture sites. When taking goniometric measurements on the limb with the amputation, use the midshaft of the femur or tibia as your moving arm. Since there is extra tissue, which is rolled and positioned distally for additional padding during weight-bearing, be sure that you identify where the shaft of the bone actually is because the excessive soft tissue may erroneously lead you away from the bone itself.

Skin Integrity

Examine the skin for abrasions, redness, and tenderness to palpation. There should be no skin flaps or dog ears on the medial and lateral side of the stump. The scar should be well-healed, nontender to the touch, and able to move well because it is not adhered to any tissue (including bone). Note areas of excessive redness, especially to areas that are not expected to bear weight. The patient should be able to independently feel the entire stump; and if sensation is an issue, visualize the entire area with a small handheld mirror.

Edema Management

Girth measurements are very helpful to determine how much swelling remains in the residual limb. Especially with lower extremity amputation, dependency increases swelling. A patient also has to have stable girth measurements before the final prosthesis can be made. As with any girth measurement, measurements should be taken in centimeters from a known landmark. For transtibial amputees, the middle of the patella is an appropriate landmark to use, and the anterior superior iliac spine is the best choice for the transfemoral amputees. Measurements are then taken five to ten centimeters above and below that site. You should be able to palpate the distal end of either the tibia or the femur. Use this as your ending point—because after the end of the bone, the shape of the stump changes to narrow to a rounded edge. Because 97% of patients with lower extremity amputations have a dysvascular disorder, do not use pen or a grease pencil on the patient's skin, as it may result in skin breakdown.

Range of Motion

Goniometry is a commonly used evaluation technique in physical therapy. How much a joint can move is dependent on the joint arthrokinematics, the ligaments, capsular integrity, and the muscles and tendons that cross the joints. Values obtained from measuring range of motion are compared to normal values to determine goals for physical therapy, or progress made toward the completion of those goals. Because active range of motion and passive range of motion impact different structures during the performance of an activity, range of motion can be used to diagnose which structures have been impacted. Range of motion is also a great tool to motivate a patient to perform better than he or she did last time. Range of motion is typically performed as a right-left comparison for

extremities and, if necessary, compared to normative data. Accessory motions occur at the end range of active and passive range. An end feel can also be assessed at that time. AROM is performed independently by the patient and requires active use of muscles and tendons. PROM is performed by the clinician, a caregiver, the patient, or by a piece of equipment. Active assistive range of motion is performed actively by the patient, who is then assisted by either equipment or the clinician.

Goniometry

Clinicians use a goniometer to measure joint range of motion. A goniometer is a protractor with extensions that are aligned with specific bony landmarks to measure joint movement. The size of the goniometer is dependent on the joint being evaluated and may range in size from very small (to assess fingers) to very large (to assess the hip). The goniometer has a central axis, which is positioned over the joint, and a stationary arm (or stable arm) as well as moving arm. The stationary arm is a nonmoving segment, and the moving arm is distal to the joint and represents the joint movement. It is vitally important that clinicians use standardized methods for identifying landmarks, taking measurements, and comparing results to normative data. Clinicians who work together and take goniometric measurements of the same patients should have no more than a five-degree inter-rater reliability. In addition to standard goniometers, bubble inclinometers have been developed to measure trunk range. Bubble inclinometers use a bubble (similar to the kind found in a carpenter's level) to determine changes in motion. It uses gravity to document changes in motion on a 360 degree scale.

Muscle Length Assessment

Two joint muscles have the advantage that they can produce motions at more than one joint but are more susceptible to losing tension and developing active insufficiency when the muscle tries to contract over both joints. Because of the nature of two joint muscles, after injury or lack of use, the muscle may no longer be sufficiently flexible to provide stability and mobility. Muscle length testing is designed to determine if loss of motion at a joint is from intrinsic muscle tightness of a two-or multi-joint muscle or if the loss is from the joint itself. Muscle length testing is based on the principles of passive insufficiency. A two-joint muscle performs at least two actions. To determine the muscle's length, it is moved opposite its own muscle actions. For example, the triceps brachii flexes at the elbow, and the long head also flexes at the shoulder. In order to put the triceps long head on passive insufficiency you must both flex the elbow and flex the shoulder. The joint that will demonstrate limited range of motion is the last joint in the series where motion was performed.

Apley's Scratch Test

The Apley's scratch test is a simple screening tool to assess whether the patient has functional movement of the glenohumeral joint. Studies have indicated that patients who do well on this test have a high correlation to being able to perform functional activities with the shoulder.

Abduction and external rotation. The patient is asked to reach and touch the superior medial aspect of his or her contralateral scapula. The patient moves into abduction and external rotation in order to demonstrate this position.

Adduction and internal rotation. The patient is asked to reach behind his or her back and touch the inferior angle of the contralateral scapula. Together, these two simple tests screen shoulder range of motion. Their results do not imply that there are no limitations in range but that the patient has the ability to perform most functional tasks involving the shoulder—including combing the hair or reaching into a back pocket to get a wallet.

Observations of Segmental Quality of Spine Motion

Trunk range of motion can often be challenging to assess because so many segments make up composite motions. A dual inclinometer is designed to use gravity to assess motion at the inferior segment, and then again at the superior segment. When the inferior segment motion is subtracted from the superior segment, the resultant range represents that segment of the spine's motion. When physicians are asked to do disability ratings for workers' compensation, long-term disability benefits, or Social Security disability benefits, and the condition involves the spine, inclinometers are required. The American Medical Association's *Guide to the Evaluation of Permanent Impairment, 5th Edition* bases impairment ratings on inclinometry measurements. Bubble inclinometers can also be used to measure spinal motion, but they cannot be used for an impairment rating.

A great deal of information can be assessed when you observe spinal motion from a posterior view. As you observe the quality of motion of each spinal segment, look at the relationship between the spinous processes. As you watch the patient move, look for a smooth, continuous line in the skin which represents the spinous processes. In areas where the joint mobility is limited secondary to muscle tightness, ligamentous tightness, or misalignment of the vertebrae, a flattened segment can be observed. This flattened segment may look different with lateral bending to the right or left or with rotation. A flattened segment that is observed in left lateral bending and not right implies limitations with left lateral bending. If right rotation is impacted, you know that the muscle that is likely limiting motion is a contralateral rotator. Although this is a nonspecific tool, it can assist you to quickly identify segments of the spine where problems exist.

Practice 2 Questions

1. You are performing manual muscle testing for the middle deltoid. In supine, your patient is able to go through full range and take minimal resistance. What would be the appropriate muscle grade to give her?
   a. 2+/5
   b. 3–/5
   c. 3+/5
   d. 4–/5

2. You are performing manual muscle testing of the elbow flexors. You would like to differentiate between the various muscles that perform elbow flexion. If you are trying to isolate the brachialis, how would you position the patient for testing?
   a. seated, with elbow flexed and forearm supinated
   b. side-lying, with elbow flexed and forearm in neutral
   c. seated, with the elbow flexed and forearm pronated
   d. seated, with the elbow flexed and forearm in neutral

3. What is the moving arm for performing ankle inversion?
   a. along the ridge of the calcaneus
   b. along the shaft of the tibia to the patella
   c. along the shaft of the second metatarsal
   d. along the shaft of the second digit

4. Which of the following tests may be performed prior to an offer of employment?
   a. preplacement screen
   b. physical agility test
   c. X-rays
   d. manual muscle testing

5. Which of the following activities is not an example of an agility task?
   a. cariocas to left and right
   b. ladder jumping forward and back
   c. vertical jumping up and down
   d. shuttle run forward and back

6. For which patient would the Faces Pain Scale be most appropriate?
   a. 7-year-old child with a fibula fracture
   b. 25-year-old male in a coma
   c. 45-year-old female with back pain
   d. 68-year-old female with shoulder impingement

7. Which postural deviations can best be observed when looking at the patient posteriorly?
   a. recurvatum, elevated L shoulder, increased lumbar lordosis
   b. scoliosis, elevated R scapula, pronated feet
   c. left lateral head tilt, anterior pelvic tilt, right high iliac crest
   d. genu varum, increased thoracic kyphosis, elevated scapula

8. Given the joint described, which end feel would be considered abnormal?
   a. hard end feel, elbow extension
   b. soft end feel, knee flexion
   c. empty end feel, shoulder abduction
   d. firm end feel, forearm pronation

Practice 2 Answers

1. **a.** The middle deltoid performs abduction. Supine is the gravity-eliminated position; and because she is able to move through full range, she has at least 2 out of 5 strength. With minimal resistance, this is 2+.

2. **c.** Seated, with elbow flexed, is against gravity. The forearm must be pronated to eliminate the use of biceps brachii and brachioradialis so that only the brachialis functions.

3. **c.** Inversion has an axis over the dome of the talus and a stationary arm along the shaft of the tibia. The moving arm is along the shaft of the second metatarsal.

4. **b.** A physical agility test is a qualifications exam and can be done prior to offering employment. The other three options are considered medical screening and can only be completed after employment has been offered.

5. **c.** Vertical jumping will work on power, but the other tasks take explosive power, tasks and have the patient quickly change direction which is necessary for agility. Vertical jumping is a plyometric task.

6. **a.** The faces scale is most appropriate for a child or an adult for whom English is not their primary language. A numeric scale or a visual analogue scale would be appropriate for C (45-year-old female with back pain) and D (68-year-old female with shoulder impingement). No scale would be appropriate for B (a 25-year-old male in a coma).

7. **b.** Scoliosis, elevated scapula, and pronated feet can all best be observed posteriorly; the other responses have combinations of postural deformities that are best observed laterally, anteriorly, and posteriorly.

8. **c.** An empty end feel implies that pain is limiting the patient before the physiological end feel is reached. The other examples are normal end feels for those joints.

Neuromuscular System

Because the neuromuscular system is complex and has a significant impact on an individual's function, the physical therapist assistant must be able to perform and understand the results of a variety of neurological tests and measures used in physical therapy. In addition, the physical therapist assistant must always be alert for clinical signs of changes in the neuromuscular system that may affect a patient's function. This section outlines the tests and measures used to assess the various aspects of the neuromuscular system.

Arousal and Attention

Arousal is the physiological readiness for activity. A certain level of arousal is needed for proper function in individuals of all ages. Arousal can be assessed by clinical observation using descriptive terms. Common terms used to describe arousal include alert, lethargic, obtunded, stupor, and coma, and they are defined in the following chart.

Measurement Tools to Assess Arousal

Arousal can also be assessed using standardized measurement tools in adults and children. Pediatric assessment involves comparing clinical presentation to age-expected norms. A physical therapist assistant should have a basic understanding of common pediatric measurement tools used to assess arousal and awareness. The Brazelton Neonatal Assessment Scale, Bayley Scales of Infant Development, and Gesell Developmental Assessment are three common tools used in pediatrics.

Brazelton Neonatal Assessment Scale

The purpose of the Brazelton Neonatal Assessment Scale is to describe an infant's interactions and behaviors within the context of a caregiver relationship. The areas tested are habituation, motor-oral, truncal, vestibular, and social-interactive. This tool is used to evaluate children from birth to two months and is administered in a dark room between the infant's feedings.

Bayley Scales of Infant Development

The Bayley Scales of Infant Development identify developmental delay in children and monitor developmental progress. This tool is used to evaluate children from 1 to 42 months. The areas tested include language and perception, gross and fine motor skills, and behavior. The test items are arranged according to degree of difficulty and are scored using a binary scoring system of pass or fail.

Gesell Developmental Assessment

The Gesell Developmental Assessment was designed to create a qualitative and descriptive profile of a child's development. There is no right or wrong answer, and this test does not result in a numerical or standardized test score. The areas tested are physical/neurological growth, language skills, and adaptive skills.

Pediatric Arousal and Awareness Assessment Tools

ASSESSMENT TOOL	AGE RANGE	PURPOSE	AREAS TESTED
Brazelton Neonatal Assessment	Newborn to two months	Describe behaviors and interactions with a caregiver	Habituation, motor-oral, truncal, vestibular, social-interactive
Bayley Scales of Infant Development	One to 42 months	Identify developmental delay and monitor developmental progress	Mental: language, perceptual; motor: gross, fine; behavior
Gesell Developmental Assessment	One month to five years	Understand characteristics of behavior relative to typical growth patterns	Physical/neurological growth, language skills, adaptive behaviors

The results of pediatric assessments are compared to age-expected norms.

Glasgow Coma Scale

Level of awareness is also measured in adults using assessment tools such as the Glasgow Coma Scale. The Glasgow Coma Scale measures the severity of injury and is considered the gold standard to document the level of coma/consciousness. The areas tested are motor response, verbal response, and eye opening. Each section receives 1–5 points. The three response scores are added together to create a total score, which is then used for classification. The possible cumulative scores range from 3–15.

Glasgow Coma Scale

EYE OPENING	SCORE
Spontaneous	4
To speech	3
To pain	2
No response	1
BEST MOTOR RESPONSE	
Follows motor commands	6
Localizes	5
Withdraws	4
Abnormal flexion	3
Extensor response	2
No response	1
VERBAL RESPONSE	
Oriented	5
Confused conversation	4
Inappropriate words	3
Incomprehensible sounds	2
No response	1

The scores in the three categories are added together to acheive a total Glasgow Coma Scale score.

Glasgow Coma Scale Score Interpretation

SCORE	INTERPRETATION
8 or less	Coma; severe brain injury
9–12	Moderate brain injury
13–15	Mild brain injury

The score on the Glasgow Coma Scale is then placed in a category that describes the level of consciousness and severity of injury.

Ranchos Los Amigos Scale

The Ranchos Los Amigos Scale is used to describe cognitive function in individuals who have experienced a traumatic brain injury (TBI) as they emerge from a coma. The eight levels of the Ranchos Los Amigos Scale are organized in progression, describing the typical behavior as an individual emerges from a coma. Note that an individual can plateau at any level or progress through all eight levels.

Ranchos Los Amigos Levels of Cognitive Function

LEVELS	DESCRIPTION	ASSISTANCE LEVEL REQUIRED
1. No Response	Unresponsive to all stimuli	Total assistance
2. Generalized Response	Inconsistent and nonpurposeful reaction to all stimuli; generalized responses may be movement, vocalization, or physiologic changes	Total assistance
3. Localized Response	Specific and inconsistent reactions; localized response to stimuli; may follow simple commands	Total assistance
4. Confused-Agitated	Heightened state of activity with bizarre behavior; unable to cooperate directly; incoherent and inappropriate vocalization; brief attention to environment	Maximal assistance
5. Confused-Inappropriate	Responsive to simple commands; gross attention to environment but highly distractible; significant memory impairment; unable to learn new information	Maximal assistance
6. Confused-Appropriate	Goal-directed behavior dependent on instruction; consistently follows simple direction; reacts appropriately to environment; some carryover for basic tasks (e.g., ADLs)	Moderate assistance
7. Automatic-Appropriate	Behavior is appropriate and patient is oriented in structured environment; shallow recall; judgment remains impaired; goes through daily routine automatically	Minimal assistance
8. Purposeful-Appropriate	Responsive to environment; shows carryover; continued difficulty with abstract reasoning; judgment in nonstructured or unexpected environments/situations	Standby assistance

This scale is used to categorize behavior as an individual emerges from a coma.

TAKE NOTE

As individuals emerge from a coma and transition between cognitive levels, some may demonstrate responses or behaviors that do not fall neatly into the Ranchos Los Amigos levels. In addition, not every individual will progress through each level during recovery.

INFORMATION IN ACTION

You are reviewing the physical therapy evaluation for a new patient you are preparing to treat. The physical therapist has noted that the patient is a Ranchos Los Amigos level IX or X. The most common form of the scale includes the traditional eight levels. However, the Ranchos Level of Cognitive Function was recently revised to include ten levels. Levels IX and X have the same name as level VIII, "Purposeful-Appropriate." These two levels indicate improving cognitive function, such as independently shifting back and forth between tasks, using assistive memory devices in level IX, and handling multiple tasks simultaneously in level X.

Orientation

The term orientation refers to an individual's awareness of person, place, and time. In order to assess orientation to self, the examiner asks questions such as, "What is your name?" or "How old are you?" Questions that can be asked to assess a patient's orientation to place include, "What city are you in?" or "Where are you?" A patient's orientation to time can be assessed by asking, "What day is it?" or "What year is it?" If these three areas of questions are answered correctly, the examiner documents that the patient is "oriented × 3," meaning oriented to (1) person, (2) place, and (3) time. There is a fourth domain that can be assessed by asking questions such as, "Why are you here?" or "What happened to you?" These questions assess orientation to circumstance, and documentation of correct answers in all four domains would be "oriented × 4."

Memory

Memory is the process of registration, retention, and recall of past experiences, knowledge, and ideas. Though there are many types of memory, the three most commonly assessed types are: immediate memory, short-term (recent) memory, and long-term (remote) memory.

Types of Memory

TYPE	DEFINITION	EXAMPLES
Immediate memory	Register and recall of information after an interval of a few seconds	Example: "repeat after me"
Short-term memory	Retrieve material after an interval of minutes, hours, or days	Example: remembering the date or what was eaten for lunch
Long-term memory	Recall of facts or events that occurred years before	Example: remembering birthdays or historical facts

The complex neurological processes involved in memory occur within the central nervous system and are not fully understood. This table offers a simplified depiction of types of memory.

Measurement Tools to Assess Overall Cognition

A common measurement tool used to assess overall cognition is the Mini-Mental State Exam (MMSE). This tool was designed to assess cognitive changes in older adults and can indicate intellectual impairment. Orientation, registration, attention/calculation, recall, and language are all assessed using the MMSE.

There are two main parts to the MMSE. The first part focuses on orientation, memory, and attention, while the second part focuses on the ability to name objects, follow verbal or written commands, and write a sentence. The maximum score possible is 30, with a score of 28 approximating normal and a score below 24 indicating cognitive impairment that is not considered normal for older persons. The score earned on the MMSE has also been shown to indicate depression. The MMSE is not sensitive to executive cognitive function.

Mini-Mental State Exam Score

SCORE	INTERPRETATION
Above 24	Normal
21–24	Mild intellectual impairment
16–20	Moderate intellectual impairment
Below 16	Severe intellectual impairment
Score of 19	Can be indicative of depression
Score of 9.7	Dementia

The MMSE is not a diagnostic tool, and it is not sensitive to executive cognitive function.

Motivation

Motivation can be defined as an inner urge that moves an individual to action. There are two main types of motivation: internal and external. Internal motivation is made up of past experiences and values, such as fears or desires. Learning about a client and his or her past allows an examiner to gain insight into what motivates a client. External motivation includes factors in the environment, such as privacy, expectations from others, temperature, or possible rewards. External motivation can be influenced by a well-designed environment and appropriate interactions with a client.

Assessment of Assistive and Adaptive Devices

Patients with neuromuscular impairments frequently use assistive or adaptive devices to augment their function. The PTA must be able to assess the fit and effectiveness of these devices.

Assessment of Activities of Daily Living

The effects of assistive and adaptive devices used during the performance of activities of daily living can be assessed using standardized tools designed for this purpose, as well as reports from the individual. There are multiple tools designed to assess independence in ADLs. However, self-report may be preferred under certain circumstances. The individual's assessment of the functionality and effectiveness of equipment used during ADLs is important, whether or not a standardized tool indicates independence. Therefore, it is best to combine the information gathered from these methods.

Functional Independence Measure (FIM)

The Functional Independence Measure assesses function from a physical, social, and psychological perspective. There are 18 items on the FIM, with levels ranging from total independence to total assistance. There are six self-care activities assessed, including feeding, grooming, bathing, upper body dressing, lower body dressing, and toileting. Functional mobility activities assessed include bed, chair, and wheelchair transfers; toilet transfers; tub or shower transfers; walking or use of a wheelchair; and stairs. The remaining items on the FIM assess sphincter control, communication, and social cognition.

The FIM uses observation to assess what the individual does, and not what *could be* done in certain

Functional Independence Measure Scores

SCORE	LEVELS	DESCRIPTION
No Helper		
7	Complete Independence	Safe and timely completion of the activity
6	Modified Independence	Safe completion of the activity with the use of adaptive or assistive devices
Helper-Modified Dependence		
5	Supervision	Individual performs 100% of the effort required to complete the activity, but requires supervision for safety
4	Minimal Assistance	Individual performs 75% or more of the effort required to complete the activity
3	Moderate Assistance	Individual performs 50% or more of the effort required to complete the activity
Helper-Complete Dependence		
2	Maximal Assistance	Individual performs 25% or more of the effort required to complete the activity
1	Total Assistance or Not Testable	Individual performs less than 25% of the effort required to complete the activity

Any clinician can administer the FIM after sufficient training in the scoring of each item.

circumstances or environments. The FIM is commonly used to show progress toward functional PT goals. It can also be used to determine whether or not it is appropriate to discharge a patient and what setting is most appropriate upon discharge. The individual can be scored from 1–7 on each item. All items must be scored, and if the individual does not perform an activity due to safety concerns, the activity is still scored as a 1 for "not testable." The previous table outlines the scores of the FIM and what each score indicates.

TAKE NOTE

An individual may be seen as independent in ADLs if physical assistance from another person is not needed. However, if an assistive or adaptive device is used to complete an activity, the FIM scores that as "modified independence," which is different than "complete independence."

Katz Index of Activities of Daily Living

The Katz Index of ADLs assesses the assistance needed to perform six basic ADLs: bathing, dressing, toileting, transferring, continence, and feeding. This tool combines the results of observation and the individual's self-report over a two-week period. No points are given if human help is required to complete an activity or if the activity is not performed. One point is given if the activity is performed without human help. If an activity is performed with the use of an assistive or adaptive device, the individual receives a point because the activity did not require physical assistance from another person.

The Katz Index of ADLs results in a letter grade from A through G, in order of increasing dependence. Explanations of each letter grade, as well as what *independent* and *dependent* mean in the context of each activity, are somewhat unique to the Katz Index and are fully explained on the test itself. For example, dressing includes getting clothes from closet and drawer; putting on the clothes; managing fasteners or buttons; and putting on any braces and outer garments, such as a jacket. With the results of this assessment, the PT and PTA can identify the areas of function in which the patient may need assistive or adaptive equipment. The assessment also indicates areas in which the patient is safely performing and which no longer need to be a focus of intervention.

Cranial and Peripheral Nerve Integrity

For individuals who present clinically with motor control impairments, assessment of cranial nerve and peripheral nerve integrity may reveal more about the cause of impairments. Assessment of cranial nerves is not commonly performed by PTAs. However, PTAs need to be knowledgeable about the cranial nerves and their functions in order to be able to recognize changes in the function of these nerves. Cranial nerve testing is based on the function of the nerve being tested and whether the tested nerve has sensory function, motor function, or both sensory and motor function. Peripheral nerve integrity is assessed using strength testing of muscles that correspond to the peripheral nerve innervations and sensation testing of areas of skin corresponding to the peripheral nerve innervations.

Cranial Nerves

There are 12 cranial nerves, with 11 distributed in the head and neck and one, the vagus nerve, distributed in the thorax and abdomen. Cranial nerves 1, 2, and 8 have sensory functions only and are responsible for the special senses. Cranial nerves 3, 4, 6, 11, and 12 have motor functions only and are responsible for eye movement, pupillary constriction, and innervations of the SCM, trapezius, and muscles of the tongue. The remaining four cranial nerves have both a motor and sensory function.

TAKE NOTE

Individuals who are suspected to have a brainstem lesion, a brain injury, or a cervical injury should undergo thorough and individual testing of the cranial nerves. Referral to another healthcare practitioner may be appropriate when possible cranial nerve deficits are discovered by the physical therapist or physical therapist assistant. For example, an individual with difficulty swallowing may need to be referred to a speech-language pathologist, or an individual who presents with a change in hearing may need to be referred to an audiologist.

Cranial Nerve Function and Testing

CRANIAL NERVES	SENSORY AND MOTOR FUNCTIONS	FUNCTION	TEST
1. Olfactory	Sensory only	Smell	Smell common odors such as lemon or coffee, one nostril at a time
2. Optic	Sensory only	Vision	Snellen eye chart, testing one eye at a time from a distance of 20 feet
3. Oculomotor	Motor only	Eye movement	Look up, down, and medially with the test eye
4. Trochlear	Motor only	Eye movement	Look down and medially with the test eye
5. Trigeminal	Motor and sensory	Facial sensation and muscles of mastication	Sensory: Detect pain and light touch sensations on forehead and cheeks Motor: Contract the muscles of mastication
6. Abducens	Motor only	Abduction (lateral movement) of eye	Look laterally with the test eye
7. Facial	Motor and sensory	Facial muscles and taste in anterior two-thirds of tongue	Sensory: Saline and sugar solution to anterior two-thirds of tongue Motor: Raise eyebrows, frown, smile, close eyes tightly, puff out both cheeks
8. Vestibulocochlear	Sensory only	Vestibular: balance and eye-head coordination Cochlear: hearing	Vestibular: Raise arm and bring finger to meet examiner's finger with eyes open and with eyes closed Cochlear: Move ticking watch away from ear until it is no longer heard
9. Glossopharyngeal	Primarily sensory	Taste in posterior one-third of tongue	Saline and sugar solution to posterior one-third of tongue
10. Vagus	Motor and sensory	Swallowing and gag reflex	Sensory: Lightly stimulate back of throat on each side Motor: Watch swallow mechanism
11. Accessory	Motor only	Muscles of the neck and trapezius	Shrug shoulders and maintain against examiner's resistance
12. Hypoglossal	Motor only	Movement of the tongue	Stick out tongue

The patient is asked to do a variety of things to test the integrity of the cranial nerves. Cranial nerve testing is most commonly performed by the PT at evaluation and may not be repeated at reexamination.

Manual Muscle Testing (MMT)

Manual muscle testing is an examination tool and grading system used to quantify muscle strength. It can provide information on the function of peripheral nerves that innervate the muscles tested. Manual muscle testing is so named because resistance is applied manually by the examiner to the body part being tested. The grading scale ranges from a numerical score of 0–5 or a named score of zero to normal.

There are several important concepts to understand in order to properly perform an MMT. The most important concept is gravity and how gravity affects the body's ability to move. The patient is asked to move the body part being tested against gravity through the full range of motion available at the joint. The patient must be positioned to be able to complete the full movement.

TAKE NOTE

When performing an MMT, be aware that full range of motion is the arc of motion the patient has available at the joint being tested—not necessarily "normal" according to the published range of motion norms.

If the patient can move through the full available range of motion against gravity, the grade assigned is at least a 3 out of 5. The examiner can then apply manual resistance in order to determine if a higher grade is possible. If the patient cannot move through the full available range against gravity, the grade assigned must be less than 3 out of 5, and the examiner will need to reposition the patient in order to decrease the effect of gravity on the movement. If the patient cannot move through the range of motion in a position where gravity is minimized (i.e., the horizontal plane), palpation of the muscle contraction becomes critical.

TAKE NOTE

For the most accurate testing, muscle substitution should not be permitted. The examiner must closely watch for muscles or muscle groups that attempt to compensate for the muscle being tested.

TAKE NOTE

In order to obtain consistent results, the patient must always be positioned appropriately, with the proximal segment stabilized. The therapist should document whether resistance was applied with a short or long lever arm for consistency on subsequent examinations.

There are two types of manual resistance that can be introduced in an MMT. The first, and most common, is a break test. In a break test, the examiner applies increasing isometric resistance until the patient's ability to resist is overcome, or maximum resistance is applied by the examiner. The second is a make test, in which maximum isotonic resistance is offered throughout the range of motion.

INFORMATION IN ACTION

A physical therapist asks you to perform an MMT in order to compare current strength to strength documented on evaluation. To ensure consistency and comparable results, you can review the PT evaluation to be certain that you perform the MMT in the same position, if standard positioning cannot be used.

Sensory Testing

Sensory testing is another way to obtain information about peripheral nerve integrity. There are various types of sensory testing, including light touch, superficial pain, temperature, vibration, and protective sensation.

Light Touch

A common test for the perception of tactile sensation is light touch. A tissue or a cotton ball can be used to conduct this test, in which the examiner lightly touches or strokes the skin. The patient should verbally, or with a hand gesture, indicate the first moment he or she recognizes that a stimulus has been applied.

TAKE NOTE

To prevent the patient from seeing when contact is made with the skin (and reacting accordingly), this test can be conducted with the patient's eyes closed.

Superficial Pain

Superficial pain can be assessed using sharp or dull stimuli and can be referred to as "sharp/dull discrimination." A clean safety pin or paper clip can be used to conduct this test. The examiner randomly and perpendicularly applies the sharp end or the dull end of the instrument to the patient's skin. The sharp end of the instrument should not be sharp enough to puncture the skin. The patient is asked to identify whether a sharp stimulus or dull stimulus was applied.

TAKE NOTE

To maintain consistent pressure with each application of the stimulus, the examiner should hold the instrument firmly and fingers should slide down the pin or paper clip once it is in contact with the skin.

Temperature

Identifying a warm or cool stimulus is another sensation test performed in physical therapy. The examiner fills one test tube with warm water and one with crushed ice. The side of each test tube is placed in contact with the skin, in random spots over the area being tested. The patient identifies whether the stimulus is hot or cold after each application.

Vibration

Vibration sense is tested using a 128 Hz tuning fork. In this test, the base of a vibrating tuning fork is placed on a bony prominence, such as the sternum or elbow. To begin, the examiner holds the base of the tuning fork between the thumb and forefinger and hits the tines of the tuning fork against an open palm. The base of the fork is then placed over the bony prominence, with care taken not to touch the fork and stop the vibration. The examiner randomly applies a vibrating tuning fork and nonvibrating tuning fork. The patient verbally responds, identifying whether he or she feels vibration or no vibration with each contact.

TAKE NOTE

It is often easy to hear the sound of the tines of a tuning fork hitting the examiner's palm, resulting in inaccurate test results. To minimize this, the examiner can hit the tuning fork with each application and touch the fork to stop vibration on those applications of a nonvibrating tuning fork. Alternatively, the examiner can provide soundproof earphones for the patient during the test.

Protective Sensation

Protective sensation of the lower extremities is commonly tested in order to screen for possible peripheral neuropathy. Monofilaments (plastic filaments of varying thicknesses) of varying sizes are applied perpendicularly to the skin until the monofilament bends. With eyes closed, the client reports whether or not the filament is touching the body part that is being tested. When a 4.17 monofilament (one gram of force) can be felt, this is considered normal sensation, and when a 5.07 monofilament (ten grams of force) can be felt, this is considered intact protective sensation.

Gait, Locomotion, and Balance

The PTA may assess several aspects of locomotion and gait, including the distance covered, equipment used, and the level of assistance required, as well as the quality of movement observed. Balance may be assessed qualitatively or with the use of standardized assessment tools.

Level of Assistance

Assessing the level of assistance required for gait and locomotion involves close observation and analysis of the individual performing these activities. Assistance levels can be labeled with descriptive terms, numbers, or a percentage of effort required for the activity. The following table outlines the various levels of assistance and multiple scales that can be used to describe assistance levels.

Levels of Assistance during Gait and Locomotion

DESCRIPTIVE TERM	DESCRIPTION
Independent	Consistent and safe locomotion without physical assistance or assistive device
Modified Independent	Consistent and safe locomotion with the use of an assistive device and without physical assistance
Supervision	Observation of locomotion as a precaution and cues (if needed) in order to ensure safety
Close Guarding	Verbal cues and physical assistance are close by and ready if needed, but no physical touch is required
Contact Guarding	Hands on the individual and cueing due to a high probability of the individual needing physical assistance
Minimal Assistance	Able to complete the majority of the effort required for locomotion
Moderate Assistance	Able to complete approximately half of the effort required for locomotion
Maximum Assistance	Able to complete a part, but less than half, of the effort required for locomotion
Total Assistance	Unable to assist and total physical assistance required for locomotion

Cueing can include verbal, visual, or tactile cues.

INFORMATION IN ACTION

You are reviewing a PT evaluation, and you notice that the PT has indicated that the patient's sit-to-stand activity requires minimal assistance. There is also a description of the patient's participation in the transfer as scooting to the edge of the chair and pushing up from the arms of the chair, which does not seem to agree with the assistance level. You consult the PT, and he explains that the patient required 85% effort to complete the task. This is a common mistake made when describing levels of assistance. You should tactfully discuss with the PT that the percentage effort used to describe levels of assistance is the effort the patient puts forth in the transfer, not the amount of effort by the PT or PTA. Therefore, this patient would require maximum assistance because the patient performs 15% of the effort.

Gait Deviations

Gait is a complex process, requiring the coordination and proper timing of muscle activation and joint movement. Superficial gait analysis may be appropriate when overall function is the primary concern, and this type of analysis may include items such as the level of assistance required, the assistive device used, the gait pattern chosen, speed and distance walked, and any gait deviations noted. Some individuals with motor and neurological impairments will require a more in-depth examination of gait, when gait analysis is the primary concern. There are various pieces of equipment and assessment tools used to analyze gait. However, observational gait analysis remains the most commonly used tool, allowing qualitative and quantitative data to be collected while an individual walks.

Observational gait analysis involves each segment of the body during all phases of a gait cycle. The gait cycle begins when the heel or other part of the foot makes contact with the ground and ends when the heel or other part of the same foot makes contact with the ground. When performing observational gait analysis, the examiner should select one joint or body segment and review the normal movements that occur at that body part during gait. Observation of that joint or body segment during all phases of the gait cycle should be complete before moving on to analyze another part of the body. Both sides of the body should be observed during gait analysis because some gait deviations cannot be seen from certain perspectives.

There are two primary systems of terminology used for qualitative gait analysis: traditional terminology and the Ranchos Los Amigos Observation Gait Analysis system. The two systems are compared in the following table:

Gait Terminology Systems

TRADITIONAL TERMINOLOGY	DESCRIPTION	RANCHOS LOS AMIGOS TERMINOLOGY	DESCRIPTION
Heel strike	Heel of reference foot contacts the walking surface.	Initial contact	Any part of reference foot makes contact with the walking surface.
Foot flat	Sole of reference lowers to the surface, and foot makes contact with the walking surface.	Loading response	Nonreference leg leaves the walking surface.

Gait Terminology Systems (*continued*)

TRADITIONAL TERMINOLOGY	DESCRIPTION	RANCHOS LOS AMIGOS TERMINOLOGY	DESCRIPTION
Midstance	Body passes directly over the reference leg.	Midstance	Body weight is directly over reference leg.
Heel-off	Body weight shifts forward, and heel of the reference foot leaves the walking surface.	Terminal stance	Heel of reference foot rises off the walking surface, and toes leave the walking surface.
Toe-off	Only the toes of the reference foot are in contact with the walking surface.	Preswing	Initial contact of non-reference leg, and body weight shifts forward over the nonreference leg.
Acceleration	Toe of the reference foot leaves the walking surface, and the reference leg moves directly under the body.	Initial swing	Reference leg leaves the walking surface, and reference knee maximally flexes.
Midswing	Reference leg passes below the body.	Midswing	There is maximal knee flexion of reference leg to vertical tibial position.
Deceleration	Reference leg decelerates and prepares for heel strike.	Terminal swing	Reference knee extends and prepares for initial contact.

The terminology of these two systems should not be combined when referring to the phases and portions of the gait cycle.

INFORMATION IN ACTION

You are reviewing the chart of a patient who was evaluated yesterday. The PT has left you a note asking you to collect qualitative data of the patient's gait. With the knowledge of the phases and portions of gait, as well as the terminology described in this section, you are able to complete this data collection. Qualitative gait analysis includes descriptions of joint angles, movements, and deviations from normal gait and is described using the terms outlined in the previous table. Quantitative gait analysis includes collecting data on temporal and spatial variables, such as gait speed, gait velocity, stride length, and step length. For a thorough analysis of gait, both forms of gait analysis can be performed.

In order for accurate measurements of spatial and temporal variables to be made, the examiner must understand what each variable is and why it is important to the analysis of gait. The following table outlines quantitative measurements and what they mean within the context of the gait cycle.

TAKE NOTE

Gait speed and walking velocity may seem like very similar terms and are often incorrectly used interchangeably. Gait speed is the speed at which an individual walks in any direction on any path. If the same path is covered more than once, the distance covered is still part of the calculation for gait speed. Speed is distance divided by unit of time. Velocity is the measurement of the forward translation of an object moving in one direction and indicates how far an individual walked in one direction over a unit of time.

Knowledge of the qualitative and quantitative kinematics occurring during a normal gait cycle can help the examiner identify deviations. In addition, knowing the muscles that are active during each phase and portion of a normal gait cycle can assist the examiner in identifying a possible source of a gait deviation if one is observed.

Quantitative Gait Variables

VARIABLE	DESCRIPTION
Gait speed	The distance walked, divided by the amount of time it takes the patient to walk that distance. The individual can walk in any direction, and the entire distance walked must be accurately measured.
Free gait speed	An individual's normal, self-selected gait speed
Walking velocity	Number of steps taken in a unit of time; can be measured by counting the number of steps taken in a certain time period

Quantitative Gait Variables (*continued*)

VARIABLE	DESCRIPTION
Stride time	Time elapsed from heel strike of one foot to the next heel strike of the same foot
Step time	Time that elapses from the moment one foot makes contact to the moment the other foot makes contact with the walking surface
Stride length	Distance measured between the heel strike of one foot to the next heel strike of the same foot
Cadence	Number of steps taken per minute
Step length	Distance measured between the heel strike of one foot and the next heel strike of the other foot
Swing time	Time during the gait cycle that one foot is not in contact with the walking surface
Double support time	Time during the gait cycle when both feet are in contact with the walking surface
Step width	Distance measured between both feet

These variables can be measured with simple equipment (such as a tape measure and stopwatch) or with complex equipment (such as force plates or pressure switches in the insole of an individual's shoe).

Muscle Activity During Gait

MUSCLE	ACTIVITY
Hamstrings	Peak activity during swing phase as the leg decelerates
Quadriceps	Peak activity during early stance phase, single leg support
Gastroc-soleus	Peak activity during stance phase and raising the heel off the ground during heel-off
Anterior tibialis	Peak activity just after heel strike when the foot is lowered to the ground by eccentric control, and during swing to clear toes

It is important to understand what muscles are working during gait in order to assist in identifying the reason for a gait deviation noted during observation.

The following is a list of some of the terms used to describe common gait deviations, and knowledge of these terms and their meanings can assist the examiner in recognizing a gait deviation and possibly identifying the source of the deviation:

- **Antalgic gait.** Weight-bearing is avoided due to pain. This avoidance often results in a shortened stance phase of the painful extremity.
- **Ataxic gait.** Wide-based gait, unsteady, with the inability to walk in tandem; the individual often staggers with eyes open or eyes closed. This type of gait can be the result of central nervous system pathologies or cerebellar lesions.
- **Steppage gait.** High knee lifting when advancing the affected extremity and slapping the foot on the ground. This type of gait may indicate weakness or paralysis of the dorsiflexor musculature.
- **Genu recurvatum gait.** Excessive or hyperextension of the knee in the stance phase of gait. This type of gait may indicate poor control of the extremity when accepting weight, such as poor eccentric quadriceps control.
- **Hip extensor gait.** Thorax thrusts posterior at heel strike in order to maintain hip extension, and the knee is fully extended. This type of gait may indicate weakness of the gluteus maximus muscle.
- **Trendelenburg gait.** Pelvis dips when the unaffected extremity is in the swing phase. This type of gait may indicate a weak gluteus medius muscle.
- **Hemiparetic gait.** Circumduction of the paretic extremity and initial contact to the floor with the forefoot. This type of gait is also present when one leg is shorter than the other.
- **Parkinsonian gait.** Minimal extension of the ankle, knee, hip, and trunk; decreased step length and reciprocal arm swing; shuffling and possible festination. This type of gait may indicate Parkinson's disease.

- **Scissoring gait.** Leg that is in the swing phase crosses over the stance leg. This type of gait may be due to excessive hip adduction.
- **Dystrophic gait.** Hips roll from side to side during the stance phase in order to shift body weight with the appearance of waddling. This type of gait can be seen with various myopathies, for example, muscular dystrophy.

TAKE NOTE

The skill of analyzing gait through observation requires a lot of training, regardless of the terminology. Observing gait and then comparing analysis with an experienced practitioner's knowledge is a good way to become comfortable with this skill.

Functional Gait Assessments
Timed Up and Go Test

The timed up and go test, which you may recall from earlier in the chapter, assesses an individual's basic mobility skills. It is made up of functional activities like standing up from a chair and walking at a self-selected pace. This test requires that an individual stand up from an armchair, walk ten meters, turn around, walk back to the chair, and return to sitting. One practice run is permitted. The examiner begins timing at the cue word "go" and stops when the individual is sitting all the way back in the chair. The individual's normal assistive device is permitted to be used during this test, and no other physical assistance can be given.

The examiner records the time of three TUG trials and averages the three times for a final score. This score is then compared to TUG norms, as seen in the following table. Included are average TUG times for healthy individuals and cutoff scores that indicate that assistance is needed.

Timed Up and Go Test Norms

AGE	TUG TIME	CUTOFF SCORES	INTERPRETATION
60–69 years old	8.1	< 10 seconds	Freely mobile
70–79 years old	9.2	> 20 seconds	May need assistive device
80–89 years old	11.3	> 30 seconds	Dependent

There are multiple interpretations of this tool that are not in perfect agreement, so the most common use of the TUG test remains to determine if individuals' function lies within the normal range for their age.

INFORMATION IN ACTION

You are asked to complete TUG trials with a patient by a PTA who had an emergency with another patient. You perform two trials of this test, and you are concerned that the times you noted are significantly different than the times the other PTA noted on the first trial and practice run. The most likely reason for the discrepancy is that you both started timing at different points in the test. Be sure to include in your instructions to the patient that the time starts when you say "go" and stops when the individual is seated all the way back in the chair. The reason for this is the desire to capture how long it actually takes an individual to initiate movement after the cue to "go"—and this may include positioning hands on the armrests or scooting forward, all of which are part of the sit-to-stand transition for that individual. Also, be sure to keep timing until the individual completes the transition to sitting and is seated all the way back in the chair.

Tinetti Performance Oriented Mobility Assessment

As you may recall from earlier in the chapter, the Tinetti tool is made up of two separate subscales: one assessing balance and the other assessing gait. The combination of these two Tinetti subscales make up the Performance Oriented Mobility Assessment, and measure an individual's gait and balance on a numerical scale. The balance subscale has ten components with a maximum score of 16; and the gait subscale has six components with a maximum score of 12. This tool is commonly used to identify a patient's fall risk. This tool focuses on functional balance activities, such as forward reach, sit-to-stand, and turning, as well as gait characteristics like trunk mobility, step length, and symmetry. The maximum score possible is 28. A score of less than 19 indicates high fall risk, and a score between 19 and 24 indicates moderate fall risk.

Dynamic Gait Index

The Dynamic Gait Index is used to assess the characteristics of gait in individuals with balance or vestibular deficits. It can also be used pre- and post-intervention to determine the effects of intervention. There is a long, eight-item version and short, four-item version of the DGI. Gait characteristics are scored from 0–3. The maximum possible score is 24 on the long version and 12 on the short version. The DGI evaluates the following items:

- gait on level surfaces
- horizontal head turns and vertical head turns
- gait with pivoting and stopping (long version only)
- gait with speed changes
- stepping over obstacles (long version only)
- walking around obstacles (long version only)
- stairs (long version only)

Dynamic Gait Index Score Interpretation

SCORE	INTERPRETATION
< 20 out of 24	Related to falls in community-dwelling older adults
< 12 out of 12	Balance deficits
< 10 out of 12	Fall risk

The measurement properties of the four-item DGI are equivalent to those of the eight-item version.

Standardized Balance Assessments
Berg Balance Scale

The Berg Balance Scale is a tool made up of 14 common functional activities that become progressively more difficult for the individual being tested. Each item is rated on a scale from 0–4, with a maximum score possible of 56. The BBS is a strong fall predictor, and it can be used to identify the functional areas in which instability or fear is present. This scale can be used to compare fall risk before and after intervention. The 13 items on the BBS are as follows:

- sitting to standing
- standing unsupported
- sitting with back unsupported and feet supported on floor
- standing to sitting
- transfer from seat without armrests to a seat with armrests
- standing with feet together
- reaching forward in standing
- picking up an object on the floor from standing position
- turning to look over left and right shoulders in standing
- turning 360 degrees
- placing alternate foot on step while standing
- tandem standing (one foot in front of the other)
- standing on one leg

The numerical score earned on the BBS is compared to predetermined cutoffs that indicate fall risk. A score of 45 or below indicates a high fall risk. The BBS can be useful in predicting falls in the elderly, evaluating change in patients who are participating in physical therapy, and measuring recovery. The organization of the BBS allows the examiner to identify the specific areas of balance deficits, allowing the PT plan of care to focus on those specific areas and related areas of balance.

TAKE NOTE

When assessing balance using the BBS, the patient is not permitted to use an assistive device. However, the patient is permitted to wear any orthosis he or she typically uses. This allows the patient's true balance to be assessed; and once true balance is determined, the appropriate assistive device can be recommended for the balance deficits noted. This may be important for individuals who are using assistive devices that are not specifically prescribed for them.

Functional Reach Test

The functional reach test measures how far forward an individual can reach while standing in one place. Standing perpendicular to a yardstick secured to the wall, the patient flexes the shoulder that is against the wall to 90 degrees, with the elbow fully extended and hand in a fist position. The tip of the third metacarpal is used for measurement purposes. With the tip of the third metacarpal at a baseline measurement of zero, the examiner instructs the patient to reach as far forward as possible without taking a step. Two practice trials are given, and the distance reached during three test trials are averaged for a final score.

The final measurement is then compared to cutoff scores that indicate fall risk, as well as published norms for certain age groups. The published norms can be a guide for creating a goal for a patient to perform within the age-related norm if appropriate.

TAKE NOTE

A common compensation technique is twisting of the trunk in order to move the arm further along the yardstick. Be sure to make the official measurement before the patient begins to twist, and measure this way consistently each time you perform the test, in order to be able to accurately compare a patient's scores.

Functional Reach Test Interpretation

REACH DISTANCE	INTERPRETATION
0 inches	Likelihood of falling twice increases eightfold.
6 inches	Likelihood of falling twice increases fourfold.
> 6 inches and < 10 inches	Likelihood of falling twice within two months increases twofold.

The results of this test can be a persuasive and motivating screening tool when an individual is aware of what the results mean, in terms of fall risk.

Functional Reach Test Averages by Age

AGE	INTERPRETATION	WOMEN'S SCORES (in inches)
20–40 years old	16.7	14.6
41–69 years old	14.9	13.8
70–87 years old	13.2	10.5

The distance reached is influenced by many factors, such as overall health, gender, age, height, and size of the individual being tested.

Multidirectional Reach Test

The Multidirectional reach test is an assessment tool similar to the functional reach test and provides information about the risk of falling forward, backward, right, and left. The patient stands perpendicular to a yardstick at shoulder height, with the shoulder flexed to 90 degrees for the forward and backward reach. The patient then stands parallel to the yardstick, with the shoulder abducted to 90 degrees for the reach to the right or left. The patient is instructed to reach as far as possible without stepping. The end of the second finger is used as the endpoint for measurement. The starting measurement is subtracted from the end measurement, to show the total distance the patient reached in each direction. The distance is measured in inches. The patient reaches forward, backward, to the right, and finally to the left. Information on how the patient is able to balance in these four directions allows for a better understanding of real-life situations, when he or she may need to lean to the side or backward.

One-Legged Stance Test

The one-legged stance test is a tool used to measure static control of posture. This test can also measure fall risk. This test is very easy and quick to perform, with a stopwatch being the only equipment that is needed. The test posture is the patient standing on his or her dominant bare foot, with arms folded across the chest and eyes open. The timing starts as soon as the non-test foot leaves the ground. There are certain conditions that stop the test including:

- The non-test, suspended foot touches the ground.
- The non-test, suspended leg supports the weight-bearing leg.
- The test foot moves from original test position.

If none of these conditions stop the test, the examiner should stop the test after 30 seconds. There are normal values to which the test individual's time can be compared and a cutoff score indicating risk for injurious fall.

One-Legged Stance Test Norms

AGE	TIME
65–74 years old	9.7 seconds
< 75 years old	5.6 seconds
All ages	< 5 seconds indicates risk for injurious fall

This test should not be performed with individuals who have lower extremity weight-bearing restrictions of any kind.

TAKE NOTE

The one-legged stance test is a quick screening tool that can be used to identify fall risk in a situation where the PT or PTA does not have time to perform lengthy balance assessments. The objective identification of fall risk may be enough to motivate an individual to seek help or intervention for balance deficits. For example, a community health fair often includes brief assessments such as vital signs, and a brief balance screening tool can be a great addition.

Sensory Organization Test (SOT)

The body uses primarily visual and somatosensory input for postural orientation. When not impaired or altered, this input allows the body to maintain accurate postural orientation. The sensory organization test measures the body's sway while the patient attempts to stand still. There are six different conditions under which body sway is measured. These conditions involve varying alterations of somatosensory and visual input. The platform under the patient can be static or moving, and the visual reference point for postural orientation is altered. The baseline condition is normal vision and fixed support. The conditions under which the patient's body sways can indicate which balance mechanisms are impaired and can help to discover the source of balance deficits. The PT intervention can then be tailored to the specific needs of the individual. The six test conditions of the SOT are as follows:

- normal vision, fixed support
- absent vision, fixed support
- sway-referenced vision, fixed support
- normal vision, sway-referenced support
- absent vision, sway-referenced support
- sway-referenced vision, sway-referenced support

Pediatric Mobility Assessment

Standardized tests exist that specifically measure elements of motor function in children.

The Gross Motor Function Measure (GMFM) is a tool used to assess change in the gross motor function of children with cerebral palsy and Down syndrome. This tool allows for the examination of change over time and is appropriate for children who perform up to the level expected of a five-year-old. The GMFM assesses rolling, crawling, kneeling, sitting, standing, walking, running, and jumping.

The Gross Motor Performance Measure (GMPM) was designed to be used with the GMFM. It assesses body alignment in space, coordination, movement dissociation, postural stability, and weight shifting.

The GMPM has 20 items and is used with the same population as that of the GMFM.

Assessment of Motor Function

Motor control involves the interaction of multiple complex body systems. Some motor responses will emerge during the process of normal growth and development, while others are learned when exploring and discovering specific environments. A physical therapist can evaluate motor control through observation, and a physical therapist assistant must be knowledgeable of the assessment techniques and how the results affect the PT intervention. Some of the possible assessment techniques are outlined in the following table:

Measurement of Motor Response

MEASUREMENT	EXAMPLES OF ACTIVITIES
Time taken to initiate a response to a command or desire for movement	Time between the commands to "go" and the initiation of the movement
Time taken to complete a given task	Time to walk a predetermined distance
Number of successful attempts	Number of successful transfers compared to total attempts at the transfer
Number of trials required for completion	Number of practice trials required before correct response is demonstrated
Time spent on/off balance	Time that center of gravity remains within base of support

These types of assessments can assist in setting goals, such as a certain desired start time or an ideal number of attempts to complete a task.

Coordination

Motor coordination can be divided into two main categories: gross and fine. The four motor tasks assessed through coordination tests are:

- **Mobility.** Initial movement that occurs within a movement pattern (example: initial muscle contraction)
- **Stability.** Ability to maintain a steady antigravity posture while bearing weight (example: increased body sway in standing)
- **Controlled mobility.** Ability to change position while remaining stable (example: inability to transition from sitting to standing)
- **Skill.** Highly coordinated movements (example: inability to stabilize proximal segments to allow distal segments to move)

The following screening tools assess motor coordination and can identify coordination impairments such as dysdiadochokinesia, dysmetria, akinesia, etc.:

Finger to nose. The individual abducts the shoulder to 90 degrees with the elbow extended and brings the tip of the index finger to meet the tip of the nose.

Pronation/supination. With elbows held at the side of the body and flexed 90 degrees, the individual alternates pronation and supination of the forearm. A similar test of reverse movements between opposing muscle groups can be performed at other joints, such as flexing/extending the knee or elbow.

Heel on shin. From a supine position, the individual slides the heel of one foot up and down the shin of the opposite leg.

Fingertip to thumb. The individual touches the tip of the thumb to the tip of each finger in sequence.

Finger to examiner's finger. The examiner sits directly across from the individual being tested. With the examiner's index finger held up, the individual's index finger touches the tip of the examiner's index finger. The examiner can change the position of the target to assess change in distance or direction.

Patients with impaired coordination have trouble controlling the speed, course, and volume of movement. The following terms describe various coordination impairments:

- **Dysdiadochokinesia.** Impaired ability to perform rapid alternating movements
- **Dysmetria.** Inability to judge distance of a movement
- **Dyssynergia.** Inability to perform movement in one smooth motion (movement is performed in a sequence of individual motions instead)
- **Asynergia.** Inability to associate muscle for complex movements
- **Akinesia.** Inability to initiate movement
- **Bradykinesia.** Decreased amplitude of movement

In addition to these impairments, muscle tone also affects movement and coordination. The following terms identify different impairments of muscle tone.

- **Dystonia.** Impaired or disordered tone which can affect one part of the body or adjacent segments of the body
- **Hypertonicity.** An increase in muscle tone seen as increased resistance to passive motion
- **Hypotonicity.** A decrease in muscle tone seen as decreased resistance to passive motion
- **Rigidity.** A form of hypertonicity that presents as uniform increased resistance throughout a range of motion and not affected by the velocity of the movement
- **Spasticity.** A form of hypertonicity which presents as velocity-dependent increased resistance to passive stretch

Assessment of muscle tone includes observation of muscles at rest and tests of passive motions.

Observation

The examiner should note the posture of the trunk, extremities, and head. Spasticity can cause fixed postures, while hypotonic extremities will appear floppy. Hypertonic muscles look and feel taut and harder than a muscle with normal tone.

Passive Motion

When performing passive motion testing, the examiner is looking for the responsiveness of a relaxed muscle when stretched. The muscle being tested should be moved in multiple directions. A hypertonic extremity feels stiff, while a hypotonic extremity feels unresponsive and heavy. The examiner must be sure to vary the speed of movement, in order to differentiate spasticity from rigidity. Comparison should be made between the left and right side.

Changes in muscle tone may be difficult to measure and quantify objectively. There is a numerical scale used to grade muscle tone, as well as the Modified Ashworth Scale that assesses spasticity.

Muscle Tone Grade

GRADE	DESCRIPTION
0	No response
1+	Decreased response
2+	Normal response
3+	Exaggerated response
4+	Sustained response

This scale is subjective, depending on the examiner's judgment of what is decreased or exaggerated.

Modified Ashworth Scale

GRADE	DESCRIPTION
0	No increase in muscle tone
1	Slight increase in tone, with minimal resistance at the end of the range of motion
1+	Slight increase in tone, with a catch or resistance throughout the remainder of the range of motion
2	Marked increase in tone through most of the range of motion
3	Significant increase in tone, with passive movement becoming difficult
4	Rigid flexion or extension

This scale is considered the gold standard for grading spasticity.

Muscle Performance

Muscle performance is the ability of a muscle to generate force and involves muscle strength, power, and endurance. Muscle strength is the measurement of the force exerted against maximal resistance. Muscle power is the product of strength combined with speed. And muscle endurance is the ability to sustain these forces repeatedly or over time. These three properties of muscle performance are all assessed with a variety of tools that will be discussed here.

Manual Muscle Testing

Muscle strength is the force exerted by a muscle to overcome resistance, and one way to assess strength is the manual muscle test. The resistance that a muscle is trying to overcome during a MMT is the manual resistance offered by the PTA. The MMT grading scale ranges from a numerical score of 0–5 or named score of zero to normal.

The most important concept in MMT is gravity's effect on the body's ability to move. The individual is asked to move the body part being tested against gravity, through the full range of motion available at the joint. The body part must be positioned to be able to complete the movement against gravity. If the patient can move through the full available range of motion against gravity, the grade assigned is at least a 3 out of 5. The examiner can then apply manual resistance in order to determine whether a higher grade is possible. If the patient cannot move through the full available range against gravity, the grade assigned must be less than 3 out of 5—and the examiner will need to reposition the patient in order to decrease the effect of gravity. If the patient cannot move through the range of motion in this gravity-minimized position, palpation of muscle contraction becomes critical.

Dynamometry

A portable dynamometer is a device that measures mechanical force. When testing muscle performance using a dynamometer, the examiner reads the amount of force being applied as the patient pushes into the dynamometer. One benefit of a dynamometer is its ability to give a more objective muscle test than the MMT scale. However, it can be difficult to position the patient appropriately for all muscle groups when using a dynamometer, and it may be difficult for some examiners to produce enough force for a break test.

Isokinetic dynamometers are not portable, and they allow for the evaluation of many additional aspects of muscle performance. Velocity of muscle shortening, peak torque produced by the muscle, and the arc of excursion can all be assessed with an isokinetic dynamometer. Concentric and eccentric contractions can be analyzed as comparisons of reciprocal muscles around a joint. These two features can be very helpful in understanding why and how a patient carries out functional activities.

Electromyography/Biofeedback

Electromyography is another tool that can be used to assess motor performance. This type of EMG is referred to as kinesiological EMG. An EMG can detect electrical potentials produced by skeletal muscle fibers and can help the examiner to understand the role of muscles in specific activities. The examiner can look at characteristics of a muscle, such as muscle response, onset and duration of muscle activity, muscle fatigue, and type of muscle contraction. This type of assessment is performed by physical therapists trained in the use of EMG biofeedback—especially the application and use of surface and percutaneous electrodes. The PTA should have knowledge of the information gathered from an EMG assessment and understand how this data relates to the PT plan of care. Electromyography also allows for objective documentation of the effects of physical therapy intervention on muscle function. EMG biofeedback can be useful in the assessment and treatment of motor function, neuromuscular dysfunction, and musculoskeletal pain.

Muscle Power and Muscle Endurance

Muscle power and endurance can also be assessed with the use of timed activity tests. The 30 second sit-to-stand test is a common functional performance measure that can reveal muscle strength and endurance of the lower extremities in adults. To perform this test, the examiner instructs the patient to sit in a chair with his or her feet a shoulder's width apart and with arms across the chest. The patient then stands as many times as possible in 30 seconds. The number of sit-to-stands is then compared to normal values by age range and gender, as seen here:

30 Second Sit-to-Stand Test Norms

AGE (in years)	NUMBER OF SIT-TO STANDS	AGE (in years)	NUMBER OF SIT-TO STANDS
Men		Women	
60–64	14–19	60–64	12–17
65–69	12–18	65–69	11–16
70–74	12–17	70–74	10–15
75–79	11–17	75–79	10–15
80–84	10–15	80–84	9–14
85–89	8–14	85–89	8–13
89–90	7–12	90–94	4–11

The ability to stand up from a standard-height chair, without assistance, is commonly lost as individuals age and become less active.

Motor Skills: Acquisition and Evolution

Primitive and postural reflexes. During normal development, certain primitive and postural reflexes emerge at predictable times. Primitive reflexes are outgrown at predictable times. Pediatric patients undergo reflex assessment in order to determine their level of development and whether or not the child is experiencing any delay in development. The emergence and disappearance of primitive and postural reflexes have a significant impact on the acquisition of motor skills because abnormal reflexes can prevent a child from being able to move into certain postures required to learn specific motor milestones.

The assessment of primitive and postural developmental reflexes is important because of the significant effects on muscle tone, movement, balance, and function. A PTA may be asked to assess reflexes in order to determine a child's functional development.

Primitive reflexes are so named because they are present at birth and are innate motor responses that assist in survival, such as the sucking reflex associated with breast-feeding. Primitive reflexes can also reappear in adults in cases of neurological insults. Postural reflexes are so named because an individual is attempting to orient the body to the environment in an upright posture. Some postural reflexes, such as protection and equilibrium reactions, emerge in childhood and are maintained through adulthood. When assessing postural reflexes, the PTA must be sure to position the child appropriately in order to observe the full reflex or reaction. The following table identifies the reflex, testing position, stimulus, and anticipated response of the child being tested.

Primitive Reflexes

REFLEX	TESTING POSITION	STIMULUS	ANTICIPATED RESPONSE
Flexor withdrawal (0–2 months)	Supine or sitting	Apply noxious stimulus to bottom of foot (example: pinprick)	Toe extension, dorsiflexion, uncontrollable leg flexion
Crossed extension (0–2 months)	Supine with one leg fixed in extension	Apply noxious stimulus to ball of foot of extended leg	Opposite leg flexion, adduction, and extension
Moro (28 weeks gestation–2 months)	Sitting	Change the position of the head in relation to trunk (for example, shift child backward while in sitting position)	Extension, adduction of arms, and opening of hands followed by flexion, adduction, and arms across chest
Startle (0–6 months)	Any position	Make a sudden, loud noise	Upper extremity extension and abduction
Palmar grasp (28 weeks gestation–4 months)	Any position	Apply pressure to palm of hand	Flexion of fingers

Primitive Reflexes (*continued*)

REFLEX	TESTING POSITION	STIMULUS	ANTICIPATED RESPONSE
Plantar grasp (28 weeks gestation–9 months)	Supine or sitting	Apply pressure to ball of foot under the toes	Flexion of toes
Asymmetrical tonic neck reflex (0–6 months)	Supine most common	Rotate head to the side	Extension of arms and legs on side the child's face is turned; flexion of arms and legs on opposite side
Symmetrical tonic neck reflex (6–8 months)	Supine most common	Flex or extend the head and neck	Head flexion: flexion of arms and extension of legs; head extension: extension of arms and flexion of legs
Babinski (0–12 months)	Supine or sitting	Touch or stroke the lateral aspect of the sole of the foot	Extension and fanning of toes
Sucking (28 weeks gestation–2 months)	Any position	Touch or stroke the cheek	Turning of head toward touch with mouth open
Rooting (28 weeks gestation–3 months)	Any position	Place an object in the mouth	Sucking

Children's primitive reflexes are controlled by the central nervous system. They are inhibited by the central nervous system as the child develops and the reflexes are no longer needed.

Postural Reflexes

REFLEX	POSTURE	STIMULUS	ANTICIPATED RESPONSE
Neck righting (0–6 months)	Supine	Passive rotation of head to one side	Whole body rotation in attempt to align body with head
Body righting (2 months–5 years)	Supine	Passive rotation of trunk (upper or lower)	Body segment not rotated follows segment that was rotated in attempt to align body segments
Optical righting (1 month–adulthood)	Upright standing or sitting	Tip body in any direction	Orientation of head to vertical position
Upper extremity protective extension (4 months–adulthood)	Sitting or standing	Displace center of gravity outside base of support	Fingers and elbows extend, and child flexes, abducts, or extends shoulders toward direction of displacement
Lower extremity protective extension (4 months–adulthood)	Standing	Displace center of gravity outside base of support	Child steps in the direction of displacement
Equilibrium reaction (5 months–adulthood)	Sitting or standing	Displace center of gravity but not outside base of support	Trunk curves toward the displacement force, extension and abduction of extremities on side of force

Many of these reflexes allow for protection and orientation of the body, so they are seen in childhood as well as throughout adulthood.

Motor Milestones

Motor development is a process common to all individuals and continues throughout the lifespan. The motor milestones most commonly tested are those demonstrated by children from birth to adolescence. These milestones are commonly used as benchmarks by which normal and timely development are measured. The timing of the development of motor milestones is unique to each individual—however, there are common age ranges in which children demonstrate certain motor behaviors. In adolescence, individuals do not learn new milestones but work on refining learned behaviors.

Different motor behaviors are seen in different positions as the child is discovering the environment from all positions, such as prone, supine, kneeling, etc. There are also fine motor milestones of the upper extremities and locomotion milestones that are identified.

Motor Milestones

AGE RANGE	MILESTONE IN PRONE POSITION	MILESTONE IN SUPINE POSITION	UPPER EXTREMITY MOTOR MILESTONES	LOCOMOTION MILESTONES
0–1 month	Lifting head and turning head to the side	Turning head side to side	Jerky arm movement	Making crawling movements
2–3 months	Lifting head to 90 degrees, bearing weight on arms, initiating rolling	Hand to foot play	Briefly holding a toy placed in the hand, moving hands to mouth and midline	Pivoting 30 degrees in prone
4–6 months	Reaching and pushing up on extended arms	Initiates rolling supine to side-lying	Grabbing objects within reach, holding objects with two hands, and bringing objects to mouth	Full pivoting in prone
7–10 months	Rocking on hands and knees, transitioning into sitting	Lifting head as in sitting	Grasp progressing from radial to inferior to lateral, spontaneously releasing objects	Moving forward on belly, pushing up to hands and knees, pulling to stand
11–12 months	Transitioning to standing		Using objects as tools	Walking with one hand held, transitioning stand to sit
13–14 months	Transitioning to standing using a half-kneel		Grasping with thumb and first two fingers	Walking without support, stooping and returning to stand, walking backward
15–18 months	Creeping up stairs, walking up stairs with support		Propelling a ball, finger poking	Carrying objects while walking, walking sideways, initiating running
19–22 months			Building towers with cubes	Ascending stairs with step-to pattern

Motor Milestones (*continued*)

AGE RANGE	MILESTONE IN PRONE POSITION	MILESTONE IN SUPINE POSITION	UPPER EXTREMITY MOTOR MILESTONES	LOCOMOTION MILESTONES
24 months				Kicking a ball, throwing a ball forward, jumping off low step
30 months			Initiating strokes with a crayon	Jumping with one foot leading
3–3½ years			Buttoning and unbuttoning, hand dominance emerging, stringing beads	Propelling self on tricycle, reciprocating arms while running, briefly balancing on one foot
4–4½ years			Grasping pencils with tripod grasp, cutting shapes from paper, dropping objects in a jar	Hopping up to three times, walking on tiptoes, catching large ball, jumping with both feet
5–8 years			Drawing letters, numbers, and shapes, placing pegs in a pegboard	Jumping forward, sideways, and over small objects; skipping, bouncing a ball
9–12 years			Handwriting developing and learning to draw	Mature running, jumping, and throwing techniques

Not every child will reach these motor milestones in the "normal" time frame, while other children will skip some milestones and move right on to more complex movements. However, this can still be considered normal development for the child if there are no functional setbacks.

INFORMATION IN ACTION

Knowledge of the common motor milestones allows the PTA to observe infants and children during normal activities, such as play, and to identify whether or not the infant or child is interacting with the environment using age-expected movements and transitions. A child's job is discovering the environment; and play is the primary way they make this discovery. The PTA working with infants and children will need to identify play activities that will promote the functional movement or transition that the child is trying to learn.

Sensory Integration

Sensory integration involves the ability of the brain to organize, interpret, and use sensory information. This sensory information is what the body uses to plan and perform its motor programs. Disorders of sensory integration can have a significant impact on an individual's motor and cognitive function. Therefore, it is an important area for the PT to evaluate and an important part of the intervention provided by the PTA.

Sensory integration disorders can often be recognized by a parent or caregiver of a child. During an interview with a parent or caregiver, the PT may be able to identify a behavior that indicates possible sensory integration impairment. For example, if a child has tactile defensiveness, the parent might mention in an interview that the child is bothered by shirts made of a certain material or the tag in the neck of shirts. This may indicate a heightened tactile sensation, leading to the defensive touch exhibited by the child. Based on a child's behavior, the PT can develop a plan of care that addresses the sensory integration impairments and allows the child to interact with the environment more effectively.

Orthotics and Supportive Devices

Lower extremity orthotics and supportive devices are valuable pieces of equipment that can drastically improve functional mobility in individuals with musculoskeletal and neurological impairments. However, the device can be a limitation if it does not fit properly or causes pain to the wearer.

Assessment of Alignment and Fit

When assessing the fit and effectiveness of orthotics and other supportive devices, the examiner should consider the following:

- comfort
- fit
- stability
- appearance
- function
- alignment

The appearance of the orthotic may be a significant factor in whether or not the wearer is compliant with its use. The wearer's ability to put on and take off the device, as well as the cosmetic effect once the device is on, can be very important to the wearer and must be considered by the examiner. The device must fit well in order to be effective, and not cause the wearer pain or discomfort. This will also affect compliance. If the device is uncomfortable, the patient will probably not wear it. The stability and alignment of the device also play a large role in the device's comfort. Finally, the device must effectively perform the function it is designed to perform. If the device is prescribed to prevent a gait deviation or to support weak muscles, then the device must actually do those things—or the other assessments do not matter.

In order to assess the fit and alignment of an orthotic, the examiner must know the proper alignment of the various components of the device. Standard alignment and fit considerations are detailed here.

Orthotic Alignment and Fit

ORTHOTIC COMPONENT	PROPER ALIGNMENT
Medial upright	Terminates below perineum
Lateral upright	Terminates below greater trochanter
Knee joint	Aligns with true knee joint axis
Thigh band and calf band	Equidistant from the axes of the knees
Ankle joint	Level with distal tip of medial malleolus

The wearer's opinion of whether or not the orthotic fits and is comfortable is very important and should be considered when assessing the fit and effectiveness of an orthotic.

The upright, or plastic shell, of the device should contour to the patient's thigh and leg, without being too tight. The patient's skin should show no signs of irritation after the device is removed. If redness is present but disappears completely within ten minutes after removal of the device, and the patient has no complaints of pain or discomfort, the device is a good fit.

Signs that the device may be misaligned include skin abrasions, blisters, distal edema, and pain. Skin abrasions may be related to the amount of time the wearer spends in the device. Blisters may be related to friction between the device and the skin. Constriction of the strap or other area of the device may cause distal edema, and pain may be related to uneven weight-bearing and pressure. With lower extremity orthotics, common pain areas include navicular tuberosity, malleoli, tibial crest, and the fibular head.

Assessment of Effectiveness

To accurately assess the effectiveness of an orthotic or supportive device, the examiner should watch the wearer walk both with and without the device. The orthotic should fix the gait deviation or other problem that was noted without the orthotic. For example, if an individual presents with foot drop during the swing phase of gait, the orthotic should prevent the foot drop and allow for proper swing on the involved side. The examiner must also be observant for gait deviations that are caused by the orthotic. For example, excessive plantar flexion during the stance phase due to an inadequate plantar flexion stop can cause hyperextension of the knee.

The following table outlines some of the deviations seen during gait with an orthotic and possible causes therein:

Gait Deviation and Orthotics

GAIT DEVIATION	ORTHOTIC CAUSES
Foot slap	Inadequate dorsiflexion assist or plantar flexion stop
Toe contact	Inadequate heel lift, dorsiflexion assist, or plantar flexion stop
Excessive lateral or medial foot contact and weight-bearing	Incorrect transverse plane alignment
Excessive knee flexion	Inadequate knee lock or dorsiflexion stop; inadequate heel lift on opposite side; often seen with solid AFO with anterior band
Knee hyperextension	Inadequate plantar flexion stop or knee lock; excessively concave calf of orthotic

Other gait changes may be seen as a result of the wearer attempting to avoid pain from an ill-fitting orthotic.

Posture

Posture is the position of the body. It can have a significant impact on physical function if not maintained properly.

Postural Assessment

There are a variety of methods to assess posture. One of the simplest methods is to compare the body's posture against a plumb line. When using a plumb line, the subject stands next to the line and the assessor determines a fixed point of reference. Typically, for anterior/posterior postural evaluation, the point is fixed equally between the two heels. Another option is to compare posture against a grid. In a grid assessment, the subject stands in front of a wall with a grid drawn on it. The lines of the grid serve as the reference points for comparison front to back and right to left. The assessor should look for the following when completing a postural assessment from anterior and posterior view:

- level head with no lateral tilt or rotation to either side
- level shoulders with dominant shoulder possibly slightly lower than the nondominant side
- no lateral curvature of the spine to the right or to the left
- level hips with neither hip more prominent than the other
- level popliteal fossae
- evenly distributed body weight between both lower extremities

Overall, when assessing posture from the anterior or posterior view, the plumb line should fall midway between the heels, knees, and thighs, and should be in line with the midline of the pelvis, chest or spine, and skull. The two halves should be close to mirror images in terms of the body's posture.

Posture can also be evaluated effectively with a plumb line or grid from the lateral view, allowing assessment of normal spinal curvature. For lateral evaluation, the point is fixed just anterior to the lateral malleolus. The assessor should look for the following when completing a postural assessment from the lateral view:

- Plumb line falls in the middle of the earlobe.
- Plumb line falls in the middle of the acromion process.
- Head should not be thrust forward compared to the body.
- Plumb line falls through the bodies of the lumbar vertebrae.
- Cervical lordosis, thoracic kyphosis, and lumbar lordosis are not exaggerated or flattened.
- Plumb line falls just posterior to the axis of the hip joint.
- Plumb line falls just anterior to knee joint but posterior to the patella.
- Plumb line falls just anterior to lateral malleolus.

Postural assessment is an important part of physical therapy, regardless of the patient's diagnosis or functional deficits. Posture can be assessed if a patient is ambulatory with an assistive device, uses a wheelchair as the primary means of mobility, or presents with any other functional deficit or physical impairment. Posture is the basis for all movement, and the energy expended during functional activities (as well as pain) can often be minimized with correct posture. Postural assessment is also appropriate in all day-to-day settings, including school, work, home, travel, and leisure activities. The PTA should be able to assess posture using both the plumb line and the grid method and have an understanding of interventions that can impact posture positively.

Postural Deviations of the Upper and Lower Extremities

Lower extremities. Effective postural assessment of the lower extremities involves appropriate exposures of the ankle, knee, and hip joints. Anterior, posterior, and lateral views are observed, with any deviations or malalignment noted. Postural deviations of the lower extremities can be unilateral or bilateral. The examiner should observe the position of the feet, knees/patellae, and hips and note whether or not the individual bears weight equally right to left. The following table outlines possible postural deviations of the lower extremities:

Lower Extremity Deviations

ANTERIOR AND POSTERIOR OBSERVATION	DESCRIPTION	ASSESSMENT
Unlevel pelvis	One side of the pelvis higher than the other	Palpate iliac crests; look for a raised iliac crest on one side.
Pelvic rotation	One hip bone rotated anterior or posterior compared to other side	Palpate bilateral ASIS; look for higher ASIS on one side.
Genu varum	Bowleg	Patient stands with medial aspect of knees and medial malleoli as close as possible; PTA observes that the ankles touch and the knees do not touch.
Genu valgum	Knock-knees	Patient stands with medial aspect of knees and medial malleoli as close as possible; PTA observes that the knees touch and the ankles do not touch (distance of 9–10 cm is excessive).
Medial/lateral orientation of the patella	Outward tilt: "grasshopper eyes"; inward tilt: "squinting patellae"	PTA observes the tilt of patellae while patient stands with patellae facing forward.
Lateral tibial torsion	Out-toeing	Patient stands with knees facing forward; out-toeing may be present due to excessive lateral tibia rotation.
Medial tibial torsion	In-toeing	Patient stands with knees facing forward; in-toeing may be present due to excessive medial tibial rotation.
Overpronation	Excessive forefoot abduction, hindfoot eversion, and collapse of the arch	PTA observes whether the arch is dropped or absent or whether there is a bulge on the inside of the foot.

Lower Extremity Deviations (*continued*)

ANTERIOR AND POSTERIOR OBSERVATION	DESCRIPTION	ASSESSMENT
Oversupination	Excessive forefoot adduction and hindfoot inversion	Observe whether patient is bearing weight on lateral edge of foot.
Lateral Observation		
Genu recurvatum	Hyperextended knee	Observe both sides to assess both legs.
Patella alta	Patella higher than normal	Observe the patellar position and tilt of the inferior pole of the patella (plane of patella and femoral condyles should be the same).
Patella baja	Patella lower than normal	Observe the patellar position.

Postural deviations of the lower extremities (such as ankle deviations affecting the knee, hip, and spine) can affect the entire body's function, such as deviations of ankle affecting knee, hip, and spinal alignment.

Upper extremities. Effective postural assessment of the upper extremities involves appropriate exposures of the wrist, elbow, shoulder, and scapula. Anterior, posterior, and lateral views are observed, with any deviations or malalignment noted. Postural deviations of the upper extremities can be unilateral or bilateral. The examiner should observe the position of the scapula, shoulder girdle, elbow, wrist, and hand in a relaxed and anatomical position. The following table outlines possible postural deviations of the upper extremities:

Upper Extremity Deviations

UPPER EXTREMITY OBSERVATION	DESCRIPTION	ASSESSMENT
Forward shoulders	Protracted scapula, internally rotated humerus, accompanying increased thoracic kyphosis	Acromion process anterior to plumb line; palms face slightly posterior
Winged scapula	Inferior angle of the scapula, projecting posterior	Inferior angle of scapula protruding posterior and raised from rib cage
Cubitus valgus	Excessive carrying angle of the elbow (normally 5–15 degrees)	Valgus angle of the elbow > 15 degrees (in anatomical position)

Postural deviations of the upper extremities may cause pain and discomfort, weakness in overstretched muscles, or compression of nerves and other tissue.

Reflex Integrity
Primitive Infant Reflexes

The common primitive reflexes assessed by a PT or PTA include:

- babinski reflex
- flexor withdrawal
- crossed extension
- asymmetric tonic neck reflex (ATNR)
- symmetric tonic neck reflex (STNR)
- palmar and plantar grasp
- rooting
- sucking
- moro reflex
- startle response
- landau response

Postural Reflexes

Postural reflexes include righting reflexes, protective reactions, and equilibrium reactions. In general, protective and equilibrium reactions emerge in childhood and are present throughout adulthood. There are righting reflexes that emerge and go away by adulthood and others that remain throughout adulthood.

Sensory Integrity

The human body has a complex sensory system, which includes senses of movement and touch. A variety of sensory tests that affect function are performed in physical therapy, and the PTA will need to be able to perform these tests—as well as know the implications of the outcomes in order to provide effective PT intervention.

Proprioception

Proprioception is the awareness of a joint at rest and the position of a joint at rest. Proprioception is assessed by moving a joint through the available range of motion and asking the patient to identify whether the joint is in the initial, middle, or terminal range of motion of that joint. To perform this assessment effectively, the PTA should grip the lateral joint surfaces over bony prominences with his or her fingertips. He or she should move the joint through the range of motion, stopping at various points throughout the range. The patient then needs to identify (either verbally or via predetermined signals) where in the range of motion the joint is resting. The brain processes proprioceptive information subconsciously in order to determine if the parts of the body are in the correct position during skilled activities.

Kinesthesia

Kinesthesia is the awareness of movement. The assessment for kinesthesia is similar to that of proprioception. The PTA uses the fingertips to grasp the bony prominences on the lateral aspects of the joint being tested. The joint is moved up, down, to the middle, or to the side, and the patient identifies which direction the joint is being moved. Common questions used for this assessment are "Is this movement up or down?" or "Is this movement in or out?" Another method to test awareness is to move the opposite side of the body to the same position. This method is known as mirroring. Similar to proprioception, subconscious processing of kinesthetic information is critical to successful completion of skilled movement.

Stereognosis

Stereognosis is the ability to identify an object by touch. To assess stereognosis, place a common item (such as a paper clip, a key, or a coin) in the patient's hand without letting him or her see what it is. Have the patient identify the object by touch only, without looking at the object. The absence of stereognosis, astereognosis, can indicate central nervous system lesions or peripheral nerve damage.

Two-Point Discrimination

A two-point discrimination test assesses the ability to perceive two points in contact with the skin at the same time. The examiner is attempting to determine the shortest distance between the two points that still allows two distinct points to be perceived. The typical testing site is the distal upper extremities, where this sensation is most pronounced. Specialized instruments for two-point discrimination are available and allow specific measuring of the distance between points. The examiner is looking for the distance at which two stimuli are no longer distinguished and the client states there is one point in contact with the skin. Abnormal results noted on this assessment may indicate central or peripheral nerve damage.

Practice 3

1. A PTA is performing observational gait analysis and notes that the patient has a Trendelenberg gait. The patient will benefit the most from which of the following interventions?
   a. dynamic balance training
   b. gluteus medius strengthening
   c. step-ups
   d. quad sets

2. A PTA is preparing to assess static posture using a plumb line. To complete a lateral postural assessment, what is the best reference point for the plumb line?
   a. midline of the ankle joint
   b. anterior to the lateral malleolus
   c. posterior to the lateral malleolus
   d. midline of the calcaneus

3. A PTA is performing gait analysis and notes that the patient has a slow gait and increased double support time. The PTA suspects it is due to the fear of falling. If fear is affecting the patient's gait pattern, what type of motivational factor is this?
   a. internal
   b. external
   c. reward
   d. environmental

4. A PTA is working with a five-month-old infant, and is testing the assymetrical tonic neck reflex (ATNR) in supine. What is the most appropriate response for a child of this age?
   a. flexion of arms and extension of legs
   b. turning head toward side of touch
   c. flexion of arm and leg on opposite side that head is turned
   d. lateral neck flexion toward side of touch

5. A PTA is performing gait training with a patient two weeks into the PT POC. The PTA moves from the left side of the patient to the right, while giving verbal cues for step length. The PTA notices that the patient is not responding when verbal cues are given from behind and to the right. The PTA should test which cranial nerve?
   a. vagus
   b. trigeminal
   c. trochlear
   d. vestibulocochlear

6. A PTA is performing manual muscle testing and finds that the patient cannot move through the full hip abduction range of motion against gravity. What is the best position for the patient to proceed with this manual muscle test?
   a. seated in a chair with arms
   b. standing with upper extremity support
   c. supine on a plinth
   d. prone on elbows

7. A patient is performing self-care activities while the PTA observes the patient's performance. The PTA observes that the patient performs feeding with the use of a weighted spoon. According to FIM scoring, what score should the PTA assign to this activity?
   a. 6 out of 7
   b. 4 out of 7
   c. 2 out of 7
   d. 0 out of 7

8. You are working at a community health fair, and your job is to screen older adults for balance deficits. You choose the one-legged stance test, and the first subject is a 67-year-old female who is able to complete the one-legged stance test for only four seconds. What is the most appropriate interpretation of this time?
   a. normal stance time for age range
   b. mild risk of falling
   c. high risk of falling
   d. fear of falling

9. The supervising physical therapist asks you, the PTA, to perform a functional gait assessment with a patient who has a vestibular diagnosis. What is the best functional tool for this patient?
   a. Dynamic Gait Index
   b. Tinetti Performance Oriented Mobility Assessment
   c. Berg Balance Scale
   d. timed up and go test

10. During a static postural assessment, you note that when instructed to put feet and legs together, the patient's knees make contact with each other while the ankles are not touching. What is this postural abnormality called?
   a. genu recurvatum
   b. genu valgum
   c. genu valgus
   d. genu hyperextension

11. A PTA is assisting a patient with a sit-to-stand transfer and needs to document the assistance level used for this transfer. The PTA estimates that the patient required approximately 15% physical assistance from the PTA. What is the most appropriate level of assistance?
   a. minimal assistance
   b. moderate assistance
   c. maximum assistance
   d. total assistance

12. A PTA attempts to assess a patient with suspected dysmetria. What is the best method to assess this patient?
   a. finger to nose
   b. finger to examiner's finger
   c. heel on shin
   d. pronation/supination

13. During gait training with a patient following a stroke, the PTA notes that the patient is having difficulty during the swing phase of gait, with the inability to control the forward swing of the lower extremity when preparing for heel strike. What is the most likely muscle weakness related to this problem?
   a. quadriceps
   b. hamstrings
   c. gastroc-soleus
   d. anterior tibialis

14. You are performing manual muscle testing with a patient who presents with unilateral upper and lower extremity weakness following a stroke. You are preparing to test hip adduction on the uninvolved side. What is the best way to position this patient in order to perform this test?
   a. supine
   b. prone
   c. sitting
   d. side-lying

15. A PTA is performing a static postural assessment from the lateral view using a plumb line. Assuming the patient has normal posture, where should the plumb line fall?
   a. posterior to the lateral malleolus
   b. anterior to the knee joint
   c. anterior to the greater trochanter
   d. posterior to the acromion

16. A PTA is completing a sensory assessment with a patient who is recovering from a motor vehicle accident. Part of this assessment includes kinesthesia testing. What is the best instruction to give the patient during this test?
   a. "Identify whether the movement is up or down."
   b. "Identify whether this is the beginning or end of the range."
   c. "Identify the item placed in your hand."
   d. "Identify the moment when you first feel touch."

17. A PTA is performing observational gait analysis and notes that the patient's stance time on the right side is significantly shorter than on the left side. What is the most likely cause of this difference?

    a. pain in the right lower extremity when bearing weight

    b. pain in the left lower extremity when bearing weight

    c. difficulty with swing phase of the left lower extremity

    d. difficulty with the swing phase of the right lower extremity

18. A PTA is working with a new pediatric patient and is performing a gross visual assessment of the patient's motor development. As the child plays in the PT clinic, the PTA observes the child jump from a high step and land on one foot. Based on this performance, the PTA estimates that this child is in what age range?

    a. 10–16 months

    b. 18–26 months

    c. 30–36 months

    d. 40–46 months

19. You are performing balance testing with a patient, and you are preparing to measure the patient's functional reach. The patient is positioned against the wall with a yardstick at shoulder level, and the average distance reached during three trials is eight inches. You inform the patient that the results of this test indicate what?

    a. The likelihood that the patient will fall twice within the next two months is increased twofold.

    b. The likelihood that the patient will fall twice within the next two months is increased fourfold.

    c. The likelihood that the patient will fall twice within the next six months is increased sixfold.

    d. The likelihood that the patient will fall twice within the next six months is increased eightfold.

20. A PTA is working with a patient who has profound weakness of the right gastroc-soleus complex. The PTA anticipates that this patient will have the most difficulty during which aspect of gait?

    a. toe-off

    b. heel-off

    c. heel strike

    d. midstance

21. The supervising PT asks you to measure the stride length of a patient's gait. What is the best way to take this measurement?

    a. measure the distance between the heel strike of one foot and the next heel strike of the same foot

    b. measure the distance between heel strike of one foot and the next heel strike of the other foot

    c. measure the time elapsed between heel strike of one foot and the next heel strike of the same foot

    d. measure the time elapsed between heel strike of one foot and the next heel strike of the other foot

Practice 3 Answers

1. b. The Trendelenberg gait is the dropping of one side of the pelvis during the stance phase of the opposite leg, and this is caused by weak gluteus medius musculature on the leg in the stance phase. Therefore, strengthening the gluteus medius is the most appropriate intervention for this patient.

2. b. When assessing static posture using a plumb line, there should always be a fixed reference point. In lateral postural assessment, that fixed point should be just anterior to the lateral malleolus.

3. a. Fear is an internal motivator that may be based on the patient's past experiences, such as knowing someone who hurt themselves in a fall. As a result, the patient may change gait patterns in order to feel safer while walking, even though altered gait patterns may be less safe.

4. c. The ATNR response is the "fencer" position. When the infant's head is turned to one side, the arm and leg on the side of the head move into extension, and the opposite arm and leg flex.

5. d. The patient is suspected to have difficulty hearing. The function of the cochlear division of the vestibulocochlear nerve is responsible for the ability to hear.

6. c. The best position for the patient to perform the hip abduction range of motion in a gravity minimized position is supine on a plinth. Standing results in hip abduction against gravity, sitting in a chair with arms may not allow full abduction range of motion, and lying prone on elbows is not as stable a position for resisted hip motion as supine.

7. a. According to the FIM, if an assistive or adaptive device is used, a patient cannot be graded as completely independent (7 out of 7). This would be rated as 6 out of 7, modified independent.

8. c. If an adult cannot balance on one leg for at least five seconds, the individual is at risk for injurious falls.

9. a. The Dynamic Gait Index is the only functional gait assessment designed to be used with patients with vestibular diagnoses.

10. b. Genu valgum is the knock-kneed position. This presents when a patient's knees are touching and ankles cannot touch when he or she is standing. Genu recurvatum is hyperextension of the knee, and genu varum is bowlegged.

11. a. Minimal assistance means that the patient is performing a majority of the effort required to complete an activity. If the PTA is performing 15% of the effort, then the patient is performing 85% of the effort, and more than 50% is a majority.

12. b. Dysmetria involves the inability to judge distance. Having the patient try to place a finger on the tip of the examiner's finger (which is placed in front of the patient) requires good judgment of distance.

13. b. Eccentric contraction of the hamstrings controls deceleration of the swing leg as it prepares to extend for heel strike.

14. d. In order to place the adductors in an anti-gravity position, the best position is side-lying. The patient can raise his or her leg into adduction against gravity, and the examiner can introduce resistance.

15. b. During static postural assessment with a plumb line, the plumb line should fall anterior to the lateral malleolus, anterior to the knee joint (but behind the patella), through the greater trochanter, and through the acromion.

16. a. Kinesthesia, the awareness of movement, is tested by moving a patient's joint through the range of motion and asking the patient if the joint is being moved up or down, laterally or medially.

17. a. Decreased stance time is often due to pain during weight-bearing. The patient attempts to stand on the affected leg for as little time as possible due to pain. This is referred to as antalgic gait.

18. c. The ability to jump from a step leading with one foot is developed at approximately 30 months.

19. a. The functional reach test indicates fall risk. If a patient has a forward reach of greater than six inches but less than ten inches, the likelihood that the patient will fall twice within the next two months increases twofold.

20. b. The gastroc-soleus complex is most active during heel-off as the foot pushes into plantarflexion in preparation for initiating the swing phase.

21. a. Stride length is defined as the distance measured between the heel strike of one foot and the next heel strike of the same foot.

Integumentary System

The physical therapist performs many tests and measures when examining a patient at risk for, or with, an open area of the integumentary system (skin). The physical therapist assistant may be called upon to assist with certain elements of data collection during the course of treatment. Tests and measures to assess circulation, sensation, wound characteristics, and other factors that affect healing are performed on patients with open wounds. For patients with burns, data is collected regarding the depth of the burn, the total body surface area involved, joint range of motion, scar quality, and pain.

Circulation

Normal circulation is essential for healthy skin. Patients with impaired circulation are at increased risk for developing open areas and for delayed healing of these open areas. Circulation of the arterial, venous, and lymphatic systems must be assessed.

Arterial Circulation

Oxygen and nutrients are delivered to the tissues of the body by arterial circulation. When arterial insufficiency is present, the epidermis and dermis are gradually deprived of oxygen and nutrients. The skin may slowly break down or be unable to heal in the event of injury. Arterial circulation may be measured by palpating pulse volume, by measuring the ankle-brachial index, by assessing capillary refill time, and by observing the color and quality of the skin.

Assessment of Pulse

Pulse is commonly assessed in the lower extremity in the femoral, posterior tibial, and dorsalis pedis arteries.

The femoral artery is palpated along the inguinal crease, midway between the anterior superior iliac spine and the pubic symphysis. The posterior tibial artery is palpated behind the medial malleolus, and the dorsalis pedis artery is palpated between the tendons of extensor hallucis longus and extensor digitorum longus. With firm palpation from the second and third digits, a normal pulse is easily palpable.

> **TAKE NOTE**
>
> Excessive pressure during palpation of the pulse may actually occlude the artery and result in no pulse being felt.

Patients with arterial insufficiency often demonstrate diminished or absent pulses. If that is the case, the Ankle-Brachial Index should be calculated.

Ankle-Brachial Index

The ABI is the ratio between the systolic blood pressure taken at the brachial artery and the systolic blood pressure taken at the posterior tibial artery. Instead of a stethoscope, a Doppler ultrasound is used to identify the pulse. The blood pressure is measured in both upper extremities, and the higher of the two is recorded. The blood pressure is then measured in the involved lower extremity and divided by the upper extremity pressure.

$$ABI = \frac{\text{systolic pressure in LE}}{\text{systolic pressure in UE}}$$

Normal values range from .95 to 1.1. Values above 1.1 indicate vessel calcification and are not valid. Values below .95 indicate arterial insufficiency.

Capillary Refill Time

To determine capillary refill time, push on the nail bed of the toe with enough pressure to cause blanching. Measure the time it takes for the color to reappear after release of the pressure. Normal refill time is three seconds or less.

Skin Color and Quality

In patients with normal circulation, limb color should not change dramatically with elevation or dependency. In a patient with arterial insufficiency, elevation will create pallor, and dependency will create a flushed appearance. This reddening of the skin is called dependent rubor, or reactive hyperemia. Skin should normally be pliable, moist, and have hair. Chronic hypoxia due to arterial insufficiency robs the epidermal and dermal structures of oxygen and nutrients.

Trophic changes include dry, thin, shiny, inelastic skin and loss of hair.

Signs of Arterial Insuffiency

Pulse volume	Diminished or absent
ABI	Less than .95
Capillary refill time	Greater than three seconds
Skin color	Dependent rubor
Skin quality	Dry, inelastic, thin, shiny; hair loss

This is a summary of results from tests and measures that may indicate arterial insufficiency.

INFORMATION IN ACTION

A PTA is working with a 58-year-old man who is coming to therapy for treatment of a degenerative disk disease of the lumbar spine. The man smokes, is moderately obese, and generally has poor fitness. His past medical history includes hypertension. The PTA notices a dry, circular wound on the crest of the patient's tibia. When asked, the patient reports that he ran into the coffee table "a month or so ago," and that the wound "just doesn't seem to want to heal up." The PTA assesses the patient's femoral pulse, which is present, but is unable to detect a pulse in either the dorsalis pedis or tibial artery. The PTA shares this information with the PT and an ABI is performed, revealing a score of .8. This score indicates mild to moderate arterial insufficiency. The wound, an arterial ulcer, was treated, and the patient's primary care physician was informed of the results of the ABI.

Venous Circulation

Normal venous circulation is required to remove less oxygenated blood and waste products from the tissues. When venous stasis occurs, the skin is at risk for breakdown. Venous circulation may be assessed by measuring edema and by observing skin color.

Assessment of Edema

Edema may be quantified through limb girth measurements or by limb volume measurements. Girth measurements are taken by placing a tape measure flat against the skin and measuring the circumference of the limb, using bony landmarks as references.

Volume measurements are taken by submersing the edematous extremity into a container of water and measuring the amount of water displaced by the limb.

Skin Color

Color changes in the skin of the lower extremities due to venous insufficiency generally occur below the knee. The skin may appear reddened if dermatitis or cellulitis is present. It often has a mottled brown appearance, due to staining from the seepage of red blood cells out of the veins and into the surrounding tissue spaces.

Lymphatic Circulation

The lymph system removes excess interstitial fluid from the dermis and filters dead cells and bacteria out of it. The presence of lymphedema increases the risk of skin breakdown. Lymphatic circulation may be assessed by measuring edema in the same manner as noted for venous insufficiency.

INFORMATION IN ACTION

A 27-year-old woman with congenital lymphedema of the right lower extremity is seen monthly in a lymphedema clinic to monitor her status. One of the goals is to minimize lymphedema to prevent open wounds. The PT has asked the PTA to perform a volumetric assessment to determine the amount of edema present in the right foot. The patient sits and places her foot into a rectangular container full to the brim with water. As she lowers her foot, the displaced water flows out of the spout of the container and into a holding receptacle. Once the patient's foot is on the bottom of the container and the water has stopped flowing, the PTA pours the displaced water into a graduated cylinder. The PTA then records the amount of water displaced as an indicator of the volume of the patient's limb and reports the information to the PT.

Sensation

Aspects of sensation that may be assessed in patients at risk for open wounds (or in those who already have open wounds) are light touch, temperature, and protective sensation. Light touch means touching the patient lightly with the fingertips or brushing the skin with a cotton ball. The patient is instructed to look away and identify the presence of the touch. The intensity of the touch can be compared to a known area of normal sensation. Light touch is assessed as being intact, diminished, or absent. Temperature sensation may be assessed by filling one glass test tube with warm water and one with cold. These are then applied to the skin, and the patient is asked to identify the temperature of the tube touching them. Protective sensation is measured with a series of monofilaments, which are plastic filaments of varying thicknesses that are applied perpendicularly to the skin until the filament bends.

Inability to detect the 5.07 (10 g) monofilament means there has been loss of protective sensation and indicates the patient will be unable to feel skin damage.

TAKE NOTE

A patient with loss of protective sensation must inspect his or her skin visually, daily, to prevent open areas.

Wound Characteristics

There are many aspects of the wound itself that must be measured to establish a baseline and to monitor healing. Wound characteristics include:

- size and depth
- stage/depth of tissue involvement
- wound bed
- drainage
- tunneling/undermining
- pain
- periwound condition

Wound characteristics are measured to establish a baseline and to monitor healing.

Size of the Wound

The surface area of the wound may be measured using a tape measure, a transparent piece of plastic with or without a calibrated grid, or by taking a photograph.

When using a tape measure, both the longest head-to-toe length and the widest aspect of the wound (perpendicular to the length measurement) should be recorded. Measurements should be made in centimeters, to the first decimal point. Wounds that are irregular in shape may be better represented by tracing their periphery on a plastic sheet. Poloroid™ or digital photographs with superimposed measurement grids provide an accurate measurement of size, as well as a visual representation of the wound bed. The depth of the wound must be recorded. So must the degree of tunneling or undermining. Tunneling is the presence of a hole between the layers of fascia in tissue. Undermining is the separation of the intact epidermis and dermis at the periphery of a wound from the tissue below the dermis. Wound depth, tunneling, and undermining can all be measured by placing the handle of a sterile cotton swab into the wound, and then removing it and measuring how far it went in with a tape measure.

TAKE NOTE

Wounds that do not decrease in size or show evidence of healing for two weeks should be reassessed by the physical therapist.

INFORMATION IN ACTION

The PT asks you to make a follow-up measurement on the size of a pressure ulcer on a patient's greater trochanter. Using a tape measure, you measure the length (top to bottom) and the width (side to side) of the ulcer. Using the handle end of a sterile cotton-tipped applicator, you measure undermining at the positions of 12 o'clock, 3 o'clock, 6 o'clock, and 9 o'clock. You document these measurements and report them to the physical therapist.

Wound Bed

The wound bed may contain both healthy and necrotic tissue. Granulation and epithelial tissue are healthy tissues. Epithelial tissue is thin and translucent. Granulation tissue is beefy red, shiny, moist, and bumpy (granular) in appearance when it is in good shape. Granulation tissue that is pale, a dull red, or dry and crumbly in nature has poor blood supply or may be infected. Necrotic tissue can be white, yellow, brown, or black. Stringy or mucouslike yellow or white necrotic tissue (also called slough), is dead connective tissue. Brown or black necrotic tissue is called eschar and may be hard or soft.

Estimate the percentage of healthy and necrotic tissue in the wound bed. The presence of other structures in the wound bed, such as exposed tendon or bone, should be noted.

Drainage

Drainage from the wound should be assessed. This is typically observed on the dressings as they are removed. It is important to know when the dressings were last changed. The color, consistency, amount, and odor of the drainage should be noted. Arterial and neuropathic ulcers typically have little to no drainage. Pressure ulcers have more drainage the deeper they are; and venous ulcers have a lot of drainage. Wounds that are infected also have a lot of drainage. This drainage is typically colored and may be foul smelling.

TAKE NOTE

Any wound that has had a dressing on it may have an unpleasant odor. Always cleanse the wound with saline to remove the dressing odor prior to assessing actual wound odor.

Parameters of Wound Drainage

	NORMAL	ABNORMAL
Color	Clear; pale yellow; pink	Red; cloudy; tan; blue-green
Consistency	Thin	Thick
Amount	Minimal/ moderate	Dry; copious
Odor	Minimal after cleansing	Moderate to strong

Examining the drainage from a wound can give information about the overall health of the wound.

Periwound Skin

The skin around the wound must be assessed, as it is critical to keep that skin healthy to prevent an increase in the wound size. Skin that is too dry may crack, and skin that is too moist may become macerated. Color of the surrounding skin should be noted. Loss of hair and/or poor nail quality may indicate long-standing ischemia. Edema may indicate venous insufficiency, lymphedema, or infection. Increased temperature may indicate inflammation or infection, and decreased temperature may indicate ischemia.

Color Changes in Periwound Tissue

Red	Inflammation; infection; ischemic damage
Pale	Ischemia; new scar tissue
Blue	Ischemia
Brown	Chronic venous insufficiency

This table describes the possible implications of color changes in the skin around an open wound.

Pain

The presence of pain (or lack thereof) associated with an open wound is often associated with the wound's cause. For example, arterial ulcers are very painful due to ischemia. Venous ulcers are generally not painful. Ulcers resulting from diabetes are not painful due to loss of sensation. Stage I and stage II pressure ulcers may be painful due to nerve irritation, but those at stage III and IV are often pain-free due to destruction of sensory receptors in the dermis.

Pain may be assessed using a number of scales, but the Visual Analogue Scale is most commonly used.

Factors That Affect Healing

Many factors apart from the status of the wound itself may affect healing.

Nutrition, hydration, and physiological status should be assessed and monitored by the physical therapist and other members of the healthcare team. The patient's ability to change positions in bed, transfer, and ambulate are important indicators of his or her risk for developing an open area and give insight into the speed with which a wound may heal. The effectiveness of pressure-relieving devices must be monitored.

> ## TAKE NOTE
>
> The Braden Scale is a valid and reliable tool used to measure a patient's risk of developing a pressure ulcer. Items assessed include the patient's ability to change body position, his or her level of physical activity, his or her sensation, the amount of moisture exposure to the skin, nutritional status, and the degree to which the skin is subject to friction and shear. Scores range from 16 to 23, and a score of less than 16 to 18 indicates substantial risk of developing a pressure sore.

> ## TAKE NOTE
>
> Pressure-relieving devices may include specialty mattresses, wheelchair cushions, and heel protectors.

Burn Depth

The depth of a burn is described qualitatively. A superficial burn involves the epidermis. A superficial partial-thickness burn involves both the epidermis and upper dermis. A deep partial-thickness burn involves the epidermis and the lower level of the dermis. A full-thickness burn involves the epidermis, the entire dermis, and part of the subcutaneous tissue. A subdermal burn penetrates to the level of muscle, tendon, and bone. A patient will usually demonstrate burns of varying depths throughout the body.

Burn Depth

DEPTH OF BURN	TISSUE INVOLVED
Superficial	Epidermis
Superficial partial-thickness	Epidermis; upper layer of dermis
Deep partial-thickness	Epidermis; upper and lower layers of dermis
Full-thickness	Epidermis; entire dermis; subcutaneous tissue
Subdermal	Epidermis; entire dermis; through subcutaneous tissue to muscle, tendon, bone

The depth of a burn is described qualitatively, and different types of burns involve different layers of muscle and tissue.

Total Body Surface Area

When a patient has extensive burns, the size of the burn is not measured. Rather, the percentage of the body involved in the burn is estimated. The quickest and most commonly used method to estimate the extent of burns is the rule of nines. The areas of the body are divided into areas of 9% of TBSA or multiples thereof. For example, the anterior aspect of the entire lower extremity is 9% TBSA for an adult. The anterior aspect of the trunk is 18% of TBSA.

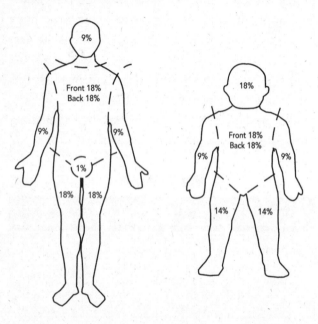

The values are modified for infants and children to reflect variations in body proportions. According to the American Burn Association, adults with full-thickness burns of more than 5% TBSA or partial-thickness burns of more than 20% TBSA are considered to have sustained a major burn injury.

INFORMATION IN ACTION

You are reviewing the chart of man who has recently been admitted with burns to the anterior aspect of the entire right upper extremity due to scalding with a hot liquid. Based on this description, you correctly estimate the TBSA involved as 4.5% using the rule of nines.

Joint Range of Motion

Burns often extend over at least one joint. As the burn heals, wound contraction and scar tissue formation may combine to limit flexibility of the joint. Initial goniometric measurement of joint range of motion is done by the physical therapist to determine a baseline. Subsequent range of motion measurement monitors the improvement in motion or the development of contractures.

Scar Quality

The remodeling of scar tissue may take up to two years. The characteristics of a scar that are assessed include the pliability of the tissue, the color of the scar, and the height of the scar. The ideal scar would look and feel exactly like the surrounding, nonburned tissue. In other words, it would be of the same pigmentation as the surrounding skin, it would be supple, and it would be flat. A severe scar would be a purple color, over 5 mm in height, with ropelike bands of tissue throughout it. With proper management, most scars are probably somewhere between these two extremes.

INFORMATION IN ACTION

A 23-year-old man has scarring in the left axillary region due to a flame burn sustained eight months ago. The PTA is working with the patient on strengthening and stretching exercises to improve the function of the left arm. The PTA notices that the scar is developing a red color, that the tissue seems more firm, and that the surface of the scar is raised and bumpy. The patient reports that he has not been wearing his compression garment due to the hot summer weather. The PTA explains the consequences of a contracted, inflexible scar on the patient's long-term function. The PTA and patient talk together with the PT to develop a plan for scar management that is acceptable to the patient.

Pain

Pain is present in all burns, due both to the injury itself and to the application of interventions to manage the burns, such as debridement or range of motion exercise. Continual assessment of pain is critical to allow the patient to participate fully in the rehabilitation program, to diminish anxiety, and to ensure optimal quality of life. The most commonly used scale is the 10 cm Visual Analogue Scale. The goal of pain management is to keep pain at a level of four or less on the VAS.

Practice 4

1. Which of the following is the best indicator of venous circulation?
   a. Ankle-Brachial Index
   b. blood pressure
   c. girth measurement
   d. temperature assessment

2. You notice that a patient's feet appear quite pale while she is lying in bed and that they become red after she has been sitting for a few minutes. Which pathology is most likely present?
   a. venous insufficiency
   b. arterial insufficiency
   c. lymphedema
   d. diabetes

3. What is the primary advantage to measuring the area of a wound with a tracing compared to using a linear measurement (e.g., a tape measure)?
   a. It more accurately reflects changes in wound size.
   b. It is quick and easy to perform.
   c. It is painless for the patient.
   d. The tracing sheets are sterile, which protects the wound from contamination.

4. A firefighter was exiting a building when a blast from behind burned the back of his head and torso and the posterior aspect of his left upper extremity. Using the rule of nines, what is the best estimate of total body surface area that was burned?
   a. 18%
   b. 27%
   c. 30%
   d. 36%

Practice 4 Answers

1. c. Venous insufficiency results in edema formation in the lower extremities and/or skin abnormalities and ulcerations. Girth measurement would be most appropriate to assess edema formation.

2. b. With arterial insufficiency, the arteries are no longer able to dilate and constrict to control blood flow. Blood flow will be affected greatly by gravity. Since oxygenated blood is red in color, elevation of the leg will drain the limb of blood and therefore of color. A dependent position will bring blood, and a red color, back into the limb.

3. a. Wounds do not always heal symmetrically. When wounds are measured by tracing their perimeter on acetate sheets, changes in size around the entire perimeter of the wound are captured completely

4. c. The posterior head is 4.5% of TBSA. The posterior torso is 18%, and the posterior aspect of one upper extremity is 4.5%. That would add up to 27%.

Metabolic and Endocrine Systems

The metabolic and endocrine systems play significant roles in many functions of the body. Therefore, when physical therapy tests and measures are performed, the metabolic and endocrine systems may be affected. The physical therapist assistant must be aware of how the results of the tests and measures identified in the *Guide to Physical Therapist Practice* and the effects of these tests and measures on the metabolic and endocrine system influence physical therapy interventions.

Tests and Measures

The testing of aerobic capacity and endurance is the category of assessment that may have the most significant impact on the metabolic and endocrine systems. Aerobic capacity and endurance testing is used to assess the body's ability to respond to increased oxygen demands. This includes how the body takes in oxygen, how the body delivers oxygen to the cells of the body, and how the body releases energy. During aerobic capacity and endurance testing, the examiner may be looking for the ability to perform functional activities or activities of daily living.

An individual's aerobic capacity during standardized exercise tests and the body's cardiopulmonary responses to these tests are also assessed. The responses monitored include (but are not limited to) heart rate, respiratory rate, cardiac rhythm, rate of perceived exertion, dyspnea, angina, and oxygen saturation.

INFORMATION IN ACTION

When working with individuals who take cardiac medication, heart rate may not be a reliable method to monitor response to exercise, due to the blunting effect some cardiac medications have on heart rate. Rate of perceived exertion is a reliable method to monitor response to exercise when other methods are not possible or reliable.

Testing Aerobic Capacity and Endurance

Aerobic capacity and endurance testing can lead to changes in the endocrine system, such as decreased blood glucose. The cells of the body demonstrate increased uptake and use of glucose during exercise; this leads to decreased levels of glucose in the blood. If an individual had normal or low blood sugar levels before beginning an endurance test, hypoglycemia may occur during testing. The examiner must be able to recognize signs of adverse reactions to testing and stop the test as appropriate. The endocrine system also reacts to exercise by increasing the secretion of epinephrine by the sympathetic nervous system, increasing the secretion of cortisol by the adrenal glands, and increasing the secretion of growth hormones by the pituitary gland. In addition, the secretion of insulin decreases while the secretion of glucagon increases. The following items are examples of tests used to assess aerobic capacity and endurance that may result in these changes in the endocrine system.

Tests of Aerobic Capacity/Endurance

TEST	DESCRIPTION
Twelve-minute walk test	Client walks at a brisk pace, and distance is recorded at the end of 12 minutes.
Six-minute walk test	Client walks at a brisk pace, and distance is recorded at the end of six minutes.
One-mile walk test	Client walks for a mile at a brisk pace, and the time it takes to walk the final quarter mile is recorded.
Modified Bruce treadmill test	Client walks on treadmill at 1.7 mph at a 5–10% incline; every three minutes the speed and incline are increased, up to 5 mph and 18% incline.
Cycle ergometer test	Client cycles continuously for six to nine minutes, with a gradual increase in intensity and speed.

These are examples of aerobic capacity and endurance tests that may be used during a physical therapy evaluation. These tests will most likely result in decreased blood sugar in the individual being tested. It is important that the PTA monitor the client for possible adverse effects of low blood sugar.

Short-Term Effects of Testing

These tests of aerobic capacity and endurance can also have short-term effects on the metabolic system. Physical activity causes an increase in the body's metabolic rate in order to provide energy to the muscles during activity. In addition, epinephrine is secreted by the adrenal glands in response to decreasing blood sugar, which can be a result of physically demanding aerobic capacity and endurance testing. Epinephrine causes increased heart rate and can prepare the body for the fight or flight response, which results in increased metabolism. The body's responses to increased metabolism and increased oxygen demand induced by exercise testing give the examiner and the PTA information about aerobic capacity and endurance. The physical therapist can then determine if aerobic capacity or endurance is limiting an individual's functional abilities. The PTA can use this information during intervention by having the patient exercise at the appropriate intensity, duration, and frequency in order to allow for improvements in aerobic capacity and endurance while preventing adverse effects of overexertion.

Other Tests

Some of the other tests and measures used in physical therapy evaluations also have potential to elicit responses from the metabolic and endocrine systems. These tests and measures require physical and aerobic activity from the individual being tested; and therefore, these tests have the same effects seen during aerobic capacity testing and aerobic exercise. The tests and measures that fall into this category include body mechanics assessment, gait and balance assessment, neuromotor development and sensory integration testing, orthotics and prosthetic assessment, reflex testing (including righting and balance reactions), self-care abilities assessment, and ventilation and respiration testing.

Tests without Physical Activity

There is also a category of tests and measures that do not require a lot of physical activity on the part of the individual being tested—but may still have effects on the endocrine system. The tests and measures that assess the integumentary system (as well as pain) are examples of tests that may cause an endocrine reaction. A wound causing pain and discomfort may cause an increased stress response in the body, and pain assessments can also elicit a stress response. Under situations of stress, the body may increase the release of cortisol, as well as epinephrine, in preparation for the fight or flight response. Fear may also be a factor affecting the endocrine system during testing, and fear can also elicit a stress response. Tests of balance, gait, pain, prosthetics, orthotics, reflexes and righting reactions, work and community reintegration, and others may induce fear in an individual who has a fear of falling or an individual who is afraid of what the results of testing may mean for his or her functional abilities.

TAKE NOTE

There are assessment tools that can objectively measure an individual's fear of falling or fear of certain activities. A baseline measurement of fear can be useful when fear is a factor that interferes with an individual's progress in physical therapy. The PTA can offer interventions that assist in decreasing fear with activity.

Tests Using Adaptive Equipment

Other tests and measures that may have an effect on the metabolic and endocrine systems include assessment of the use of assistive and adaptive equipment, cranial and peripheral nerve integrity testing, assessment of environmental barriers, motor function and muscle performance testing, postural assessment, and work or community reintegration assessment, because these tests may involve the individual's performing physical and aerobic activity. For example, an individual demonstrating the use of adaptive equipment during functional activities may present with signs of low blood sugar during testing, due to the physical demands of the test. The individual may present with dizziness, lightheadedness, or excessive fatigue. Testing should be stopped if any of these signs are present. If the cause of these symptoms is likely low blood sugar, then the individual should be given sugar and the individual's blood sugar should be tested. These tests also have the potential for causing fear, stress, or pain with the associated endocrine responses previously discussed.

Tests with Little Impact on the Metabolic and Endocrine Systems

There is also a group of tests and measures performed in a physical therapy evaluation that have little to no direct effect on the metabolic and endocrine systems. For example, anthropometric measurements that assess body composition and body dimensions do not require a lot of physical exertion by the individual being tested and are typically not emotionally stressful tests or tests that elicit fear. In addition, testing of attention and cognition, circulation testing, joint integrity and range of motion assessments, and sensory integrity testing do not typically cause significant changes or reactions from the metabolic and endocrine systems. Although these tests and measures do not typically elicit strong reactions from the metabolic or endocrine systems, any test or measure that is emotionally stressful, requires uncomfortable or frequent changing of positions, or causes physical pain can lead to endocrine responses.

Effects of Physical Therapy Tests and Measures

TEST	EFFECTS ON THE METABOLIC AND ENDOCRINE SYSTEMS
Aerobic capacity/endurance	Decreased blood sugar; increased secretion of epinephrine, cortisol, and growth hormone
Anthropometrics	Minimal direct effect; epinephrine and cortisol secretion if stressed or fearful
Arousal, attention, and cognition	Minimal direct effect; epinephrine and cortisol secretion if stressed or fearful

Effects of Physical Therapy Tests and Measures (*continued*)

TEST	EFFECTS ON THE METABOLIC AND ENDOCRINE SYSTEMS
Assistive and adaptive devices	Epinephrine and cortisol secretion if stressed or fearful; decreased blood sugar if physically demanding
Circulation (arterial, venous, or lymphatic)	Minimal direct effect; epinephrine and cortisol secretion if stressed or fearful
Cranial and peripheral nerve integrity	Epinephrine and cortisol secretion if stressed or fearful; decreased blood sugar if physically demanding
Environmental, home, and work barriers	Epinephrine and cortisol secretion if stressed or fearful; decreased blood sugar if physically demanding
Ergonomics and body mechanics	Epinephrine and cortisol secretion if stressed or fearful; decreased blood sugar if physically demanding
Gait, locomotion, and balance	Decreased blood sugar; may elicit stress or fear response
Integumentary integrity	May elicit pain, fear, or stress response
Joint integrity and mobility	Minimal direct effect; epinephrine and cortisol secretion if stressed or fearful
Motor function (motor control and motor learning)	Epinephrine and cortisol secretion if stressed or fearful; decreased blood sugar if physically demanding
Muscle performance (strength, power, or endurance)	Epinephrine and cortisol secretion if stressed or fearful; decreased blood sugar if physically demanding
Neuromotor development and sensory integration	Epinephrine and cortisol secretion if stressed or fearful; decreased blood sugar if physically demanding
Orthotic, protective, and supportive devices	Epinephrine and cortisol secretion if stressed or fearful; decreased blood sugar if physically demanding
Pain	May elicit pain, fear, or stress response
Posture	Epinephrine and cortisol secretion if stressed or fearful; decreased blood sugar if physically demanding
Prosthetic requirements	Epinephrine and cortisol secretion if stressed or fearful; decreased blood sugar if physically demanding
Range of motion	Minimal direct effect; epinephrine and cortisol secretion if stressed or fearful

Effects of Physical Therapy Tests and Measures (*continued*)

TEST	EFFECTS ON THE METABOLIC AND ENDOCRINE SYSTEMS
Reflex integrity	Epinephrine and cortisol secretion if stressed or fearful; decreased blood sugar if physically demanding
Self-care and home management (ADLs and IADLs)	Epinephrine and cortisol secretion if stressed or fearful; decreased blood sugar if physically demanding
Sensory integrity	Minimal direct effect; epinephrine and cortisol secretion if stressed or fearful
Ventilation and respiration/gas exchange	Epinephrine and cortisol secretion if stressed or fearful; decreased blood sugar if physically demanding
Work, community, and leisure integration and reintegration	Epinephrine and cortisol secretion if stressed or fearful; decreased blood sugar if physically demanding

Physical therapy tests and measures can result in valuable information about an individual's metabolic and endocrine response to various conditions and environments.

Practice 5

1. A PTA is working with an individual immediately after the physical therapy evaluation that focused on gait and balance. The PTA looks at the past medical history and notes that the patient has been diagnosed with diabetes. During the assessment, the PT had asked the patient to participate in extensive gait and standing balance analysis. The PTA notices that the patient appears fatigued and that she complains of being light-headed. After the PTA stops the intervention, what is the most appropriate response?

   a. The patient should lie down and rest.

   b. The patient should take sugar and test blood sugar levels.

   c. The patient should monitor heart rate using rate of perceived exertion.

   d. The patient should reschedule the treatment session.

Practice 5 Answer

1. b. After the PTA stops the intervention, the patient should take sugar and test his or her blood sugar levels because the most likely cause for the light-headedness and fatigue during the gait and balance evaluation is low blood sugar.

Assessing Multi-System Involvement

The PTA must often assess individuals whose functional disability is due to the interaction of more than one pathology (or the interaction of symptoms in multiple systems). The evaluation of individuals with multi-system involvement must include the same tests and measures that are performed for all physical therapy clients, with additional attention given to the effects of those tests and measures on each system and symptom.

Environmental, Work, and Home Barriers

For individuals with multi-system involvement, functional disability may be due to the effects of one pathology or the interaction of the symptoms of multiple systems. Physical therapy tests and measures are directed at the sequelae (or aftereffects) of multiple diagnoses and the functional presentation of the individual, not the pathologies themselves.

Gathering Information

There are three common ways to assess self-care, activities of daily living, and independence in community, work, and leisure activities.

Self-Report

Self-report is a quick and easy way to gather information about function. This method can provide valuable information about an individual's perception of function. The drawbacks of self-reporting are the subjective nature of the information and the various influences on an individual's answers. The questions may be answered with the goal of pleasing the therapist, or the individual may be fearful of losing his or her freedom.

Observation

Another common method of assessment is rating performance from observation of an individual's overall function. This kind of assessment can serve as a quick screening tool to get a picture of overall function. For example, a PTA may gather information about ADL status from a nursing screen based on the nurse's observation of the individual in the hospital room. The final method is a detailed and objective observation of functional activities by a PT or PTA. Performance-based assessments can reveal information about the progression of disease and the resulting disability.

Evaluating Work Barriers

It is very important that work activities are evaluated in order for an individual to carry out all job responsibilities. Job analysis or a functional capacity evaluation tool can give the PTA information about the requirements and physical duties of a job that may be limiting. Simulated work environments can allow for assessment of specific tasks within the confines of the real job. Specific functional activities can be learned and practiced, or the work environment can be modified to allow for easier access. If adaptive devices are needed, functional training should include the use of those devices; assessment following this training to ensure safety and ability is essential.

Evaluating Environmental Barriers

Environmental barriers and challenges must be identified in order to train an individual to be functional and independent at work and in the community. Many of the barriers encountered during an environmental assessment can be modified; however, some cannot. For example, an individual's route to work may include stairs, and the individual may need to climb the stairs daily in order to perform his or her job. This may be an obstacle that cannot be modified. Physical therapy intervention will need to focus on stair training or training in the use of adaptive equipment that will allow the individual to safely use the stairs in the community. In addition, during and after training, the client's ability to safely use adaptive equipment must be assessed in order to ensure safety. Some obstacles or barriers may allow for modifications such as the arrangement of equipment, floor surfaces, or desk heights. For individuals with multi-system involvement, every modification must be evaluated for the effects on all the systems. A modification for one functional limitation may create a barrier due to an unrelated pathology.

Evaluation of an individual's community can guide functional training for regular daily activities. For example, simulated community environments, such as a crosswalk or model car, can be used to assess whether or not an individual can cross the street within a safe time frame or can access transportation such as a car or bus. If an individual must take a bus to the grocery store, functional training must include stepping up on a bus, maintaining balance while standing on a moving bus, and sitting or standing for a bus seat. Access to the community may require locomotion or adaptive devices, and training should include the devices that the individual anticipates will be used regularly for mobility. Functional training in desired leisure activities is critical, and training of these activities in real-world environments can be motivating and encouraging.

Cognition

Another aspect of the evaluation of the work, community, home, and leisure activities is cognition. An individual may present with the physical ability to perform a job or hobbies, but if the individual does not know enough about an activity or have the cognition to safely perform an activity, this can be disabling. Tests and measures in the area of work, home, and community independence must include the physical aspects of function such as strength, range of motion, coordination, and endurance but must also assess awareness and cognition, especially for individuals with multi-system involvement.

INFORMATION IN ACTION

You are working with a patient who has experienced a spinal cord injury and has limited use of his lower extremities. The patient's medical history includes cardiac involvement. In this situation, a wheelchair seems appropriate as the primary means of mobility; but because of his heart condition, the patient may not have the endurance to allow a wheelchair to be functional. As a result, energy conservation may be a focus of intervention for this patient. This patient's cognitive status may not allow for understanding of the concept of energy conservation, and he may not know when to rest. The interaction of all of the involved systems leads to the need for creative problem solving and complex intervention techniques.

Self-Care and Home Management

The evaluation of self-care and home management is more complex for individuals with multi-system involvement. The modification of the home for one aspect of mobility may have negative impacts on other systems. For individuals with multi-system involvement, every modification must be evaluated for the effects on all the systems.

INFORMATION IN ACTION

You are working with an individual who has undergone a hip replacement, and the physical therapist's evaluation reveals the need for a rolling walker to be used in the home. After assessment of the home, it is determined that furniture will need to be rearranged in order for the walker to be safely negotiated throughout the house. You determine that there is enough room to rearrange the furniture in a more effective layout, and this appears to be the best solution to the problem.

You know that it is important to have the client involved in these kinds of decisions. Therefore, you discuss the changes with the client and evaluate the new layout idea from the perspective of how it will affect other systems involved. The client is apprehensive about moving the furniture and admits that she uses the furniture to steady herself when walking around the house. This is because of impaired balance due to peripheral neuropathy. You discuss the fact that the walker will now be what the client uses for balance. She goes on to tell you that with her significantly impaired vision, due to retinopathy as a result of her diabetes, the only reason she has been able to be independent in her home prior to her hip replacement is because of her knowledge of where everything in the house is located. Moving the furniture will rob the client of this safety measure. You begin to realize the impact of home modifications on all systems involved. Modifications that solve one problem create problems based on other pathologies. A reevaluation of the situation is clearly warranted.

Home Modifications

The evaluation of the home environment may reveal the need for home modifications or adaptive devices that are needed in order for the individual to be independent. Adaptive devices can be prescribed by the physical therapist, and intervention provided by the PTA should include any adaptive or supportive devices that will be used in the home.

TAKE NOTE

Some adaptive equipment and home modifications, such as rearranging floor rugs, can be performed by the PT or PTA. Keep in mind, however, that some modifications may require the skills of a third party—for example, the installation of a ramp. In addition, some adaptive equipment may also need the skills of a third party—for example, the installation of grab bars in the bathroom.

Evaluation of the bathroom is an important aspect of self-care and ADLs. The height of the toilet, type of bathtub, and height of the vanity are examples of aspects of the bathroom that must be evaluated in order to allow for appropriate PT intervention. In addition, evaluation of the furniture in the home is important; for example, the PTA should determine if the bed is too high for the patient to safely get in and out, or if the mattress is too soft for the patient to safely transfer, or if chairs are so low that they impede independent transfers. Evaluation of the home should also include door widths, counter heights, lighting, safety of floor surfaces, and general accessibility to the home from outside. Bed mobility, transfers, gait, balance, bathing, dressing, and home management are examples of specific skills that can be evaluated in order to determine safe and effective self-care and home management.

TAKE NOTE

During environmental evaluations, barriers to function may not be immediately obvious. Although an individual may be able to access the home, reach the countertops, and stand from chairs safely during the assessment, real life often poses greater challenges. For example, these activities may need to be performed multiple times throughout the day. The demand of the environment combined with decreased functional ability can be a barrier. The individual must have the endurance and cognitive ability to safely navigate the home.

Assessment Tests and Tools

There are many self-report and screening tools available, and it is important to use a tool that is appropriate for individuals with multi-system involvement. There are also a variety of standardized assessment tools that can be used to assess an individual's ADL and IADL status. These standardized tests allow the clinician to have a baseline evaluation of an individual's independence with self-care, as well as objectively track progress. In addition, there are standardized assessment tools that have been created to evaluate the aspects of self-care that best capture true functional ability or accurately predict the level of assistance an individual may need following a disease or injury.

The Barthel Index

The Barthel Index is a standardized assessment tool that was designed to gather information on self-care from medical records as well as from direct observation of mobility. This tool measures the level of assistance required for an individual to perform certain activities. There are ten activities observed for the Barthel Index: feeding, toileting, transferring on/off toilet, bathing, walking or wheelchair ambulation on a level surface, stair climbing, transferring between a chair and bed, dressing, maintaining bowel continence,

and maintaining bladder continence. Each item is graded on a three-point scale and given a score of 0, 5, 10, or 15. More weight is given to mobility and continence activities. Possible scores range from 0 to 100, with 0 meaning that the individual is completely dependent for the ten activities and 100 indicating that the individual is completely independent in all ten activities. This tool is commonly used in inpatient rehabilitation settings in order to measure independence before, during, and after physical therapy intervention. In addition, the Barthel Index is used to guide discharge planning including whether or not an individual can return home or needs another level of care and whether or not an individual needs assistance at home. Although a score of 100 indicates that an individual is completely independent with the ten activities, this does not automatically mean that individual will not need help at home. The real-life expectations of continuous and repetitive functional activities, cognition, and high-level tasks, such as financial issues, are not captured in this tool.

TAKE NOTE

There is a modified Barthel Index that evaluates the same items and is weighted in the same way as the original but includes detailed operational definitions and different scoring. Each item is graded on a five-point scale, with 1 meaning unable to perform an activity independently and 5 meaning independent.

The Katz Index

The Katz Index of activities of daily living is another standardized assessment tool that is commonly used in the area of self-care and home management. The Katz Index assesses the level of assistance needed to perform six basic ADLs, including bathing, dressing, toileting, transferring, continence, and feeding. This tool combines the results of observation and the individual's self-report over a two-week period. No points are given if human help is required to complete the activity, including supervision or direction, or if the activity is not performed. One point is given if the activity is performed without human help. If an activity is performed with the use of an assistive or adaptive device, then the individual receives one point because the activity did not require physical assistance from another person.

The Katz Index results in a letter grade from A through G in order of increasing dependence. Explanations of each letter grade, as well as the operational definitions of *independent* and *dependent* are somewhat unique to this tool and are fully explained within the tool. For example, dressing includes retrieving clothes from a closet and drawer, putting on the clothes, managing fasteners and buttons, and putting on any braces or outer garments such as a jacket. With the results of this assessment, the PT and PTA can identify the areas of function in which an individual may need assistive or adaptive equipment, as well as areas of function in which the individual is safely performing activities independently.

Practice 6

1. Identify one drawback of the self-report method of assessment.
   a. The patient's family may not agree with the patient's self-report.
   b. The patient may not perform certain tasks that are on the questionnaire.
   c. The patient may try to please the therapist with certain answers.
   d. The self-report does not allow for demonstration of improvement over time.

2. When treating individuals with multi-system involvement, the PTA should focus on which of the following?
   a. the number of systems involved
   b. the most severe pathology
   c. how each system affects function
   d. the most severe symptom

3. Which of the following is one aspect of participation in leisure activities that is important to evaluate in addition to physical ability?
   a. how long the individual has been participating in the activity
   b. the patient's family's approval of the leisure activity
   c. the degree to which the patient enjoys the activity
   d. the patient's ability to understand the activity

4. One benefit of standardized ADL assessment tools is
   a. the ability to see function from the patient's perspective.
   b. the ability to objectively track progress during therapy.
   c. the ability of the patient to use the tool independently.
   d. the subjective information gathered by using this kind of tool.

5. The physical therapy evaluation indicates that the PT recommends the use of a walker for ambulation in the home. The PTA performs gait and balance training with the walker for two weeks, and then discusses with the PT that the patient may be ready to discharge from therapy due to the good progress he has made. Which of the following is the best course of action?
   a. Order a walker for home use.
   b. Reevaluate the patient's function with the walker.
   c. Discharge the patient from physical therapy services.
   d. Recommend progression to ambulation without assistive device.

6. The Katz Index of activities of daily living assesses all of the following EXCEPT
   a. feeding.
   b. ambulation.
   c. dressing.
   d. transferring.

7. The Katz Index of activities of daily living gathers information through
   a. the physical therapist's observations only.
   b. patient self-report only.
   c. both observation and self-report.
   d. neither self-report nor observation.

8. The Barthel Index assess all of the following EXCEPT
   a. grooming.
   b. transferring.
   c. stairs.
   d. driving.

9. The range of possible scores on the Barthel Index is
   a. 0 to 10.
   b. 0 to 25.
   c. 0 to 75.
   d. 0 to 100.

10. A perfect high score on the Barthel Index means
    a. the patient can return home independently with no assistance required.
    b. the patient can return home but may need assistance with high-level activities.
    c. the patient can return home but requires a minimum of two hours of assistance per day.
    d. the patient can return home but requires 24-hour supervision and assistance.

11. The results of a direct examination by the physical therapist indicates that a patient is independent in all community, home, and leisure activities—including his favorite hobby, bowling. However, the patient states that he does not have the upper extremity strength he needs to bowl well. Which of the following is the best course of action for the PTA to take?
    a. Recommend that the patient find a new leisure activity that does not require as much strength.
    b. Provide additional physical therapy. intervention to increase upper extremity strength.
    c. Discharge the patient and refer him back to his primary care physician.
    d. Train the patient's son on how to assist the patient to be a better bowler.

12. The PTA communicates to the supervising physical therapist that the patient has achieved all of his physical therapy goals. The home evaluation indicated that the patient was safe and independent in the home and community, the PTA has completed all patient and family education indicated, and the patient is satisfied with his functional ability. The physical therapist performs the final assessment for the discharge summary and asks the PTA if she is sure that the patient has met all of his goals because the Katz Index of ADLs revealed little progress in functional independence. Which of the following is the best course of action for the PTA to take?

   a. Recommend 24-hour supervision at home for the patient, and discharge the patient from physical therapy.

   b. Refer the patient back to his primary care physician for approval of the discharge home.

   c. Continue physical therapy intervention with the goal of improving the Katz score.

   d. Discharge the patient with a home exercise program.

13. When scoring the Katz Index of ADLs, how would the PTA describe a patient who requires supervision and direction for daily activities?

   a. completely independent

   b. requiring human help

   c. unable to perform the activity

   d. completely dependent

14. Performance-based assessments are beneficial for patients with multi-system involvement because these assessments can identify

   a. which system is causing a functional limitation.

   b. the progression of a disease.

   c. the severity of symptoms for all systems.

   d. the symptoms that are unrelated to function.

Practice 6 Answers

1. c. One drawback of self-report by a patient is the fact that the patient's answers might be influenced by the patient's wanting to please the therapist.

2. c. When treating patients with multi-system involvement, intervention should focus on the functional presentation of the patient, not the pathologies.

3. d. In addition to physical ability, an important aspect of assessing leisure activities is cognition and the ability for the patient to understand the activity.

4. b. Standardized assessment tools allow the PTA to objectively track a patient's progress.

5. b. It is important to reevaluate patient's functional independence after training with a new assistive device in order to ensure safety and understanding of the new device.

6. b. The Katz Index of activities of daily Living does not assess ambulation.

7. c. The Katz Index of activities of daily living gathers information through self-report and observation.

8. d. The Barthel Index does not assess driving. The Barthel Index does assess grooming, transferring, and the use of stairs.

9. d. The possible range of scores on the Barthel Index is 0 to 100.

10. b. A perfect high score of 100 on the Barthel Index indicates that the patient can return home but may need assistance for high-level daily activities.

11. b. The PTA should provide additional physical therapy intervention to increase upper extremity strength for this patient. It is important that self-report and patient goals are recognized and addressed in treatment. Because this patient would like to continue bowling and is not able to do so due to upper

extremity weakness, therapy intervention should continue until the patient is independent in bowling, assuming that the goal of independence is reasonable.

12. d. The best course of action for the PTA to take is to discharge this patient from physical therapy services due to the fact that the physical therapist, the PTA, and the patient agree that the patient has reached functional independence with all goals met. Standardized assessment tools can be helpful but may not always be the best indication for continuing or discharging physical therapy services.

13. b. The Katz Index of activities of daily living would describe a patient with the need for supervision and direction as a patient who requires human help.

14. b. Performance-based assessments are beneficial for patients with multi-system involvement because these assessment can identify the progression of a disease. Performance-based assessments may be able to follow progression of a pathology based on the patient's functional status.

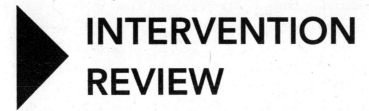

CHAPTER

7 ▶ INTERVENTION REVIEW

CHAPTER SUMMARY

The majority of the PTA's time is spent in applying physical therapy interventions to patients as directed by the physical therapist. The physical therapist assistant must be proficient in applying interventions related to the cardiovascular and pulmonary systems, the musculoskeletal system, the neuromuscular system, and the integumentary system in a safe and effective manner.

I n order to demonstrate proficiency, the PTA must be knowledgeable about the indications, precautions, and contraindications of each intervention; the application of the intervention; the effect of the intervention on other systems; and any complications that may arise from the intervention. This chapter will review intervention application by body system. Modalities, equipment, and assistive, orthotic, and prosthetic devices will be covered in separate sections, as those interventions are applied to all body systems.

Cardiac, Vascular, and Pulmonary Systems

The physical therapist assistant must apply interventions for the cardiac, vascular, and pulmonary systems to a variety of populations. In fact, the principles of aerobic exercise can be applied to any patient whose goal is to improve his or her activity tolerance and aerobic fitness level.

For those patients with acute cardiac pathologies, the PTA must be able to implement the specific phases of a cardiac rehabilitation program. The PTA also must be able to apply interventions at an appropriate intensity to those with chronic cardiac conditions. Finally, the PTA must be equally knowledgeable about interventions for patients with acute and chronic pulmonary and vascular pathologies.

Coordination, Communication, and Documentation

Coordination, communication, and documentation form a set of interventions that apply to all physical therapy encounters. Both the PT and the PTA have responsibilities related to these areas of care. Coordination is simply the working together of all parties involved with a patient, communication entails exchanging information with these parties, and documentation is any entry into the patient record. To provide optimal service to patients with problems in the cardiac, pulmonary, and vascular systems, the PTA will often coordinate care and communication with nursing staff, social services and discharge planners, and other rehabilitation disciplines.

These are some specific examples of interventions related to coordination, communication, and documentation for patients with cardiac, pulmonary, or vascular pathologies in which a PTA might participate:

- advance directives
- individualized education plans (IEPs)
- informed consent
- care conferences
- patient care rounds
- family meetings

Principles of Aerobic Conditioning

In the United States, approximately 26% of adults and 17% of children are obese. Many do not get the recommended amount of 30 to 60 minutes of physical activity per day. Virtually every patient seen in physical therapy can benefit from aerobic conditioning exercise.

If a patient is exhibiting any of the conditions listed below, aerobic exercise is contraindicated and the PTA should contact the supervising PT immediately:

- unstable angina
- symptomatic heart failure
- uncontrolled arrhythmias
- moderate to severe aortic stenosis
- uncontrolled diabetes
- acute systemic illness or fever
- uncontrolled heart rate over 100 bpm
- resting systolic blood pressure over 200 mm Hg
- resting diastolic blood pressure over 110 mm Hg

TAKE NOTE

Formal cardiac rehabilitation programs for patients with acute cardiac events contain all interventions described in this section, provided in an interdisciplinary atmosphere. However, cardiac rehab is not available in all communities nor are all patients referred to cardiac rehab when it is available. All PTAs must understand the principles of a cardiac rehab program and provide cardiac rehab to patients who cannot participate in a formal program.

Types of Aerobic Exercise Activities

Aerobic exercise must be rhythmical and sustained and use the large muscle groups of the body. It should not require special skill by the patient, and the intensity should be easy to modify. Factors such as the amount of joint impact, the ability to be outdoors, and the equipment and financial resources available to the patient must be considered. Choose an aerobic activity that is enjoyable to the patient. Examples of common aerobic activities include walking, swimming, biking, and running, with the possible use of treadmills, elliptical walkers, stair climbers, exercise bikes, and rowing machines.

Intensity of Exercise

Ideally, the intensity of exercise should be 50 to 85% of VO_2max or 65 to 90% of the maximum heart rate, both as determined by a graded exercise tolerance test. The challenge is that many patients have not had a formal exercise tolerance test. To estimate VO_2max and maximum heart rate, the PT or PTA can perform a submaximal stress test in the clinical setting. Alternatively, maximum heart rate can be estimated by using the equation 220 – age. However, this does not account for factors related to the person's current level of conditioning. Finally, the Borg Rate of Perceived Exertion Scale can be used to assess intensity of aerobic exercise. An RPE of 12 to 17 corresponds to an appropriate target zone intensity.

INFORMATION IN ACTION

A PTA is working with a 45-year-old man who is coming to therapy for a low back injury sustained at work. The patient is overweight and has poor aerobic physical fitness. He expresses a desire to improve his fitness level. The PT asks the PTA to explore the types of activities that the man enjoys and to design an aerobic exercise program for him. The PTA and patient decide that the elliptical trainer would be the most enjoyable, accessible, and comfortable exercise option for this patient at this time. The patient is instructed to perform seven minutes on the elliptical trainer at an RPE of 10 (light), and then to increase his speed until the RPE is at 13 (somewhat hard). He is to sustain this level for 25 minutes, and then decrease back to an RPE of 10 for another eight minutes, for a total workout time of 40 minutes. After two weeks, the PTA instructs the patient to increase the time he spends at target intensity by 5 minutes per week, up to 45 minutes. Six weeks after the initiation of the patient's aerobic exercise program, the patient is able to maintain a total workout time of 60 minutes every other day.

Patients with Cardiac and Pulmonary Pathologies

Patients with acute or chronic cardiac pathologies, or chronic pulmonary or vascular disease, may benefit from aerobic conditioning, provided that they do not have any of the contraindications to these types of activities. However, intensity, duration, and progression of exercise must be modified to make it safe for the patient.

Acute Cardiac Pathologies

Deciding when aerobic exercise can be started following an acute cardiac event depends on the nature of the event and numerous patient factors. Two to four weeks following a myocardial infarction, an angioplasty, or a coronary artery bypass graft (CABG) would be typical for the initiation of aerobic exercise training. Prior to that, the patient should participate in exercise and activities designed to prevent deconditioning and other complications, such as pneumonia, contractures, and pressure sores. Patients should have clearance from a physician before aerobic activities are initiated. Once the patient is cleared to participate, the starting intensity and subsequent progression will be more conservative than it would for a person without cardiac problems. Vital signs should be measured before, during, and after activity. Target intensity initially may be around 11, or fairly light, with no more than a 20 bpm increase in heart rate from baseline (assuming heart rate response is not blunted by medication). Frequency begins at 10 to 20 minutes, twice per day. Once the person can tolerate exercising at an RPE intensity of 13 (somewhat hard) for 20 minutes, frequency can be declined to every other day, and the time spent at target intensity can be gradually increased to 30 to 40 minutes.

INFORMATION IN ACTION

A 56-year-old man is eight weeks status post CABG. He presents to the outpatient therapy clinic with a referral for aerobic conditioning. The patient has completed a postsurgical exercise stress test and has a documented maximum heart rate and VO_2 max. He has been taking two to three slow walks of 20 minutes each day around his subdivision. The PT performs an initial examination and evaluation and develops the exercise program. The patient has elected to use the stationary bike. He will begin biking at low resistance for ten minutes, with an RPE of 9 (very light). He will increase resistance until the RPE is 12 and maintain that for 20 minutes. The cool-down will be for ten minutes, again at an RPE of 9. The physical therapist will monitor the patient's heart rate during the aerobic portion to ensure that it approximates 70% of his maximum heart rate as determined by the stress test. The patient will attend therapy three days per week.

INFORMATION IN ACTION

An 83-year-old resident of a skilled nursing facility returns to the facility one week after sustaining an acute MI. She had been undergoing therapy for a hip fracture sustained seven weeks earlier. The patient had been ambulating with a wheeled walker for 150 feet and was weight-bearing as tolerated (WBAT). In the hospital, she received bedside exercise and transfer training for two days prior to discharge back to the SNF. The PT determines that it is too early to begin aerobic conditioning. The PT has the patient perform active exercise of the upper and lower extremities in supine with her head elevated, transfer training in and out of bed, and ambulation with the wheeled walker from the bed to the bathroom. The patient is mildly confused and unable to understand the concept of the RPE scale. Because she is also on a beta blocker, heart rate cannot be used to determine tolerance to treatment. Therefore, the physical therapist monitors the patient's pulse oximetry, her rate of respiration, her skin color, and her verbal expressions of fatigue to determine her tolerance to the activities. The patient is seen for 25 minutes, twice daily.

Frequency and Duration of Exercise

Each exercise session should consist of a 5 to 10 minute warm-up period to prepare the muscles, joints, and cardiovascular system for exertion; 20 to 60 minutes of exercise at the target intensity; and a five to ten minute cool-down period to prevent hypotension. Exercise must be done at least every other day. It takes 6 to 12 weeks before significant improvements in cardiovascular health occur but only 5 weeks for all gains to be lost once exercise is discontinued. Therefore, patients wishing to make sustained improvements in their cardiovascular fitness must commit to a lifelong program of aerobic activity.

Phases of Cardiac Rehabilitation

PHASES	GOALS	INTENSITY	DURATION/FREQUENCY
Phase I (inpatient)	Prevent deconditioning; prevent complications; assess cardiovascular response to activity; pt/family education	1 to 5 METS	10 to 20 minutes/BID
Phase II	Functional activities; promote positive lifestyle changes	5 to 9 METS	60 minutes/three to five times per week
Phase III	Maintain function; promote lifelong commitment	7 to 10+ METS	60 minutes/three to five times per week

Goals and intensity evolve as the patient progresses through the phases of cardiac rehabilitation.

Chronic Cardiac and Pulmonary Pathologies

Patients with chronic conditions such as congestive heart failure, coronary artery disease, and chronic obstructive pulmonary disease can certainly improve their endurance through aerobic exercise. The program must be initiated and progressed with careful attention to signs of exercise intolerance and adverse effects. The PTA must take note of heart rate, RPE, and clinical signs such as pallor and diaphoresis. Adverse effects include chest pain, excessive shortness of breath, excessive fatigue, and oxygen saturation below 90%.

Guidelines for Aerobic Exercise for Patients with Chronic Conditions

	ARRHYTHMIAS	CAD	CHF	COPD
Intensity	50% to 85% max HR 11 to 16 RPE	40% to 80% max HR 10 to 15 RPE	40% to 70% max HR 11 to 16 RPE	11 to 13 RPE O_2 sat $\geq$ 90%
Frequency	3 to 7 days per week 20 to 60 minutes daily	3 to 7 days per week 20 to 60 minutes daily	3 to 7 days per week 20 to 40 minutes daily	3 to 7 days per week 30 minutes BID

Patients with chronic conditions participating in aerobic exercise should start at the low end of the guidelines and be progressed gradually as their tolerance and medical status permits.

Chronic Arterial Insufficiency

The goal of aerobic exercise for patients with chronic arterial insufficiency is to improve endurance by making the muscles more efficient at using oxygen and increasing the collateral circulation of the muscles. A target heart rate or RPE level must be established by one of the methods described earlier. Once established, the patient should perform at that target level as long as possible without causing claudication once or twice a day, three to five days per week. Proper footwear for aerobic exercise is essential for patients in this population in order to prevent open areas. Over a 12-week period, the patient's pain-free walking distance can double and blood flow to muscles can increase tenfold.

INFORMATION IN ACTION

A 69-year-old man comes to physical therapy with a diagnosis of chronic arterial insufficiency. His goal is to walk six blocks to the local playground with his grandchildren without experiencing leg pain. The PT determines that the patient can currently ambulate two blocks before experiencing symptoms. The PTA instructs the patient to walk one block from his house, rest for two minutes, and return home. The rest allows the patient to get home without leg pain. He does this twice a day for two weeks. The PT reassesses him and adjusts his ambulation distance to three blocks. After eight weeks, he is able to walk to the park with his grandchildren and back again, with a rest while the children play. The patient continues to progress his ambulation independently after discontinuing formal therapy sessions.

Lymphedema

If the amount of lymphedema the patient is experiencing is not stabilized, aerobic exercise should be done at an intensity of 40 to 50% of maximum heart rate. Once stable, intensities of up to 80% of maximum heart rate may be performed.

Strength Training

Resisted exercise is critical to allow patients who have become deconditioned to regain the strength needed to be independent in all their desired activities. Ideal strength training would involve using the amount of resistance that the patient could lift through 8 to 12 repetitions (8 to 12 repetition maximum). This may be appropriate for patients with chronic venous insufficiency and lymphedema, provided that these patients do not experience pain for more than 24 hours following exercise, that they do not have increased edema, and that they do not lose strength following the exercise. If these problems occur, strengthening should continue with the patient utilizing a 15 to 25 repetition maximum level of resistance. This level of resistance should also be used for patients with chronic cardiac, pulmonary, and arterial disorders.

Flexibility Exercises

Patients with chronic pulmonary disorders exhibit characteristic postural changes that often lead to muscles and joints around the thorax becoming less mobile. The PTA may apply active and passive stretching techniques to improve muscle flexibility. The PTA may also perform segmental breathing to improve lateral costal expansion. In this technique, the PTA's hands are placed on the lateral aspect (bilaterally) of the patient's rib cage. The PTA then compresses the ribs during expiration and gives a quick stretch to facilitate medial/lateral expansion just prior to inspiration.

The PT may perform joint mobilization to improve rib cage mobility and increase thoracic extension.

Patients with COPD tend to exhibit a thoracic kyphosis with a forward head and to use accessory muscles of respiration, causing the muscles listed to become shortened:

- pectoralis major
- pectoralis minor
- sternocleidomastoid
- scalenes

INFORMATION IN ACTION

A 71-year-old man with emphysema is receiving outpatient physical therapy. He exhibits an increased kyphosis and barrel chest, stiffness of the rib cage, and weakness of the rhomboids and lower trapezius muscles. The PT does mobilization of the rib cage and asks the PTA to instruct the patient in a home exercise program for stretching and strengthening of the postural muscles. The PTA instructs the patient in a corner stretch for the pectoralis major and in Thera-Band® exercises to strengthen the rhomboids and lower trapezius. The PTA has the patient do two stretches of 30 seconds duration, once daily, with an emphasis on relaxed expiration. The PTA instructs the patient to perform two sets of 20 repetitions of each of the strengthening exercises every other day.

Airway Clearance Techniques

Many types of pulmonary pathologies result in the inability of the patient to clear secretions from the airways. Airway clearance is made difficult by increased secretions, decreased bronchiole size, and chest wall pain. The main ways that physical therapy assists in airway clearance are postural drainage, improving the effectiveness of the cough, and providing an assisted cough.

Postural Drainage

In postural drainage, the body is positioned so that lung secretions may drain along the bronchioles toward the main stem bronchus through the force of gravity. Percussion in the form of cupping and vibration are often added. While the patient is in the postural drainage position, cupping is applied over the involved segment for two to four minutes. The therapist applies vibration two to three times during exhalation. The patient is allowed to sit up and cough if needed and the sequence is repeated. The treatment is effective if sputum is produced. The PTA should note the amount, color, and consistency of the sputum and note any odor present. The patient should be advised to monitor sputum production over the next few hours, as production may be delayed.

Postural drainage and percussion can be applied to one or multiple segments as long as vital signs remain stable and treatment time does not exceed 45 to 60 minutes. The general sequence for application of postural drainage is as follows:

1. Gather tissues and positioning aids.
2. Measure vital signs.
3. Position patient.
4. Apply percussion over affected segment for two to four minutes.
5. Do vibration two to three times.
6. Encourage patient to cough.
7. Repeat for treatment time of five to ten minutes per segment.
8. Can do multiple segments for total treatment time of 45 to 60 minutes.
9. Assess vital signs and characteristics of any sputum produced.

Contraindications to Postural Drainage and Percussion

POSTURAL DRAINAGE	PERCUSSION
Untreated acute pulmonary conditions	Osteoporosis
Cardiovascular instability	Chest wall pain
Severe hemoptysis	Over fractures
Recent neurosurgery	Over tumor
	Patient hemorrhages easily

Contraindications to postural drainage relate primarily to the stress of placing patients in various positions, including head-down positions. The contraindications to percussion relate primarily to the force of the cupping and vibration on the thoracic cage area.

Improving Cough Effectiveness

Airway clearance may be impaired if the patient has a poor cough. Causes for this may include inability to take a deep breath due to pain or poor rib cage flexibility or inability to forcefully expel air due to pain or abdominal weakness. For example, after a rib fracture, the patient will experience pain during both deep inspiration and forced expiration, resulting in a poor cough. If pain prevents forceful exhalation during the cough, patients are advised to splint the painful area by tightly holding a pillow or firm pad against the painful area while coughing. The PT and PTA may apply flexibility exercises as described previously to improve the patient's ability to take a deep breath. The PTA may also help the patient to take a deep breath by improving the patient's breathing pattern. If the patient uses accessory muscles to breathe instead of using the diaphragm, then the volume of inspiration will be reduced. The PTA may also review the sequence of an effective cough with the patient.

Instructions in Diaphragmatic Breathing

- Place patient in semi-reclined position.
- Instruct patient to breathe in through nose and out through mouth.
- Place hand firmly over patient's diaphragm.
- Encourage patient to feel and watch abdomen rise during inspiration.
- Patient puts own hands over diaphragm to feel movement.
- Instruct patient to sniff in quickly to engage diaphragm.

Teaching patients to improve their breathing pattern through diaphragmatic breathing can improve efficiency of breathing and increase cough effectiveness.

Instructions for an Effective Cough

- Patient should be sitting or leaning forward.
- Ensure or teach diaphragmatic breathing with deep inspiration.
- Demonstrate sharp, deep double cough.
- Have the patient huff or make K sound to engage abdominals.
- Put it all together: Have the patient take a deep breath in and make a sharp, double cough.

Improving the effectiveness of a patient's cough will increase airway clearance and improve ventilation.

Assisted Cough Techniques

Patients with weak abdominal musculature may require physical assistance to improve the expulsion phase of the cough. This is common with patients with weakened abdominal muscles following spinal cord injury.

INFORMATION IN ACTION

A 73-year-old woman is recovering from pneumonia involving the anterior apical segments of both lungs. She demonstrates use of accessory muscles during breathing and a weak cough. The PTA begins by facilitating diaphragmatic breathing. He continues by demonstrating and having the patient practice an effective cough. He then has the patient sit in a slightly reclined position and applies percussion directly under the clavicle on both sides. He alternates percussion with vibration, and after eight minutes, the patient is able to produce an effective cough. The PTA notes the amount, color, and consistency of the secretions and also notes any odor. The patient is instructed to monitor any further sputum production over the next few hours.

Relaxation Techniques

Patients with cardiac and pulmonary pathologies may experience anxiety, particularly when the patient is frequently short of breath. For example, patients with asthma often experience a great deal of anxiety during an asthma attack because they feel as though they cannot breathe. The anxiety can worsen the asthma attack, and the cycle is difficult to break. Those with cardiac pathologies may become short of breath with exertion and fear that they are bringing on a heart attack. Therefore, patients with both cardiac and pulmonary pathologies may benefit from learning relaxation techniques to manage the inevitable episodes of shortness of breath.

Diaphragmatic Breathing

A common symptom associated with anxiety is rapid, shallow respiration. Having a person consciously perform diaphragmatic breathing can assist in bringing respiration under control, thereby decreasing the anxiety response. The PTA can train the patient in this breathing pattern by having the patient start in a semi-reclined position. The PTA and/or the patient places his or her hands over the diaphragm and gives gentle pressure so that the patient has something to breathe against as he or she inhales. Exhaling through pursed lips to achieve a two-to-one inhalation to exhalation ratio can help pace the breathing. Pacing can also diminish the sensation of shortness of breath for patients with emphysema, which in turn decreases anxiety.

Progressive Relaxation

While continuing the controlled, paced breathing, the PTA may direct the patient to contract the muscles in the hands or feet for 5 seconds, then relax for 20 to 30 seconds. The PTA then tells the patient to feel how heavy and warm the relaxing muscles feel. This sequence is repeated with more proximal muscles and then with the entire extremity. After contracting and relaxing the muscles in the extremities and trunk, the PTA tells the patient to feel the heaviness and warmth permeating their entire body.

Compression Therapies

The hallmark symptom of both venous insufficiency and lymphedema is edema. Management of the edema prevents skin breakdown, fibrosis of the tissue, contractures, and ultimately functional mobility and gait limitations.

Bandaging and Pressure Garments

Bandaging and garments promote venous and lymphatic return by placing an external compressive force on the vessels. Bandaging is generally done until the limb size has stabilized and a permanent garment may be ordered for long-term use. Short-stretch elastic bandages are used by compressing the limb when the muscles are contracting and releasing the limb when the muscles are relaxed. In this way, they complement the natural compressive forces of the working muscles and do not constrict the limb during periods of relaxation. Bandages are layered to provide enough compression, with padding over bony prominences to prevent skin breakdown. Pressure garments may be custom-fit or off-the-shelf and are more cosmetic and easier to apply than the bandages. They serve to maintain the degree of edema reduction achieved by the bandaging.

Manual Lymphatic Drainage (MLD)

For patients with lymphedema, manual lymphatic drainage is another component of edema control. It is a manual therapy technique that uses short, superficial strokes to stimulate lymph vessel contraction. The skin and superficial fascial layer is stretched, then quickly released and allowed to snap back. The strokes are generally applied to proximal areas first, moving distally as central lymph channels are opened. Total treatment time may be 30 to 60 minutes.

Exercise

Active exercise of the distal extremities is effective in moving edema proximally. For patients with venous insufficiency, the exercises consist of active or resisted exercise of the lower extremities, with the extremities elevated above the level of the heart. Patients with lymphedema progress through a more specific sequence of lymphatic drainage exercise. Bandages or a compression garment are worn during the exercises. The exercises are done with the limb elevated. Repetitions are done slowly and rhythmically and excessive fatigue is avoided. The exercises are done twice daily for 20 to 30 minutes.

Intermittent Pneumatic Compression Pump

Mechanical compression pumping creates external compression on the limb to facilitate venous and lymphatic return. Compression progresses from distal to proximal and includes a period of relaxation. The on-to-off time ratio is generally three to one. The pressure ranges from 20 to 50 mm Hg for the upper extremity and 30 to 60 mm Hg for the lower extremity but should not exceed 45 mm Hg when applying compression for lymphedema.

INFORMATION IN ACTION

A 34-year-old woman is recovering from a mastectomy and reconstruction to treat breast cancer. She has developed lymphedema in the left upper extremity as a consequence. The PT begins the session by performing manual lymphatic drainage. The PTA then assists the patient in donning her compression garment and conducts the lymphatic drainage exercises.

Functional Training

Many people would say that the ultimate purpose behind all physical therapy interventions is to return the patient to independent functioning in the patient's home and community. Training in activities of daily living, instrumental activities of daily living, community, work, and leisure activities will comprise a large portion of the therapy provided to patients with cardiopulmonary and vascular disorders.

Activities of Daily Living and Instrumental Activities of Daily Living

Functional training related to self-care (ADLs) and home management (IADLs) generally focuses on safety and energy conservation. Patients with significant aerobic capacity impairments can save energy and prevent falls by sitting while they brush their teeth or apply makeup. Taking a shower while seated on a shower bench instead of standing may be another strategy. Facilitating proper posture during ADL activities will improve ventilation and enhance endurance.

Examples of energy conservation during IADLs would include planning the day to avoid multiple trips up and down the stairs, taking breaks between cleaning chores instead of trying to do everything at once, and using paced breathing during yard work to prevent shortness of breath. Home management may also include learning to plan healthy menus or buying home exercise equipment.

Community/Work/Leisure

The direction of training in community, work, and leisure activities will vary widely from patient to patient depending upon the patient's age, interests, physical abilities, and working status. One patient may need to incorporate more active leisure activities into his or her schedule, such as playing softball instead of cards two nights a week. Another may need guidance in order to gradually progress from a part-time to a full-time work schedule. Yet another person may need volunteer opportunities that provide social interaction and mild physical activity, such as passing out the mail at the local skilled nursing facility.

Education of Patient and Caregivers

The PTA can provide patients and caregivers with education regarding which types of risk factors will increase the likelihood that a patient will develop a problem or make existing ones worse. Many of the disorders covered in this section are chronic in nature. Patients need to be empowered to manage these disorders to maximize their health and function and to feel as though they have a measure of control over the disorder. The PTA should also give detailed descriptions of how a patient should do exercises or engage in other activities related to their care.

Cardiac Pathologies

The PT and the PTA together are responsible for helping a patient understand the effect of smoking, high blood lipid levels, obesity, inactivity, and stress on the cardiac system. The PT and the PTA should direct patients toward resources for smoking cessation, healthy food choices and meal planning, and stress management. They should instruct the patient in activity guidelines and energy conservation techniques, as described in the functional training section of this chapter. They will additionally instruct each patient in how to take his or her own pulse and in the RPE scale so that the patient may monitor exertion appropriately. The patient must also recognize symptoms, such as angina or lower extremity edema, which may signal an exacerbation. Overall, the PT and PTA team need to educate and support the patient in making necessary lifestyle changes to promote ongoing health.

Pulmonary Pathologies

The main risk factors associated with COPD are smoking and obesity. Key symptoms to look for include dyspnea, weight gain, or needing more pillows to sleep. Learning to monitor exertion and conserve energy are also important concepts to discuss with patients with pulmonary pathologies. Patients with ongoing airway clearance issues may need to learn how to do postural drainage independently at home. Instruction in relaxation strategies as described earlier in this chapter may also be beneficial.

Peripheral Vascular Disease

The PT and the PTA must educate the patient about many of the same lifestyle issues covered for patients with or at risk for cardiac pathologies. Smoking is primary among them, as well as elevated glucose levels. The key symptoms to recognize are claudication pain in arterial disorders and edema in venous and lymphatic disorders. Instruction in proper skin care is also critical, as is edema management for those with venous and lymphatic disorders.

TAKE NOTE

A long-handled, gooseneck mirror can help a patient independently perform visual skin inspections.

Elements of Proper Skin Care

Proper skin care is essential for patients with or at risk for cardiac pathologies. Elements of proper skin care are as follows:

- Wash, dry, and moisturize skin.
- Avoid restrictive clothing.
- Do visual skin inspection daily.
- Wear proper footwear.
- Avoid sunburn.
- Avoid nicks, cuts, abrasions, and burns.
- Avoid blood pressure measurements on involved extremity.

INFORMATION IN ACTION

Mrs. Jennings is a 66-year-old woman with chronic bronchitis living alone in her own home. She is recovering from a bout of pneumonia. The PTA works with Mrs. Jennings on energy conservation techniques. The PTA instructs Mrs. Jennings in proper posture while stooping and reaching to dust furniture. The PTA and Mrs. Jennings work together to rearrange the kitchen cupboards so that the most frequently used items are at thigh-to-chest level. They create a list of A.M. and P.M. chores and apportion them across the days of the week. Finally, the PTA tells Mrs. Jennings to use a rolling cart to take objects from one room to the next instead of carrying them.

Practice 1

1. Mr. Hayes is referred to physical therapy for aerobic conditioning. His past medical history includes diabetes mellitus, hypertension, and mild atrial fibrillation. He takes an oral medication for the diabetes, and his blood sugar was 102 this morning. He takes medication for the hypertension, and his blood pressure as measured by the PTA is 180/116. His heart rate is 84 bpm. Based on this information, which of the following is the most likely reason that the PTA decides not to do aerobic exercise with Mr. Hayes at this time?
   a. His diabetes is out of control.
   b. His atrial fibrillation is out of control.
   c. His blood pressure is too high.
   d. His pulse is too high.

2. Mrs. Jones is a 58-year-old woman who is deconditioned due to a sedentary lifestyle. She comes to physical therapy to develop a safe and effective aerobic exercise program. What would be the most appropriate rate of perceived exertion at which to begin her conditioning program?
   a. 7
   b. 12
   c. 16
   d. 20

3. A patient is participating in phase I of a cardiac rehabilitation program following an acute myocardial infarction. Which of the following is the most appropriate goal of treatment?
   a. preventing deconditioning
   b. improving aerobic capacity
   c. returning to work
   d. quitting smoking

4. A patient with COPD is participating in aerobic conditioning exercises, and the PTA is periodically monitoring oxygen saturation. At what minimum level should oxygen saturation be maintained?
a. 100%
b. 95%
c. 90%
d. 85%

5. A PTA is instructing a patient with chronic arterial insufficiency in an ambulation program to improve his walking distance. What is the most important sign of intolerance for the patient to use to limit ambulation distance?
a. shortness of breath
b. increased heart rate
c. increased blood pressure
d. pain in the legs

6. The PTA is performing strength training exercises for the quadriceps with a patient with chronic heart failure. Which of the following is the most appropriate level of resistance?
a. 1 repetition maximum
b. 5 repetition maximum
c. 10 repetition maximum
d. 20 repetition maximum

7. A patient with COPD needs to mobilize her upper chest. Which of the following would be the best exercise to achieve this?
a. seated wheelchair push-ups
b. bilateral PNF upper extremity D2 flexion pattern, done actively
c. posterior pelvic tilts in supine
d. diaphragmatic breathing

8. A patient recovering from bronchitis has accumulated secretions in the posterior apical segments of both lungs. The patient has severe osteoporosis. Which of the following statements is true?
a. Postural drainage may be performed, but percussion is contraindicated.
b. Percussion may be performed, but postural drainage is contraindicated.
c. Both postural drainage and percussion may be performed.
d. Both postural drainage and percussion are contraindicated.

9. A patient underwent a coronary artery bypass graft and has a weak cough due to pain. What would be the most effective way to help this patient produce a more effective cough?
   a. Perform an assisted cough technique with the patient in supine.
   b. Have the patient sniff in to engage the diaphragm.
   c. Have the patient practice the hard "K" sound.
   d. Have the patient hold a pillow over his or her chest incision while coughing.

10. The PTA is progressing a patient with lower extremity lymphedema through lymph drainage exercises. What would be the best sequence to follow?
    a. ankle pumps, hip range of motion, pelvic tilts
    b. total body relaxation, pelvic tilts, knee flexion and extension
    c. knee flexion and extension, knee to chest, scapular protraction and retraction
    d. hip rotation, cervical rotation, total body relaxation

11. Education about which of the following risk factors would be appropriate for patients with cardiac, pulmonary, and arterial vascular disease?
    a. smoking
    b. high blood sugar
    c. high lipid levels
    d. alcohol use

12. A 48-year-old man is at home recovering after a four-day hospital stay for a myocardial infarction. Which of the following would be the most appropriate suggestion to help this patient reenter his home and work roles?
    a. Do all household chores in the morning before he gets fatigued.
    b. Do all the lawn chores in the evening when it is not so hot.
    c. Space activities throughout the day.
    d. Return to work full-time to avoid depression from staying at home.

Practice 1 Answers

1. c. The PTA most likely decides not to do aerobic exercise with Mr. Hayes at this time because his blood pressure is too high. A patient with a systolic blood pressure over 200 mm Hg or a diastolic pressure over 110 mm Hg should not participate in aerobic exercise. Mr. Hayes's blood sugar and heart rate values are within normal limits, and there is no evidence that his atrial fibrillation is not controlled.

2. b. The most appropriate rate of perceived exertion at which to begin Mrs. Jones's conditioning program is 12. An RPE between 12 and 17 is the appropriate target range for most age groups. Because Mrs. Jones is just beginning her conditioning program, staying at the bottom of the range would be most appropriate for her.

3. a. The most appropriate goal of treatment for this patient is to prevent deconditioning. Phase I of cardiac rehab occurs in an inpatient setting and emphasizes prevention of deconditioning and other complications of the acute myocardial infarction. Improving aerobic capacity, returning to work, and making long-term lifestyle changes (such as smoking cessation) are done in the outpatient phases of cardiac rehab.

4. c. Oxygen saturation should be maintained at a minimum level of 90%.

5. d. The patient should be encouraged to walk as far as possible without intermittent claudication.

6. d. The most appropriate level of resistance for this patient is 20 repetition maximum. Strengthening exercises should be done with high repetitions and low resistance.

7. b. The best exercise for a patient with COPD who needs to mobilize her upper chest is bilateral PNF upper extremity D2 flexion pattern, done actively. The upper extremity D2 flexion pattern will bring both arms up over the patient's head into flexion, abduction, and external rotation. This will open the thorax anteriorly and extend the spine.

8. a. Osteoporosis is a contraindication for percussion, due to the risk of fracture from the force applied. The patient may still be placed into the postural drainage position.

9. d. The most effective way to help this patient produce a more effective cough would be to have the patient hold a pillow over his or her chest incision while coughing. If pain is restricting the cough, then the patient should splint over the painful area during coughing.

10. b. The exercises should begin with total body relaxation, progress to proximal lymph channel clearing, and then move down the extremity from proximal to distal.

11. a. Smoking is the one risk factor common to all the diseases listed.

12. c. This patient should space activities throughout the day in order to alternate periods of activity with periods of rest.

Musculoskeletal System

Physical therapy plays a central role in managing musculoskeletal conditions. The intervention focus is to help patients resume functional movement and to optimize the potential to restore, maintain, or enhance performance.

Types and Applications of Interventions

Treatment interventions vary depending on the stage of rehabilitation, the extent of the injury, and the specific goals identified for the patient. An important aspect of the interventions must include education of the patient and in some cases family members or caregivers to ensure that specific instructions are being carried out and that the patient is continuing to work outside of the rehabilitation facility on the home exercise program. Interventions are not complete without thorough documentation that details the activities provided and describes the need for skilled services. This chapter summarizes physical therapy interventions that are commonly used to address musculoskeletal conditions.

Coordination, Communication, and Documentation

Although clinical documentation is usually completed at the end of physical therapy interventions, it is appropriate for us to begin with it here. Clinical documentation is the foundational communication tool between and among the physical therapist and the physical therapist assistant, the primary care physician and other specialists, the insurance carrier, and in some cases the employer. Clear communication regarding the patient's progress, current treatments, response to treatment, and barriers that interfere with successful progress all may be communicated with a clinical note.

Medical Documentation

The most common format is the problem-oriented medical record or SOAP note, where subjective and objective information is combined to determine an assessment of how well the patient is managing the current level of treatment, and then a plan is made as to how to proceed with the patient's care.

Billing and Clinical Documentation

Coordinated with the medical documentation is the billing documentation. For each billable CPT code considered, there must be adequate documentation noting that the service was performed, was skilled in nature, and was delivered by the appropriate personnel. Clinical documentation is both a medical and legal document that can be used to measure the extent of disability, terminate or continue benefits, and support the need for additional services. It is being used more frequently to assess or measure the quality of care received by a patient as a part of outcome measures. Clear, concise, and thorough communication requires clinicians to speak and write in a functional manner so that all who read the documentation will understand it.

In an orthopedic setting, it is common to find a flow sheet, in addition to the clinical note, which summarizes all therapeutic exercise interventions as well as applicable modalities and educational topics. Using a grid or flow sheet allows the clinician to see at a glance what was done during the previous session, allowing appropriate progression or regression as needed. It is important to note that the flow sheet is not in and of itself complete documentation but simply a tool used to streamline documentation. It is an ancillary component so that in each note a narrative summary of the activities need not be written down.

Clinical documentation must be made with each patient visit, with a progress or summary note completed as often as weekly but in some cases every two weeks or in time for the next physician follow-up visit. In the managed care arena and with patients who are being treated under workers' compensation benefits, there may be an additional need to contact the case manager on a weekly basis for an update.

It is important that each note describes the patient's current functional levels and puts them in perspective with regard to the short- and long-term goals established at the initial evaluation. At a minimum, there should be updated measurements relating to specific impairments which may include range of motion, muscle strength, lifting ability, girth, grip strength, sensation, aerobic capacity. Additionally, notes may document the progress of any other test or measurement that might be repeated in the course of treatment. Each note also should describe the need for the skilled services of a physical therapist or physical therapist assistant in order for the patient to achieve the stated goals. Clinicians should also remember to include information related to the quality of the performance observed. A simple way to think of it is to describe quality of movement, quantity of movement, speed, and symptoms. These four factors will encompass most of the PTA's observations. For example, a patient who is having difficulty with an activity may demonstrate tremoring, substitution patterns, or accessory muscle recruitment, or require verbal or tactile cues to perform the activity correctly—all examples of quality measures. The patient may not be able to complete the established sets, reps, or time that was requested, or if completed, may have required more frequent rest breaks—all examples of quantity of movement. A patient who is uncomfortable may rush through an activity to complete it sooner or move very slowly because of fatigue; these observations suggest issues with speed. Finally, changes in subjective reports of symptoms—especially to the injured area—complete the documentation.

Timeliness Counts

Documentation needs to be timely. Waiting until the end of the day to do one's documentation may often result in mistakes because it can be difficult to remember each patient and the myriad number of clinical observations a PTA might make in a treatment session.

The PTA should document during the treatment session and then summarize at the end of the treatment; if he or she is in a setting where the charts cannot be moved, the PTA should carry a small notebook to keep track of important observations until he or she can complete the documentation.

Standards for Documentation

APTA's guidelines include seven specific elements required for appropriate documentation: (1) patient/client self-report, as appropriate; (2) identification of specific interventions provided, including frequency, intensity, and duration, as appropriate; (3) equipment provided; (4) changes in patient/client status as they relate to the plan of care; (5) adverse reaction to interventions, if any; (6) factors that modify frequency or intensity of intervention and progression toward goals and outcomes, including patient/client adherence to patient/client-related instructions; and (7) communication/consultation with providers/patient/client/family/significant others. These standards will help to ensure that the documentation be legally defensible. They may also help to ensure prompt payment for skilled services and good communication with healthcare providers.

Instruction, Education, and Training of Patients/Clients and Caregivers

Education of the patient or client and appropriate family members or caregivers is appropriate at any stage of rehabilitation. The educational topic may vary depending on the stage of rehabilitation; however, the need for the education does not. In the acute stage of rehabilitation, the focus of education is on protection of the injured area, how to safely use protective equipment or assistive devices, special precautions, and how to manage symptoms most effectively. The educational topics may also include best positions for sleeping or resting, possible side effects of medication, and how to perform basic activities of daily living with or without assistance. In the subacute phase of rehabilitation, which is where controlled motion begins, the focus of the educational topic shifts to encouraging the patient or client to become more active and how to do that without causing harm or re-injury. Additional guidelines for how the patient or client should add increasingly demanding activities to his or her daily life are also included at this stage. Finally, in the chronic stage of rehabilitation, the patient is ready to resume many or all of the premorbid activities and is moving toward discharge. Education in this stage of rehabilitation is guidance as to how the patient or client will gradually resume activities and what to watch for which might indicate an adverse effect.

Educating Families and Caregivers

Family members or caregivers may also be included in the educational aspects of rehabilitation. If the client or patient is at an age or mental state where he or she might need reminders to perform activities on a schedule or how to perform activities correctly, it is appropriate to include the family or a caregiver in the educational aspects of rehabilitation. Family and caregivers can also act to help motivate a patient or client to continue a home exercise program. "Use it or lose it" is a phrase that is frequently quoted in physical therapy centers because patients who do not continue to show gains achieved through rehabilitation services in their home exercise program are bound to lose them.

Summaries and Handouts

When providing a patient or client with a home exercise program, it is important to provide a written summary of the program. In many cases, the name of the exercise; a picture or drawing of the exercise being performed; the weight or resistance used; and the number of sets, repetitions, or sessions per day and hold time are provided on a handout. These handouts provide a visual reminder for patients should the exercise be forgotten and can be reviewed and cue the patient to perform the activities properly. It is important that these exercises be reviewed with the patient or client prior to sending them home with the handouts.

Understanding the Program

Education is more than a one-way street in which the PTA provides all the information and the patient passively receives it. Part of the PTA's clinical documentation should include how the physical therapist assistant knows that the patient or client understands what has been taught. The PTA must ask whether or not the patient/client or caregiver can verbalize an understanding of the information, can correctly demonstrate performance of the activity, or can appropriately cue the patient to perform the activity correctly. This information (along with the subject matter of the educational topic) should be documented in the objective portion of the daily note.

Feedback during the Stages of Learning

Feedback is another important consideration when educating a patient or client. As the patient is learning to perform a new skill, there are three stages of learning: the cognitive stage, the associative stage, and the autonomic stage. The cognitive stage is the first stage where the patient requires the most feedback. This feedback will be concurrent (or given while the activity is being performed) and very frequent. It might include reminders or verbal or tactile cues to signal by touch what the patient should do. At this stage, the patient is easily distracted, makes frequent mistakes, and requires a lot of feedback. In the second stage, or the associative stage, the patient no longer needs constant feedback. The performance of the skill is better, with fewer mistakes, and feedback is used to fine-tune the performance. Feedback is still necessary in the associative stage; however, the focus is on the quality of the performance. Feedback is generally given after the patient has performed the task and is a summary of overall quality or quantity of performance rather than an attempt to identify every mistake. Finally, the autonomic stage is the stage in which the motor task becomes almost automatic and very little conscious thought goes into the performance. Errors are rare, and the focus is to maximize the patient's or client's potential for the task. Feedback for the most part is now internalized, as the patient or client can feel when the task is being performed correctly. Feedback from the clinician is more general guidance and progression, as this process will continue with the patient after discharge.

The educational part of a clinician's job cannot be underestimated. There are many hours in the day when the patient is not under the direct care of the physical therapist or physical therapist assistant. The more the patient and/or the family understands the importance of what needs to be done and how it can be performed correctly, the more they will be able to help the patient to maximize the benefits of physical therapy intervention and speed up the recovery process.

Therapeutic Exercise

Therapeutic exercise is an important element of physical therapy interventions designed to restore, improve upon, or prevent functional deficits. Therapeutic exercise encompasses a broad scope of activities and includes muscle performance, cardiopulmonary endurance, mobility and flexibility, balance, stability and neuromuscular control, and coordination.

Balance and Agility Training

Balance is a complex coordination of sensory information with muscular performance to maintain the body within a stable base of support. Visual, proprioceptive, and vestibular are the three primary systems which influence balance. The visual system provides information to supplement sensory information from proprioceptive and vestibular systems to improve stability. It provides information as to where the head is relative to the environment to maintain a level gaze as well as notes the speed and position of the head. The somatosensory system provides sensory information from the mechanoreceptors and proprioceptors to orient a body part to its support surface. The vestibular system provides information about the position and movement of the head relative to gravity, sensing both speed and position. All three systems work in concert to ensure that one is oriented to the ground

and can move in a coordinated fashion. Deficits to one system can usually be compensated by the other two. This integration of the three systems is the basis for many physical therapy treatment strategies in that PTs and PTAs reduce the feedback from one system so that the other two will provide greater feedback to maintain balance.

Ankle, Hip, and Stepping Strategies

Ankle, hip, and stepping strategies are the three primary strategies used by the body to maintain the body's center of gravity over its base of support. Each person has a cone of stability. This cone is narrow at the base and wide as he or she moves cranially, representing the limits of where the body can move without loss of balance if the feet remain fixed. Small perturbations or slow speed movements within the limits of stability are usually accommodated through ankle strategies. These are small amplitude shifts and compensations made in the anterior and posterior as well as lateral directions to maintain the center of gravity over the base of support. With an anterior sway, one would see muscle activation beginning distally to proximally. This would recruit the ankle plantar flexors first, then the hamstrings, and finally, the paraspinals. The posterior sway would recruit first the ankle dorsiflexors, then the quadriceps, and finally, the abdominals.

A hip strategy is used for larger amplitude or faster movements that move the patient to the limits of the cone of stability. These are accommodated by rapid hip flexion or extension to move the center of gravity quickly within the base of support. Hip strategies are observed when the support surface moves out from underneath the base of support. Therefore, if the support surface is moved backward, the body will sway forward, recruiting first the abdominals and then the quadriceps. The paraspinals and hamstrings are activated to accommodate for a backward sway. The stepping strategy is incorporated when the perturbation is so large that it shifts the center of gravity beyond the cone of stability, or is so fast that the other strategies are not successful. The body steps out in the direction of the center of gravity deviation and places a contact point (usually the foot but sometimes the hand) so that the base of support is enlarged and the center of gravity is once again within the base of support.

Safety First

When incorporating balance activities as part of a therapeutic exercise plan, safety is an important consideration. Ensure that obstacles are removed from the patient's path and that equipment is in good working order. Guard the patient as he or she transitions on and off equipment or while performing activities. Use a gait belt to facilitate guarding and perform more challenging tasks within the parallel bars or near a railing so that the patient has something to grasp if necessary.

Range of Complexity

Balance activities range from simple static tasks to complex functional activities. Aside from the acuity of a patient's condition, most patients can tolerate some level of balance activity. Contraindications are limited to acute inflammation and such impaired balance that the patient requires maximum support to assume postures or perform transitional movements. Keep in mind that static activities are typically easier than dynamic activities, and purposeful dynamic activities that can be anticipated are easier than reacting to a sudden change in the environment. Progression of balance tasks may range from reducing the base of support, making the support surface unstable, occluding vision, or having the patient perform reaching tasks or react to external perturbations. As the tasks become more dynamic and functional, changes in head position or changes in the environment—such as an obstacle course, adding a cognitive task, or carrying an object—can be added to increase difficulty. Functional tasks—such as a golf swing or reaching to the floor to pick up an object—are examples of activities that require dynamic balance at each moment and throughout the movement. Ideally, the patient is challenged with the task presented. When a patient is challenged, you will see evidence of the patient trying to stabilize against another body part or surface. The patient may move into a low- or high-guard position with his or her upper extremities, and there will be evidence of larger amplitude compensations with ankle or hip strategies. Activities that are performed with resistance bands can be made easier by increasing the level of resistance. Although increasing the level of resistance in most therapeutic exercise scenarios makes the activity more challenging, for balance activities, resistance provides greater stability and therefore reduces the challenge.

Aerobic Capacity and Endurance Conditioning or Reconditioning

Aerobic conditioning involves sustained total body movements over a period of 20 minutes or more designed to improve cardiac muscle function, reduce body fat, and reduce risk factors related to heart disease and high cholesterol. Because many people in the general population have several risk factors associated with the development of heart disease, patients should be screened prior to beginning an aerobic exercise program.

Screening for Readiness

There are several options for screening; however, one of the more simple options is to complete the PAR-Q. The PAR-Q, or Physical Activity Readiness Questionnaire, was developed in Canada as a screening tool. It is appropriate for those between 15 to 69 years old. This simple questionnaire contains seven questions, asking things such as, "Do you feel pain in your chest when you do physical activity?" Patients who have a positive response to any of the questions should have medical clearance prior to beginning an aerobic exercise program. Those that answer negatively to all seven questions should be able to tolerate a conditioning program.

Guidelines during Aerobic Exercise

Once a patient has been medically cleared to perform an aerobic activity, there are a few precautions to observe while the patient is exercising. A patient's heart rate should be limited to 85% of maximum heart rate, and if the PTA is staying in the target heart rate, he or she should be able to do that without difficulty. Blood pressure will increase 7 mm Hg to 10 mm Hg for every increase in MET level. Maximum ceilings for blood pressure should be that systolic does not exceed 220 mm Hg and diastolic should not exceed 120 mm Hg. Patients should be monitored for a drop in blood pressure as the activity intensity rises, and the PTA should watch for lightheadedness, dyspnea, and extreme shortness of breath. These guidelines can be used to determine if an aerobic exercise should be terminated.

Picking Training Levels Based on Heart Rate and Age

Determining the appropriate training level is an additional step. If the patient has not undergone a stress test to determine his or her maximum VO_2 (maximum oxygen capacity), then an estimated training heart rate can be calculated based on age and resting heart rate. The simplest method of determining an estimated training heart rate begins with determining the maximum heart rate—220 minus the patient's age. This number is then multiplied by 0.6, and that number is then multiplied by 0.8. This represents 60 to 80% of maximum heart rate. This is quick and easy and works well for young, healthy individuals as a training heart rate range. In order to reduce body fat, the patient would be encouraged to work closer to the 60% end of the training heart rate. If cardiac fitness is the goal, working toward the 80% is more effective. It is important, however, that the patient stay within the target heart rate because too low a heart rate will not result in any changes, and too high a heart rate may result in injury.

An alternative method for determining a training heart rate is through Karvonen's formula. This has been shown to be more accurate because it incorporates the resting heart rate into the formula. Karvonen's formula begins by determining the maximum heart rate by taking 220 minus the patient's age. From that number, 60 and 80% is taken. Then, from those two resulting numbers, the resting heart rate is added back into the equation. As with the first method, patients should work within the training heart rate range and avoid working outside of the range because too low a heart rate will not result in any changes, and too high a heart rate may result in injury.

It is important to remember that patients that are on certain types of blood pressure medications, especially beta blockers, have an artificially limited heart rate. A training heart rate will not be accurate for these patients because the patient's heart rate will not rise the same way as that of someone not on the medication. The patient who is on blood pressure medication will have to work harder to increase the intensity of the exercise in order to get to the training heart rate. This may result in injury because the exercise may become too intense.

In addition to measuring heart rate, the PTA can use the Borg scale, which is a scale of perceived exertion. If the PTA desires the training heart rate to be 150 bpm, for example, then a Borg rating of 15 plus or minus 1 is a good approximation. Another heart rating test the PTA can use is the functional talk test. At lower intensities, the patient will be able to sing; at moderate intensities, the patient will be able to talk; and at a high intensity, the patient will not be able to talk consistently without resting. These results are excellent ways to cross-check the heart rate with the patient's perception of intensity. It can be used from an educational standpoint to help the patient recognize when activities are either too intense or inadequate.

Intensity and Duration of Training

According to the American Heart Association, aerobic exercise should be performed for 20 to 60 minutes, three to five days per week, at 65 to 90% of maximum heart rate. As the intensity of the exercise increases, so too should heart rate, respiration rate, and systolic blood pressure. Diastolic blood pressure should rise 7 mm Hg to 10 mm Hg for the entire exercise period. If the patient does not tolerate sustained activity for 20 to 60 minutes, interval training or a work circuit can be developed to assist with increasing sustained tolerance. Generally, the longer the work interval, the more the aerobic system is stressed. Initially, a rest interval of one to one-and-one-half times the work interval is necessary for adequate recovery, but as the work interval becomes longer, the rest time can decrease until continuous activity is performed.

Modes of Exercise

The mode of aerobic exercise may vary considerably depending on the equipment available, the interests of the patient, and the activities to which the patient desires to return. Activities that allow for sustained total body movement may be in the form of interval training, circuit training for functional activities, or the traditional bike, treadmill, or elliptical cycle. Aerobic activities may also be performed in the pool. It is important to remember, however, that hydrostatic pressure increases the pressure on the peripheral vascular system. Therefore, training heart rates will be 7 to 20 beats less in the water than on land.

Body Mechanics and Postural Stabilization

Patients can be easily overwhelmed with too many instructions when it comes to body mechanics education. Keeping it simple and focusing at first on one or two problem areas allows the patient to master them before moving on to other areas that need improvement.

Identifying the neutral spine position is the initial step. Neutral spine is the position of the spine that puts the least amount of stress on the joints and is usually most comfortable and stable for the patient to maintain. Neutral lumbar spine is best identified through the drawing-in maneuver, which is a cocontraction between the multifidus and the transverse abdominus. Through the use of biofeedback techniques, visual and tactile cues, and visual imagery, patients can identify this posture. It may take more than one treatment session to be consistently successful with the identification of neutral spine. However, once identified, body mechanics training is a matter of maintaining this posture while moving the body.

Body mechanics training often identifies strength deficits in the large muscles groups to which the patient desires to shift the load. Care needs to be taken not to overtax these new areas, which can result in additional injury. Remember that proper body mechanics for one individual may be different for another because of strength, flexibility, or stabilization issues. Sometimes, "ideal" is not possible, and "best fit" for the patient's lifestyle and activity should be the goal.

Best Methods for Lifting Loads

The ideal method for lifting loads has not been definitively identified. Kinesiological studies identify advantages and disadvantages that are beyond the scope of this manual. Some principles can be extrapolated to the general population:

- Keep loads close to the body and close to the center of gravity.
- Push or pull rather than lift.
- Develop a diagonal base of support (modified lunge) for greatest stability.
- Minimize trunk rotation and instead shift weight or pivot feet.
- Change postures frequently.

Sustained Postures

Sustained body postures such as prolonged sitting or sleeping also require individual analysis rather than a "one method suits all" approach. Sleeping postures are often among the first areas identified for education so that the patient will rest comfortably. Whether it is best to sleep supine, side-lying, or prone is dependent on the patient's premorbid sleeping posture and on the nature and acuteness of the injury. Patients benefit from sleeping in midrange without significantly stressing supporting structures. The use of pillows or bolsters can often achieve these two goals. The firmness of a mattress or pillow may also increase or decrease stress, and the focus should once again be on supporting structures.

Sitting postures will also vary depending on whether the patient is driving, sitting and working, or relaxing while watching television. When possible, the lumbar support or a small pillow or rolled towel can help to reinforce spinal neutral. Chair height and depth should allow for feet to be comfortably positioned on the floor without reducing circulation in popliteal fossa or moving away from back support. Desk and armrest height as well as the height of the work itself should be such that the body can remain comfortably supported without creating undue stress in the neck, shoulders, elbows, wrists, or hands.

Flexibility Exercises

Flexibility is defined as the extensibility of soft tissue structures in and around the joint. It impacts muscles, tendons, fasciae, and joint capsules, as well as ligaments, nerves, blood vessels, and skin. Adequate flexibility allows the patient or client to achieve unrestricted pain-free movements of the body while performing functional tasks and leisure activities. Stretching is a general term that is used to describe interventions that address improvement in flexibility. In addition, mobilization techniques and range of motion activities are often performed in conjunction with stretching to achieve goals.

Avoiding Negative Repercussions

It is important not to overstretch tissues. Overstretching will trigger the golgi tendon organ and result in reflexive activation of the muscle spindle to prevent overstretching from occurring. Failure to recognize this can result in muscle tearing and, in the case of high speed and high intensity stretching, muscle or tendon rupture. In order to prevent these negative repercussions, stretching should be performed at a low

intensity for a relatively long duration of 15 to 60 seconds for a single stretch. The low intensity is best described to the patient as tension in the muscle, and no pain should be elicited. Studies suggest that stretching of at least two repetitions performed at least twice per week will result in improvement in range of motion. Three to five repetitions, repeated several times per day, may do more to encourage consistency of performance on the part of the patient than result in any additional change in flexibility. The frequency of stretching should be geared toward reducing the experience of delayed onset muscle soreness. While flexibility does decrease with age, improvements in flexibility can be seen at any age.

When working with an injured population, static stretching, which is performed at a low intensity for a sustained period of time, should be used. For patients with soft tissue contractures, mechanical devices may sustain the stretch for several hours to several weeks. Manual stretches performed by the physical therapist assistant or self-stretches performed by the patient are usually held for 15 to 60 seconds and are repeated several times. Ballistic or quick stretching is typically observed with athletes prior to athletic competition to help prepare the elasticity of the muscles for rapid contractions. This is not typically done with patients except in the more chronic phases of rehabilitation.

Stretching Facilitation Techniques

Proprioceptive neuromuscular facilitation techniques can be used to promote stretching and are designed to use neurological principles to allow for greater changes in range of motion to occur.

Hold-relax techniques use the principle of autogenic inhibition to stretch the tight muscle. The tight muscle is first taken to its most elongated position. An isometric contraction is performed with the tight muscle for three to five seconds, and then the muscle is passively repositioned to its new elongated position. This may be repeated three times and ends with a static stretch in the new elongated position for 15 to

60 seconds. This technique is most effective when it does not hurt to contract the tight muscle.

Agonist-contraction technique uses the principle of reciprocal inhibition to stretch the tight muscle. The tight muscle is first taken to its most elongated position. Then an isometric contraction of the agonist muscle (the muscle that produces the motion that is limited) is performed for three to five seconds. Next, the patient is asked to actively move to the new elongated position. This may be repeated three times and ends with a static stretch in the new elongated position for 15 to 60 seconds. This technique is most effective when the patient experiences pain when contracting the tight muscle and when large changes in motion are necessary.

Slow-reversal hold technique uses both the principles of autogenic and reciprocal inhibition to produce the greatest changes in range of motion. Slow-reversal hold technique is a combination of the hold-relax technique and the agonist-contraction technique. The patient is first passively moved to the elongated position of the tight muscle. An isometric contraction is performed using the tight muscle for three to five seconds. Next, the patient is asked to actively move the muscle to the new elongated position.

These three techniques usually make it more comfortable for patients to tolerate manual static stretching than just the static stretching alone. Heating the structures with a heat modality or actively through a warm-up exercise will facilitate the ease with which stretching is performed. Icing the stretched tissues at the new end range after stretching helps to maximize the retention of the new range and minimize the creep back to the old range.

Gait and Locomotion Training

Gait training is not the same as ambulating with a patient; it is a skilled service that requires the knowledge and expertise of a physical therapist or a physical therapist assistant. Before beginning gait training, it is important to determine what assistive device (if any) is needed. Determining the need for an assistive device requires knowledge of the client's weight-bearing status, level of stability, and cognitive abilities. Walkers, bilateral axillary crutches, or Loftstrand (Canadian) crutches are for those who have significant weight-bearing restrictions. A walker is best for a patient that needs significant support for balance, while axillary crutches or Loftstrand crutches provide less support. Unilateral crutches or canes, which are positioned opposite the affected limb, are for those who have at least partial weight-bearing through both limbs or need some additional balance support. Upper extremity support devices, such as a platform, also require at least partial weight-bearing through both extremities.

Once the device has been identified, the appropriate gait pattern is determined. During normal gait, one limb is in swing phase while the opposite is in stance. During that same period, the contralateral upper extremity is swinging forward while the lower extremity in the swing phase is doing the same. The limb in swing phase also swings past the limb in stance. This smooth, coordinated pattern should be mimicked as much as possible, even when working with an assistive device.

Gait patterns requiring three or four points to sequence are slower patterns than those that only require two. Typically, the slower gait patterns are taught initially because they are more stable, with the patient progressing to faster patterns. Further, the advancing swing leg can either be positioned at the same level as the injured leg (swing-to gait pattern) or move past it (swing-through gait pattern). With any gait training endeavor, the goal is to normalize the gait pattern as much as possible.

Proper Demonstrations

Instruction should begin with a demonstration of the proper gait pattern. The physical therapist assistant can demonstrate the pattern while the patient observes. It is important to clearly identify the weight-bearing status to the patient and also be aware of any specific precautions which might exist. Once the patient verbalizes understanding of the pattern, then the patient can try it. After placing a gait belt on the patient, the therapist assistant shows the patient how to rise with and correctly position the assistive device. The PTA should guard the patient by standing on the involved side and slightly behind the patient because he or she is more likely to lose balance to the involved side. The patient is cued for the correct sequence until he is able to consistently demonstrate it independently.

Performing Turns

Turns should be performed at a slower pace using the same sequence. There are advantages and disadvantages to turning right or left, toward or away from the injured side. The advantage of turning toward the injured side is that the patient does not have to take as large a step with the injured leg. The disadvantage is that the patient may tend to twist on the injured extremity, which may be contraindicated for healing. Turning away from the injured side necessitates a larger step, but because it is a larger step placement of the foot, it can be more easily controlled. For patients with specific precautions, such as those with a posterior approach total hip replacement, the rotation of the foot can be more easily controlled. Either way, the PTA should be consistent with instructions and ensure that the patient does not twist on the injured leg.

Ascending and Descending Stairs

The patient should also learn how to ascend and descend stairs. Determine if the patient will have at least one handrail, and identify on which side the handrail will be. Then make sure that the training is done consistently following that pattern. If a handrail is available, the patient should always use it because it is more stable than the assistive device itself. If there is a single assistive device, and it would normally go on the side of the handrail, the patient should switch it to the other hand until he or she reaches the top or the bottom of the stairs.

When guarding the patient, the PTA should be on a lower stair than the patient. If the patient is going up the stairs, then the PTA should be to the side and slightly behind the patient so that the PTA would be available to help control a fall. If going down the stairs, the PTA should be slightly to the front and to the side of the patient. When the patient is going down the stairs, the injured extremity should always remain with the assistive device. Therefore, if the patient is descending the stairs, the assistive device is moved to the next step, and then the injured extremity advances forward on to the next step. Next, the patient should use the handrail (if available) and the assistive device to slowly lower the body to the next step and position the uninjured leg next to the injured leg. The patient should keep repeating this process until at the bottom of the stairs. When ascending the stairs, the patient should lead with the uninjured leg first. In order to advance this leg up, the patient should put weight through the handrail and through the assistive device and push up until the uninjured leg is on the next step. Then, leaving the assistive device where it is, the patient should push up until the injured leg joins the uninjured leg and finally have the assistive device follow last. Curbs are negotiated similar to the stairs.

When possible, gait training should address all environmental challenges that the patient may face. If the patient is going to his or her home, then a home visit may be beneficial so that the PTA may better understand the nature of the obstacles. Later on in this chapter, you will find information on home visits and specific items to be addressed that will increase the risk for falls. Whenever possible, these items should be eliminated. Those challenges that cannot be eliminated should be addressed and an action plan identified to ensure safety and success.

Relaxation Training

Relaxation training is designed as an adjunct tool to help patients better manage their symptoms and reduce muscle tension associated with stress and anxiety. Patients with chronic pain conditions, headaches, hypertension, and respiratory conditions may also benefit from relaxation strategies. Relaxation requires conscious effort to reduce muscle tension and control respiration. Patients in acute as well as chronic pain may benefit from these strategies, as well as those who become emotionally distraught.

Relaxation Strategies

The clinician who is providing the relaxation education must speak in a relaxed, calm, and soothing voice. Often, it is helpful to have soft music or background noises of waves or rain showers playing when working with a patient on relaxation training. The patient will be taught to diaphragmatically breathe and slow down respirations, while either visualizing a peaceful place or actively contracting and relaxing muscles. It is important to note that falling asleep is not the goal. Instead, the patient should attempt to achieve a deep relaxation, although conscious awareness remains. There are several relaxation strategies that can be used.

Progressive relaxation was developed by Jacobson and uses systematic isometric contractions of muscles from distal to proximal to release voluntary control of tight muscles. By actively tightening the muscles, the patient receives feedback on what the muscle is like when contracted, and then actively and consciously relaxes the muscles to reduce tension.

Guided imagery uses techniques developed through self-hypnosis to allow the patient to visualize a calm or peaceful scene. The patient is encouraged (through a series of cues) to use as many senses as possible to perceive the scene that he or she is imagining. Once he or she is deeply immersed in the scene, the patient is able to relax and become refreshed before returning to day-to-day activities.

Breathing strategies are often helpful during an acute flare-up of symptoms. Calmly encouraging the patient to breathe in through the nose and out through the mouth, or "smell the roses and blow out the candles," can help the patient separate himself or herself from the situation until the PTA can remove the source of the symptoms.

The Feldenkrais method is awareness through movement. Although many of the other aspects of relaxation are incorporated into this method, the focus is on identifying imbalances within the muscular system in order to self-correct these imbalances and achieve harmony.

Strength, Power, and Endurance Training for Head, Neck, Limb, Pelvic-Floor, Trunk, and Ventilatory Muscles

Muscle performance is composed of muscle strength, endurance, and power, and each of these can be improved through the use of resistance training. Muscle strength is the ability of the muscle to produce tension while muscle endurance is the ability of the muscle to repeatedly contract over a period of time and resist fatigue. Muscle power is the ability of the muscle to perform a quick, powerful contraction. The goal of muscle power is to improve the contractility of the muscle over a shorter period of time.

Progressive resistance exercises (PREs) are guided by three principles—overload, specific adaptation to imposed demands (SAIDs), and reversibility. These principles guide both the progression and regression of resistance exercises. The overload principle states that in order for the muscle strength to improve, the muscle must be challenged at a level that is greater than it is currently able to perform. Either the load or the number of sets and repetitions must be great enough that the muscle becomes challenged. If the focus of the intervention is to improve strength, then increasing the load the muscle is able to lift will be the target. Conversely, if it is muscle endurance, the number of sets and repetitions will be increased. With patients, it is important to remember that the underlying pathology dictates how much the muscle can be overloaded. When the muscle is overloaded, the resulting microtears must be repaired. It often takes 48 to 72 hours to repair these fibers. Therefore, there are usually two to three days between sessions where the muscle is brought to this fatigue point.

Wolff's law states that the body system adapts over time to the stresses placed upon it. Specific adaptation to imposed demands capitalizes on this law and causes the body to make specific changes by design. This is most readily seen with sports-related activities. For example, in order to become a more powerful linebacker, a faster sprinter, or a stronger boxer, one must perform the activities specific to that sport. The mode and the intensity and volume of exercise are all geared to accommodate this principle.

The reversibility principle and the phrase "Use it or lose it" are often used to encourage patients to keep up with a home exercise program. The reversibility principle states that once gains have been achieved they must be maintained through regular use of the muscles at that intensity, or there will be a gradual decline beginning as quickly as one to two weeks after the cessation of exercise, and the muscles will continue to decline over several weeks to premorbid levels.

Developing a PRE Program

When a PTA is developing a progressive resistance training program for a patient, it is important to know what specifically he or she wants the patient to achieve. If the focus is on strength, then the PTA will go about the program differently than he or she would if the emphasis were on endurance or power. The intensity of the exercise relates to the load the muscle must move. If the emphasis is on improving strength, then the load will be high and repetitions relatively low. If the emphasis is on endurance, then the load will be relatively low and the repetitions will be high. Finally, with power, the focus is on higher loads but moving them over a specific range in a shorter period of time. Most patients with injuries will be working with submaximal loads at least early on in the rehabilitation phase. Maximal loads are most appropriate in the chronic phase of rehab or for healthy adults who are preparing to return to high physical demand jobs or activities. Although most patients will not be working with maximal loads, most exercise prescriptions use the one repetition or ten repetition maximum as a starting point. Taking 60 to 70% of the one or ten repetition maximum is an appropriate load for developing strength for an injured individual, with the range being 30 to 40% up to 80 to 90%, depending on the patient's premorbid conditioning. The volume of exercise relates to the number of sets and repetitions performed. The current philosophy for strength training is that three sets of 6 to 12 repetitions are optimal. For endurance training, three to five sets of 10 to 20 repetitions are optimal, or a time goal of 30 seconds to five minutes may be established.

There are two schools of thought regarding applying progressive resistance concepts to achieve maximum gains. DeLorme suggests progressive loading beginning with 50% of ten repetition maximum, then 75% of ten repetition maximum, and finally 100% of ten repetition maximum, with each set being ten repetitions. Sixty to 90 seconds of rest is suggested between sets to allow for adequate recovery. The Oxford plan suggests a regressive strategy beginning with 100% and progressively reducing to 75 and then 50%. The DeLorme plan allows for a warm-up within the series and maximal effort at the end of the series. If fatigue is an issue, then this can be problematic. The Oxford plan, on the other hand, allows for maximal output early on; however, injured tissues may have more difficulty adapting quickly to maximal loads. Studies have not found a significant difference between the two plans.

Types of PRE Exercises

There are a myriad number of choices when determining the mode or type of exercise chosen for progressive resistance exercise. The mode also influences the type of muscle contraction that is identified and how and when the external load is applied. The mode will also influence whether external stability or internal stability is required when performing the task. The mode may require the use of equipment, such as weight or Thera-Band® or even a specific exercise machine. For patients who are significantly deconditioned or injured, just moving the body weight through a specific range of motion may be challenging enough. The mode can allow for variety and changes in stabilization, which can increase or reduce the intensity of the activity.

Exercises may incorporate an isometric muscle contraction, in which there is no movement of the body segments but a cocontraction around a joint. Isometric exercises are simple and easy to perform. In a submaximal capacity, they can be initiated in the acute phase of rehabilitation and can improve strength at any point in range so they are good for stability. The disadvantage of using isometric contraction exercises is that they are often associated with a Valsalva maneuver and increases in blood pressure that are not appropriate for patients with heart disease or hypertension. A Valsalva maneuver increases the intra-abdominal and intrathoracic pressures and results in an increase in blood pressure. This is most commonly seen with isometric exercises, but patients frequently need to be cued for any type of exercise. Patients are encouraged to breathe in through the nose and out through the mouth when exercising. The exhale should be associated with the exertion portion of the exercise. For those at increased risk for cardiovascular disease, a Valsalva maneuver may increase risk for an ischemic incident. Postsurgical patients and post-fracture patients are at increased risk for the development of deep venous thrombosis (DVT). Also, because isometric exercises only improve strength at a single point in the range, they have limited benefit.

Dynamic exercises may have both a concentric or shortening contraction and an eccentric or lengthening contraction. The eccentric muscle contraction requires one-and-one-half times the force of a concentric muscle contraction. Eccentric muscle contractions are important for shock absorption or rapid deceleration and are often the type of contractions encountered when athletes become injured. Concentric muscle contractions, on the other hand, are more traditional muscle contractions and are associated with a wide variety of functional tasks. Dynamic activities are very functional; however, the primary limitation with dynamic activities is that the load that the patient is able to move is limited to the weakest point in the range. The resistance may be constant or variable. Constant resistance is a load that does not change, such as a cuff weight or a dumbbell or even a weight stack on a machine. Variable resistance changes depending on how large a range you move with the load—the larger the range, the greater the resistance.

Isokinetic exercises are based on a consistent speed or velocity. The advantage to isokinetic exercises is that the muscle can work maximally throughout the entire range. The disadvantage is that isokinetic equipment is both expensive and cumbersome and therefore not available as part of a home exercise program.

Speed is also a factor with plyometric exercises. Plyometric exercises are designed to rapidly alternate between concentric and eccentric muscle contractions. The speed is based on the alternation rather than the speed of the activity itself. Agility drills are designed to use this principle to help athletes and others to quickly change direction, gain vertical height, or quickly initiate a start or stop of an activity.

Activities may also be designed as either open- or closed-chain activities. Open-chain activities allow the distal segment in the chain to be free to move even if it is attached to a piece of equipment. In closed-chain activities, the distal segment is fixed. Open-chain activities allow the patient to focus on a single muscle or muscle group, closed-chain activities necessitate more internal stabilization because muscles around the joint must all participate. Closed-chain activities (especially of the lower extremities) are performed in weight-bearing postures. Open-chain activities are usually performed in non-weight-bearing postures or a combination of weight-bearing postures and non-weight-bearing postures (as is observed with gait). Closed-chain activities require that muscles work in a reverse action. This can be very functional, particularly for the lower extremities, because this is how the muscle generally works. When weight-bearing precautions need to be observed, closed-chain activities may need to be delayed or significantly modified.

TYPE OF EXERCISE	TYPE OF CONTRACTION	BENEFITS	LIMITATIONS	PRESCRIPTION	OPTIONS
Stabilization	Isometric	Safe, easy, and can begin in acute phase	Strength gains limited to one point of range; no eccentric work performed; watch Valsalva maneuver; high risk for cardiovascular patients	Hold of 6–10 seconds, 6–12 reps, and 2–3 sets for strength; or 30 seconds to 3 minutes for 3–5 sets	Muscle set—acute maximal; open-or closed-chain
Strength	Dynamic concentric; dynamic eccentric	Functional	Limited by weakest point in the range	6–12 reps, and 2–3 sets	Constant resistance; variable resistance; open-or closed-chain
Endurance	Dynamic concentric; dynamic eccentric	Functional	Limited by weakest point in the range	20–50 reps, 3–5 sets, or 30 seconds to 3 minutes for 3–5 sets	Constant resistance; variable resistance; open-or-closed chain
Power	Plyometrics; agility	Functional; rapid; alternating between concentric and eccentric	High risk for injury if not ready for activity	Strength or endurance (depending on goals)	Own body weight or with equipment; open-or closed-chain
Speed	Isokinetic concentric; isokinetic eccentric	Maximize strength throughout range	Expensive, cumbersome equipment; speed is not at functional level	Strength—peak torque; endurance—sustained activity until 50% of peak; power—peak torque in shorter burst	Speeds determined by degrees per second, 30–300 degrees per second; open-chain

Different types of exercises have different benefits, limitations, and uses.

Getting Started

When developing strength and endurance in small postural muscles or the pelvic floor, initiating the movement is often the most difficult part of the process. For many patients, even identifying the correct muscle contraction becomes a challenge. For example, with spinal stabilization activities for the lumbar spine, when a dynamic contraction of the multifidus and the transverse abdominus is expected, the physical therapist assistant may need to incorporate other muscles initially, such as when performing a pelvic tilt or abdominal tensing before the patient is able to correctly contract the muscle and achieve a drawing-in maneuver. Biofeedback devices, such as a blood pressure cuff in the lordosis of the lumbar spine, visualizations of "tilting the bowl" of the pelvis or "drawing up and in like an elevator," as well as direct palpation to the impacted muscles, can help achieve the correct contraction. The pelvic floor is also another group of muscles that patients may have more difficulty contracting properly. Using activities that the patient has done before, such as stopping the flow of urine midstream, can help connect the cognitive with the volitional muscle control. These techniques all necessitate the use of a skilled clinician providing appropriate feedback so that patients may achieve their treatment goals.

Injury Prevention or Reduction

Although most people interact with physical therapists and physical therapist assistants after injury, injury prevention is a growing service area. There are three levels of injury prevention in which PTs and PTAs may be involved—primary prevention, secondary prevention, and tertiary prevention. Primary prevention is generally in the form of education to specific populations that are at risk for the development of a specific disease. For example, educational sessions to postmenopausal women may address prevention of osteoporosis or fall risk prevention strategies. Secondary prevention is designed to catch individuals early in a disease process and implement strategies to reduce or prevent the negative effects of the disease. For example,

if a patient is diagnosed early on with osteoarthritis, then the patient may become involved in low-impact water aerobics or learn about appropriate exercises to reduce the impact on the joints or increase the strength of the surrounding muscles. Finally, tertiary prevention is for patients who already have a chronic, irreversible disease. Here, prevention strategies are designed to slow down the progression of the problem. A patient who is diagnosed with ankylosing spondylitis, for example, may be shown how to perform self-stretching activities and given assistive devices, such as sock aids and reachers, to allow the patient to maintain normal ADLs and IADLs as long as possible.

Therapeutic Massage

Therapeutic massage may serve a variety of purposes throughout the course of rehabilitation. In the acute stage of rehabilitation, during a period of acute inflammation, tissues are swollen and edematous and there is often muscle guarding. Gentle massage may serve to mobilize fluid out of the injured area where it can be absorbed by lymphatic and venous tissues in the body. It may serve the additional purpose of limiting adhesion formation and relaxing surrounding muscles to reduce guarding and muscle splinting. Gentle effleurage techniques are appropriate to reduce muscle tension while gentle movement of edematous tissue in a distal to proximal direction can assist with fluid management.

In the subacute or proliferative phase of rehabilitation, controlled motion is the hallmark of this phase. Therapeutic massage at this juncture may move in many directions. Cross-friction massage is appropriate to mobilize scar tissue and reduce adhesions between ligaments and across incision sites so that free range of motion can occur over the joint. Deep tissue massage may be used to increase blood flow to trigger points and other areas of restricted blood flow. Massage may also be used as an adjunct to relaxation techniques. As acute symptoms come under control, the patient moves away from more passive techniques to active self-management of stress and muscle relaxation. Effleurage and petrissage are appropriate techniques to improve localized circulation, reduce the impact of lactic acid buildup, and minimize delayed onset muscle soreness after stretching.

Although sometimes referred to as soft tissue mobilization, myofascial massage, or myofascial release are deep massage techniques that are designed to move adhesions between the layers of muscle and fascia. By performing deep sustained strokes, adaptive changes in the scar tissue or alignment of collagen fibers can occur. These techniques are most appropriate for patients with restricted mobility.

Manual Traction

Manual traction is designed to stretch surrounding muscle tissue and distract the joint capsules while widening the intervertebral foramen. Manual traction has the benefit of allowing the therapist assistant maximum control of the position to direct forces to the area most needed.

Manual Traction of the Cervical Spinal Cord

Prior to beginning manual traction of the cervical spine, it is important to clear the spine using a vertebral artery test. The vertebral artery test places the patient first in full extension and then extension, lateral bending, and rotation to one side, effectively cutting off the vertebral arteries on that side. A positive response will result in reports of lightheadedness, nausea, and possibly nystagmus. No interventions to the cervical spine should be performed without medical clearance from a physician if there is a positive vertebral artery test.

Once the vertebral artery test is cleared, manual cervical traction is generally performed in supine. The PTA's hands support the occiput or one hand is on the occiput, while the other is on the forehead. The force for providing the distraction should come from weight shifting posteriorly and the weight of the clinician pulling on the head and neck rather than the force being generated by the small muscles of the hand.

Generally, it is easiest to begin in a neutral position and then move into various degrees of flexion or extension, lateral bending or rotation, depending on which provides the most relief for the patient. Constant monitoring should occur to ensure that any radiating symptoms into the arm should move proximally, not distally. Distal movement implies worsening of symptoms. The force is applied gradually with smooth ramping up of the force as well as gentle release. The length of the treatment will vary depending on the tolerance that the PTA has for supporting the head and neck and applying the force.

Manual Traction of the Lumbar Spine

Manual traction may also be applied to the lumbar spine, however it is not as easy to do as to the cervical spine. In the cervical spine, the PTA applies approximately 15 to 20 lb. of force to achieve distraction, which equals the approximate weight of the head. In the lumbar spine, the forces need to be as high as 50% of the patient's body weight. When working with the lumbar spine, the physical therapist assistant will be applying force to the lower extremities to have a resulting effect on the lumbar spine. If the PTA is trying to distract both facets at a particular level, then the patient should be positioned supine. The lower extremities are flexed, and force can be applied directly through the thighs or through a belt.

Finally, manual traction can also be used to encourage extension of the lumbar spine. The patient is positioned prone, and the pull is exerted on the ankles. Depending upon the type of surface on which the patient is lying and the type of clothing worn, belts may need to be used to stabilize the upper body while stretching is being applied to the lower body.

Manual traction may also be used for peripheral joints. The joint must be positioned in the open packed position. This is the position of the joint on which there is the least amount of stress, and the joint surfaces are separated. The hands are then positioned close to the joint, one on the proximal segment and one on the distal segment, and then the points are distracted. With the large lower extremity joints, it is helpful to use a belt to stabilize the proximal segment while both hands are being used to distract the distal segment.

Application of Adaptive, Assistive, Supportive, and Orthotic Devices

Patients are often prescribed supportive or assistive devices during the acute phase of rehabilitation to protect the injured area. The use of adaptive devices may be temporary during the acute phase, or it may be long-term for a chronic or progressive condition. Regardless of the temporary or permanent nature of the device, there are several key areas that should be assessed before and during its use.

Correct Fit and Use

First and foremost is the correct fit of the device. Assistive devices should be adjusted so that they are consistent with the patient's height and can be held comfortably in the patient's hand during use. Adaptive, supportive, and orthotic devices should fit without causing redness or rubbing the skin. When the patient wears the device it should not piston inside a shoe (if one is worn), nor should the shoe become excessively tight so that the use of the device results in diminished circulation to the affected body part. Once proper fit has been assured, the patient should be instructed in correct use and care of the device.

Correct use should cover proper putting on and taking off of the device as well as how often or how long it should be worn. Functional use of the device should include rising and sitting, ambulation, dressing, toileting, or eating as well as any other ADLs or IADLs that may need to be addressed with the application of the device. The patient should be comfortable while wearing the device and should be aware of whom to contact should problems arise. Finally, the device should do what it was intended to do. Devices that are worn on the lower extremities that impact gait should improve the efficiency and reduce the energy expenditure associated with gait and hopefully will act to normalize the pattern. Patients should not only understand what they should do with assistive or adaptive devices, but they should also understand how to use these devices correctly.

Proper fit of assistive devices is critical. For example, axillary crutches that are positioned too low can pop out from underneath the axilla while the patient is ascending or descending stairs; this may result in a fall. Patients should also be aware to check the wing nuts on wooden axillary crutches to ensure they are tight; and if possible, the patient should keep all the wing nuts facing forward so that he or she is reminded to check them.

Patients should learn what to do in case of a fall in order to prevent more severe damage from occurring, as well as how to rise from the floor should that become necessary. Upper extremity devices are sometimes designed for resting and sometimes designed for protection while performing activities. Depending on the nature and fit, if the patient were to attempt to perform activities within the device, he or she might irritate already inflamed tissue if the device is acting as a resistance load. Patients benefit from knowing how to keep assistive devices clean and how to wash them if needed. Many items need to be washed by hand and air-dried or should not be worn when damp. This is critical information that patients should have prior to beginning routine use with any device.

Functional Training in Self-Care and Home Management

Discharge planning should begin early on in the rehabilitation process. Gaining insight into the activities that a patient will need to perform at home, how much help will be available, and the layout of the environment are key pieces of information to gather when beginning to work on functional activities.

Home Evaluations and Interviews

When possible, a home evaluation should be conducted to observe the types of floor surfaces, number of steps, and the presence and absence of handrails as well as the width of doorways and types of showers, baths, and commodes present. If a home evaluation is not possible, then a detailed interview with the patient and/or family member is helpful. This conversation may lead to the identification of adaptive or supportive equipment that the patient may need prior to discharge and will give the staff the opportunity to work with the patient so that the patient will be comfortable with the use of the adaptive or supportive equipment prior to discharge.

While in the clinic, functional simulations can be developed which mimic the environment to which the patient will return. For example, the patient may practice walking sideways with a walker in order to enter a bathroom door to use the commode. The patient may also need to practice with a tub shower bench and mimic the movements necessary to safely sit down and transfer into the shower. Dressing with the use of a reacher or other adaptive device should be practiced until the patient is comfortable. The patient may need to practice going up and down ramps should he or she have a sloped driveway. This may need to be progressed from a slight incline to an incline that represents the true nature of the driveway over a period of several days. Additionally, if the patient's home is covered with wall-to-wall carpeting, gait training should incorporate this surface.

A home safety evaluation will likely identify potential hazards such as throw rugs, narrow passageways, stairs, and obstacles. Whenever possible, these should be reduced or eliminated in the home environment. However, some obstacles may not be removed, or hazards such as small animals or toys may be unexpected or difficult to control. Patients benefit from not only participating in obstacle courses but also learning strategies to successfully negotiate them.

Functional Training in Work, Community, and Leisure

Like functional training for self-care and home activities, functional training for work, community, and leisure activities begins with an understanding of the issues that the patient is likely to encounter. With work activities, it is helpful to speak with the employer or case manager to identify a functional job analysis. It is also useful to observe the work being performed. If the facility works with many patients from a particular employer, it is well worth the time and energy to go on a site visit and see and measure the work in progress. Physical therapists and PTAs are often asked to perform job analyses in the work setting to assist employers with managing injuries. This partnership is often rewarding and allows clinicians to use their knowledge of kinesiology and functional movement in new and exciting ways. Although community, sports, and leisure tasks do not often require a specific analysis, videotapes or observation of the activities are helpful to develop functional training programs for these patients.

Simulation in a Clinical Environment

Once the elements of the various activities are identified, they can be simulated in a clinical environment. If repetitive lifting is a job component, then repetitive squatting or lunges may be incorporated into the treatment plan. Lifting, pushing, or pulling loads may be replicated with boxes or weights to simulate the functional task. As the patient becomes more adept in the individual components of work, sports, or leisure activities, they can be put together into a circuit. In the case of sports activities, such as golf, the circuit may consist of going to the driving range and hitting a bucket of balls or playing 3 holes instead of 18. This an example of a gradual reentry into activities to which the patient desires to return; the patient is often motivated to participate in these tasks because he or she realizes achieving the functional goal is getting closer.

The use of functional patterns of movement, such as proprioceptive neuromuscular facilitation

(PNF) patterns, can simulate the complete muscles and joints needed to perform a wide variety of functional tasks. Even if the pattern is not an exact replica of the movement necessary, if it focuses on working the joint or muscles necessary for the activity, this is often an excellent addition to a rehabilitation program. Patients who need to work on speed and power may incorporate agility drills or plyometrics into their rehabilitation. Working on quick changes in direction or hopping, skipping, and sidestepping are all ways to incorporate higher intensity activities. Finally, increasing the eccentric load of a muscle to maximal levels will put the patient at the highest intensity of exercises. These must be closely supervised, as the patient is at high risk for injury if not protected throughout. As the patient masters these higher-level functional tasks, he or she can also begin low intensity return to regular activities, either for a limited period of time or under specific conditions. As the patient tolerates these lower activity tasks, he or she can progress to returning to full work duty or resume sports or leisure activities at premorbid levels.

Responses to Treatment and Potential Complications

The goal of physical therapy intervention is to reduce pain and inflammation and to assist the patient in returning to premorbid functional levels. Careful application of the discussed principles can help to achieve these goals, but occasionally a patient regresses or has difficulties that are unexpected.

Healing after Trauma

Patients that sustain a musculoskeletal trauma from surgery or injury proceed through the three phases of healing. The initial acute phase is associated with the four cardinal signs of inflammation—pain, swelling, redness, and heat. During this phase, efforts are made to protect the injured area and reduce these signs of inflammation. In addition, patients are often taking medications such as analgesics to manage pain or nonsteroidal anti-inflammatory medications to reduce

the signs of inflammation. Moving the patient too quickly or not taking these medications as prescribed or not resting appropriately during this phase may prolong the phase for extended periods. Analgesics may also result in constipation and excessive drowsiness. NSAIDs have an anticoagulation effect, and care must be taken to avoid excessive bruising and bleeding when taking these medications. In a small percentage of cases, there may be evidence of complex regional pain syndrome in which the patient's initial sympathetic response to trauma continues and the patient becomes hypersensitive to pain and poorly tolerates any weight-bearing.

The subacute stage of rehabilitation is associated with controlled motion. Once again, if progression of activities occurs too quickly, the patient may return to the acute stage with increased evidence of inflammation. If, however, the patient is not moved or progresses too slowly, adhesions may result limiting range of motion and soft tissue extensibility. Later in the subacute stage, vigorous and unaccustomed resistance training or overexertion with functional tasks may produce delayed-onset muscle soreness (DOMS). DOMS has also been associated with high levels of eccentric exercise. It typically develops in the muscle belly or musculotendinous junction of involved muscles 12 to 24 hours after activity and peaks 48 to 72 hours after activity. There is tenderness to palpation, evidence of edema, and warmth in the muscles. This may result in diminished strength to the muscle for one to two weeks after the onset of DOMS. DOMS is prevented by gradually increasing exercise amounts. Active cooldowns and ice are effective in reducing the impact of DOMS.

Other Complications

Pathological fractures are a negative side effect for patients with osteoporosis or those who have been placed on a high level of steroid medications for prolonged periods of time. Osteoporosis and osteopenia are associated with bone loss and increased fragility of bone tissue. Although weight-bearing exercises and resistance training are essential elements for the treatment of these conditions, excessive loads, high velocity exercise, and high impact activities may result in pathological fractures. Ideally, the load is greater than what the bone is normally exposed to, but not so great that a fracture occurs.

Patients who may be at increased risk for cardiovascular disease should be careful to avoid Valsalva maneuver. A Valsalva maneuver increases the intra-abdominal and intrathoracic pressures and results in an increase in blood pressure. This is most commonly seen with isometric exercises, but patients frequently need to be cued for any type of exercise. Patients are encouraged to breathe in through the nose and out through the mouth when exercising. The exhale should be associated with the exertion portion of the exercise. For those at increased risk for cardiovascular disease, a Valsalva maneuver may increase risk for an ischemic incident. Postsurgical patients and post-fracture patients are at increased risk for the development of deep venous thrombosis. Total knee replacement patients are at the highest risk for development of DVT. Patients with DVT will present with calf pain, especially with weight-bearing, and pain with dorsi-flexion of the ankle. A secondary complication is that the DVT will become a pulmonary embolism, which could result in dyspnea, shortness of breath, and possibly death.

When patients have been exposed to excessive exercise, either in one session or cumulatively, they will typically demonstrate decline in functional abilities, progressive weakness, loss of mobility, and increased subjective reports of stiffness and soreness. Pain does not begin to subside until approximately four hours after exercise and may not resolve within 24 hours, or pain may occur earlier than it did in previous sessions. These are all indications of therapeutic exercise interventions that may result in reinjury or new injury.

Effects on Musculoskeletal System from Interventions Used on Other Systems

The most significant factor that impacts the musculoskeletal system is immobilization from bed rest. Immobilization results in decrease in muscle mass, decrease in strength, diminished cardiovascular functioning, orthostatic hypotension, and decreased bone mineral density. The more prolonged the immobilization or bed rest, the greater the impact on these aspects. The reversibility principle also supports that within one week, exercise tolerance, cardiac output, and strength will decline, resulting in impaired functional mobility.

These factors will also impact the other systems of the body. Prolonged bed rest will diminish tissue integrity, increasing the risk for the development of pressure ulcers. A decline in the gastrointestinal system may result in diminished appetite and diminished ability for the body to draw necessary resources from digested food as it passes through the alimentary canal. Increase in orthostatic hypotension impacts both the cardiovascular system as well as balance in the neuromuscular system. Sustained postures may result in adhesions or, with prolonged immobility, adaptive shortening of tissues forming contractures. Diminished mobility will also result in decreased air exchange and increased likelihood of developing pneumonia. Finally, the urinary system is at increased risk for the development of urinary incontinence.

Although the musculoskeletal system may not be the primary system being treated, it is vital to keep patients as mobile as possible so that the secondary effects of immobilization do not occur.

Practice 2

1. The patient is a 42-year-old male who is medically cleared to begin an aerobic exercise program. His cholesterol level is 175 mg/dL, his blood pressure is 135/84 mm Hg, his respirations are 16 rpm, and his resting heart rate is 72 bpm. The PTA is asked to determine a training heart rate based on Karvonen's formula for a normal healthy adult. Which choice represents the training heart rate for this patient?
   a. 84 to 135 bpm
   b. 107 to 142 bpm
   c. 136 to 157 bpm
   d. 178 to 220 bpm

2. The PTA is working with a patient who was working on highly repetitive exercises and suddenly draws up and complains of a muscle cramp. The patient is very upset, her breathing is erratic, and she is grasping her leg in pain. Which of the following is the best response for the PTA to take first with this patient?
   a. Tell the patient that she needs to work through the pain; everyone gets a muscle cramp now and then.
   b. Take the patient through a guided imagery sequence and hope that she falls asleep.
   c. Tell the patient to breathe slowly in through her nose and out through her mouth while the PTA shows her how to stretch the muscle.
   d. Tell the patient to breathe slowly in and out through her mouth while saying "ohm."

3. A PTA is treating a 67-year-old man who recently sustained a fall and sustained a contusion to his left hip and knee. Part of the plan of care is to work on balance strategies to prevent future falls. Which of the following positions would most challenge his balance?
   a. standing on a foam block with eyes closed
   b. sitting with the upper extremities at end range of shoulder flexion
   c. sitting in a chair with eyes closed
   d. standing on the floor with narrow base of support

4. A physician orders a program of closed chain strengthening exercises for a patient recovering from knee surgery. Which of the following would be contraindicated?
   a. weight-shifting activities on a rocker board
   b. seated isokinetic terminal knee extension
   c. bridges with weights over abdomen
   d. partial squats with ball behind back

5. A PTA is instructing a patient in a home exercise program. Of the following information, what is not necessary to include in the instruction?
   a. intensity of exercise
   b. volume of exercise
   c. time of day to exercise
   d. frequency of exercise

6. Which of the following changes will NOT make a partial squat exercise more challenging?
   a. performing squats with ball held adducted between both thighs
   b. placing theratubing under both feet and holding the end in each hand while performing the squat
   c. standing with one foot on a foam disk while performing the squat
   d. positioning therapeutic ball behind lower back while performing the squat

7. The PTA is asked to work on dynamic spinal stabilization activities for a patient with spondylolisthesis in the early subacute phase of rehabilitation. Which of the following activities is contraindicated for this patient?
   a. hook-lying dead bug activities with a short lever arm
   b. prone rapidly alternating leg and arm elevation with long lever arm
   c. seated on a ball performing alternating knee extension and shoulder flexion with a long lever arm
   d. quadruped alternating arms and legs with short lever arms to neutral extension

8. The PTA is presenting an in-service on the advantages and disadvantages of various forms of resistance exercises. The PTA informs the group about some of the disadvantages of a particular type of exercise: Muscle strength is limited to a point in the range of motion, there is no improvement in muscle endurance, and no eccentric work is created. Which of the following is the type of exercise characterized by the disadvantages that the PTA describes?
   a. dynamic variable resistance
   b. dynamic constant resistance
   c. isokinetic
   d. isometric

9. The patient is a 72-year-old female who underwent a total knee replacement three weeks ago. She is doing well with her home exercise program, performing three sets, ten reps of ankle pumps, heel slides, quad sets, glut sets, SAQ, and SLR every day. As the PTA observes the patient performing the SLR, the patient's knee bends as she lifts it up in the air. The PTA measures a five-degree extension lag. After explaining to the patient how important it is to keep the knee fully extended during this exercise, what is the most appropriate next action by the PTA?

   a. Have the patient perform a quad set, and then passively raise the extended leg up six to eight inches. Next, have the patient lower the leg on her own, keeping her knee extended.
   b. Tell the patient to increase to four sets of ten. The sooner the quads get stronger, the less extension lag she will have.
   c. Have the patient stop doing SLR completely. Have the patient do heel slides and short arc quads. Try the SLR again in a few days.
   d. Place a rolled towel under the calf of the affected knee. Place a three-pound weight above the knee, being careful not to put the weight directly on the patella.

10. The PTA is working with an 87-year-old female patient who is a resident of a skilled nursing facility. The patient sustained a compression fracture of T12 vertebra when she inadvertently sat down forcefully on a hard chair. The patient has been diagnosed with osteoporosis. Which of the following activities would NOT be an appropriate activity for this patient?
    a. biceps curls and lateral shoulder raises with a load that is 60% of one repetition maximum
    b. abdominal crunches with rotation with body weight
    c. walking 1.5 miles on the treadmill
    d. standing hip abduction, flexion, and extension with a load that is 80% of ten repetition maximum

11. The physical therapist assistant is observing a patient perform three sets of a long arc quad exercise for the right knee. Which of the following observations is NOT consistent with evidence of localized muscle fatigue?
    a. muscle tremoring in the quadriceps
    b. trunk extension when concentrically contracting quadriceps
    c. reports of numbness in right foot
    d. multiple starts and stops with movement

12. A PTA is observing a patient who sustained a right ankle sprain which is resolving. The assistant notes that when the patient is asked to lean forward, he has no trouble keeping his balance. However, when he leans backward, he does not respond appropriately when correcting a backward sway of the body. Which list is the correct firing order for muscles to correct a backward sway?

   a. bilateral tibialis anterior, quadriceps, and abdominals

   b. bilateral flexor digitorum longus, hamstrings, paraspinals

   c. abdominals, quadriceps, and bilateral tibialis anterior

   d. paraspinals, hamstrings, and bilateral flexor digitorum longus

13. The patient is a 47-year-old male with mechanical lower back pain. He has tight erector spinae muscles bilaterally. Which of the following is the best choice to perform a self-stretch for this muscle group?

   a. prone on extended elbows keeping ASIS on the table

   b. long sitting with an anterior pelvic tilt and reaching to touch toes

   c. doubling knees to chest

   d. prone raising both arms in the air

14. The physical therapist assistant has been asked to provide massage to reduce joint and tissue swelling after an acute injury. Which of the following is the most appropriate application of the massage technique?

   a. gentle pressure along the direction of the muscle fibers

   b. deep pressure perpendicular to the direction of the muscle fibers

   c. deep pressure along the direction of the muscle fibers

   d. from distal to proximal following the direction of venous return

15. The patient is a 19-year-old male basketball player who sustained an inversion sprain to his ankle. He is performing an isometric exercise. The PTA asks the patient to sit with his ankles crossed and instructs the patient to press the lateral borders of his feet together. Which muscle is the patient strengthening?

   a. fibularis (peroneus) longus

   b. tibialis posterior

   c. soleus

   d. tibialis anterior

16. A muscle is considered more powerful than another muscle when which of the following conditions is met?

   a. It can perform work at the same intensity for a longer period of time.

   b. It has a shorter lever arm.

   c. It can perform the same amount of work over a shorter period of time.

   d. It produces less resistance.

17. The PTA is implementing a treatment program for a patient who needs to improve her gait pattern. The PTA reevaluated the patient's gait and noticed that the patient is having difficulty initiating the swing phase of gait. Which of the following muscles would be most appropriate to emphasize in this patient's rehabilitation?

   a. biceps femoris

   b. iliopsoas group

   c. gastrocnemius

   d. tibialis anterior

18. The PTA is working with a patient who is performing resistance exercises. The PTA desires to correctly cue the patient to avoid a Valsalva maneuver. Which of the following is NOT a good strategy to employ?

    a. Have the patient exhale with each resistive effort.

    b. Have the patient inhale with each resistive effort.

    c. Have the patient count the number of repetitions for each exercise.

    d. Caution the patient to avoid holding his breath.

Practice 2 Answers

1. c. Karvonen's formula is based on the formula [(MHR − RHR) 0.6 − 0.8] + RHR. 220 − 42 = 178 MHR − RHR (72) = 106 × 0.6 = 63.6 106 × 0.8 = 84.8 and add back RHR 63.6 + 72 = 135.6. 84.8 + 72 = 156.8. Therefore, the training heart rate for this patient (rounded up to the nearest whole number) would be 136 to 157 bpm.

2. c. The PTA should tell the patient to breathe slowly in through her nose and out through her mouth while the PTA shows the patient how to stretch the muscle. Slowing down the patient's breathing while showing her how to stretch the cramped muscle is the most effective strategy. Guided imagery is appropriate for overall relaxation but is not appropriate with acute pain. Ignoring pain is also not an appropriate strategy because the PTA should remove the source of the patient's discomfort. Mouth breathing encourages hyperventilation, which the PTA should try to reduce. Although it is fine to have the patient say "ohm" and to slow her exhalation, the PTA

who chooses this tactic is not addressing the primary source of the patient's discomfort.

3. a. Standing on a foam block with his eyes closed will challenge this patient's balance the most. Foam with vision occluded limits feedback from the visual and proprioceptive systems and will challenge the patient's balance the most. Sitting postures have a lower center of gravity and a wider base of support because of contacts. Standing with a narrow base of support is also challenging, but because in choice **d** the patient's eyes are open, this choice is not as challenging as choice **a** and is therefore not the best answer.

4. b. Seated isokinetic terminal knee extension would be contraindicated because isokinetic terminal knee extension is an open chain activity. Weight shifting on a rocker board, bridges with weights over abdomen, and partial squats with ball behind back are all closed chain in nature because the distal segment (the foot) is fixed.

5. c. It is not necessary to indicate to the patient the time of day to exercise. The intensity or amount of resistance, volume or numbers of sets and repetitions, and the frequency or number of exercise sessions per day or per week are all necessary components that the PTA should address with the patient.

6. d. Placing the therapeutic ball behind the patient's back may improve the patient's squatting technique, but it does not increase the intensity of the exercise and will therefore not make the exercise more challenging. Performing squats with a ball held adducted between both thighs or placing theratubing under both feet and holding the ends of the theratubing in each hand increases the intensity of the squat. Standing with one foot on a foam disk while performing the squat requires greater stabilization, which also makes the activity more challenging.

7. b. Patients with spondylolisthesis should avoid extension past neutral. Positioning a patient prone and performing rapid alternating long lever arm activities is challenging in the sub-acute stage, is posturally beyond neutral, and should therefore be avoided. The other postures mentioned—hook-lying and sitting—accommodate the precaution of avoiding extension past neutral. Although the client is working into extension in quadruped, there is a limit to neutral posture.

8. d. The disadvantages that the PTA describes are all characteristic of isometric exercises. Isometric exercises are limited to strengthening to a specific point in range of motion, they do not improve muscle endurance, and no eccentric work is performed.

9. a. The PTA should have the patient perform a quad set, and then passively raise the extended leg up six to eight inches. Next, the PTA should have the patient lower the leg on her own, keeping her knee extended. By modifying the SLR so that the patient performs just the eccentric component of the SLR with some assistance, the patient should be able to minimize the extension lag quickly. Increasing the demand for more SLR does not address the problem; with fatigue the extension lag will likely worsen rather than get better. Placing a rolled towel under the calf of the affected knee and then placing a three-pound weight above the knee focuses on improving passive extension, not active extension, of the knee. Having the patient stop SLR for a few days may be appropriate if, after the PTA modifies the SLR, he or she finds that that approach is not successful.

10. b. Abdominal crunches consist of trunk flexion with rotation; this may increase risk for anterior compression wedge fractures and increase the load to the disk. The other activities listed are all in weight-bearing positions with either light weights or focusing on increasing contraction of muscles in the lower extremities for better stabilization.

11. c. Reports of numbness in the patient's right foot are not consistent with evidence of localized muscle fatigue. A temporary loss of sensation is not expected with resistance training and fatigue. Muscle tremoring, substitution patterns, slowing of movement, and jerky or hesitant motions are all consistent with localized muscle fatigue.

12. a. Bilateral tibialis anterior, quadriceps, and then abdominals lists the firing order for correcting backward sway. Flexor digitorum longus, hamstrings, and paraspinals lists the correct firing order for forward sway. If hip strategies are initiated to correct a backward sway, the order should be abdominals, quadriceps, and then dorsiflexors. For hip strategies with a forward sway the order should be paraspinals, hamstrings, and then plantar flexors.

13. c. The best choice for this patient to perform a self-stretch of the erector spinae muscles is double knees to chest. This will self-stretch the bilateral erector spinae and can be modified to stretch the entire length of the spine. Prone on extended elbows stretches abdominals. Prone with arms extended is a strengthening exercise for the erector spinae. Seated with anterior tilt and reaching toward toes will stretch hamstrings. With anterior tilt of pelvis, the erector spinae will still be tight.

14. d. In order to reduce joint and tissue swelling after an acute injury using massage, the PTA should massage from distal to proximal following the direction of venous return. To address edema using massage, the stroke direction must be from distal to proximal along the venous and lymphatic pathways. Massage with gentle pressure along the direction of the muscle fibers represents effleurage used for relaxation. Massage with deep pressure perpendicular to the direction of the muscle fibers is cross-friction massage. Massage with deep pressure along the direction of the muscle fibers is petrissage used for deeper tissue massage.

15. a. The patient is strengthening the fibularis (peroneus) longus. Fibularis longus is an everter. The description of the isometric exercise is for eversion. Tibialis anterior is a dorsiflexor and an inverter. Tibialis posterior is a plantar flexor and an inverter. Soleus is a plantar flexor.

16. c. A muscle is considered more powerful than another muscle when it can perform the same amount of work over a shorter period of time. Power is equal to work divided by time. The same amount of work over a shorter period of time makes a muscle more powerful. A muscle with a shorter lever arm or reduced resistance is a weaker muscle. A muscle that can work over a longer period of time is less powerful and has more endurance.

17. b. The PTA should emphasize the iliopsoas group in this patient's rehabilitation. The iliopsoas group are hip flexors, and hip flexors initiate the swing phase of gait. The biceps femoris is a hamstring muscle, the tibialis anterior is a dorsiflexor, and the gastrocnemius is a plantar flexor.

18. b. The patient should not inhale with each resistive effort but rather should exhale with each resistive effort. Having the patient count while performing the exercises and cautioning the patient to avoid holding his or her breath during exercise are both appropriate recommendations.

Neuromuscular System

Individuals with neuromuscular diagnoses can present with a variety of signs and symptoms, and each will experience a different severity of these symptoms. Physical therapy intervention can be very effective in improving function for these individuals. The physical therapist assistant must be able to identify and implement a wide variety of physical therapy interventions for appropriate treatment of the effects of neuromuscular pathologies.

Types and Applications of Interventions

Intervention refers to the techniques and activities that make up a treatment plan. The PTA's role in the physical therapy plan of care falls primarily in the area of intervention.

Coordination, Communication, and Documentation

Providing PT intervention for adults and children with neuromuscular diagnoses requires coordination and communication between the PT and PTA, as well as among all providers involved in the care. Documentation is a primary mode of communication among healthcare providers and third-party payers. Accurate and thorough documentation is vital to effective patient care.

Communication: A Common Framework

In addition to comprehensive documentation, a common conceptual model for healthcare assists in communication between therapists and assistants and among providers. The American Physical Therapy Association outlines clinical guidelines in the *Guide to Physical Therapist Practice*, which describes accepted physical therapist practice and helps to bridge the gap between concept and clinical practice. The guide is based on the Nagi Disablement Model, which allows for standard terms to be used in physical therapy. This promotes better communication within physical therapy. Also, other disciplines and third-party payers can more effectively understand and evaluate PT documentation knowing that the profession of physical therapy has a common framework and standard definitions of terminology.

TAKE NOTE

The APTA has recently endorsed the World Health Organization's International Classification of Functioning, Disability, and Health (ICF) model. This model replaces the Nagi Disablement Model that is currently seen in the *Guide to Physical Therapist Practice*. The PTA will still see the Nagi Disablement Model used in practice and must be familiar with the model and terminology used. The ICF model contains different terminology and instead describes individuals in terms of function.

Coordination and Teamwork

Physical therapists and physical therapist assistants work together to verify that effective communication is taking place throughout any plan of care. This requires an open line of discussion. Both the PT and PTA must be approachable and receptive to suggestions for treatment. Common abbreviations must be established within an organization to be sure that there is no misinterpretation. Written communication must be legible and documentation must also be timely.

Documentation of Treatment

The PTA provides intervention and documents the treatment session. Documentation of treatment should be comprehensive, clearly written, and very specific. Another PTA or PT should be able to read a treatment note and know exactly what was done, and why, during the treatment session. This requires thorough documentation of the intervention provided, including patient education, assistance given, number of repetitions, physical agent parameters, time of intervention, patient positioning during treatment, and patient response. Documentation should also be clearly linked to functional PT goals in order for other healthcare providers, as well as third-party payers or auditors, to recognize why each intervention was performed. Effective collaboration between the PT and PTA requires that both people effectively carry out their responsibilities within the scope of practice.

Primary PTA Responsibilities When Providing Physical Therapy Services

- Review the PT plan of care with the PT whenever possible.
- Discuss patient goals and expectations with the PT.
- Be aware of precautions, contraindications, or other unique circumstances that apply to the plan of care.
- Carry out agreed-upon interventions within the plan of care.
- Modify or progress the intervention within the plan of care to ensure patient safety and comfort.
- Communicate frequently and openly with the PT.
- Provide information on patient response to care.
- Document thoroughly and clearly following all intervention and patient interaction.
- Provide information and data for progress notes and other PT documentation.
- Discuss modifications to the plan of care that may be appropriate with the PT.
- Discuss recommendations for discharge planning with the PT.

Instruction, Education, and Training of Patients and Caregivers

In today's healthcare environment, patients are taking increasing control of their own health, healthcare decisions, and preferences for treatment. Physical therapists and physical therapist assistants are encouraged to actively involve patients and caregivers in treatment options and treatment decisions. This active involvement by patients and caregivers requires education on the healthcare issues in order for informed decisions to be made. Patient education must be a logical and systematic process that is unique to each patient's needs. Education and instruction must be personalized depending on a patient's cultural background, level of education, communication style, and physical therapy goals.

Patient-Centered Instruction

The patient should always be the primary focus of education and instruction. However, there are times when a family member or caregiver will receive more training and instruction than the patient. The family member or caregiver may be educated because of the patient's cognitive or physical status. If the caregiver is assisting a patient with significant receptive and expressive aphasia, for example, then the caregiver may be the most logical person to receive detailed instruction about the patient's care. Regardless of the level of participation by the caregiver, however, the patient must remain the focus of education about his or her care. The patient should be addressed during education and asked to participate as appropriate. All decisions regarding the patient's care should be made for the well-being of the patient. The education needed for the caregiver to provide the best care while not neglecting his or her own needs is also an important part of education. The caregiver must learn how to safely and effectively assist the patient and allow the patient to participate in his or her own care as much as possible.

Effective teaching and instruction requires a comprehensive assessment of an individual's needs, an environment conducive to learning, and confirmation of understanding. Patient instruction needs a plan of care similar to the plan of care needed for treatment. The following should be included in a plan of care: an evaluation of the patient's preferred mode of communication, educational level, preferred instructional methods, and an assessment of the frequency of instruction required for continuous understanding and compliance with the plan of care.

A thoughtful discussion with the patient or caregiver regarding these issues can go a long way in developing an effective plan of care for patient instruction. This kind of communication regarding patient education and intervention will allow the patient to feel empowered and to assist the healthcare team in the decision-making process.

Communicating Effectively

A patient-centered teaching approach is vital to effective communication. The PTA must know the best language and terms to use to effectively communicate. For example, if an interpreter is needed, the PTA should ensure that an interpreter is available. The PTA should also attempt, when possible, to use laymen's terms and appropriate vocabulary for the patient's level of understanding. There are various technologies that can assist the PTA in creating appropriate instruction, such as software that will create material at a specified reading level, in a specified language, or in a specified print size. There are also technologies that will allow the patient to listen to instruction at desired volumes or see pictures of exercises. The PTA must be aware of any communication impairments that the patient may have, such as visual or hearing impairments, in order to create the best method to offer instruction to the patient.

The PTA must also consider the patient's values when creating a plan of care for patient instruction. Some patients value active participation in healthcare decisions, while others may value a more passive approach to healthcare for cultural or generational reasons. An assessment of the patient's desired role will guide the PTA in teaching the patient the appropriate level of information regarding the plan of care. If the patient values a more passive role in healthcare, the PTA must respect this perspective and adjust patient education accordingly. The PTA should also assist the patient by providing patient education using various teaching styles—including written and verbal instruction—and by assisting the patient in problem solving.

Confirmation of Instruction

After patient education is complete, the PTA must evaluate the patient's understanding. A good way to do this is to have the patient demonstrate what has been taught. If the patient needs a lot of cueing or repetition of instructions, then the PTA may want to readdress the material in a different way. The patient can also demonstrate understanding by verbalizing the instructions given and discussing the information and how it specifically applies to his or her situation. A comprehensive patient education plan and active communication between the patient and the PTA are vital to successful outcomes in physical therapy.

Therapeutic Exercise

Individuals with neuromuscular diagnoses may react differently to exercise, experiencing prolonged weakness and fatigue long after the exercise has stopped. The PTA must be aware of preventing overexertion that could be detrimental to functional activities in the following hours or days.

Aerobic and Endurance Training

Endurance is an important part of function. Without endurance, an individual is limited to short, low energy activities which may prevent a person from completing all required daily activities. Individuals with neurological or motor function impairments may present with poor muscle as well as poor overall endurance. Aerobic training will have central benefits to the cardiovascular and pulmonary systems.

Poor endurance and fatigue involve the inability to sustain an activity over time. When overall physical fatigue sets in, an individual will be unable to sustain the exercise needed to increase endurance. This can lead to a cycle of no progress due to overexertion. Conditioning programs must initially be carefully monitored by the PTA in order to avoid overexertion and injury.

TAKE NOTE

The PTA must be knowledgeable about diagnoses and conditions that have specific exercise recommendations and precautions. Some diagnoses, such as multiple sclerosis, require temperature monitoring due to intolerance of heat or cold. A decreased ability to regulate temperature may also be present with advanced age. Patients with neurological diagnoses or advanced age may not be able to recover from exercise as easily as younger, healthier individuals. Patients also may not be able to perform all modes of exercise.

For example, a patient who sustained a spinal cord injury may be limited to upper extremity exercises, and a patient who experienced a stroke may have high-energy demands and decreased motor initiation with the presence of hemiparesis. These patients may not be able to sustain exercise for long periods of time, and they may fatigue more quickly. In addition, some conditions, such as muscular dystrophy, were once thought to worsen due to exercise. Although this is no longer the accepted approach to treating patients with muscular dystrophy, what can be detrimental to patients with this diagnosis is high resistance eccentric training and exercising at maximum levels. The PTA must be knowledgeable about the appropriate role of exercise in the course of neurological diagnoses.

Type of Exercise

When creating an aerobic endurance training program, there are many factors to consider. The mode or type of exercise must be appropriate for each individual and must be an activity that can be sustained for the time and intensity recommended. Possible activities for endurance training include walking, jogging, cycling, swimming, or athletics (including wheelchair sports). Ideally, exercise should not only be enjoyable but also easily accessible, or compliance may be diminished due to boredom and inconvenience.

Intensity and Frequency of Exercise

The intensity and frequency of exercise are two other factors to consider. The intensity should begin low enough that the individual is encouraged and not completely worn out. It is better to begin with a low intensity and increase it rather than to begin with a high intensity and risk injury or frustration from poor performance.

The frequency of exercise must be realistic but occur often enough to result in positive outcomes. A frequency of three times per week or every other day is appropriate when exercise is sustained for at least 15 to 20 minutes. This allows for adequate rest and recovery. However, exercising every day is more beneficial for cardiovascular fitness if an individual exercises for less than 15 minutes per day, and it still allows for adequate recovery.

The final factor to consider is time. Again, the time to exercise must be realistic but also allow for progression toward the established goals. For an individual who is very deconditioned, five to ten minutes may be a good starting point. Once the individual can sustain ten minutes of exercise without signs of overexertion, the time can be increased in five to ten minute increments. Once an individual can sustain the desired level of exercise for 30 to 60 minutes, the intensity can be increased with a corresponding decrease in time until endurance can be built up to maintain the new intensity for 30 to 60 minutes. Monitoring response to exercise in order to know when to increase or decrease time and intensity is very important.

Monitoring

There are a variety of ways to monitor an individual during exercise, and some are more appropriate than others in certain circumstances. Heart rate is a popular method to monitor response to exercise in individuals of all ages. Heart rate can be affected by many factors. Heart rate at rest, or resting heart rate, can be affected by age, level of cardiopulmonary fitness, and the presence of cardiovascular disease. Improving cardiovascular fitness results in a lower RHR. Maximum heart rate can also be affected by similar factors. Maximum heart rate decreases with age and cardiovascular disease. An individual's maximum achievable heart rate is determined by the equation 220 − age = maximum achievable heart rate. For example, a 45-year-old female would have a maximum achievable heart rate of 175 beats per minute. Knowing an individual's maximum achievable heart rate allows the PTA to determine what heart rate an individual needs to maintain in order to be exercising at the right intensity. If the PTA instructs an individual to exercise at 60 to 65% of maximum heart rate, then that individual should maintain a heart rate of 105 to 114 bpm.

INFORMATION IN ACTION

You are working with a patient and beginning an exercise routine. You are monitoring heart rate in order to determine the level at which the individual is working. The patient's heart rate responds as you expect as she begins walking on the treadmill, but you become concerned when the patient's heart rate seems to level off even though she is obviously increasing the intensity of her workout. You ask the patient to stop the activity, and you consult the PT about the unexpected heart rate response.

The PT asks you to review the patient's medical record, and you read that the patient has cardiovascular disease and is on blood pressure medication. You remember that cardiovascular disease can alter heart rate response to exercise and that blood pressure medication can blunt the heart rate response despite increasing exercise intensity. Because this makes sense with what you are observing clinically, you instruct the patient to continue the exercise routine and use a different method to monitor response to exercise.

With the presence of cardiovascular disease or cardiovascular medication, the heart rate may not reach expected levels regardless of the intensity of exercise. Therefore, another form of monitoring must be used. Another common measure of exercise intensity is the Borg Rate of Perceived Exertion Scale. During exercise, the PTA asks the individual to indicate on the scale the level of exertion required for the exercise. Once an individual is comfortable with using the scale, it is a convenient method to independently monitor exercise intensity.

Maximum heart rate and the RPE scale are both used for determining exercise intensity. When creating a new exercise program, 60 to 80% MHR ("somewhat hard" on the RPE scale) is a common place to start. If this intensity is recommended, that is the heart rate or the perceived exertion rating that should be maintained throughout exercise. With continued exercise, the cardiovascular system demonstrates increased endurance. This means that it will take more intense and longer bouts of exercise to maintain this goal intensity. Therefore, the intensity, duration, and possibly frequency will need to be increased in order to maintain 60 to 80% MHR. The goal of endurance programs is to increase intensity and duration while maintaining safe exercise parameters, demonstrating improved fitness and cardiovascular endurance.

INFORMATION IN ACTION

When using the Borg RPE Scale, it can be helpful to note that the number the patient indicates on the 15 grade scale can be correlated to an estimated heart rate. By multiplying the score on the scale by ten, the PTA can estimate the heart rate of young, healthy patients. However, the correlation to heart rate weakens in patients with comorbidities or advanced age.

Additional techniques to monitor exercise response include blood pressure, respiratory rate, and oxygen saturation. The PTA can monitor blood pressure before, during, and after exercise. The PTA can use a talk test to determine breathlessness based on whether or not the patient can carry on a conversation during exercise, or the PTA can use a pulse oximeter to measure O_2 saturation. A normal response to increasing activity is a linear increase in systolic BP with the diastolic BP not significantly changing. If an individual's systolic BP is below 80 mm Hg or above 180 mm Hg, then exercise is contraindicated. Similarly, if an individual's diastolic BP is above 110 mm Hg, then exercise is contraindicated. While exercising, BP should not drop, and a drop of greater than 20 mm Hg is an indication to immediately stop exercise. During exercise, if an individual can easily carry on a conversation, then the exercise intensity is very low; if the individual is unable to talk, then the intensity is too high. An individual's oxygen saturation monitored with a pulse oximeter should not fall below 5% of the resting saturation.

Balance and Agility Training

Maintaining balance requires accurate input to the three major balance systems: the somatosensory system (in the muscles and joints), the visual system, and the vestibular systems (located in the inner ear). It also requires accurate balance reactions from the body, such as the ankle, hip, or stepping strategy. Based on the assessment of an individual's balance, the cause of balance deficits may be determined as impairments in any or all of these systems. As a result, balance intervention can be focused on retraining or compensating for the systems involved in balance impairments.

Three Balance Strategies

There are three primary balance strategies that are normally elicited during a loss of balance:

- ankle strategy—the primary balance strategy used in response to a minimal perturbation when the feet are on the ground
- hip strategy—elicited with a moderate perturbation

- stepping strategy—elicited when a step is required to maintain balance in response to a maximum perturbation, causing the center of gravity to shift outside the base of support

Balance intervention may involve the PTA's retraining the patient in these balance strategies if an individual's reactions to perturbations are impaired. Training a person's balance systems involves placing the individual in situations where a balance strategy would normally be elicited and consciously practicing these strategies. The following table outlines the circumstances under which balance strategies can be elicited and practiced.

Use It or Lose It

Following a period of decreased activity or immobility, balance strategies and balance systems may be impaired due to nonuse. The idea of "use it or lose it" applies to many aspects of the human body, and balance systems and strategies are no exception. In order to retrain or improve balance, a PTA must introduce situations that challenge an individual's balance in order to elicit the strategies.

Effective balance training maintains the individual's safety with proper guarding or assistance to prevent falling. For example, if an individual has a fear of falling, he or she may begin to use a walker and

Balance Strategies

STRATEGY	STIMULUS	RESPONSE
Ankle strategy	Perturbations with a small base of support	Shifting the center of mass forward or backward at the ankle joints
Hip strategy	Larger or fast perturbations or standing on narrow base of support	Shifting the center of mass by flexing or extending at the hips
Stepping strategy	Larger or faster perturbations	Realigning base of support under the center of mass by stepping in the direction of the displacement force

These balance reactions can be distinct movements based on the displacement force, or they can be used in combination.

increase double support time during gait. When the walker is taken away and the individual has to walk up stairs (which requires single-leg stance), the individual's balance on one leg would most likely be impaired because the individual has not practiced or been exposed to true single-leg balance. After immobility due to a lower extremity fracture, for example, the single-leg stance balance on the involved lower extremity will be impaired due to muscle atrophy, decreased proprioception, and lack of balance challenges during immobility. Individuals can also see changes in balance as a result of neurological diagnoses, neurological lesions, or aging.

Direct Impairment

Direct impairments to one of the balance systems can also lead to decreased balance. For example, in an individual who has progressive vision loss or inner ear infections affecting the vestibular system, balance will be altered due to inadequate visual and/or vestibular input. The individual's balance responses are not impaired, but the accurate input that balance responses rely upon are.

An individual can also have a combination of these concerns. For example, as vision loss progresses, an individual may begin to change gait characteristics in fear of falling due to poor visual input. Regardless of the reason for a balance deficit, PT intervention for balance retraining must challenge balance systems and teach individuals how to maintain balance through refining balance reactions, using assistive devices, or altering the environment in order to maintain safety.

Input and Information

Balance systems can be challenged in a variety of ways, depending on the balance deficit demonstrated. The somatosensory system gives the body input about proprioception and where the body parts are relative to each other and to the support surface. This information is received from receptors in the muscles and joints. The visual system provides information about the surrounding environment and the location of the body relative to the environment. The vestibular system, found in the inner ear, provides information about head position relative to gravity. The vestibular system is more sensitive to head movement than body sway.

These three balance systems give specific information to the body about orientation. Therefore, if one of these systems is impaired, balance will be impaired. There are specific environments and surfaces that can reveal what balance system is affected and can also be used to challenge the balance systems during treatment. Balance training can become more and more challenging for high-level balance and agility training by changing the environment to challenge all balance systems.

The following table outlines the environmental conditions that will challenge balance by altering input from one or more of the primary balance systems.

Body Mechanics and Postural Stabilization

Because postural muscles are type I muscle fibers, they can maintain low-intensity, long-duration contractions that are needed to perpetrate posture of the body. Type I muscles respond to different kinds of training than type II muscles. In order to maintain body mechanics, an individual must know the best position in which to hold the body and must also have the postural muscle endurance to maintain the best body position.

Body mechanics during static and dynamic activities involve maintaining the most neutral posture possible during the activity. For example, for individuals who sit and work at a computer during the workday, neutral spinal posture with maintenance of

Challenging Balance

CHALLENGING ENVIRONMENT	BALANCE SYSTEM AFFECTED	REAL-LIFE EXAMPLES	INTERVENTION POSSIBILITIES
Unstable surface	Somatosensory system	Walking on a moving bus or standing on an escalator	Bosu ball, BAPS board, or trampoline
Unlevel surface	Somatosensory system	Walking across the lawn to the mailbox	Grass, pebbles, or shaggy carpet
Decreased base of support	Somatosensory system	Tandem stance, single-leg stance	Walking on a straight line or balance beam, stair training, or obstacle courses
Altered lighting	Visual system	Walking at night or in bright sunshine or glare	Low lighting, blind fold, or saran wrap over eyes or glasses
Scanning environment	Vestibular system	Walking down the aisle in a theater looking for an open seat	Scan environment while walking
Moving objects in environment	Vestibular system	Walking through a crowded shopping mall	People walking by while walking; walking past moving images on TV screens

Challenging an individual's balance, with appropriate guarding, allows for balance systems to be activated. Keep in mind that a patient's safety must always be the PTA's first priority.

the lumbar lordosis, as well as avoiding a forward or excessively extended cervical posture, is important in order to prevent pain and injury. For individuals with a job that requires physical activity, it is important to maintain a neutral spine and keep extremities close to the trunk when lifting or bending in order to prevent strain on the spine. Maintaining these neutral postures requires good fitness and endurance of postural musculature.

Postural Stabilization Training

Once a PTA has instructed an individual on proper body mechanics during static and dynamic postures

and movements, the PTA must then focus on increasing strength and endurance of postural muscles. Postural stabilization training involves low-intensity, high repetition exercises performed more often than type II strength training exercises.

The primary postural muscles are those of the spine and abdomen. Abdominal muscle training can be achieved through a variety of therapeutic exercises, including abdominal crunches, pelvic tilts, and isometric abdominal exercises. Training of the spinal musculature can be accomplished with trunk extension, bridging, or controlled extremity movement while maintaining a neutral spine. Cervical spine stabilization exercise is always effective for maintaining cervical posture and can include axial extension, eye-head coordination activities, and deep cervical flexor training. All of these activities must be performed with greater than 30 repetitions and can be performed multiple times, every day. This allows the frequent, high repetition training that is required of type I aerobic postural musculature.

Flexibility Exercise

Muscle length and joint range of motion play a large role in the function of the body. Without adequate muscle and joint flexibility, the body is restricted and normal movement may not be possible. There are many things that can have a negative effect on muscle and joint flexibility, such as prolonged immobility, prolonged disuse, and aging.

Following a prolonged period of immobility or disuse, muscle fibers become tight and contractures can result. In addition, ligaments and joint capsules can shorten or tighten, leading to decreased range of motion available at the joint, regardless of muscle length. As the body ages, synovial fluid becomes more viscous and articular cartilage can calcify, limiting joint mobility.

Exercises to maintain flexibility as well as gain flexibility include passive and active range of motion, muscle stretching, and joint mobilization. The application of heat or low-intensity exercise for warm-up prior to any of these techniques allows for increased muscle and soft tissue extensibility.

Range of motion can be passive, active assisted, or active and is performed through the full available range of motion at a joint. The movement should be slow and controlled at all times. The PTA should ensure stable posture and provide adequate support to the limb being moved. Range of motion exercises performed regularly will help the patient maintain flexibility and prevent the shortening or tightening of tissues that can result from prolonged immobility and disuse. The three types of ROM are outlined in the following table:

Range of Motion

TYPE	DESCRIPTION
Passive ROM	Performed and controlled by the PTA
Active-assisted ROM	Requires external assistance from the PTA
Active ROM	Performed and voluntarily controlled by the patient

The type of range of motion performed is based on the patient's ability to actively control movement while also considering possible restrictions to active muscle contraction.

Stretching

Stretching is a technique that can increase flexibility by elongating the tissue being stretched. Static stretching involves slowly elongating a muscle to the point of tolerable tension or stretching sensation. Stretches should be held for a minimum of 30 seconds with a 30 to 60 second hold (if tolerated) recommended for elderly individuals. Low-load prolonged stretching (LLPS) is a very safe and effective form of stretching and refers to the application of a minimal force, or low load, to an elongated muscle in order to maintain the position of elongation over a prolonged period of time. This type of stretching can be maintained for different lengths of time—from 30 minutes at a time up to hours at a time. An example of a low load could be a cuff weight, a pulley, or a positioning device such as an orthotic device.

Ballistic stretching involves a high-load, short duration stretch, such as a bouncing movement while reaching to touch the toes in sitting. This type of stretching is most appropriate for young, healthy individuals because it has a higher risk of muscle tearing and injury compared to static stretching.

Facilitated stretching is another option, and this type of stretching involves the use of an inhibitory technique to relax and elongate tissue during static or ballistic stretching. An example of facilitated stretching is the contract-relax technique in which the target muscle is placed in an elongated position, and then the individual performs a maximum isometric contraction of that muscle. The contraction causes reflex inhibition and relaxation of the muscle, allowing the muscle to be moved into a more elongated position. Contract-relax is also an example of a facilitated stretching technique.

Joint Mobilization

Joint mobilization is a manual therapy technique used to increase mobility at a joint that is limited due to a tight capsule or ligament at the joint. There are progressive grades of joint mobilizations outlined in the following table:

TAKE NOTE

The American Physical Therapy Association prohibits performance of joint mobilizations by PTAs because it requires continual evaluation of the patient. However, the PTA should understand the theory, procedure, and benefits to the patient.

Gait Training

Gait training can be a critical part of a PT plan of care because ambulation is the primary means by which individuals move through the environment in order to

Joint Mobilization

JOINT MOBILIZATION GRADE	DESCRIPTION	BENEFITS
Grade I	Small amplitude rhythmic oscillation at the beginning of range of motion	Manage pain and spasm
Grade II	Large amplitude rhythmic oscillation at the midrange of motion	Manage pain and spasm
Grade III	Large amplitude rhythmic oscillation up to the point of limitation in motion	Gain motion by stretching the joint capsule
Grade IV	Small amplitude rhythmic oscillation at the end of range of motion	Gain joint mobility
Grade V	Small amplitude quick thrust at the end of range of motion	Gain joint mobility

Proper joint mobilization requires that the PTA understands joint kinematics and the relationship of the articulating surfaces.

perform daily activities. Motor control of the gait cycle is a complex interaction of maintaining upright posture, balancing the trunk in all directions, and controlling the lower extremities in order to maintain standing while advancing with safe ground clearance. When an individual has lost the ability to effectively ambulate, the PTA can play a critical role in retraining the complex processes that allow for safe and effective gait.

A central issue that must be addressed for each patient is identification of the overall goal of gait training. The goal may be that the patient be able to move safely and effectively from point A to point B. For example, if an elderly individual is facing ADL limitations due to the inability to cross a street fast enough, the goal should be safely increasing gait speed. This can be achieved through muscle strengthening, balance training, or the introduction of an assistive device for safe intersection crossing. Note that the primary goal is safely crossing the intersection and not necessarily proper gait kinematics during each phase of the gait cycle.

However, there are times when the goal for a patient in gait training may be more complex and involve correct performance of each gait cycle phase with correct muscle timing and movement amplitude. There are individuals who have experienced a lower extremity injury, for example an ankle sprain, and whose long-term goal of gait training is to return to an agility sport. Intervention for these individuals may include retraining the timing and amplitude of muscle contraction which may have been lost due to muscle atrophy during weeks of immobility.

Six Approaches to Gait Training

There are six general approaches to gait training. These are possible components that can be used based on the needs of the individual. For example, an individual who has experienced a stroke may need to begin with bodyweight-supported treadmill training, while an individual with balance deficits may need to begin with foundational postures that challenge balance before training in standing.

In addition, within each of these components, the focus on specific joint and muscle performance will be unique to the individual depending on the physical therapy goals. Because PTAs understand the muscle activity that is required during each phase of normal gait, a PTA can provide intervention that targets specific gait deviations or impairments noted during the gait assessment. The plan of care can include therapeutic exercise to address specific muscle weakness or lack of coordination; balance training; or practicing the actual gait cycle while refining various aspects of performance.

Gait Intervention

LEVEL OF TRAINING	EXAMPLE ACTIVITIES
Preparation for locomotor training	Bridging, quadruped, sitting, kneeling or half-kneeling, modified plantigrade, standing
Parallel bar training	Standing, balance and weight-shifting training, stepping and side-stepping, forward progression and gait pattern training, assistive device training

Gait Intervention (*continued*)

LEVEL OF TRAINING	EXAMPLE ACTIVITIES
Indoor overground training	Walking forward and backward, side-stepping, braiding, stair training, resisted forward progression
Outdoor overground training	Opening and closing doors, walking over thresholds, curb and ramp negotiation, crossing an intersection, elevator and escalator training
Bodyweight-supported treadmill training	Treadmill training with bodyweight supported, slow progressing to fast speed, reciprocal stepping training
Indoor overground training	Walking on level surface with bodyweight supported, assistive device training, stair training, opening doors and crossing thresholds

Gait training within a real-world environment allows for accurate assessment and training for situations that the individual will experience outside of the physical therapy setting.

Assistive Devices

Assistive devices may be used during gait training in order to make gait more functional. The PTA must be able to provide proper instruction for gait with a variety of assistive devices such as those identified below:

- rolling walker
- front-wheeled walker
- four-wheeled walker
- straight cane
- quad cane
- axillary crutches
- Lofstrand crutches

Relaxation Training

The relaxation response is one that can be very beneficial to individuals who are unable to participate or progress in physical therapy due to tension. This tension can be present for a variety of reasons, including headaches, hypertension, anxiety, or depression. One important goal of relaxation training is to equip the individual with the ability to relax independently in order to maintain functional mobility and independence.

Relaxation Techniques

Relaxation training can decrease heart, breathing, and metabolic rates and can help to bring the body back to a relaxed and balanced state. With these effects, the body will be able to more effectively respond to PT intervention. There are a variety of relaxation training techniques, including repetition, diaphragmatic breathing, guided imagery, and desensitization, which can be used by a PTA during treatment, as well as cognitive-behavior therapy, which requires skilled health professionals in the area of cognition or behavior therapy. This discussion focuses on relaxation techniques that can be used by the PTA.

- **Repetition.** Relaxation training using repetition involves choosing a phrase that can be easily remembered and that does not elicit an emotional response such as the phrase "I am calm." Then the individual is instructed to find a comfortable position with eyes closed, to relax all muscles of the body, to breathe slowly, and to repeat the phrase out loud or silently.

- **Diaphragmatic breathing.** Diaphragmatic breathing allows an individual to focus on and decrease the rate of respiration with the focus on the diaphragm controlling breathing. The PTA should instruct the individual to avoid using accessory respiratory muscles as much as possible and allow the diaphragm to relax and contract.

- **Guided imagery.** Guided imagery is another technique that can assist in relaxation. This technique involves guiding the individual to think of a special place such as a garden, an open field, or a calm lake and to focus on the details of the image in his or her mind. Guided imagery can reduce pain, blood pressure, stress, and uncertainty.

- **Desensitization.** If fear or phobias are interfering with an individual's progress, desensitization can be used to help the individual deal with these fears. Desensitization allows the individual to face his or her fear in a calm and safe environment in order to cope with the fear.

A PTA may work with individuals who cannot overcome anxiety and fear despite the relaxation techniques used. In these cases, the PTA will need to refer back to the supervising PT and recommend a referral to the appropriate healthcare provider.

NAVIGATION TIP

For further information on relaxation techniques, see the Therapeutic Exercise section of this chapter.

Strength, Power, and Endurance Training

Individuals with neurological diagnoses may present with different types of strength and endurance deficits. Following a stroke, for example, an individual may present with hemiplegia and be unable to voluntarily move against gravity. However, it is critical that the muscles on their uninvolved side be strengthened as much as possible. Other individuals may present with generalized upper or lower extremity deconditioning or weakness as a result of a progressive neurological diagnosis. The principles of strength, power, and endurance training must be applied, and possibly modified, to prevent overwork in this population.

Approaches to Training

There are many approaches to strength and endurance training that can be used. Free weights, elastic bands, weight machines, aquatic exercises, or powder boards are examples of equipment that can be used to improve strength. For individuals who cannot perform active movements against gravity, a gravity-eliminated position will be needed. Positioning the body part in the appropriate position in relation to gravity and using equipment such as a powder board can allow for strength training in very weak muscles. Aquatic therapy may also be beneficial to individuals with significant weakness due to problems such as spinal cord injury or multiple sclerosis because of the support the water offers. Water can assist a body part during active exercise or act as resistance to active movement as strength increases. For individuals with the ability to strength train against gravity and with external resistance, free weights, bands, and weight machines can be used.

Critical Components

Regardless of the equipment or exercises chosen for a strength training program, there are five critical components that must be addressed: mode, intensity, frequency, rest, and duration.

Critical Components of Strength Training

COMPONENT	DESCRIPTION
Mode	Type of exercise—including type of muscle contraction and type of resistance
Intensity	Load or level of resistance
Frequency	Number of repetitions and sets
Rest	Time between sets and exercise sessions (to allow for recovery)
Duration	Total time of training

Within these critical components of strength training, the PTA also must be aware of correct alignment and appropriate stabilization.

Four Principles of Strength Training

Specific components must be addressed in order to create a comprehensive strength training program that an individual will be able to accurately carry out and sustain on his or her own. The mode and frequency of exercise should be convenient and realistic in order to encourage compliance. In addition, the initial intensity and duration of the strength training program should not be so difficult that discouragement sets in. However, it must also be difficult enough to result in strength gains. In order to determine the appropriate mode, frequency, and intensity of a strength training program, the following principles must be recognized: overload, specificity, cross-training, and reversibility.

In order to determine the correct load to use during strength training, the principle of a one repetition maximum is used. One repetition maximum (1 RM) is the amount of weight that can be lifted through full range of motion one time only. In order to determine an individual's one repetition max, the PTA begins with a weight that is the PTA's best estimate of a one repetition max for the individual's target muscle. Based on the number of full repetitions the individual can

Strength Training Principles

PRINCIPLE	DEFINITION	APPLICATION
Overload	Load placed on muscle must be greater than loads normally placed on muscle.	Progressive resistance should achieve at least 80% of maximum strength.
Specificity	Training effects will be specific to the mode of exercise.	Effects of training from one activity do not carry over to other ones.
Cross-training	Training program should include a variety of training.	Variety in strength training includes concentric, eccentric, isometric, and endurance training.
Reversibility	Failure to sustain benefits of training will occur if muscles do not regularly participate in resistance exercise.	An ongoing functional exercise program must include resistance.

These four principles must be addressed in all strength training programs.

perform with the estimated one repetition max weight, the one repetition max weight can be determined.

The PTA should then create a strength training program based on a minimum of 80% of the individual's one repetition max. The one repetition max must be determined for each muscle involved in the strength training program. The number of repetitions should be approximately 8 to 12 reps. When the individual can easily accomplish 15 repetitions, the weight must be increased. In addition, the last repetition completed for each muscle should be so difficult to complete that another repetition would not be possible. Therefore, when the individual is able to perform greater than 15 repetitions before reaching the last repetition possible, the weight should be increased according to the new 1 repetition max.

TAKE NOTE

The type of contraction used is an important aspect of a strength training program and is based on a patient's individual needs and abilities. Because isometric training involves no joint movement, this type of training can be effective if an individual has pain with movement or movement restrictions. Abnormal muscle activation may be seen in individuals with neurological or motor control impairments. For these individuals, beginning with isometric and eccentric contractions will allow the individual to maintain a contraction more easily during training.

One Repetition Maximum

MUSCLE	WEIGHT	NUMBER OF FULL REPETITIONS PERFORMED	CALCULATION	ONE REPETITION MAX	80% ONE REPETITION MAX
Biceps	45 pounds	3	One rep max = $[(r/30) + 1] \times w$	49.5 pounds	40 pounds for strength training the biceps
Quadriceps	75 pounds	7		92.5 pounds	74 pounds for strength training the quadriceps

This process can be repeated as strength improves in order to determine the new one repetition max.

Muscle Endurance Training

Muscle endurance is also an important factor to consider in the rehabilitation of patients with neurological problems. Low endurance is a hallmark symptom of many neurological diseases, such as multiple sclerosis and Guillain-Barré. Poor muscle endurance is also an impairment following a CVA. Muscle endurance training must be part of a comprehensive program that includes muscle facilitation, strength training, and aerobic activity.

Strengthening Muscle Groups for Normal Function

Muscles of ventilation and pelvic floor muscles are examples of other muscle groups that need strength, power, and endurance to carry out normal function. These muscles can be trained using the same principles, but the specific exercises used may be different. Kegel exercise is a common recommendation for strengthening the pelvic floor. The pelvic floor supports several internal organs including the bladder. Weakness of the pelvic floor can lead to prolapse of organs and can also contribute to low back pain due to lack of intra-abdominal support.

Strengthening Pelvic Floor Muscles

To contract the pelvic floor muscles, the PTA should instruct the individual to contract the muscles that stop the flow of urine without contracting the buttock or abdominal muscles. The pelvic floor muscles must be trained with high repetitions and high frequency. These exercises can be performed 10 to 20 repetitions at a time, multiple times a day, starting with a four to five second hold and progressing to a ten second hold. This will help build strength and endurance of these muscles. If sufficient strength and endurance is not gained from these exercises, there are additional interventions that can be applied. Biofeedback will inform the individual about when the correct muscles are contracting and how long the contraction is maintained. This visual feedback may be enough to train for correct Kegel exercises. In addition, vaginal weights can be used to build strength in the pelvic floor. A weight is inserted into the vagina and must be held with the contraction of the pelvic floor. The weight can be progressed as strength increases.

Strengthening Muscles of Ventilation

Muscles of ventilation may be impaired in a variety of neuromuscular conditions. Expiratory muscle weakness may be related to a weak coughing mechanism, which can prevent secretions from being expelled. An effective cough requires the contraction of the abdominals, intercostals, and pelvic floor muscles. Therefore, strengthening these muscle groups may assist in an effective cough. Inspiratory muscles may also be affected, resulting in hypoxemia or hypercapnia.

Ventilation muscle strength can be measured using specialized equipment that prevents the movement of air and measures the pressure generated during inspiration and expiration. When ventilator muscle strengthening is indicated, the individual will be asked to move air through resistive loading or threshold loading. Resistive loading requires the movement of air through a small space, and threshold loading requires reaching a certain pressure before air will flow.

Whether the physical therapy goals focus on strength or endurance, it is important to always incorporate gains in these areas into functional activities. The type of muscle contraction used is an important consideration. Functional activities can allow for strengthening using various types of contractions as well as all muscle groups, including the pelvic floor and ventilator musculature. Strength and endurance gains in many muscles can be achieved with the use of functional activities. Gravity, body weight, or external forces such as weights or manual resistance activities are used for specific body regions that would benefit. This allows the individual to improve strength, coordination, postural control, and balance within functional activities. Using a combination of a strength training program and task-specific training is an effective way to maximize an individual's progress toward functional independence.

Developmental Activities Training

Developmental activities training involves training within developmental postures and can assist an individual in bridging the gap between disordered movement and independent control of active movement. These postures are used for training because it is believed that the brain and body can relearn mobility and skills in the same progression that the brain and body originally learned them as an infant. The developmental postures place progressively more demands on the body; the goal is for the individual to gain freedom to move within these postures. Achieving motor control in one development posture creates the foundation needed to progress to the next demanding posture.

Developmental Postures

POSTURE	MOTOR CHALLENGES	TREATMENT RESULTS	FUNCTIONAL BENEFITS
Rolling	Trunk and extremity muscle activation and coordination	Trunk rotation and lower extremity coordination	Preparation for bridging and scooting
Prone on elbows	Weight-bearing through upper extremities and head control with a wide base of support and a low center of gravity	Strengthening shoulder and neck stabilizers, upper trunk and head/neck control	Preparation for bed mobility and sit-to-stand
Hook-lying	Cocontraction of lower extremity and trunk musculature to maintain position	Weight-bearing through feet and co-contraction of trunk and lower extremity muscles	Preparation for bridging and scooting
Bridging	Multiple muscle group activation and balancing low center of mass with wide base of support	Strengthening hip stabilizers, hip extensors, and lower trunk and lower extremity control	Preparation for bed mobility and sit-to-stand
Quadruped	Stabilization of shoulder and hip girdle musculature with a wide base of support and an increasingly higher center of gravity	Strengthening trunk, upper and lower extremities, head control; hip and shoulder stabilizers	Preparation for lower extremity weight-bearing and weight shifting through hip girdle

Developmental Postures (*continued*)

POSTURE	MOTOR CHALLENGES	TREATMENT RESULTS	FUNCTIONAL BENEFITS
Sitting	Trunk and head control with moderate base of support, moderate height of center of mass	Weight-bearing in upright posture, improve trunk, lower extremity, and head control	Functional posture important for reaching and ADLs
Kneeling and half-kneeling	Kneeling: trunk control and hip stabilization with narrow base of support; half-kneeling: trunk control and hip stabilization with wide base of support	Weight-bearing through hips in upright posture, strengthening hip and trunk stabilizers	Maintaining balance in upright posture with decreasing base of support
Modified plantigrade	Stabilization of shoulder and hip girdles with wide base of support and high center of mass	Weight-bearing through extended upper and lower extremities; improve balance reactions	Preparation for standing, stepping, and reaching
Standing	Trunk control: balance in upright posture with narrow base of support and high center of mass	Weight-bearing through lower extremities in full, upright posture; improve balance reactions	Preparation for gait training

Intervention in these stages will be based on the individual's ability. As a result, not all individuals will need to begin in the first stage.

Neuromuscular Facilitation Techniques

While maintaining these postures, the individual can participate in neuromuscular reeducation that is guided and facilitated by the PTA. This progression of developmental postures is most appropriate during treatment for individuals with insufficient central nervous system (CNS) recovery and voluntary control of movement. These individuals may also present with abnormal muscle tone that prevents control of movement. Abnormal muscle tone involves an overactive or underactive neuromuscular system, resulting in firing of a muscle that cannot be voluntarily controlled, or lack of muscle firing preventing voluntary movement. For example, muscle spasms may interfere with neuromuscular communication, preventing accurate cues from being received by the body. This leads to inappropriate motor responses. There are techniques the PTA can use to help promote a normal muscle tone in preparation for movement. Additionally, there are facilitation techniques and inhibition techniques that can be applied by the PTA.

Neuromuscular Facilitation Techniques

TECHNIQUE	DESCRIPTION	RESPONSE	APPLICATION
Quick stretch	Brief stretch applied to the agonist muscle	Facilitates contraction of the agonist muscle	With the agonist muscle in the lengthened range, apply a quick stretch and encourage the patient to contract the target muscle.
Resistance	Exertion of force on a muscle	Facilitates agonist muscle contraction and can inhibit antagonist muscle contraction	Manual resistance of the muscle being facilitated
Joint approximation	Compression of joint surfaces	Facilitates postural muscles and stabilizers surrounding the joint	Weight-bearing through a joint; for example, weight-bearing through shoulder when using a walker
Manual contact	Firm pressure	Facilitation of muscle contraction directly under the pressure	Applying pressure to agonist muscle—with or without resistance
Vestibular stimulation	Head and body movements	Facilitation of postural muscles and improvement of motor coordination	Fast spinning or bouncing up and down on a therapy ball

The PTA must be aware that facilitation techniques may also have adverse effects in muscles that are in spasm or joints that are unstable.

Inhibition Techniques

TECHNIQUE	DESCRIPTION	RESPONSE	APPLICATION
Prolonged stretch	Slow, maintained stretch at maximal available range	Inhibits muscle contraction and tone through the stretch-protection reflex	Positioning, inhibitory splinting or casting, low-load weight using traction
Inhibitory pressure	Deep, maintained pressure across the longitudinal axis of tendon or muscle	Inhibits muscle tone	Manual maintained pressure through positioning or weight-bearing
Slow stroking	Slow strokes applied to paravertebral spinal region	Calming effect and generalized inhibition	Firm, alternating strokes in a downward direction over paravertebral region
Neutral warmth	Retention of body heat	Generalized inhibition of tone, relaxation, and decrease in pain	Wrapping body or body segments with towel, ace, or other wrap
Prolonged icing	Application of ice to area requiring inhibition	Decreases neural and muscle spindle firing; inhibits muscle tone	Immersion of body part in cold water, ice towel, ice massage
Slow vestibular stimulation	Slow, rhythmic vestibular stimulation	Generalized relaxation; inhibits muscle tone	Slow, repetitive rocking (such as in a rocking chair)

These techniques inhibit muscle tone or provide general relaxation in preparation for normal movement.

When an individual has impaired voluntary control of movement due to increased or decreased tone, the techniques outlined in the previous table can be used to normalize tone. Once tone is normalized, the PTA can begin training new motor tasks and offering appropriate guidance and feedback so that the body can learn new motor programs.

Neuromuscular Reeducation

Neuromuscular reeducation involves motor learning and motor control. Motor learning refers to the ways in which motor patterns are acquired, modified, and retained so that they can be used and reused by the body during appropriate activities. A learned motor pattern is a result of the interaction between the need for a certain action and the environment in which the action will take place. An example of a motor pattern would be the process of sit-to-stand or walking. These patterns are combinations of simple and complex motor programs and are coordinated by the body into an effective movement.

Complex motor patterns can be broken down into individual motor programs and practiced individually or as a whole with different types of feedback from the PTA helping correct and refine movement. There are many things that can affect motor learning, including the stages of motor learning, the type of practice, and feedback. There are three stages of motor learning—the cognitive stage, the associative stage, and the autonomous stage.

Stages of Motor Learning

STAGE	CHARACTERIZATION	DESCRIPTION
I: Cognitive stage	Acquisition of a motor skill	Practice of the skill, external feedback, and self-correction are needed.
II: Associative stage	Refinement of a motor skill	Skill is completed in a specific environment, needs fewer corrections, and requires less energy.
III: Autonomous stage	Retention of a motor skill	Skill can be transferred to different environments and is more automatic.

Determining the stage of motor learning for each patient and task can help guide the treatment intervention.

Stages of Motor Learning

In the cognitive stage of motor learning, external feedback as well as self-correction are both important. The skill needs to be practiced often. A lot of initial external feedback may be required for the skill to be performed without error. However, once an individual knows how to perform the skill correctly, the PTA needs to allow for self-correction by not offering as much external feedback. Once an individual can self-correct and practice the skill after self-correction, the second stage, or the associative stage, of motor learning can be achieved. The associative stage involves the ability to perform a skill correctly within certain environmental conditions. In this stage, the PTA will keep the environment the same in order to allow for refinement of the skill as well as increased self-correction. Upon reaching the third stage, or the autonomous stage, the patient will have achieved total control of the skill and will have the ability to transfer it to various environments.

An example of the stages of motor learning can be seen in a patient learning to stand from a chair. In the first stage, the PTA instructs the patient in the mechanics of sit-to-stand and allows practice of the skill while offering verbal or tactile feedback to correct. This feedback should be reduced progressively, allowing for self-correction. The patient will begin to recognize when an error has occurred in the movement and will self-correct. As the patient continues to practice the skill, it will become more refined and the patient will enter the associative stage. The environment, for example a firm, standard-height chair with arms, will remain constant. In the last stage, the skill can be transferred to other environments such as softer chairs and chairs of varying heights. There is little error, so practice is no longer needed as the skill becomes automatic and part of everyday life.

Types of Feedback

The type of feedback given can affect how a skill is learned. Intrinsic feedback is feedback from the body that provides sensory information about motor performance such as where the body is in space during an activity. Sensory impairments can lead to inadequate intrinsic feedback, and the PT can delegate specific activities to the PTA that assist in regaining sensory awareness during an activity or identify a compensatory technique. Extrinsic feedback is given from an outside source, such as auditory cues from the PTA or the use of a mirror for visual feedback. This type of feedback is important as a skill is initially learned, but extrinsic feedback must be decreased in order for an individual to use more intrinsic feedback and self-correct. An individual cannot become functionally independent if extrinsic feedback is still needed for safe and correct performance.

Types of Practice

The type of practice is another consideration for the PT and PTA. An individual can learn different parts of a skill and practice each individual part or learn a whole task and practice the task as a whole. Part learning is used for complex activities that have discrete parts and motor programs. For example, when learning supine-to-sit, the PTA may first instruct an individual on how to obtain the hook-lying position. Then, the PTA would teach the individual how to reach to the side and roll into side-lying. Finally, the PTA would instruct how to bring the legs off the edge of the bed and push the trunk into sitting. Each of these parts can be practiced separately, but eventually the parts must be put together in the correct order, which is the basis for another type of learning called progressive learning. Some skills are made up of sequential parts, and each part can be practiced in sequential order. For tasks such as dancing, individuals who are taught the separate parts may inadvertently put them together in a different sequence. In order for the parts to equal the whole, there is a proper sequence and practice should progress in sequential order. Whole learning involves practicing a skill as a whole task. Tasks such as rolling are best practiced as a whole task. The final type of practice is a combination of whole and part practice. The first step is practicing the whole task in order to allow for task analysis. The PT can then direct the PTA to practice the parts of the task that are missing or difficult for the individual to perform.

Practice Schedules

The schedule of practice is also an important consideration. There are three main types of practice schedule—mass, variable, and random. Each type of practice is indicated in the following table based on the physical therapy goals:

Practice Schedules

SCHEDULE	DESCRIPTION	APPLICATION
Mass	Entire motor pattern must be practiced as a whole and practiced frequently.	Patient repetitively practices a motor pattern with few interruptions in order to make sure that the motor program is learned by the central nervous system.
Variable	Practice progresses from very often to less often.	The central nervous system is capable of the motor program, but errors still occur in the execution; the skill is refined as independence increases, and practice can be less frequent.
Random	Practice is done without a set schedule of frequency.	Once the skill can be performed independently, the skill should be practiced as part of daily life.

Practice schedules can vary depending on the skill being practiced and the patient's diagnosis.

Motor Control

Motor control is the means through which an individual controls movement already acquired. Analyzing motor control of specific movements requires observation of the multiple motor programs that are working at the same time to complete the task. The central nervous system must be able to control and modify all of these motor programs in order to successfully carry out a movement. Individuals with neurologic impairments may lose the ability to complete a motor program. Physical therapy intervention will be focused on refining the motor programs available as well as training the body in the missing programs. For example, during walking there are multiple motor programs working such as balance, postural control, stepping, and arm swing. If an individual lacks balance, an assistive device can be used to allow for training and refinement of the available motor programs. As these aspects of walking improve and balance training has progressed, the assistive device can be removed, demanding more control of the balance system during walking.

Functional Training

Intervention that focuses on the ability to perform specific functional activities is the focus of functional training. An individual will need to learn how to perform activities safely and effectively, and then continue to practice those activities in order to incorporate them into daily life. The goal of functional training is for automatic performance of daily activities. Functional training is not appropriate with individuals who lack sufficient voluntary motor control or who lack the cognitive ability to understand the training.

Functional training is an approach that can be effective with individuals of any age with a variety of neurological and musculoskeletal diagnoses. For individuals who have experienced an injury, functional training is best initiated as early as possible in order to avoid nonuse or wrong-use habits and motor patterns. For individuals who present with motor control impairments that are not the result of injury, functional training can be effective throughout the physical therapy plan of care. It is important that functional training involve activities that are interesting to the individual and directly related to daily activities.

An assessment of what is limiting an individual's ability to complete a task is an important first step. Poor endurance, weakness, impaired motor control, or decreased range of motion are examples of possible limitations and will guide intervention. Functional training in combination with specific intervention for the deficits noted will give the best opportunity for progress.

Effective functional training begins by minimizing the use of compensatory strategies and focusing on restoring the use of the affected body segments. Repeated practice is important for motor learning, as is participation of affected body segments. The PTA can initially offer guidance, assistance, and supervision of activities. The patient then progresses to independent activity performance in order to reduce dependence on the PTA for cueing or encouragement. In addition to increasing task independence, tasks should initially be practiced in a supportive and controlled environment and progress to real-world environments. If an individual is unable to regain the ability to perform a functional task, compensatory training may be needed. This can involve the use of adaptive equipment or use of another body part to complete a task.

Functional Training in Self-Care and Home Management

Evaluation of the bathroom is an important aspect of self-care training. The height of the toilet, type of bathtub, and height of vanity are bathroom examples that must be evaluated in order to allow for appropriate training. In addition, evaluation of the furniture itself is important, for example determining if the bed is too high, if the mattress is too soft for effective mobility, or if chairs are too low to allow independent standing.

Evaluation of the home including door widths, counter heights, and outdoor home access are some of the important aspects that will guide functional training. If the opportunity to work with an individual in the home is available, this can allow for specific and appropriate self-care and home management training. Bed mobility, transfers, gait, balance, bathing, dressing, and home management are examples of specific skills that can be evaluated in the home in order to determine safe and effective self-care and home management.

The evaluation of the home may lead to identification of home modifications or adaptive devices that may be needed in order for the individual to be independent in the home. These modifications may require a third party. Adaptive devices can be prescribed by the physical or occupational therapist, and functional training should include any adaptive or supportive devices that will be used in the individual's daily life. Examples of devices used during self-care and home management are identified in the following table:

Functional Training in Work, Community, and Leisure

In addition to evaluation of the home environment, the work, community, and leisure environments must also be evaluated in order for the individual to carry out all desired life roles. Job analysis or a functional capacity evaluation can give the PTA information about the areas of work that need training. Specific functional activities required for the patient's job can be learned and practiced, or the work environment may need to be modified to allow for access. If adaptive devices are needed, functional training should include the use of those devices. Evaluation of an individual's community can guide functional training for daily community activities. For example, if an individual is required to take a bus, functional training of stepping up on a bus, maintaining balance while standing, and sitting or standing from a bus seat will be a focus of treatment. Access to the community may require that the patient walk or use adaptive devices, and training should include the devices that the

Adaptive Devices for Self-Care

SELF-CARE ACTIVITY	DEVICE
Meal preparation	Suction devices to stabilize plates, rocker knife, universal cuff for utensils, and weighted utensils
Bathing and dressing	Long-handled sock aid and shoe horn, long-handled sponge, shower chair, and grab bars in bathroom
House cleaning	Long-handled reacher and duster, self-propelled vacuum, and self-wringing mop

These devices can be used by individuals with neurological diagnoses that result in hemiplegia, decreased coordination, or decreased upper extremity range of motion and strength.

individual is anticipated to use daily. Functional training in desired leisure activities is also very important. Identification of an individual's leisure activities is critical, and practicing the leisure activities in real-world environments can be motivating and encouraging. Adaptive devices that can be used during work, community activities, or leisure include electric wheelchairs or scooters, vehicle steering wheel adaptations, and work stations designed specifically for an individual's needs, such as lowered desk height or larger keyboards.

Application of Adaptive, Assistive, and Orthotic Devices

There are a variety of adaptive, assistive, and supportive devices that have been identified to assist with different areas of function. The application of these devices is a critical component of effective treatment and is unique for each individual with proper sizing, fit, and training.

Other adaptive devices used to support function include orthotics and are recommended based on specific muscle weakness or impairment identified during

Common Assistive Devices Used for Gait

DEVICE	FIT	USE OF DEVICE
Standard walker	In an upright posture with arms at side, height of walker at level of ulnar styloid process, 20 to 30 degree elbow flexion when walker handles are grasped	Walker is advanced approximately arm's length by picking it up followed by advancement of involved extremity, then uninvolved extremity; weight is transferred through upper extremities if NWB
Front-wheeled walker	In an upright posture with arms at side, height of walker at level of ulnar styloid process, 20 to 30 degree elbow flexion when walker handles are grasped	Walker is advanced approximately arm's length by rolling it forward; involved extremity advances followed by uninvolved extremity
Straight cane	With point of cane six inches in front of and lateral to little toe, height of cane at level of ulnar styloid process, elbow flexed 20 to 30 degrees when cane handle is grasped	Cane placed opposite the involved side; should not be advanced further than toes of involved foot; cane and involved extremity advance simultaneously
Quad cane	In an upright posture with arms at side, height of cane at level of ulnar styloid process, 20 to 30 degree elbow flexion when walker handles are grasped	Cane placed opposite the involved side; should not be advanced further than toes of involved foot; four feet should touch the ground together; cane and involved extremity advance together

Common Assistive Devices Used for Gait (*continued*)

DEVICE	FIT	USE OF DEVICE
Axillary crutches	In standing position, height of crutches two inches below axilla with tip of crutch six inches in front of and lateral to little toe, 20 to 30 degrees of elbow flexion when crutch handles are grasped	Body weight through hands, not axilla; keep crutches at least four inches in front and side of feet; crutches advanced with NWB or PWB extremity followed by uninvolved extremity
Lofstrand crutches	In standing position with crutch handles grasped, 20 to 30 degree elbow flexion	Body weight through hands; keep crutches at least four inches in front and side of feet

There are many varieties of walkers, canes, and crutches with various attachments to make the device more specific to the patient's needs.

evaluation. Application of these devices includes training the functional activity with the device.

Airway Clearance Techniques

Individuals with neurological diagnoses or lesions may present with overproduction of pulmonary secretions as well as ineffective airway clearance techniques such as coughing. PTAs can provide training in a variety of interventions to assist with airway clearance including positional, manual, and breathing techniques.

Postural Drainage

Postural drainage is a positioning technique that involves placing the involved bronchus perpendicular to the ground in order to allow gravity to assist with drainage. Once the secretions drain, the individual can perform airway clearance techniques to expel the secretions and clear the lungs. The positions for postural drainage are based on the area of the lung involved. Each body posture targets a different area of the lungs and allows gravity to assist drainage.

Orthotic Devices

DEVICE	APPLICATION
Ankle-foot orthosis	Control ankle motion by limiting plantar flexion and/or dorsiflexion or assisting motio
Knee-ankle-foot orthosis	Control ankle and knee motion; medial-lateral and hyperextension control while allowing flexion
Hip-knee-ankle-foot orthosis	Control hip abduction, adduction, rotation; stabilizes hip in extension for standing and walking

The orthoses listed above (used for the lower extremity) are those most often used for physical therapy. Orthoses for the upper extremities are available but are not used often in physical therapy.

The PTA can also use manual techniques to assist in loosening secretions in the pulmonary system. Percussion and shaking are two primary techniques used. Percussion is performed with the clinician's cupped hands applying force to a specific area on the chest wall. This can be applied during inspiration and expiration and can be performed for five to ten minutes at a time.

Shaking, or vibration, follows a deep inhalation with a vibratory force applied to the rib cage during expiration. Shaking is also applied to a specific area of the chest wall and is commonly performed after percussion.

Both of these techniques can be performed in the appropriate postural drainage position. Following these techniques, the individual is encouraged to perform airway clearance techniques such as coughing in order to expel secretions.

Effective Coughing

Coughing is a reflex that prevents inhalation of foreign particles or gases and also expels foreign objects or secretions in the lungs. A weak coughing mechanism can result in the buildup of excessive secretions in the lungs which can lead to infection. A productive and effective cough requires strong abdominal, intercostals, and pelvic floor musculature, as well as appropriate mobility of the rib cage and thorax to allow effective muscle contraction for coughing.

Ventilatory Muscle Training

Ventilatory muscle training can assist with strengthening the coughing mechanism. In addition, there are assisted coughing techniques that are effective with weak expiratory muscles. For example, an individual who has experienced a spinal cord injury affecting innervations of the abdominal muscles can be assisted by having the PTA place a hand on the upper abdomen and push upward and inward during the expulsive phase of a cough. Coughing more than once following inspiration can improve cough strength.

Responses to Treatment and Potential Complications

The goal of neuromuscular physical therapy intervention is functional motor recovery in all aspects of life. Once an individual can independently carry out motor programs, it is important that this function is used and practiced frequently in order to be maintained. Nonuse can result in the loss of function or injury and a need for repeated physical therapy intervention.

There is always a risk of complications with physical therapy interventions. It is critical that the PTA recognize all contraindications and precautions to treatment. The physical therapy evaluation should identify all relevant medical history and restrictions, and the PTA must ask questions for clarification if needed. It is the responsibility of the PTA to provide safe and effective treatment. Possible complications of treatment are identified in the following table:

Possible Treatment Complications

TREATMENT	CONTRAINDICATIONS AND PRECAUTIONS
Aerobic and endurance training	Unstable angina; high or low resting BP, HR, RR; or hypotension during activity
Balance training	Insufficient guarding or impaired cognitive status
Stretching	Muscle guarding, patient intolerance, or fracture

Possible Treatment Complications (*continued*)

TREATMENT	CONTRAINDICATIONS AND PRECAUTIONS
Joint mobilization	Advanced osteoporosis, fracture, acute inflammation, active disease, or infection
Gait training	Weight-bearing restrictions, insufficient guarding, impaired cognition, or orthostatic hypotension
Strength training	Severe osteoporosis, fracture, or Valsalva maneuver
Neuromuscular reeducation	Impaired cognition, pain, or fracture
Airway clearance	Fracture, site of fusion, severe osteoporosis, pulmonary embolism, angina, or significant pulmonary edema

In addition to these contraindications and precautions, if the patient is unable to tolerate the treatment due to pain, fear, or injury, then the treatment is not appropriate at that time.

Practice 3 Questions

1. The PTA is working with a patient who reports balance concerns while walking down her dirt and gravel driveway to retrieve the mail in the afternoon. Which of the following activities should the PTA have the patient use to train for improved balance?
   a. scan the environment while walking
   b. balance on a trampoline
   c. walk in an environment with low lighting
   d. practice single-leg stance

2. The PTA is reviewing the physical therapy plan of care for a new patient and reads that the PT has recommended grade III joint mobilizations of the right glenohumeral joint. Which of the following is the best application of a grade III joint mobilization?
   a. large amplitude rhythmic oscillations in midrange
   b. small amplitude rhythmic oscillations at end range
   c. large amplitude rhythmic oscillations up to the point of limitation
   d. small amplitude rhythmic oscillations at beginning range

3. The PTA is currently performing postural drainage with a patient and will progress onto a new lung segment based on the PT's reassessment. Which of the following is the best position for the patient for drainage of the posterior segments of the upper lobes?
   a. supine on flat surface with pillow under knees
   b. sitting and leaning back against a pillow at a 30 degree angle
   c. prone with two pillows under the hips
   d. sitting and leaning over a pillow at a 30 degree angle

4. The PTA is working with a child who has vestibular impairment resulting in poor balance during play. Which of the following is the best intervention to stimulate the vestibular system?
   a. assisted walking through an obstacle course
   b. guarded bouncing up and down on a therapy ball
   c. putting together a puzzle in standing with assist
   d. assisted walking on a balance beam

Practice 3 Answers

1. b. The PTA should have the patient balance on a trampoline for improved balance. Training balance on a trampoline targets the somatosensory system, which is the most likely system involved if the patient has difficulty walking on an uneven surface.

2. c. The best application of a grade III joint mobilization is large amplitude rhythmic oscillations up to the point of limitation. Grade III joint mobilization is defined as large amplitude rhythmic oscillations up to the point of limitation.

3. d. The best position for the patient for drainage of the posterior segments of the upper lobes is sitting on a flat surface and leaning over a pillow at a 30 degree angle. The clinician then stands behind the patient and performs manual techniques over the upper back.

4. b. Guarded bouncing up and down on a therapy ball will stimulate the vestibular system due to the movement of the head in relation to gravity.

Integumentary System

Physical therapist assistants must be able to apply safe and effective interventions for open wounds and burns. This requires the physical therapist assistant to know about prevention of open areas, the application of debridement techniques, the application of dressings, and adjunct treatments to promote wound repair. It is also critical for the PTA to understand the impact on the integumentary system, or skin, of interventions applied to other body systems (for example, normal and abnormal skin response after application of superficial heat).

Prevention of Open Areas

Many of the patients seen in physical therapy are at risk for development of open areas. These include, but are not limited to, patients with diseases like diabetes, lymphedema, and peripheral vascular disease and patients with limited mobility due to problems such as spinal cord injury, multiple sclerosis, or surgery.

Proper skin care is a key component of prevention for every at-risk patient. Skin should be kept clean, dry, and moisturized. Management of incontinence is necessary to prevent maceration.

Daily visual inspection of skin can catch problem areas early. Pressure relief devices, such as wheelchair cushions and overlay mattresses, will diminish pressure, shear forces, and friction for patients who are limited in mobility. Pressure relief activities, including frequent turning in bed and wheelchair push-ups, are an important adjunct to those devices. Proper positioning in bed or chair will further protect patients from developing open areas. Of course, functional mobility training to improve a patient's ability to change positions is a mainstay of physical therapy interventions.

Edema management is critical for those with lymphedema and venous insufficiency. Properly fitting footwear with socks distributes forces equally on the plantar aspect of the foot, accommodates for deformities, and prevents trauma. Clothing should be nonrestrictive and provide coverage to shield vulnerable areas from trauma, insect bites, and sunburn.

Finally, care should be taken during activities of daily living and instrumental activities of daily living to prevent skin trauma. Suggestions include use of an electric razor, having nails trimmed professionally, measuring the temperature of bath and dishwashing water, and use of silicon mitts while cooking.

Bony Prominences and Positioning

POSITION	BONY PROMINENCES
Supine	Occipital tuberosity Vertebral spinous processes Scapula Sacrum Posterior calcaneus
Prone	Forehead Lateral ear Patella Dorsum of foot
Side-lying	Lateral ear Acromion process Greater trochanter Medial and latral femoral epicondyles Medial and lateral malleoli
Sitting	Vertebral spinous processes Scapula Olecranon process Ischial tuberosities Sacrum

These bony prominences are at risk for increased pressure in various body positions.

Summary of Prevention Activities

The activities below may help prevent open wounds from occurring:

- skin care/inspection
- pressure relief activities/devices/positions
- functional mobility training
- proper footwear/clothing
- edema management
- care during ADLs/IADLs

Debridement Techniques

Debridement is defined as the removal of necrotic tissue, foreign material, and debris from the wound bed. The overall goal is to enhance wound healing by creating a warm, moist, and clean bed of granulation tissue. Debridement will decrease the risk of infection, speed progression of the wound through the inflammatory phase of healing, facilitate epithelial migration over the wound bed, and decrease odor. Debridement techniques should not be used on wounds with primarily healthy tissue, in the presence of gangrene or osteomyelitis, on electrical burns, or on subdermal tissues.

Selective Debridement

Different methods exist to debride an open wound. Selective sharp debridement is beyond the scope of work of a physical therapist assistant and will not be discussed here. However, other forms of selective debridement are autolytic debridement, enzymatic debridement, and low frequency (20–100 KHz) ultrasonic debridement.

Autolytic Debridement

With autolytic debridement, a moisture-retentive dressing is used to trap drainage in the wound. The drainage softens necrotic tissue, and the macrophages and natural enzymes digest it. The presence of white blood cells helps prevent infection, but this method should not be used on wounds that are already infected. This method is noninvasive, pain-free, and easy to apply.

Enzymatic Debridement

With enzymatic debridement, a medication containing an enzyme that will break down protein, fibrin, or collagen is applied to the wound bed once or several times a day. It is pain-free and easy to apply and can be used on infected wounds. However, the cost of the medication may be prohibitive.

Low Frequency Ultrasonic Debridement

Low frequency ultrasonic debridement rapidly removes fibrin from the wound bed while sparing granulation tissue. It will also kill bacteria. It can be used on tunneling and undermining and is pain-free and easy to apply.

Nonselective Debridement Techniques

In contrast to forms of selective debridement, which remove only necrotic tissue, nonselective debridement techniques will remove all tissue with which they come into contact. Therefore, these techniques should be used judiciously and with great care, to prevent damaging healthy tissue. Nonselective debridement techniques include wet-to-dry dressings, chemical cleaners, hydrotherapy (whirlpool), and pulsed lavage.

Wet-to-Dry Dressings

Wet-to-dry dressings are aptly named, as the gauze dressing is applied to the wound after being soaked in saline solution and then allowed to dry and adhere to the wound. It is removed briskly, along with the adherent tissue. It should only be used in wounds with 100% necrotic tissue, as this method damages fragile healthy tissues and dries the wound bed, which retards healing.

Chemical Cleaners

Wound cleansing with chemicals designed for intact skin (e.g., Betadine™, hydrogen peroxide, Chlorazene™) should not be used in any concentration on open wounds, as they kill cells, including healthy ones. The rule of thumb is to not put anything in an open wound that you would not put in your eye.

Whirlpool, or Hydrotherapy

Hydrotherapy (also called whirlpool) is an appropriate debridement method for some open wounds, though it is frequently overused. Whirlpool temperature may range from 92°F–99°F. Time of immersion should not exceed 20 minutes.

INFORMATION IN ACTION

A patient with Parkinson's disease has a pressure ulcer on the lateral malleolus that is completely covered with hard eschar. The PT asks the PTA to apply whirlpool to the patient's foot in order to soften the eschar prior to the PT performing sharp, selective debridement. The PTA cleanses a small, portable foot whirlpool, fills it with water at 95°F, and places the patient's foot into it. The agitators are adjusted to create a moderate amount of turbulence and the treatment is applied for 15 minutes. At the conclusion of the whirlpool, the PTA dries the patient's foot and wraps it in a clean towel to await the PT. The PTA then cleanses the whirlpool.

Whirlpool Application

Whirlpool application may promote wound healing through a variety of mechanisms, such as:

- loosening tissue and debris
- softening necrotic tissue
- promoting a moist wound bed
- promoting circulation
- decreasing pain

There are several contraindications to whirlpool use. Taking note of the following conditions will prevent the overuse of whirlpool application to open wounds:

- wounds due to venous insufficiency
- wounds with less than 75% necrotic tissue
- incontinence if perineum submerged
- presence of tunneling or extensive undermining
- macerated skin surrounding the wound
- patient confusion

Pulsed Lavage

Pulsed lavage delivers saline solution or tap water into the wound at low pressure (4–15 psi) via a handheld device.

Pulsed lavage is appropriate for wounds of all types, including those with tunneling or undermining, as long as muscle, tendon, nerve, and bone are not exposed. Treatment can be administered at a patient's bedside and lasts 15 to 30 minutes.

Topical Dressings

As noted in the section on debridement, wound healing is optimally enhanced by creating a warm, moist, clean bed of granulation tissue while keeping the skin around the wound dry and intact. In addition, all spaces within the wound must be filled—no dead space should remain. Topical dressings play an integral role in accomplishing these things.

A moist wound bed promotes healing. Benefits of a moist wound bed are:

- It facilitates autolytic debridement.
- It promotes growth of blood vessels.
- It enhances epidermal cell migration across wound bed.
- It optimizes immune system function.
- It increases patient comfort.

Semi-Permeable Film and Semi-Permeable Foam Dressings

Semi-permeable film dressings are transparent membranes that look like plastic wrap. They allow moisture into the wound but not onto the surrounding skin. They cannot absorb any drainage. Semi-permeable film dressings are best for superficial, minimally draining, uninfected wounds, ranging in depth from the dermis to muscle/tendon/bone. They act like sheets of small-celled sponges, ranging in thickness from razor-thin to a quarter inch thick. The thicker the dressing, the more drainage it will absorb. Semi-permeable foam dressings promote autolytic debridement and protect the skin around the wound from maceration. They additionally can be used on infected ulcers.

Calcium Alginate

Calcium alginate is a natural fiber made from brown seaweed. It comes in sheets and ropes. When it absorbs drainage, it turns into a nonadherent gel, which promotes autolytic debridement. Calcium alginate can be packed into a wound to fill dead space. It must be covered by another dressing. It is best for wounds ranging in depth from the dermis to muscle, with moderate to large amounts of drainage.

Hydrocolloid Dressings

Hydrocolloid dressings contain particles of gelatin or pectin which are attached to a very strong film backing. These particles gel as they slowly absorb drainage, facilitating autolytic debridement. The film backing is impermeable to urine, stool, and bacteria. As such, hydrocolloid dressings protect the wound from contamination. They are best for wounds ranging in depth from the dermis to subcutaneous tissue with mild to large amounts of drainage. Some sources state that, due to their occlusive nature, hydrocolloid dressings are contraindicated with infected wounds. Other sources report that use of hydrocolloid dressings on infected wounds does not increase the amount of bacteria in the wound. The PT and physician should be consulted prior to use of a hydrocolloid dressing on an infected ulcer.

Hydrogel

Hydrogel is available as a gel that can be squirted into a wound to fill dead space and add moisture to a dry wound. It also comes in sheets and can be laid onto a wound bed. The sheets are best for wounds ranging in depth from the dermis to subcutaneous tissue with minimal to moderate drainage. They are not indicated for infected wounds.

Characteristics of Dressings

DRESSING	ABSORPTIVE ABILITY	WOUND DEPTH	INFECTION
Semi-perm film	None	Superficial	No
Semi-perm foam	Minimal to maximal	Dermis to muscle/tendon/bone	Yes
Calcium alginate	Moderate to maximal	Dermis to muscle	Yes
Hydrocolloid	Minimal to maximal	Dermis to subcutaneous tissue	Controversial
Hydrogel	Adds moisture	Dermis to muscle	No

This chart compares the ability of various wound dressings to absorb or add moisture, the appropriate depth of wound for which dressings should be used, and whether or not dressings are indicated for an infected wound.

TAKE NOTE

All wounds need a moist wound bed in order to heal. While dry wounds require a dressing that will add and retain moisture, wounds with drainage require a dressing that will absorb and retain moisture.

Adjunct Treatments

There are many physical therapy interventions other than direct wound care that are important to promote healing of an open wound. Therapeutic exercise increases strength, range of motion, and endurance to improve mobility skills. Proper positioning techniques reduce pressure, friction, and shear forces. The application of mattresses, seating cushions, elbow pads, and heel protectors reduce pressure and protect the patient from trauma. Therapeutic massage increases circulation to the skin. Vacuum-assisted closure applies negative pressure to the wound bed, which increases local blood flow and removes drainage. Training of both patients and caregivers is done to promote carryover of treatment activities and improve patient participation during care.

INFORMATION IN ACTION

An elderly woman has developed a pressure ulcer on the posterior aspect of the calcaneus following surgical repair of a hip fracture. She is referred to physical therapy for management of the ulcer. The examination reveals it to be a stage III ulcer, with 70% slough and 30% granulation tissue. There is minimal drainage and it is not infected. A thin semi-permeable foam dressing is applied to facilitate autolytic debridement. A heel protector is applied and worn by the patient at all times except when she is ambulating. Therapeutic exercise and functional mobility training focus on improving the patient's ability to reposition herself independently. Closure of the wound is obtained in four weeks.

Modalities for Wound Care

Modalities such as ultrasound, electrical stimulation, ultraviolet light, and pulsed diathermy enhance healing in a variety of ways

Ultrasound for Wound Care

The therapeutic effects of ultrasound on wound healing are hypothesized to occur due to its nonthermal qualities. The physical effect of the ultrasound waves penetrating into tissue is termed acoustic streaming. This describes the increased flow of fluids around cell membranes, which allows ions and nutrients to enter the cell and waste products to exit the cell more readily. This increased permeability makes the cell more active. Increasing the activation of key cells can facilitate the healing process.

During the inflammatory phase of wound repair, cells that are stimulated include the mast cells, macrophages, and fibroblasts. The result is to enhance the cleanup of cell debris and bacteria and to facilitate the production of connective tissue. The length of time it takes the tissue to pass through the inflammatory phase is shortened, speeding the healing process.

During the proliferative phase, ultrasound can stimulate fibroblasts to produce more collagen, creating the connective tissue scaffold for tissue repair and enhancing wound contraction. The activity of endothelial cells is increased, which hastens formation of new capillaries. This improves blood supply to the tissue, facilitating wound repair.

During the maturation/remodeling phase of wound repair, ultrasound continues to affect collagen formation and distribution, resulting in a stronger, more pliable scar.

The ability of ultrasound to speed wound healing has been demonstrated mainly in animal studies. There have not been many well-designed studies performed on human subjects, so much more research needs to be done to show the clinical effectiveness of ultrasound on wound repair.

Electrical Stimulation for Wound Care

Electrical stimulation accelerates wound repair through at least five different mechanisms. There is very strong research showing the clinical effectiveness of electrical stimulation for wound repair.

- **Restored current of injury.** One mechanism by which electrical stimulation accelerates wound care is by restoring the normal current of injury. Damaged tissue produces an electrical current which is believed to activate the body's healing response. Chronic wounds can lose this current of injury and become inactive. That is, the wound stops progressing through the normal stages of wound repair. Electrical stimulation restarts the healing process by once again activating the current of injury.

- **Attraction of cells.** Another mechanism of wound repair is through the attraction of positively or negatively charged cells to the wound. Macrophages and neutrophils, which help clean the wound and fight infection, are negatively charged. Epidermal cells are also negative. They produce the epithelial cells that cover the wound. These cells would be drawn to a wound receiving positive electrical stimulation. Fibroblasts, which produce collagen, a major building block of connective tissue, are positive and are drawn to a wound receiving negative electrical stimulation.

- **Increased cell activity.** Electrical stimulation increases cellular activity, enhancing DNA synthesis. This results in quicker cell replication and speeds wound repair. Collagen synthesis is also increased, which results in faster production of connective and granulation tissues.

- **Antibacterial effects.** Electrical stimulation may directly kill bacteria. It may attract other cells, like neutrophils, that kill the bacteria. Electrical stimulation generates heat and alters the pH of tissues, which may also destroy bacteria. The effect of electrical stimulation on bacteria seems greatest at the negative electrode, which is why it is usually recommended to place the negative electrode into an infected wound.

Ultraviolet Light for Wound Care

Ultraviolet treatment of open wounds is thought to stimulate wound healing by causing vasodilation and increased capillary permeability. This enhances delivery of oxygen and nutrients to tissues and removal of waste products, speeding the healing process. UV light also kills bacteria, which may eliminate infection. There is moderately strong clinical evidence supporting the use of UV light for wound care, though more studies are needed.

Pulsed Diathermy for Wound Care

Pulsed diathermy can be delivered in either a thermal (heat producing) mode or a nonthermal mode. The rationale for applying thermal pulsed diathermy to a wound is to increase blood flow to the tissue. Increased circulation should enhance healing. The rationale for applying nonthermal pulsed diathermy is to induce current flow into the tissues, much like electrical stimulation. There are few clinical studies to provide evidence of effectiveness for either form of pulsed diathermy.

INFORMATION IN ACTION

A PTA in a skilled nursing facility has been working with a 55-year-old man who sustained a C5 spinal cord injury 20 years ago. The patient was recently hospitalized with pneumonia and was admitted for rehabilitation prior to returning home. He also has an open area on his right ischial tuberosity that has been present for eight months. Wound care has consisted primarily of dressing changes, with no increase or decrease in wound size. The PTA suggests a trial of electrical stimulation for wound repair to the physical therapist. The PT agrees, and electrical stimulation is applied with a twin-peak monophasic waveform at a frequency of 100 pulses per second, a duration of 40 microseconds, and an intensity of 100 milliamps. Treatment is applied for one hour, five times per week. Within seven weeks, wound closure is obtained.

Interventions for Burns

Many of the wound care principles previously discussed may apply to wounds caused by burns. However, due to the typically large amount of skin surface involved, the systemic effects of burn injuries, and the long periods of rehabilitation, interventions in addition to wound care are necessary.

Goals for burn patients address both impairments and functional limitations. Goals of physical therapy intervention for burn injuries include:

- enhance wound healing
- decrease pain
- prevent contractures/increase ROM
- prevent muscle atrophy/increase strength
- prevent deconditioning/increase endurance
- minimize scar formation
- independence in mobility activities
- independence in ADLs/IADLs

Wound Care

One of the primary physical therapy interventions for patients with burns is the debridement of eschar and the removal of foreign material from the burn wound. Medications are commonly applied to the burns to soften eschar and enhance debridement, as well as to fight infection. Gentle cleansing of burn wounds in a whirlpool may help soften eschar, remove medication, and decrease the pain experienced during debridement. Many of the same types of topical dressings previously discussed for other types of open wounds are also applied to burn wounds.

Positioning and Splinting

Since wounds contract as they heal, it is critical to begin proper positioning immediately. In general, patients are positioned so that the involved tissues are elongated. When a burn surrounds a joint, the joint is placed in the close pack position to prevent development of joint capsule contractures. Splints are mainly used at night to maintain joint positions and after skin grafting procedures to protect the graft site. Positioning a limb in an elevated position can prevent edema formation, to which the person with a burn is prone. Finally, proper positioning can enhance respiratory function and prevent pressure sores from developing.

Positioning after Burn Injury

JOINT	DESIRED POSITION
Anterior neck	Neck extension
Shoulder and axilla	Flexion, abduction, or external rotation
Elbow/forearm	Extension and supination
Wrist/hand	Wrist extension; MCP flexion; IP joint extension
Hip	Extension and abduction
Knee	Extension
Foot/ankle	Dorsiflexion; toe extension

Positioning after a burn injury emphasizes the close pack position of the joint to prevent contractures.

Therapeutic Exercise

Therapeutic exercise includes passive ROM, active-assisted ROM, active ROM, stretching, resisted ROM, and aerobic exercises. Performance of these exercises will assist in meeting virtually every goal for the burn patient.

Passive/Active-Assisted/Active Range of Motion Exercise

Active exercise is initiated on the day of admission as long as the person is medically stable. Passive exercise may be done to maintain range of motion, but if the patient can participate, active-assisted or active exercise is preferred. Active exercise will not only maintain motion but will also prevent muscle atrophy, increase circulation, and diminish edema. Doing the active exercise when the bandages are off will allow the therapist

to see the burns and ensure there is no undue stress placed on the tissue. It also prevents chafing from the bandage and allows full range of motion without the bulk of the bandage interfering. If the exercise is done in the whirlpool during dressing changes, the warmth of the water may help the patient relax, which will increase ROM and decrease pain. In addition, the buoyancy may assist with performance of the activities. Movements that occur during the performance of functional activities—such as bathing, dressing, and eating—will help preserve gains made during therapy sessions, and participation in these activities should be encouraged. Exercises should not be done after graft placement until cleared by the surgeon.

Stretching

Stretching can be applied to grafted and healing areas once the tissue is deemed stable. Stretching should be applied gradually, with a low-load prolonged stretch. Mild heat may be applied to the tissue to make it more flexible.

Resisted Range of Motion

Resisted exercises may be applied to uninvolved muscles as soon as the patient is medically stable. The physician and physical therapist should decide when resisted exercise may begin in areas that were burned. The exercises should include a combination of isometric, concentric, and eccentric muscle activation. Resistance can be provided by a variety of means, including manual resistance, Thera-Band, free weights, or exercise equipment. Vital signs should be monitored closely, and the exercises should be progressed conservatively to prevent overwork.

Aerobic Exercise

For patients who are severely deconditioned or ill, performance of active and resisted exercise may also provide aerobic benefits. In addition, activities such as walking to the restroom or daily bathing may challenge the cardiovascular system. As the patient progresses, a variety of aerobic activities should be included to improve function and optimize patient interest and compliance. These may include stairclimbing, upper and lower extremity cycling, or rowing. Initially, heart rate should not rise more than 20 beats per minute above resting level. Ultimately, the target heart rate will be between 50 and 70% of the maximum predicted heart rate.

INFORMATION IN ACTION

A 38-year-old man sustained a combination of superficial and deep partial-thickness burns to the anterior aspect of the neck, thorax, and left upper extremity three weeks ago. He has had skin grafts applied and all are healing well. The PTA has been assisting the PT in the care of this patient by applying the exercise interventions. The patient is independent with resisted exercises for the right upper extremity, and completes three sets of ten repetitions, once per day. The PTA assists the patient in performing closed-chain lower extremity exercises consisting of squats, lunges, toe-raises, and side-stepping. An aerobic component is included by performing stair-climbing at a pace raising the patient's heart rate 20 beats over resting heart rate and by sustaining that pace for 15 minutes. The PTA also guides the patient through active exercises for neck extension, lateral flexion, and rotation; shoulder flexion, abduction, and external rotation; elbow extension; wrist extension; and opening and closing of the hand. With the patient's elbow extended and palm up, the PTA places a three-pound weight around the wrist for ten minutes for a low-load prolonged stretch of the anterior elbow. The PTA manually stretches the left arm into the PNF D2 flexion pattern. Finally, even though the patient is right-handed, the PTA encourages the patient to use the left hand as

Information in Action (continued)

much as possible. The PTA places the patient's bedside tray on the left side of the bed so the patient has to reach for desired items.

Functional Mobility and Gait Training

The patient must be instructed in safe bed mobility and transfer practices as soon as he or she is medically stable. A patient with burns to the back, for example, should not push himself or herself up in bed, as the friction and shear forces may damage the wound. Proper execution of mobility activities will increase independence and enhance, rather than disrupt, the healing process. Gait training, with an assistive device as needed, is also initiated as soon as possible. Patients with lower extremity involvement should have compression garments or wraps applied to promote venous return and diminish edema formation.

Scar Management

Scar tissue takes anywhere from six months to two years to mature. Early in this process, the scar will be flat, soft, and pink and susceptible to injury. Later in the process, the scar may be white, raised, and hard. It may contract and restrict range of motion. Good scar management is essential to a cosmetic and functional outcome.

Skin Care

The basics of skin care are to wash, dry, and moisturize. Wash the skin with a nonperfumed, gentle soap. Hypoallergenic products are a good choice. The skin must be dried thoroughly to prevent maceration. Adding a moisturizer is important for all scar tissue, but especially after full-thickness burns, as this tissue will have lost the sebaceous, or oil, glands that normally keep skin supple. The moisturizer, like the soap, should be nonperfumed and have a low alcohol content. Applying it frequently throughout the day can prevent dryness and cracking and relieve pain and itching.

The patient should protect the scar from trauma by wearing clothing that is not restrictive and that does not chafe. For example, fleece or nylon exercise pants are preferred to denim jeans. Additionally, wearing long sleeves and pants (when outdoors) offers the skin protection from cuts, insect bites, and sunburn.

Pressure

Pressure applied to a developing scar while it is still pink can help prevent hypertrophic scarring and keloid formation. In general, burns that heal in less than two weeks could have pressure applied, but wounds that require longer healing must have pressure applied. Pressure can be applied using compression wraps, self-adherent wraps, tubular stockinette, or customized compression garments. A clear plastic mask applied firmly can be used for facial burns. Compression must be maintained at all times except during bathing until the scar remodeling is complete, which can be up to two years after wound closure. Patient compliance is generally less than 50%, so excellent patient education about the importance of pressure application is critical.

Scar Mobilization

Massage along the length of the scar can be done during range of motion exercises to lengthen connective tissue and prevent contractures. Friction massage applied perpendicularly to the scar fibers can loosen adhesions to underlying tissue, improving texture and pliability of the scar.

INFORMATION IN ACTION

A 34-year-old woman sustained a superficial partial-thickness burn to the right anterior thigh 12 weeks ago when she knocked a cup of scalding tea onto her lap. The PTA recommends a number of hypoallergenic lotion products to the patient for home use. The PTA teaches the woman how to massage the scar during lotion application as part of her normal daily skin care. Together, they discuss the importance of wearing the compression garment to prevent hypertrophic scarring.

Patient Education

Rehabilitation after a burn is a long, physically painful, and emotionally arduous process. The patient and the patient's family need to be educated from the start about the importance of the PT interventions to result in an optimal outcome. Healing will continue long after the patient is discharged home. The patient will need to be independent in a home exercise program, in skin care, in scar mobilization, and in application of his or her pressure garments.

Impact of Other Interventions on the Skin

A physical therapist assistant must always keep in mind the impact of other physical therapy interventions on the skin. Therapeutic massage, modalities, and the application of orthotic and prosthetic devices all affect the integumentary system.

Therapeutic Massage

The effects of massage on the skin are a consequence of the pressure that is applied to structures within the epidermis and dermis. Pressure on the vascular and lymphatic capillaries will increase arterial circulation and promote venous and lymphatic return. The effect of touch on the nerves is to diminish anxiety and decrease pain. Pressure on the mast cells promotes the release of histamine, giving the skin a pink appearance. The connective tissue responds to massage by becoming less stiff. Overall, after massage, the skin will be warm, pink, and more pliable.

Modalities

The effect of thermal modalities on the skin depends on the depth to which the heat or cold is able to penetrate the skin. Heat that penetrates to the dermis will create vasodilation, resulting in a pink appearance. It may also cause mild edema. Heating that exceeds normal body temperature locally will stimulate the release of perspiration. Excessive heat will cause a reddened area that does not blanch to pressure. Cold that penetrates to the dermis will create vasoconstriction, resulting in a pale appearance. The skin may appear red if the cold becomes excessive as blood flow increases in an attempt to warm the tissue. The skin may also appear red upon removal of the cold due to a histamine reaction. Excessive cold will cause a chalky white, frosted area.

Resistance at the electrode/skin interface during electrical stimulation creates heat, which may result in the skin looking pink after electrode removal. Excessive ionization can cause tissue hardening or softening under the electrodes, but that is unlikely, as use of direct current is rare except in cases of iontophoresis.

Orthotic and Prosthetic Devices

It is common for physical therapist assistants to apply and monitor orthotic and prosthetic devices for the lower extremities. PTAs often provide gait training to patients wearing orthoses or prostheses and must be able to assess if the devices are functioning appropriately. One critical area to assess is the impact of the device on the skin. Excessive pressure from a tight fit or friction and shear forces from a loose fit can cause skin breakdown. The skin must be examined frequently for reddened areas or blisters, as these can develop within minutes. The fit of a device may vary from one day to the next as the patient's edema fluctuates or if the patient wears different shoes.

Summary

Many physical therapy interventions are directed at preventing or managing open areas. One of the reasons that physical therapy is begun as soon as possible after surgery or illness is to prevent pressure sores from occurring due to immobility. Proper positioning, skin care, and footwear assessment are all done to prevent skin problems. PTs and PTAs provide education about wound prevention to those at high risk, including those with diabetes, circulatory problems, and sensory loss. If open wounds or burns are present, physical therapy interventions such as debridement, dressing application, exercise, and modalities are critical to speeding the healing process and obtaining wound closure.

Practice 4

1. Your patient has deep and superficial partial-thickness burns to the shoulder and axilla. What combination of positions would be most beneficial to prevent contractures?
   a. flexion, abduction, and external rotation
   b. flexion, adduction, and internal rotation
   c. extension, adduction, and internal rotation
   d. extension, abduction, and external rotation

2. Which of the following forms of debridement would be considered selective?
   a. whirlpool
   b. wet-to-dry dressings
   c. pulsed lavage
   d. autolytic debridement

3. Your patient has a venous ulcer on the left lower extremity that penetrates to the dermis. The wound bed is mostly healthy granulation tissue. The wound has a large amount of drainage. What would be the best combination of topical dressings?
   a. hydrogel with a semi-permeable film cover
   b. semi-permeable film alone
   c. wet-to-dry dressing
   d. calcium alginate with a semi-permeable foam cover

Practice 4 Answers

1. **a.** Adduction and internal rotation of the shoulder is a common deformity that develops. The patient should be positioned in the opposite motions to prevent contracture.

2. **d.** Autolytic debridement uses the body's own enzymes to break down necrotic tissue. The enzymes will attack only the necrotic tissue, not the healthy tissue. The other three choices are nonselective forms of debridement.

3. **d.** Calcium alginate with a semi-permeable foam cover will absorb a large amount of drainage. Choice **a** would add moisture, and choice **b** would not absorb moisture. Choice **c** may damage the wound bed.

Metabolic and Endocrine Systems

The metabolic and endocrine systems affect every aspect of the function of the body. The interventions provided by a physical therapist or physical therapist assistant can affect the metabolic and endocrine systems in a variety of ways. In addition, pathologies of the endocrine or metabolic systems may be a factor in why a patient or client is under the care of a PT and PTA. The skilled PTA must be aware of the effects of physical therapy interventions on these systems, both positive and negative.

Metabolic System

The metabolic system is affected by several factors. Many of these factors, which are identified in the following list, play a role in physical therapy intervention and must be recognized by the PTA.

- exercise
- age
- body composition
- levels of sex hormones
- temperature

Exercise and Age

Metabolism increases with increased physical activity and exercise. This is due to the contraction of skeletal muscles causing more energy expenditure. As the body uses energy, more must be produced by the metabolic system, which speeds up the metabolic rate. Age is another factor that affects metabolism. After the body stops growing, the body does not require as much energy, and the metabolic rate decreases over time. When working with clients of advanced age, the PTA must recognize the need for increased activity in order to raise the metabolic rate and maintain physical function.

TAKE NOTE

While regular and frequent exercise is beneficial to the body, it must be done in moderation. For most people, moderate exercise is not a problem. However, some adolescents and young adults engage in intense exercise for prolonged periods of time. This can be harmful to the body. When the body is subjected to chronic intense exercise, nonessential functions shut down so that nutrients and energy can be directed to the active muscle. An example of a nonessential function is reproduction.

Body Composition

Body composition can also affect the body's metabolic rate. Tall individuals have increased surface area compared to their body weight, which offers increased surface for heat to be lost. Therefore, metabolism is higher in these individuals in order to maintain body temperature. Interventions performed by PTs and PTAs cannot significantly affect height; however, activity that leads to weight loss can change the surface area to weight ratio and may affect overall metabolism.

Sex Hormone Levels

Sex hormones, such as testosterone, can have an effect on metabolism. Men tend to have a higher metabolism than women because of higher levels of testosterone and more muscle tissue. Muscle is an active tissue while adipose tissue is an inactive tissue. Women have more adipose tissue compared to men, and therefore have a lower metabolism. The interventions performed by PTs and PTAs cannot significantly affect sex hormone levels; however, activity can change the muscle-adipose ratio, leading to an increased overall metabolism.

Temperature

Both the temperature of a person's environment as well as the application of different temperatures to the skin can affect metabolism. Interventions performed by PTs and PTAs, such as thermal modalities, can affect an individual's metabolism. Metabolic rate decreases with the application of cold, such as an ice pack. With the application of heat to the skin, metabolism increases because the higher temperature stimulates chemical activity in the cells of the body. This phenomenon can be readily understood by examining the effect of heat and cold on food. Cooking facilitates rapid chemical changes in food. Putting food in the refridgerator or freezer preserves it by diminishing chemical activity. Aquatic therapy and whirlpool therapy can also affect the body's temperature and lead to an increase or decrease in metabolism depending on the temperature of the water.

Factors That Affect Metabolism

INCREASES METABOLISM	DECREASES METABOLISM
Application of heat to skin	Application of cold to the skin
Testosterone and increased muscle mass	Increasing age
Body composition (tall and thin individuals have higher metabolism)	Body composition (shorter individuals have lower metabolism)
Stress	Lower muscle to adipose tissue ratio

Endocrine System

Exercise is one of the factors that can have significant short- and long-term impacts on metabolism, resulting in a variety of changes in the endocrine system. When the body is active, fuel—from blood glucose, fatty acids, and glycogen from muscles—must be made available to provide energy to maintain muscle contraction. The liver supplies glucose used during exercise by glycogen breakdown and the process of gluconeogenesis.

TAKE NOTE

Gluconeogenesis is the formation of glucose by the liver or kidneys from noncarbohydrate substances, such as fats and proteins.

Fueling the Muscles

There are three primary providers of fuel to muscles during exercise—triglycerides, fatty acids, and glycogen. Exercise stimulates the breakdown of triglycerides, and this breakdown results in the release of fatty acids into the bloodstream. Fatty acids in the blood stream are then available to serve as fuel to exercising muscles. The glycogen found in muscles is an immediate source of glucose to use as fuel for active muscles.

TAKE NOTE

Athletes who perform intense exercise for prolonged periods of time, such as marathon runners, can deplete the body's glycogen stores. This can lead to the athlete being unable to continue intense exercise. This can be prevented by the process of carbohydrate loading—a process of preparing for long periods of intense exercise, beginning approximately one week before an event, via a period of consuming large amounts of carbohydrates.

Exercise and the Nervous System

Exercise also stimulates increased activity of the sympathetic nervous system, resulting in increased secretion of the hormone epinephrine. Secretion of cortisol by the adrenal glands and growth hormones by the pituitary gland also increase during exercise. The secretion of hormones by the pancreas is also affected by exercise. While it may seem that the body would increase the secretion of insulin during exercise in order to increase the transport of blood glucose into the cells, this is not true. During exercise, the secretion of insulin decreases while the secretion of glucagon increases. The presence of cortisol, growth hormone, and decreased presence of insulin all lead to decreased glucose uptake from skeletal muscle.

Active skeletal muscle must have glucose transported for use by another mechanism. Exercised muscles require more glucose than resting muscles. Exercising muscles contract, causing the migration of intracellular glucose transporters that bring glucose to the muscles. This process counters the fact that insulin levels decrease while exercising.

Below are some of the body processes and hormones that are affected by exercise:

- Glucose production by the liver increases.
- Breakdown of triglycerides increases.
- Fatty acid utilization increases.
- Secretion of epinephrine increases.
- Secretion of cortisol and growth hormone increases.
- Levels of glucagon increase.
- Secretion of insulin decreases.

Benefits of Exercise

Exercise decreases blood sugar due to the increased uptake of blood glucose by active skeletal muscle cells. As mentioned, exercise has the short-term effect of stimulating the intracellular glucose transporters. However, it also increases the body's insulin sensitivity and improves cellular glucose uptake while the body is at rest. Frequent and consistent exercise allows the body to see these short-term and long-term benefits.

Exercise can play a significant role in preventing diseases of the metabolic and endocrine systems. Diabetes mellitus is a common disease of the endocrine system. Because exercise has a direct effect on blood sugar, exercise can benefit those with diabetes as well as help prevent its onset. Obesity is a major contributor of insulin resistance—the primary cause of type II diabetes mellitus. Exercise increases the body's metabolism, which results in increased burning of calories. Therefore, exercise can help with the goal of weight loss. Exercise that leads to weight loss can help prevent diabetes and manage existing diabetes.

In addition, regular and frequent endurance exercises can increase insulin sensitivity regardless of whether or not there is accompanying weight loss. The increased utilization of glucose by the body during exercise as well as the long-term increased insulin sensitivity can help in the prevention and management of diabetes. Exercise can play a significant role in management of blood sugar levels in those with and without diabetes.

INFORMATION IN ACTION

When working with a client during endurance exercise, it is important to monitor blood sugar. A normal resting blood sugar is 80–100 mg/dL. If a client has low blood sugar prior to exercise, instruct the client to eat something. Clients may also experience low blood sugar during activity even if blood sugar levels were normal prior to exercise. Therefore, it is a good idea to always have some high carbohydrate foods available such as orange juice or sugar candies. If a client becomes lightheaded, dizzy, or short of breath, stop the exercise and check vital signs and blood sugar as appropriate.

The metabolic and endocrine systems are complex systems that control almost every function of the human body. These systems can be affected by many factors and some can be influenced by physical therapy interventions. It is important for the PTA to be aware of any metabolic or endocrine pathology present when working with a patient or client, as well as to recognize any adverse effects of these interventions to the individual.

Practice 5

1. Which of the following factors that affect metabolism relate most to PT intervention?
   a. age
   b. body composition
   c. levels of sex hormones
   d. temperature

Practice 5 Answer

1. d. Temperature is the factor most easily affected by such PT interventions as aquatic therapy or application of a cold pack.

Managing Multi-System Involvement

The following case studies introduce patients who are experiencing multi-system involvement. Each case demonstrates the possible interactions and effects of multiple systems on physical therapy intervention. The PTA must be aware of all systems involved and their possible role in treatment. With this awareness, despite the presence of multiple diagnoses, the PTA can provide appropriate and effective care to patients and positively impact the patient's functional mobility.

Multi-System Involvement: Case Study 1

A 78-year-old woman is admitted to a skilled nursing facility for a short-term rehab stay following an open-reduction internal-fixation (ORIF) for a left hip fracture. She sustained the fracture falling off a step stool in her kitchen. Her past medical history includes diabetes mellitus, hypertension, and chronic obstructive pulmonary disease. She takes insulin for diabetes, a beta blocker for hypertension, and is currently on two liters of oxygen via nasal cannula, although she did not require oxygen prior to admission. She has a weight-bearing limitation of 30# in the involved leg.

The PTA is going to see this patient today. The plan includes lower extremity strengthening exercises, transfer training, and gait training with a wheeled walker.

The Session

The PTA begins the session by checking to make sure that the portable oxygen tank is full and properly set. The PTA measures the patient's oxygen saturation using a pulse oximeter. The PTA also asks the patient when she last ate, whether or not her blood sugar has been tested that day, what the results were, and when she last had insulin. The patient reports normal blood sugars and that she had lunch 45 minutes prior to treatment. The PTA also reviews the weight-bearing status with the patient.

The PTA assists the patient in transferring to a mat and lying in a semi-supine position. The PTA positions the patient's head and trunk at a 45-degree angle using a wedge. The PTA begins with quad and gluteal sets and then moves into active-assisted hip abduction exercises. The patient is doing well with this exercise, and the PTA asks the patient to perform hip abduction and heel slides without assistance. The patient performs both exercises to fatigue with fewer than ten repetitions and is able to complete two sets of each. The PTA monitors the patient's oxygen saturation before and after therapeutic exercise with the patient's saturation remaining between 91 and 92%. The PTA then progresses the treatment to transfer training. The first transfer performed is supine-to-sit with reports of increased hip pain with movement. The patient denies any dizziness and says that she feels fine. She performs long arc quads and knee flexion, with yellow resistive bands, to fatigue with 12 repetitions each and two sets tolerated. Sit-to-stand training is then performed from the edge of the mat. Five repetitions of the transfer are performed before the patient fatigues and requires a rest break.

After the rest break, the patient performs standing left hip extension and hip flexion exercises (12 repetitions of each before fatiguing). The PTA reinstructs the patient on the weight-bearing status of 30# on the left lower extremity. The patient independently repeats the weight-bearing precaution to the PTA and states that she understands. Prior to initiating gait training, the patient complains of feeling lightheaded. The PTA checks blood sugar, blood pressure, and oxygen saturation, and all are within normal limits for this patient. The PTA suggests a rest break and talks to the patient about her grandchildren for five minutes while the patient rests. The patient feels better and agrees to proceed with gait training. She ambulates with a wheeled walker and is able to maintain correct weight-bearing for approximately 15 minutes of training before fatigue

prevents her from being able to maintain the weight-bearing status correctly. At this point, the PTA assesses the patient's overall condition, and the patient states that she is okay to continue pre-gait activities on the parallel bars for an additional 15 minutes. The PTA checks all vital signs at the end of treatment.

Case Study 1: Discussion

The PTA should begin by checking the status of the oxygen tank. Any equipment used by the patient should be assessed to make sure that it is in proper working order and that it is being administered properly. The PTA should never assume this has been done, even if it should have been performed by someone else. Oxygen saturation is an indication of the current physiological status of a person with COPD. For example, if the patient's oxygen saturation at rest is 93%, this indicates that the patient is doing fine at rest and should be able to tolerate mild to moderate exertion. If the patient's oxygen saturation was only 88% at rest, then the patient is already at the lower end of an acceptable level and will probably tolerate little activity.

Heart rate should not be used as an indicator of activity tolerance for this patient, because beta blockers would blunt the heart rate response, making it an unreliable measure. It is important to get a sense of whether or not the patient's blood sugar is within acceptable ranges. Many patients have a poor appetite after surgery, which may lead to decreased intake of food. If this leads to low blood sugar, then the patient may have poor activity tolerance, which can limit therapy.

If the patient is not reliable enough to check for this information herself, the PTA should check with the nursing staff for blood sugar levels prior to initiating the session. Finally, a review of the weight-bearing status is critical to protect the fracture repair.

Challenge without Fatigue

The patient is placed on a mat for the lower extremity exercises to allow optimal range of motion and muscle activation around the hip. The patient's head and trunk are elevated because a flat supine position can result in more labored breathing in a patient with COPD, as the abdominal contents push against the diaphragm.

The PTA instructs the patient in active-assisted exercise on the mat and should judge whether or not the patient is receiving appropriate assistance or resistance. Therapeutic exercise should be challenging without hurting or overly fatiguing the patient. The PTA feels that she was offering too much assistance and has the patient perform the exercises without resistance but in a gravity-neutral position. The patient is able to perform the exercises to fatigue in two sets. This is an appropriate strength training guideline for this patient. If the patient were able to perform 15 or more repetitions, then the PTA should realize that the patient would be performing endurance exercises. If increased strength is a goal for therapy, then the PTA must have the patient perform exercises that challenge his or her muscles by adding more resistance or, in this case, by decreasing the assistance provided.

The patient may have discomfort with these exercises, which is expected after surgery. The PTA should assess the patient's pain before, during, and after intervention in order to determine if the intervention is leading to a significant increase in the patient's pain. Without the pain rating at rest before beginning exercise, there is no way to compare if the patient's pain is increasing with activity. If there is a tolerable level of pain or discomfort in the patient's hip from surgery before treatment, this should not prevent therapy.

The PTA should ensure that the patient is not holding her breath during exercise and should continue to monitor the patient's oxygen saturations and rate of perceived exertion periodically throughout treatment, including during nonendurance type exercises, such as strengthening exercises. Rate of perceived exertion is a good alternative to heart rate monitoring with a patient who is taking a beta blocker.

Progression of Treatment

The PTA plans the progression of treatment well, taking advantage of the patient's position. When the patient has completed the supine exercises, the PTA takes advantage of the fact that the patient needs to transfer to sitting for seated exercise and uses that time to perform supine-to-sit training. When the patient completes the seated exercise and is moving on to standing exercise, the PTA uses that transition time to train sit-to-stand. While this may not be appropriate for all patients, it is a time management tool that is often overlooked.

After completing seated exercises and sit-to-stand training, the patient performs strengthening exercises in standing. The patient performs left hip exercises, but not right hip exercises due to the weight-bearing restriction on the left lower extremity. If there are no restrictions against this exercise, hip extension should not be overlooked because it is an important component of standing and walking, and it is often weak in sedentary patients. Because it is often difficult to have patients lying prone or side-lying for hip extension exercises, standing is a good alternative. The PTA should be sure that the extension motion is happening at the patient's hip and not at the trunk, pelvis, or knee.

Ensure Understanding

Prior to gait training, the PTA should verify that the patient understands the weight-bearing restriction. Simply telling the patient the restriction does not ensure that the patient understands. The PTA should have the patient independently verbalize or demonstrate the weight-bearing status. With the patient's report of light-headedness, vital signs should be checked, with appropriate action taken if vital signs are out of normal range. For example, if the patient's blood sugar is too low, then the patient needs to have something to eat. Blood sugar testing indicates the amount of sugar available to be used by the body as energy during exercise. During activity, the body uses the sugar in the blood efficiently. Without the introduction of additional sugar from food, this can lead to symptoms of low blood sugar, such as being lightheaded or dizzy. When the patient complains of lightheadedness, the PTA allows the patient to rest and talks to the patient about a topic other than therapy. After a short period of rest and focus on a positive conversation, the patient is able to continue gait training. It is important that the PTA allow for both physical and emotional breaks during intervention because anxiety and fear can affect other systems, such as the cardiopulmonary system, and can affect performance in therapy. This patient had surgery as a result of a fall and may have a lot of fear about standing and walking.

Once the patient is unable to maintain the correct weight-bearing status, the PTA should stop the activity. However, if the patient is able to continue other activities, pre-gait activities can be performed. Weight shifting, lower extremity advancement, and heel strike can be practiced in a more controlled setting, such as in the parallel bars with a scale to monitor weight-bearing.

Concluding Treatment

At the conclusion of the treatment, the PTA should check the patient's vital signs to ensure they are in normal ranges. The PTA should not assume that because the physical therapy treatment is over and the patient feels well, that the patient's blood sugar or other vital signs are within normal range. The patient may not be presenting with symptoms immediately, and it is a risk to the patient to be unaware of possible symptoms that may occur.

Multi-System Involvement: Case Study 2

A 69-year-old man presents to outpatient physical therapy with complaints of recent onset of fatigue, decreased endurance, increased freezing episodes, and difficulty standing up from his favorite chair. His past medical history includes a two-year history of Parkinson's disease, OA, left rotator cuff surgical repair approximately one year ago, coronary artery disease managed with medication, right knee replacement at age 49 secondary to an athletic injury, and asthma. The patient states that he was a smoker for the majority of his life and has had asthma as long as he can remember. The patient does not use oxygen at home, does not complain of shortness of breath, and states that his breathing does not limit his activity. The patient is on medication for Parkinson's disease and coronary artery disease.

The PTA reviews the medical records and physical therapy evaluation. The plan for the day includes transfer training, neuromuscular reeducation, endurance and gait training, and therapeutic exercise.

The Session

The PTA begins the session by checking the patient's vital signs while the patient rests. The patient's heart rate is 68 beats per minutes, his respiratory rate is 18 breaths per minute, his oxygen saturation is 96 %, and his blood pressure is 116/75. The patient reports that these are normal for him. The PTA explains the rate of perceived exertion scale to the patient and ensures understanding. The PTA then proceeds to gait activities with a focus on creating strategies to decrease freezing episodes. The PTA uses a metronome during gait training to encourage regular cadence, and step indicators on the floor to encourage good step length. The PTA instructs the patient on verbal and visual cues that he can use at home to prevent freezing. The PTA also lets the patient know that rocking back on his heels during a freezing episode can assist with step initiation. The patient practices this technique and reports pain in his left knee, which prevents him from performing the technique safely.

The patient then participates in gait activities for 15 minutes at a time and requires seated rest breaks between episodes. The PTA monitors the patient's rate of perceived exertion throughout the treatment, and it remains within an acceptable range. The patient's respiratory rate with activity is 28 breaths per minute.

The PTA also monitors the patient's oxygen saturation throughout the treatment, due to the patient's respiratory history.

After gait training, the PTA proceeds to transfer training, specifically sit-to-stand transfers. The PTA focuses on sit-to-stand from chairs of various heights. The patient is able to stand from chairs that are 18 and 20 inches with standby assistance, no use of the upper extremities, and no difficulty with initiation. As the chair height decreases below 18 inches, the patient relies significantly on his arms in order to stand. The PTA begins training with verbal cues to aid in initiation of standing. The patient is grimacing, and he states that his left knee hurts when he stands and that this is why he cannot stand from low chairs. The PTA stops the transfer training due to pain.

Next, the patient performs lower extremity strengthening activities. The PTA determines the patient's one repetition maximum and has the patient exercise at 60% of his one repetition maximum with good tolerance. The patient reports no pain with strengthening activities.

Case Study 2: Discussion

This patient presents with multiple pathologies that are playing a role in his physical therapy treatment session. The PTA begins by monitoring the patient's vital signs with focus on the patient's diagnoses of coronary artery disease and asthma. The rate of perceived exertion scale is used with this patient because of the patient's use of cardiac medications. These medications may blunt the heart rate response to exercise, leading to an inaccurate heart rate reading. However, the PTA does monitor his heart rate prior to activity in order to determine if his resting heart rate is in an acceptable range for exercise. The PTA also has the patient rate his perceived exertion before activity in order to ensure that the patient understands the scale, as well as to have a baseline number to which to compare the patient's exertion during activity.

The patient participates in gait training activities with no signs or symptoms of distress, with the PTA allowing adequate rest breaks during treatment. Vital signs and perceived exertion are monitored with no noted adverse reactions. As the patient's knee pain, perhaps due to OA, is preventing him from performing certain techniques, the PTA must find other techniques for this patient until the patient's pain is no longer limiting. The patient's pain decreases when the activity stops and does not appear to be interfering with his overall function.

Monitoring Treatment

The treatment session moves on to sit-to-stand training. The PTA is instructing the patient on verbal cues to assist with initiation of standing, which is often a problem for patients with Parkinson's disease. The patient appears to be doing well with the initiation techniques in the higher chairs, but the patient is unable to stand from lower chairs. The PTA monitors the patient's reaction to treatment and is aware of body language. The patient's grimace is a sign that he is in pain. Upon further questioning, the PTA realizes that the patient is not having difficulty with initiation; it is the pain in the patient's knee that is preventing him from standing independently. It is important that the PTA's focus on the effects of Parkinson's disease does not result in decreased awareness of the possibility that other systems are playing a part in the patient's decreased function.

The PTA moves on to strengthening exercises and appropriately uses the patient's one repetition maximum to guide strength training for optimal gains. The PTA should not simply stop all activities related to transfer training because of pain. Strengthening of the lower extremities is a step that can be taken to help decrease knee pain while also increasing strength for transfers.

Reassess

After strengthening exercises, the PTA can readdress transfers and assess pain. If the patient's pain continues to be a problem, then the PTA will need to refer back to the physical therapist and see if the addition of pain management interventions is appropriate for this patient's plan of care.

Practice 6

1. Identify one advantage of using rate of perceived exertion rather than heart rate to monitor an individual's activity tolerance.
   a. Rate of perceived exertion is a more accurate indicator of activity tolerance.
   b. Rate of perceived exertion is a good alternative when medications interfere with heart rate.
   c. Rate of perceived exertion is easier for the patient to understand.
   d. Rate of perceived exertion is easier for the PTA to administer.

2. A PTA is working with a patient who states he has not had anything to eat for a few hours prior to therapy. The PTA should
   a. continue with the therapy session because the patient should not eat immediately before therapy.
   b. instruct the patient to take insulin before beginning activity in order to maintain blood sugar levels.
   c. recommend that the patient not participate in physical therapy and tell him that he needs to eat.
   d. check the patient's blood sugar levels prior to determining whether or not activity is appropriate.

3. A PTA is working with a patient with a diagnosis of osteoarthritis during his first physical therapy session. The patient is being seen for generalized deconditioning following a hospitalization for pneumonia, and the physical therapy plan of care includes therapeutic exercise, gait training, therapeutic activity, and neuromuscular reeducation. During gait training, the patient reports knee pain that increases with activity. The PTA should
   a. stop all gait-related activities and refer the patient back to the supervising physical therapist.
   b. place a hot pack on the patient's knee and resume gait training when the pain has decreased.
   c. stop the activity that causes pain and determine whether or not any other gait-related activities are tolerated.
   d. end the session for the day and schedule a makeup treatment session when pain is gone.

Practice 6 Answers

1. **b.** One advantage of using rate of perceived exertion rather than heart rate to monitor an individual's activity tolerance is that rate of perceived exertion is a good alternative when medications interfere with a patient's heart rate. Many medications, most commonly cardiac medications, can blunt a patient's heart rate response to exercise.

2. d. Before making a judgment about the patient's ability to participate in therapy, the patient's blood sugar should be checked. The patient may be experiencing extremely low blood sugar and may need to address it regardless of whether or not he is going to exercise. Or, the patient's blood sugar may be normal. Because blood sugar levels are anticipated to decrease with exercise, the PTA can have a sugar source available for the patient in this situation, or the patient can have something to eat and return to therapy later.

3. c. When the patient reports increased pain with gait training, it is an indication to stop that activity. Given the patient's diagnosis of osteoarthritis, pain with gait is not a significant adverse reaction. Therefore, the PTA should stop the aggravating activity and find a gait-related or other activity that does not cause increased pain.

Adaptive, Orthotic, and Prosthetic Equipment

Because physical therapist assistants work with patients with all manner of problems and impairments, the PTA will often find that the patient is using, or would benefit from using, some form of equipment. For example, a patient with hemiplegia following a CVA may need a rocker knife to cut food independently or an ankle foot orthosis to improve gait. Someone who has had a hip replacement must use a raised toilet seat to prevent dislocation of the replacement. Also, many patients utilize a prosthesis following an amputation. The PTA must be able to suggest appropriate equipment to the PT, monitor the effectiveness of the equipment, and ensure safety and fit of any device used by the patient.

Levels of Lower Extremity Amputation

TYPE OF AMPUTATION	LOCATION
Transmetatarsal	Through the shaft of the metatarsals
Lisfranc	Disarticulation at the tarsometatarsal joint
Chopart	Disarticulation at the transverse tarsal joint
Symes	Disarticulation at ankle joint
Transtibial (below knee) (BK)	Through the shaft of the tibia and fibula
Transfemoral (above knee) (AK)	Through the shaft of the femur
Hip disarticulation	Disarticulation of head of femur from pelvis
Hemipelvectomy	Removal of all or part of the ilium

The surgical goal for lower extremity amputation is generally to preserve all possible joints and the greatest bone length distal to the last preserved joint.

Residual Limb Care and Pre-Prosthetic Management

RESIDUAL LIMB CARE	PRE-PROSTHETIC MANAGEMENT
Edema control and shaping • rigid dressing • semi-rigid dressing • elastic bandage wrap • shrinker socks • intermittent compression pumping	Positioning to prevent contractures • BK: knee extension; hip extension • AK: hip extension; hip adduction
Skin care	Strengthening and conditioning General UE strengthening BK: hip extensors; hip abductors; knee extensors AK: hip extensors; hip abductors Aerobic conditioning
Scar massage	Bed mobility training
Desensitization activities	Transfer training
	Gait training with assistive device
	Patient education • residual limb care • positioning • risk factor management • exercise program • emotional adjustment

Physical therapy prepares the residual limb to fit into a prosthesis and develops the patient's range of motion, strength, endurance, and functional mobility so that he or she can eventually use the prosthesis effectively and efficiently.

Components of Lower Extremity Prostheses

Foot-ankle assembly	Non-articulated Solid ankle cushion heel (SACH) Stationary attachment flexible endoskeleton (SAFE) Dynamic response foot (e.g., Seattle foot™; Flex-Foot™) Articulated Single axis in sagittal plane Multi-axis
Shank	Endoskeleton Exoskeleton
Below-knee socket	Patellar tendon bearing (PTB)
Knee mechanism	Sliding friction mechanism Fluid friction mechanism Pneumatic cylinder Hydraulic cylinder Microchip controlled hydraulic cylinder

Above-knee socket	Quadrilateral
	    Ischial containment (contoured adducted
	    trochanter-controlled alignment method: CATCAM)

Suspension	BK only: supracondylar wedge Suction Neoprene or silicon sleeve Interlocking pin mechanism Belt

Selection of the appropriate prosthetic components depends upon many factors, including but not limited to the patient's strength, functional abilities and goals, and resources. The PT and PTA may work with the prosthetist and patient in selecting or modifying these components.

Ultimate functional ability with a prosthesis will depend upon the patient's overall physiological status, strength, flexibility, endurance, interests, and motivation. Elements of lower extremity prosthetic training are as follows:

- donning and doffing the prosthesis
- transfer training
- gait training
  - weight shifting onto the prosthesis
  - knee control during stance (esp. AK)
  - knee control during swing (esp. AK)
- balance and coordination
- stair-climbing
- running
- driving
- sports activities
  - running
  - swimming
  - biking
  - skiing

Orthoses for the Lower Extremity

TYPE OF ORTHOSIS	COMMON USES
Shoe inserts • longitudinal arch support • metatarsal pad • heel pad	Flexible flat foot Diabetic (Charcot) foot Arthritis
Shoe modification • heel wedge • metatarsal bar • rocker bar • shoe lift	Calcaneal inversion or eversion Diabetic (Charcot) foot Arthritis Leg length discrepancy
Ankle-foot orthosis (AFO)	Dorsiflexion weakness or paralysis Plantar flexion weakness or paralysis Excessive foot varus Foot/ankle hypertonicity
Knee-ankle-foot orthosis (KAFO)	LE paralysis Knee varus or valgus deformity
Hip-knee-ankle-foot orthosis (HKAFO)	LE paralysis
Trunk-hip-knee-ankle-foot orthosis (THKAFO)	Trunk and LE paralysis

Orthoses are named for the joints they cross and are used to provide support, stability, and alignment to those joints.

Orthoses are often used for the spine, and there are many different types used for this purpose. Spinal orthoses vary in the degree to which they limit motion at various spinal segments.

Orthoses for the Spine

TYPE OF ORTHOSIS	COMMON USES
Lumbosacral corset	Low back pain
Knight-Taylor brace	Limits trunk flexion, extension, lateral bending
Cruciform anterior spinal hyperextension (CASH) brace	Limits lower trunk flexion and extension
Jewett® hyperextension brace	Limits lower trunk flexion and extension
Custom thoracolumbosacral orthosis (TLSO)	Limits all trunk motions
Custom lumbosacral orthosis (LSO)	Low back pain
Milwaukee brace	Thoracolumbar scoliosis
Boston brace	Thoracolumbar scoliosis
Wilmington brace	Thoracolumbar scoliosis
Charleston bending brace	Thoracolumbar scoliosis
Soft cervical collar	Relieves muscle spasm and decreases full cervical ROM
Hard cervical collar	Relieves muscle spasm and limits cervical ROM more than soft collar
Short Philadelphia collar	Limits two-thirds cervical flexion, extension and rotation ROM, limits one-third cervical lateral flexion ROM
Long Philadelphia collar	Restricts cervical ROM in all planes
Four-poster brace	Restricts cervical motion in all planes
Halo brace	Most restriction of cervical motion in all planes

Spinal orthoses vary in the degree of motion limitation at various spinal segments.

Elements of Orthotic Assessment

Static fit
- alignment of orthosis with appropriate joints or landmarks while at rest
- skin inspection after wearing device

Dynamic fit
- alignment of orthosis during functional activities
- effectiveness of orthosis during functional activities
- identification of gait abnormalities caused by lower extremity orthosis
- skin inspection after using device

- Patient can don/doff brace with or without assistance

The safe and effective function of the orthosis must be assessed with the person at rest, as well as during all appropriate functional activities.

Adaptive Devices and Their Functions

Raised toilet seat	Easier getting up and down from toilet
Tub transfer bench	Ability to sit while showering
Hand-held shower attachment	Better control of water when showering while seated
Long-handled sponge	Ability to bathe lower extremities or posterior trunk
Rocker knife	Enable one-handed cutting of food
Plate guard	Prevent food from sliding off plate
Built-up handles on eating utensils, grooming items, writing utensils	Easier to hold; joint protection
Universal cuff	Holds eating or writing utensils for those with poor grip
Long-handled reacher	Retrieves items from floor or shelf

A great variety of adaptive devices exists to assist patients in performing ADLs and IADLs.

Practice 7

1. A patient has an amputation in which the talus is disarticulated from the tibia and fibula and the heel pad is attached to the end of the tibia. What is this patient's amputation classified as?
   a. Chopart amputation
   b. Lisfranc amputation
   c. Symes amputation
   d. transtibial amputation

2. A patient underwent an amputation in which the right lower extremity and pelvis were removed. What is this amputation classified as?
   a. hemicorporectomy
   b. hemipelvectomy
   c. hip disarticulation
   d. short transfemoral amputation

3. A patient who underwent a right transtibial amputation has a shrinker sock applied to his residual limb. What is the key purpose of a shrinker sock?
   a. to prevent skin breakdown
   b. to diminish edema
   c. to prevent skin contracture
   d. to desensitize the residual limb

4. A PTA is treating a patient with a left transtibial amputation. In an attempt to prevent contractures, the PTA should instruct the patient to position his hip in _____ and his knee in _____.
   a. extension; extension
   b. extension; flexion
   c. flexion; extension
   d. flexion; flexion

5. Which of the following choices is an example of an articulated prosthetic foot?
   a. Flex-Foot
   b. multiple-axis foot
   c. solid ankle cushion foot
   d. stationary attachment flexible endoskeleton foot

6. In which of the following types of amputation is a quadrilateral socket in a prosthetic appropriate?
   a. ankle disarticulation
   b. Symes
   c. transfemoral
   d. transtibial

7. Which of the following choices would be the next appropriate functional activity progression, following dynamic balance exercises, for a patient with a left below-knee amputation as part of her prosthetic training?
   a. donning and doffing the prosthetic
   b. gait training
   c. stairs, ramps, and curb training
   d. transfer training from bed to wheelchair

8. Which type of shoe insert or modification is appropriate for an individual with a leg-length discrepancy greater than one-half inch?
   a. heel wedge
   b. metatarsal bar
   c. rocker bar
   d. shoe lift

9. Which type of cervical orthosis below provides the maximum control of cervical motions?
   a. four-post brace
   b. halo brace
   c. hard cervical collar
   d. short Philadelphia collar

10. Which spine orthosis is NOT used to treat thoracolumbar scoliosis?
    a. Boston brace
    b. Knight-Taylor brace
    c. Milwaukee brace
    d. Wilmington brace

11. Which of the following activities is an element of a static assessment of an orthosis?
    a. assessing ground clearance of the foot during gait
    b. identifying delayed weight transfer from one extremity to the other while ambulating
    c. inspecting the skin after removing the orthosis
    d. observing for foot slap

12. Which of the following choices is part of an orthotic functional assessment for a patient with an orthosis?
    a. assessing the patient's ability to don and doff the orthosis
    b. identifying any areas of redness on the skin after removing the orthosis
    c. manual muscle testing the knee extensors
    d. measuring the patient's active range of motion of the knee

13. Which of the following is NOT a feature seen on a tub transfer bench?
    a. adjustable height legs
    b. back rest
    c. wheels on the bottom of the legs
    d. wide base of support of legs

14. Rocker knives, plate guards, and universal cuffs are all adaptive devices that assist with which of the following activities that a patient may perform at home?
    a. dressing and undressing
    b. house cleaning
    c. laundry
    d. meal preparation

Practice 7 Answers

1. c. A patient who has an amputation in which the ankle is removed and the heel pad is attached to the end of the tibia has had a Symes amputation. A Lisfranc amputation is a disarticulation at the tarsometatarsal joint. A transtibial amputation runs through the shafts of the tibia and fibula. A Chopart amputation is a disarticulation at the transverse tarsal joint.

2. b. An amputation in which the right lower extremity and pelvis were removed is classified as a hemipelvectomy. A hemicorporectomy amputation involves both lower extremities and the pelvis below the L4–L5 level. A hip disarticulation involves the removal of the entire femur and hip joint. A short transfemoral amputation is an above-knee amputation that occurs through the shaft of the femur.

3. b. An Unna's dressing is classified as a semi-rigid dressing. Rigid dressings are hard. Unna's boot is not hard. Shrinkers are cotton garments reinforced with rubber and resemble a large sock. A compression/elastic wrap is an example of a soft dressing.

4. a. The PTA should instruct the patient to position his hip and knee in extension. Hip and knee flexion contractures are common contractures for a patient with a below-knee amputation.

5. b. The multiple-axis foot is an example of an articulated prosthetic foot. The Flex-Foot, solid ankle cushion foot, and stationary attachment flexible endoskeleton foot foot are all examples of non-articulated prosthetic feet.

6. c. The quadrilateral socket is used in prostheses for above-knee amputations.

7. c. The next appropriate functional activity progression following dynamic balance exercises for a patient with a left below-knee amputation as part of her prosthetic training would be stairs, ramps, and curb training. Donning and doffing of the prosthesis and transfer training from bed to wheelchair are usually performed early in a treatment protocol. Stairs, ramps, and curb training begins after the patient is safe with ambulation and requires dynamic balance skills.

8. d. A shoe lift (also called a shoe insert) is an appropriate modification for an individual with a leg-length discrepancy greater than one-half inch. A heel wedge is used to alter the alignment of the calcaneous. A metatarsal bar and rocker bar are used to transfer stress from the metatarsal shafts to the metatarsal heads.

9. b. The halo brace provides maximal control of cervical motions because the superior band is fixated into the cranium and also connects inferiorly to a thoracic orthosis. Hard cervical collars provide minimal control of motion. The four-post brace provides moderate control.

10. b. The Knight-Taylor brace is not used to treat thoracolumbar scoliosis; it is used to limit trunk flexion, extension, and lateral bending. The Boston brace, the Milwaukee brace, and the Wilmington brace are used to treat thoracolumbar scoliosis.

11. c. Inspecting the skin is a static assessment of an orthosis. Assessing ground clearance, identifying weight transfer between extremities, and foot slap are assessed while the patient is performing a dynamic activity.

12. a. Assessing the patient's ability to don and doff the orthosis is an orthotic functional assessment for the patient. Skin assessment, manual muscle testing, and measuring range of motion are all objective measurements.

13. c. A tub transfer bench would not have wheels on the bottom of the legs. A transfer bench should not be easily movable once a patient is on it. Therefore, having wheels on the bottom of the legs of the bench is not appropriate. Adjustable height legs, backrest, and a wide base of support all contribute to safety with patient transfers.

14. d. Rocker knives, plate guards, and universal cuffs are adaptive devices that assist with meal preparation.

Therapeutic Modalities

Therapeutic modalities, or physical agents, are forms of treatment that cause physiological effects on the body. This section reviews the types of physical agents used in patient care. Descriptions, effects on the body, indications, contraindications, precautions for use, and procedures are presented.

Modalities consist of energy and materials that are applied to patients in order to facilitate the healing or inflammatory process and include the use of cold, heat, water, pressure, sound, electromagnetic radiation, and electrical current. More specifically, therapeutic modalities are placed into three categories—thermal, mechanical, and electromagnetic. Thermal modalities consist of deep heating agents (such as ultrasound and diathermy), superficial heating agents (such as hot pack), and cooling agents (such as ice pack). Mechanical modalities are made up of traction (such as mechanical traction), compression (such as intermittent compression pumps), water (whirlpool), and sound (ultrasound). Electromagnetic physical agents consist of electromagnetic fields (ultraviolet) and electrical currents (transcutaneous electrical nerve stimulation: TENS).

The purposes of using modalities are to decrease pain and to allow the patient to begin therapeutic exercise. Modalities accomplish this by decreasing the various types of pain (acute, chronic, referred, and spinal radicular), decreasing motion restrictions, changing tone abnormalities, and muscle reeducation.

Inflammation and Healing

Inflammation and the healing process are broken down into three phases—inflammatory-response (acute stage), fibroplastic-repair (subacute stage), and maturation-modeling (chronic stage). These three phases will occur in order but overlap during the sequence.

Healing Time

Factors that determine the length of time of inflammation are the specific tissue that is damaged, the severity of damage to the tissue, and the overall health of the patient. The inflammatory-response phase lasts approximately four to six days. At this time, there is vasodilation, an increase in capillary permeability, a growth of new capillaries, and the formation of a clot. During this time, a patient will exhibit the classic signs of acute inflammation—swelling, redness, pain, heat, and loss of function. In this phase, modalities are used to decrease pain, break the pain-spasm cycle, and progress the inflammatory process. The fibroplastic-repair stage lasts about 10 to 17 days. At this time, a scar begins to form and the clot begins to resolve. In addition, the signs and symptoms of acute inflammation are decreased. However, the patient may have pain at the end ranges of the available range of motion or develop shortening of soft tissue that can lead to motion restrictions. For this phase, modalities are used to promote collagen formation and progress the healing process. The maturation-remodeling stage of inflammation is a long-term process (up to one year). In this stage, there is a realignment of the collagen fibers. There should be no signs of inflammation, but the patient may continue to have decreased strength and/or range of motion. Modalities in this stage are used to improve the alignment of new collagen fibers.

Phases of Healing, Treatment Goals, and Effective Modalities

STAGE OF HEALING	TREATMENT GOALS	EFFECTIVE MODALITY
Inflammatory-response	Prevent further injury Control pain Control edema	Compression Cryotherapy Hydrotherapy (nonthermal only) Ultrasound (nonthermal only) Shortwave diathermy (nonthermal only) Electrical stimulation for pain relief
Fibroplastic-repair	Prevent stiffness Control pain Increase circulation Facilitate healing progress	Superficial heat Neuromuscular electrical stimulation Whirlpool Compression Ultrasound Shortwave diathermy
Maturation-remodeling	Increase strength Increase flexibility Control scar tissue formation	Neuromuscular electrical stimulation Superficial or deep heat Ice massage Compression

The stage of healing of a soft tissue injury must be determined in order to choose an appropriate modality and apply it effectively.

Modes of Heat Transfer

The transfer of heat can occur in several ways:

Conduction. With conduction, the transfer of heat takes place when there is direct contact between materials of different temperatures. Heat transfers from the warmer substance to the cooler one. Examples of modalities that transfer heat through conduction are hot packs and cold packs.

Convection. Heat is transferred through convection when there is direct contact between two substances of different temperatures and one of the substances circulates around the other. Whirlpool is an example of a therapeutic modality that uses convection as its mode of heat transfer.

Conversion. Conversion uses a nonthermal form of energy (such as electricity) and transforms it to heat. The transfer of heat depends on the amount of power generated, not the temperature of the modality. Examples of modalities that use conversion as their mode of heat transfer are ultrasound and shortwave diathermy.

Radiation. Heat transfer through radiation occurs when energy of one material with a higher temperature is transferred to one of a lower temperature without the need of direct contact or a medium (gel). The amount of heat transfer is dependent on the distance between the two substances, the intensity of the heat source, and the angle of incidence of the radiation. An example of a modality that uses radiation as its mode of heat transfer is infrared.

Evaporation. Vapocoolant sprays are an example of a physical agent that uses evaporation as a mode of heat transfer. The spray (liquid) absorbs the heat energy from the skin. The liquid is then changed to a gas and evaporates. This evaporation then cools the skin.

Physiological Effects of Superficial Heat

Following are the effects of superficial heat on the body:

- vasodilation
- increased nerve conduction velocity
- decreased sympathetic activity
- increased metabolism
- increased collagen extensibility
- sedated nerve endings

Indications

The following are the indicators for superficial heat application to the body:

- soft tissue restrictions
- preheating prior to exercise and passive stretching
- preheating prior to traction and soft tissue mobilization
- pain
- muscle spasms
- joint stiffness
- promotes relaxation
- promotes healing (after acute stage of inflammation)

Contraindications

The following are the contraindications for superficial heat application to the body:

- acute injuries and inflammation
- potential thrombophlebitis
- patients with impaired sensation
- patients with cognitive deficits
- areas of malignancy
- active bleeding
- fever
- patients with impaired thermoregulation (very young or elderly)

Precautions

Precautions must be taken in the following cases when using superficial heat on the body:

- individuals with cardiac insufficiency
- over abdomen and low back of pregnant women
- impaired circulation
- peripheral vascular disease
- edema
- superficial implanted metal
- over open wounds

Hot Packs

Hot packs are stored in a hydrocollator in water that is maintained at 158°F to 170°F. The position of the patient determines the number of layers of towels used during treatment. Treatment time for hot packs can range from 10 to 30 minutes. The advantage for using hot packs over other superficial heat modalities is that they are relatively safe because the temperature of the pack decreases as the treatment time progresses, thus decreasing the chances of burns to the patient. They are effective at treating local areas, and the treatment site is easily accessible during treatment. One disadvantage of hot packs is that the weight of the hot pack can be too heavy to place on a patient. In addition, the involved area is not visible during treatment, and there is a risk of infection when a hot pack is placed on an open wound.

Patient Setup

In applying hot packs, the PTA follows these procedures:

1. Inspect the treatment area and remove any jewelry.
2. Check to see if the temperature of the hydrocollator is between 158°F and 170°F.
3. Wrap the hot pack in six to eight layers of towels.
4. Explain the procedure to the patient regarding the purpose of the treatment and explain what the patient should feel during treatment. The

patient should notify the PTA if the hot pack becomes too warm.

5. Place the hot pack on the treatment area and secure it.

6. Give the patient a bell to ring if the hot pack becomes too warm.

7. After five minutes of treatment, inspect the treatment area and ask the patient how the hot pack feels.

8. After the treatment is complete (about 10 to 30 minutes), remove the hot pack, inspect the treatment area (it should be slightly red and warm to the touch), and document the treatment.

Paraffin Bath

Paraffin bath is a form of superficial heat that consists of wax that is melted and mixed with mineral oil. The wax has a safe and low specific heat, which allows it to be applied directly to a patient's skin. Paraffin treatment is typically used on the distal extremities (hands and feet) because it allows for easy contact with the contours of the small joints. Disadvantages of paraffin include:

- The temperature of the wax may be too high for many patients.
- The patient's movement must be minimized during treatment so that the wax does not crack.
- It is not appropriate for open wounds.

The PTA follows specific procedures when utilizing the paraffin bath intervention.

Patient Setup

When setting up the paraffin bath, the PTA should follow these procedures:

1. Check to see if the temperature of the paraffin bath is between 125°F and 127°F.

2. Remove jewelry, clean and dry the skin, and inspect the treatment area.

3. Have the patient relax the hands, keeping the fingers slightly parted.

4. Dip the entire hand in the bath, instructing the patient not to touch the bottom and sides of the bath.

5. Remove the hand and allow the wax to stop dripping.

6. Repeat this step six to ten times.

7. Wrap the patient's hand in a plastic bag and towel.

8. Elevate the body part.

9. Allow treatment time of 10 to 20 minutes.

10. After treatment, remove the towel and plastic bag, and discard the wax.

11. Inspect the treatment site (should be warm, slightly red, and smooth), and document the treatment.

Fluidotherapy

Fluidotherapy is a dry heat modality that transfers heat by convection. Warm air is circulated through an organic granular material (e.g., ground corn cobs) contained within a small machine. There are openings through which the distal extremities may be placed. Advantages for this modality are that the patient can move during the treatment. Also, the temperature of the treatment can be precisely set and remains constant throughout the session and can be used for desensitization of hypersensitive areas. In addition to the potential of being messy, other disadvantages are that the body part is not visible during treatment and that proximal extremities and trunk are very difficult to treat using this method.

Patient Setup

The PTA follows specific procedures when utilizing fluidotherapy interventions:

1. Remove jewelry and clothing from the treatment area.

2. Inspect the treatment area.

3. Cover any open wounds.

4. Explain the treatment procedure to the patient.

5. Place the body part in the unit.

6. Secure the sleeve so that no particles fall from the unit.

7. Set the unit for the desired temperature (105°F to 125°F).

8. Adjust the fan speed according to the patient's comfort level.

9. If desired, instruct the patient to exercise during treatment.

10. Set a timer for the prescribed treatment time (15 to 20 minutes).

11. After treatment, remove, clean, and inspect the body part.

12. Document the treatment.

Infrared Treatment

Infrared is a superficial heat that is transmitted by a luminous (lamp) or nonluminous (wires) source. The effects of infrared treatment on the body include:

- increased local metabolism
- muscle relaxation
- sensory nerve-ending sedation
- increased core temperature if applied long enough
- increased capillary pressure and cell permeability

Advantages of infrared treatment are that the body part is visible during treatment and that there is no contact between the patient and the lamp, which decreases the chances of a possible infection. Disadvantages of infrared treatment include the fact that it is difficult to treat a local area using this method. In addition, the body part being treated using this method must be treated in a dependent position, and if a luminous lamp is used, then the light can irritate a patient's eyes.

The most common indication for infrared is to treat subacute and chronic inflammatory conditions.

Other indications may be to dry moist wounds and increase perspiration to enhance conductivity during electrical stimulation treatment.

Patient Setup

The PTA follows specific procedures when utilizing infrared interventions:

1. Instruct the patient about the modality, the procedure, and his or her responsibilities during treatment.

2. Instruct the patient to remove any clothing and jewelry near the treatment site.

3. Position the patient appropriately, and drape the patient so that only the treatment area is exposed.

4. Assess the patient's integrity to differentiate temperature differences.

5. Try to position the lamp so that it is perpendicular to the treatment area (cosine law) and at the recommended distance from the patient (inverse square law).

6. Set treatment time for 15 to 30 minutes.

7. Assess the patient throughout treatment.

8. Turn off the machine, assess the patient's skin, and evaluate his or her response to the treatment.

Superficial Cold

When a patient receives superficial cold as a treatment, the individual will experience four stages—intense cold, burning, aching, and numbness. Physiological effects of superficial cold include:

- vasoconstriction
- decreased nerve conduction velocity
- increased pain threshold
- decreased spasticity
- decreased metabolism
- decreased edema

Indications

Indications for superficial cold include:

- inflammation control
- pain control
- edema control
- spasticity
- acute and chronic pain and inflammatory conditions
- muscle facilitation
- deep friction massage, joint mobilization, and strenuous exercise

Contraindications

Contraindications for superficial cold include:

- insensitivity to cold
- intolerance to cold
- Raynaud's disease
- anesthetic skin
- regenerating peripheral nerves
- decreased circulation
- cardiac dysfunction and angina pectoris
- arterial insufficiency

Precautions

When using superficial cold interventions, precautions should be taken in the following cases:

- open wounds
- hypertension
- patients with impaired thermoregulation (very young and elderly)
- patients with impaired cognitive function

Gel Packs

Commercial gel packs are semi-solid packs that are kept at 0°F to 5°F and used for treatment. Some of the advantages of using gel packs include providing good contour to the treatment area, availability in a variety of sizes and shapes, reusability, and being tolerated generally well by patients. The disadvantages of using gel packs include the weight of the pack being too heavy for some patients, lag time to re-cool the packs, and the treatment area not being visible during application.

Patient Setup

The PTA follows specific procedures when utilizing gel pack interventions:

1. Explain the treatment procedure to the patient.
2. Position and drape the patient appropriately.
3. Cover the treatment areas with a damp towel, place the ice pack on the damp towel, and secure it if needed.
4. Set treatment time for 10 to 20 minutes.
5. Remove the ice pack, dry area, and inspect the skin.
6. Document the treatment.

Ice Massage

Ice massage uses a large cube of ice that is applied directly to the skin, usually moved in a small, circular motion. Advantages of using ice massage over other methods of cryotherapy include that it cools the body part being treated quickly, that the treatment areas are visible, that it is a cost-effective, readily available treatment, and that it is effective for treating small areas. Disadvantages of using ice massage are that the very cold temperature may not be well tolerated by the patient and large body parts are difficult to treat using this method.

Patient Setup

The PTA follows specific procedures when utilizing ice massage interventions:

1. Describe the treatment process (including the cooling process) and expectations with the patient, and make sure that the patient understands his or her responsibilities during treatment.
2. Position and drape the patient appropriately. Remember to use extra towels because of the dripping of the melting ice.
3. Expose the ice from its container and apply it to the body part in a small, circular pattern.
4. Continue the treatment until the patient reports numbness or is unable to tolerate the treatment. This usually takes approximately five to ten minutes.
5. Dry the skin and inspect the skin's response to treatment.
6. Document the treatment.

Cold Immersion Baths

Cold immersion baths entail immersing the involved body part in cold to very cold water. The temperature of the water depends on the specific condition of the patient. As a general rule, the more acute the injury, the colder the water temperature is. Temperature ranges are between 80°F (27°C) to 32°F (0°C).

Patient Setup

The PTA follows specific procedures when utilizing cold immersion bath interventions:

1. Describe the treatment process (including the cooling process) and expectations with the patient, and make sure that the patient understands his or her responsibilities during treatment.
2. Check the integrity of the skin and the patient's ability to recognize temperature differences.

3. Fill a container with water at the appropriate temperature.
4. Place the patient in a comfortable position, and put the involved body part in the water. (Remember to keep the patient warm.)
5. Set a timer for 10 to 20 minutes.
6. After treatment, dry the body part being treated, and inspect the skin for response to treatment.
7. Document the treatment.

Vapocoolant Spray

Vapocoolant sprays use ethyl chloride or fluoromethane to produce significant cooling of the skin through evaporation. These sprays are typically used in therapy for treatment of isolated areas of muscle spasms or trigger points. Advantages for the use of vapocoolant sprays are that they numb the skin very quickly, and they allow for stretching without decreasing soft tissue extensibility. The main disadvantage of using vapocoolants is that the numbed area remains that way for only a very short period of time.

Patient Setup

The PTA follows specific procedures when utilizing vapocoolant spray interventions:

1. Describe the treatment process (including the cooling process) and expectations with the patient, and make sure that the patient understands his or her responsibilities during treatment.
2. Check the integrity of the skin and the patient's ability to recognize temperature differences.
3. Protect the patient's eyes if spraying near the face.
4. Hold the container approximately two feet away from the treatment area, and spray so that it comes in contact with the body part at an angle at the rate of about four inches per second.
5. Make sure all of the liquid is evaporated before spraying again.

6. Repeat the process two to three times.
7. Perform appropriate treatment (i.e., spray and stretch).
8. Document the treatment.

Contrast Baths

Contrast baths are used to stimulate peripheral blood flow. Contrast baths entail alternating submersion of a body part in warm (100°F to 110°F) then cold (55°F to 65°F) water. As a general rule, the patient places the involved area in warm water for six minutes, and then places it in cold water for four minutes. This process continues for 20 to 30 minutes. Typically, the treatment begins and ends with the extremity in warm water.

Indications

Indications for contrast baths include:

- venous circulation impairment
- subacute and chronic conditions
- chronic edema
- sinus and congestive headaches

Contraindications and precautions follow the same descriptions as for superficial heat and cold.

Patient Setup

The PTA follows specific procedures when utilizing contrast bath interventions:

1. Describe the treatment process and expectations to the patient, as well as his/her responsibilities during treatment.
2. Position and drape the patient appropriately. Remember to keep the patient warm.
3. Fill two containers with water to the appropriate temperatures and to a depth to cover the treatment area.
4. Place the body part in the warm water for the prescribed length of time, and then in the cold water for the prescribed length of time. (Note:

the treatment can start and end with cold, depending on the treatment goals.)
5. Repeat the process for 20 to 30 minutes.
6. After treatment, dry the body part, and inspect the skin for response to treatment.
7. Document the treatment.

Ultrasound

Ultrasound is defined as an inaudible (cannot be heard by the human ear) sound wave that can produce therapeutic thermal and nonthermal effects on the body. It incorporates conversion as its mode of heat transfer because electrical energy is converted into mechanical energy by a crystal in the sound (transducer) head. The vibration of the sound head creates the energy that moves through body tissue. Once in the body, the energy scatters and is absorbed. As the frequency of the crystal increases, the faster the molecules are absorbed. For this reason, there is an inverse relationship between the frequency of the waves and the penetration depth of the energy. Accordingly, ultrasound is classified as a deep-heating modality, with penetration of the energy up to five centimeters (approximately two inches). Clinically, the two most common frequencies used with ultrasound treatment are 1 MHz and 3 MHz. A 1 MHz sound head penetrates deeper, so would be most appropriate for the treatment of structures that are deeper in the body. The 3 MHz sound head penetrates more superficially, so it is more appropriate for structures that are located closer to the body surface. In addition, the heat produced through ultrasound is absorbed better by tissue that has a high content of collagen, such as tendons, ligaments, joint capsules, and fasciae. Thus, tissue low in collagen—such as skin and subcutaneous fat—absorb very little of the energy produced through ultrasound.

Treatment Tips

When using ultrasound:

- Treatment is typically documented in watts per centimeter squared (w/cm^2).
- Typical treatment intensity ranges from 0.5 to 3.0 w/cm^2.
- The intensity of the treatment remains the same throughout the treatment, specifically with continuous ultrasound. This produces heat in the tissues being treated.
- Factors contributing to rise in tissue temperatures are the rate and amount of time the energy is applied to the tissue, the thermal conductivity of the tissue, and the rate of blood flow to the tissue being treated.
- Pulsed (intermittent) ultrasound does not produce heat. It is based upon a duty cycle.
- Duty cycle (percentage of time ultrasound is delivered) ranges from 5 to 95%, with 20 and 50% the most common.

The thermal effects of ultrasound are:

- increased metabolic activity
- increased blood flow
- increased tissue temperature
- decreased muscle spasm
- decreased inflammation
- increased extensibility of collagen

Nonthermal effects of ultrasound include:

- destruction of calcium deposits
- relief of deep adhesions
- separation of collagen
- increase in cell membrane permeability
- increase in enzyme activity

Additional biophysical effects of ultrasound not discussed previously include:

- increased pain threshold
- increased fibroblast activity
- increased nerve conduction velocity
- cavitation (the vibrational effect on gas bubbles in the body). Cavitation results in an expansion and contraction of the gas bubbles in the blood and tissue fluids. If this effect is intense enough, it can result in changes in the cellular activity and can cause cell damage.

One of the main advantages of using ultrasound is that it produces a significant temperature change in deep tissues. This is not possible with superficial heat modalities. Another advantage is that the treatment time is relatively short. In contrast, the disadvantage is that the patient may experience very little sensation during treatment. Another is that the pressure of the sound head on the body during treatment can cause discomfort to the patient. This can often be resolved by performing ultrasound underwater.

Indications

Indications for ultrasound include:

- soft tissue and joint contractures
- arthritis
- capsulitis
- plantar warts
- subacute and chronic painful conditions
- open wounds (ulcers)
- strains and sprains
- contusions
- surgical skin incisions
- chronic edema
- unresolved hematomas
- low back pain
- sinusitis
- muscle spasms
- bursitis

- carpal tunnel syndrome
- neuromas
- complex regional pain syndrome
- calcific bursitis
- fractures

Contraindications

Contraindications include:

- the area over the eyes
- the area over an unprotected spinal cord (such as a postsurgical laminectomy)
- the area over cancerous lesions
- the area over the carotid sinus
- the area over an open wound with active bleeding
- the area over an infected area
- the area over the heart
- the area over the genitals
- the area over the brain
- the area over any abnormal growth
- the area over arterial insufficiency
- the area over a cemented joint replacement
- the area over a pregnant woman's uterus, abdomen, and lower back
- the area over a thrombus
- the area over impaired sensation
- the area over a superficial medical device (pacemaker or metal implant)
- an undiagnosed patient

Additional Tips for Using Ultrasound Treatments

Keep the following in mind when using ultrasound interventions:

- The effective radiating area (ERA) is roughly the size of the transducer head. Because of this, the treatment area that can be effectively treated with ultrasound is no more than twice the size of the sound head.
- Keep the sound head moving, especially if using continuous ultrasound.

- Always use a coupling medium (gel, water, lotion, gel pack).
- Maintain even contact with the sound head and the body part being treated.
- Try to remove air bubbles from the patient and sound head.
- Avoid bony prominences.
- Add 0.5 w/cm^2 to the intensity when performing ultrasound underwater.
- Keep the sound head one-half to one inch away from the body part being treated when underwater.
- Chronic and/or deeper conditions require a longer treatment time.
- Thicker tissue requires a higher intensity than thinner tissue.
- Allow five minutes of treatment for every 25 square inches of treatment area.
- The recommended treatment duration range is five to ten minutes.
- Average intensity should be greater than 1.0 w/cm^2 for thermal effects and less than 1.0 w/cm^2 for nonthermal effects.
- The average intensity is determined by multiplying the set intensity by the duty cycle.
- Frequency should be 1 MHz for deep tissues (piriformis, etc.) and 3 MHz for superficial tissues (lateral epicondyle, etc.).

Phonophoresis

Phonophoresis is the process of driving medicine through the skin and into deeper tissue using ultrasound. This process introduces medicine to a local area without puncturing the skin like an injection would. It is painless and safer than a physician's injection. Once the medicine is in the body, it has the same effect as it would if it were injected.

Patient Setup

The PTA follows specific procedures when utilizing ultrasound interventions:

1. Instruct the patient about the treatment and what it should feel like (pressure from sound head contact and slight warmth) and not feel like (pain, intense heat, or abnormal sensation).
2. Position the patient comfortably and drape appropriately.
3. Set up the ultrasound machine (appropriate frequency, duty cycle, and treatment time).
4. Apply coupling medium.
5. Place the sound head on the treatment area, and begin to move it slowly (rate of four inches per second) in a rhythmic manner.
6. Turn up the intensity to the prescribed w/cm^2.
7. At the end of the treatment, turn off the machine and remove the coupling medium from the sound head and from the patient.
8. Inspect the treatment area and evaluate the patient's response to treatment.
9. Document the treatment.

Diathermy

Shortwave diathermy is a deep-heating modality—up to three to five centimeters—that uses conversion as its mode of heat transfer. Specifically, it converts electromagnetic energy into heat. The frequency for treatment can range from 10 to 100 MHz, with the most common frequency being 27.12 MHz. The key factor that determines the change in tissue temperature is the amount of energy absorbed by the tissue being treated. This amount is determined by the intensity of the machine's electromagnetic field, the type of tissue being treated (electrical and magnetic properties), the amount of energy penetration, the density of the tissue, and the frequency of the diathermy waves. In general, tissues with a high content of water (such as muscles) absorb the electromagnetic energy better than ones lower in water content (such as fat).

In addition, the strength of the magnetic field is determined by the distance of the treated tissue from the diathermy. Therefore, the inverse square law applies.

There are two methods of diathermy—capacitive plates and inductive coil. While both methods are effective, there are several differences between the two treatment approaches. The capacitive plates are made of metal encased in a plastic housing. The capacitive plates method uses an electric field and the treated body part is part of the electrical circuit. Also, tissues that have low electrical conductivity will heat up, such as fat, ligaments, tendons, and cartilage. The inductive coil is a cable that may or may not be housed in a hinged drum. Unlike in the capacitive plate method, in the inductive coil method, the body part is not part of the electrical circuit. In contrast, parts of the body with high conductivity (such as blood, muscle, or sweat) will heat up during treatment. The capacitive plates method produces heat more in superficial structures, and the inductive coil method produces heat in deeper tissue.

General Effects of Diathermy

The general effects of diathermy include:

- increased metabolism
- muscle relaxation
- sensory nerves sedation
- decreased pain
- decreased joint stiffness
- increased tissue temperature

Thermal Effects of Diathermy

The thermal effects of diathermy include:

- increased tissue temperature
- increased local vasodilation
- increased tissue extensibility
- increased blood flow
- increased nerve conduction velocity
- increased pain threshold

Nonthermal Effects of Diathermy

The nonthermal effects of diathermy include:

- increased phagocytosis
- change in cell membrane function
- removal of muscle waste products

Indications

Indications for diathermy include:

- joint contractures
- muscle spasms
- pain
- arthritis
- bursitis
- musculoskeletal inflammatory conditions
- hematomas
- trigger points

Nonthermal Indications of Diathermy

Nonthermal indications for diathermy are:

- pain
- edema
- wound, bone, and nerve healing
- neuropathies

Contraindications

Diathermy is contraindicated in the following instances:

- identical to other heat modalities
- when there are metal implants
- when there are any implanted stimulator
- over the eyes
- over the testes

Precautions

Precautions should be taken around the following when utilizing diathermy interventions:

- electronic or magnetic equipment in the treatment vicinity
- obesity
- pregnancy
- growing epiphyses

Patient Setup

The PTA follows specific procedures when utilizing diathermy interventions:

1. Instruct the patient about the treatment and what it should and should not feel like.
2. Remove all clothing and jewelry from the surrounding treatment site.
3. Inspect the skin for integrity and sensation.
4. Position the patient comfortably and drape appropriately.
5. Instruct the patient not to move during treatment because movement may affect the spacing between the body part and the machine.
6. Select an appropriate treatment method (capacitive plates or inductive coil).

Capacitive Plates Method

The PTA should follow these procedures for the capacitive plates method:

1. Place the body part to be treated between the plates.
2. Space plates one to three inches from the treated body part (spacing should be equal between each electrode).
3. Inductive method (drum): The drum houses the coil.
4. Place the drum directly over the area being treated.
5. Place a towel between the patient and the drum.
6. Explain the procedure to the patient.
7. Turn on the machine and allow it to warm up.
8. Turn on intensity to the appropriate level.
9. Set treatment time for 20 to 30 minutes.
10. Turn off all controls at the end of the treatment session.
11. Inspect the treated body part.

12. Assess the patient's response to the treatment.

13. Document the treatment.

Hydrotherapy

Hydrotherapy uses the properties of temperature, water, and agitation to bring specific effects to the patient. There are several principles of hydrotherapy which are considered when developing a treatment program for a patient.

Buoyancy is the power of a fluid to exert a force on a body in it. Buoyancy enables an object to float or to seem lighter when in liquid. In addition, a body immersed in water is more supported than if the patient were on land. This support allows a patient to exercise and walk more easily when he or she is in water than when on dry land.

Center of buoyancy is the center of gravity of displaced fluid by an immersed object in water. It is the point at which the buoyant force acts on the body.

Specific gravity, also called relative density, compares the density of one substance against an equal volume of water (1.0). Any object that has a specific gravity less than 1.0 will float in water. (The human body, for example, will float in water.) An object with a specific gravity over 1.0 (such as, for example, a sand-filled weight) will sink in water.

Hydrostatic pressure follows the premise that as an object is immersed deeper in water, the density of the liquid increases. This can assist in venous flow. It is relevant in therapy because if a body part is immersed deep enough in water, the pressure on it may be sufficient enough to decrease edema.

Drag is the water's resistance to an object moving through it. Drag is determined by size and shape of the objects moving. Therefore, objects that are more stream-lined (and have less drag) move through the water more easily than those that are large and broad (and have greater drag). One type of drag is form drag, which is the resistance that an object encounters in water.

This is directly related to the turbulence of the water; the greater the drag, the greater the turbulence. Because water is significantly more viscous than air, it provides more resistance to movement than air does. When a patient tries to move quickly in the water, it becomes increasingly harder for the patient. This allows the patient to perform resistive exercise in water.

Wave drag, however, is the water's resistance as a result of the turbulence. As the speed of an object in the water increases, so does the wave drag. This is why exercises performed in turbulent water are harder to perform than those performed in calm water, and it is why running in water is more difficult than walking in water.

Hydrodynamics is the movement of an object through water, which is regulated by the speed, size, and surface area of the moving object in the water and the fluid's resistance to movement of the submerged object.

Heat transfer through hydrotherapy occurs through conduction (water in contact with the body part) and convection (movement of water around the body part). Besides the transfer of heat, there are numerous clinical effects of hydrotherapy:

- cleansed wounds
- decreased weight-bearing
- strengthening
- slowed bone mineral density loss
- decreased exercise-induced asthma
- decreased vital capacity
- increased venous circulation
- increased cardiac output
- decreased heart rate
- decreased systolic blood pressure
- relaxation
- identical modalities as superficial heat and cold
- resistance for exercise
- desensitization of a hypersensitive body part from the agitation of the water

Indications

Indications for hydrotherapy include:

- pain relief
- wound care
- muscle spasms
- inflammation
- burns
- peripheral nerve injuries
- contractures
- scars
- arthritis
- generalized weakness

Contraindications

Hydrotherapy is contraindicated for:

- acute edema
- acute injuries
- fever
- infections
- malignancy
- maceration (softening) around a wound
- cardiac and respiratory instability
- wounds with granulation tissue

Precautions

Situations requiring precaution include:

- confused patients
- impaired thermal sensations
- full body immersion (can increase core temperature)
- urinary incontinence.
- pregnancy (full-body immersion with hot to very hot water)
- multiple sclerosis (hot to very hot water)

Hydrotherapy Safety Tips for PTAs

The PTA should heed the following tips when utilizing hydrotherapy interventions:

- Make sure that all hydrotherapy devices are plugged in to a ground fault interrupter (GFI) receptacle.
- The PTA should never leave a patient who is receiving hydrotherapy unattended.
- The PTA should always give a patient receiving hydrotherapy a bell (so that the patient may call the PTA for help if needed).
- The PTA should make sure the hydrotherapy area is well ventilated.

Patient Setup

The PTA follows specific procedures when utilizing hydrotherapy interventions:

1. Fill the whirlpool with water to the appropriate level and temperature for treatment, making sure that the water covers the intake hole at the bottom of the shaft of the turbine.
2. Instruct the patient about what to expect from the treatment and what is expected from the patient.
3. Allow the patient to change into appropriate clothing for the treatment so that no clothing comes in contact with the water.
4. Place a chair next to the whirlpool to allow the patient to sit.
5. Place the body part to be treated into the whirlpool.
6. Turn on the turbine and adjust the intensity and direction of the turbulence to the patient's tolerance.
7. Set timer for 20 minutes and give the patient a call bell.
8. After treatment, turn off the turbine, remove the patient from the whirlpool, dry the patient, and assess the treatment site.

Common Temperature Ranges Used for Hydrotherapy

NAME	TEMPERATURE RANGE (°F/°C)	INDICATIONS	WHIRLPOOL TYPES
Very hot	104°F to 110°F (40°C to 43°C)	Increase soft tissue extensibility; chronic conditions; small treatment area	Extremity tank: This tank is tall and narrow in shape. It allows an entire upper or lower extremity to be submerged, without using a significant amount of water.
Hot	99°F to 104°F (37°C to 40°C)	Pain relief; arthritis	Low boy: This whirlpool looks similar to the size and shape of a bathtub. It is large enough to allow the patient to sit in it and low enough to the ground so that transfer in and out of the tank is fairly easy.
Warm	96°F to 99°F (35.5°C to 37°C)	Open wounds; patients with circulatory, sensory, or cardiac disorders	High boy (also called hip tank): This tank is similar in shape to the low boy, but the sides of the tank are higher off the ground, making it significantly deeper than the low boy.
Neutral	80°F to 92°F (27°C to 33.5°C)	Range of motion for patients with burns	Foot tank: This whirlpool is small and is used to treat hands and feet. It does not use a lot of water, is portable, and does not take a significant amount of time to clean.
Cold	32°F to 79°F (0°C to 26°C)	Exercise; acute inflammation if colder temperatures are not tolerated	Hubbard tank: The Hubbard tank is a butterfly-shaped whirlpool that is large enough to allow a patient to lie in it and move both the upper and lower extremities. The clinician can assist the patient from outside the tank. The patient is lowered into the tank on a stretcher, and the turbine can be moved around the tank so that the turbulence is directed to specific body parts.

9. Apply any dressing that may be indicated.
10. Clean the whirlpool according to the protocol of the facility.
11. Document the treatment.

Compression

Mechanical compression is the application of a mechanical force which places external pressure on a body part. Two methods are commonly used in physical therapy to perform this function. The first is the

Common Temperature Ranges Used for Hydrotherapy (*continued*)

NAME	TEMPERATURE RANGE (°F/°C)	INDICATIONS	WHIRLPOOL TYPES
	79°F to 97°F (26°C to 36°C)	Acute inflammation; spasticity; arthritis; balance impairments; weakness; pain	Therapy pools: Therapy pools are small pools that allow patients to exercise more easily than they would be able to if they were on land. The therapy pool's depth does not have the typical slope that is seen in many swimming pools. This allows the patient to walk and exercise. In addition, the temperature of a therapy pool is warmer than that of the average swimming pool. A swimming pool is usually kept between 79°F and 97°F. Most therapy pools are kept between 90°F and 97°F. This warmer temperature is better tolerated by the elderly and by arthritis patients. However, because much of the body is submerged, cooling via sweating will not occur, and the exercising patient's body temperature will not decrease during hydrotherapy.

use of intermittent compression pumps. These devices provide pressure through a pneumatic device or one that pumps cold fluid. The pressure from the compression can either be static or intermittent. Intermittent compression can be general, where the appliance increases pressure evenly throughout inflation, or it can be sequential, where the pressure increases from distal to proximal. The second method is to provide low-level, static pressure by having the patient wear shrinkers, elastic bandages, support hose, postoperative rigid dressings, or fitted compression garments.

Both methods of compression are used to improve venous and lymphatic circulation, modify scar tissue formation, shape residual limbs after amputation, decrease edema, and increase tissue temperature.

Indications

Indications for compression include:

- edema
- lymphedema
- deep vein thrombophlebitis prevention
- venous insufficiency
- venous stasis ulcers
- control scarring after burns
- residual limb shaping
- renal insufficiency

Contraindications

Compression is contraindicated with:

- congestive heart failure
- acute pulmonary edema
- kidney failure
- deep vein thrombophlebitis
- pulmonary embolus
- peripheral arterial insufficiency
- displaced fracture
- infection
- obstructed lymphatic channels
- heart failure

Precautions

Precautions should be taken with the following:

- impaired sensation
- uncontrolled hypertension
- cancer
- cerebral vascular accident

Patient Setup

The PTA follows specific procedures when utilizing compression interventions:

1. Explain the procedure to the patient, as well as the treatment expectations, and discuss expectations of the patient.
2. Assess the skin and patient's ability to perceive pressure.
3. Perform girth measurements at predetermined landmarks.
4. Measure patient's blood pressure.
5. Apply stockinette to the involved extremity. (Note: Be sure to tell the patient that wrinkles in the skin after this treatment are a normal response.)
6. Put the appliance on the patient and connect tubing.
7. Allow the appliance to inflate, and inform the patient that he or she should feel pressure but that he or she should not feel pain, tingling, numbness, or a pulse.
8. Do not allow pressure in the appliance to exceed the patient's diastolic blood pressure. (General rule: 60 mm Hg for lower extremities and less than 50 mm Hg for upper extremities)
9. If performing intermittent compression, set the on/off cycle for a three to one (3:1). This is typically 45 to 90 seconds on and 15 to 30 seconds off.
10. Instruct the patient to move their digits during the off cycle.
11. Treatment duration should be two hours, twice per day.
12. Stay with the patient for the first few cycles of the treatment, and provide a call bell.
13. After treatment, remove the appliance and stockinette, assess skin integrity, and retake girth measurements and blood pressure.
14. Document the treatment.

Traction

Traction is the application of an external force to the body that produces joint surface separation or stretching of soft tissue. Most often in the clinical setting, the force is applied by a traction machine or by the clinician. The types of traction available for patient treatment are continuous, positional, and self traction. The most common site for traction is the cervical and lumbar spine. Continuous traction is a long-term traction (10 to 14 days) in which a small amount of force is applied (10 to 20 pounds). With positional traction, pillows are used to place the patient in a position that places a stretching force on the soft tissue. When a patient performs self traction, she is using her body weight to place a distraction force on the involved structures. Soft tissue stretching, rather than joint surface separation, is the treatment objective of these three methods.

During manual traction, the distraction force is supplied by the clinician. Manual traction has several advantages over mechanical. First, it is a relatively safe treatment. The force used in manual traction can be changed quickly and requires little, if any, equipment to perform. It is also an appropriate mode of traction for a patient who does not tolerate the traction harnesses. However, manual therapy has some drawbacks. First, it is difficult to quantify the amount of traction force being applied. In addition, manual therapy requires a certain level of skill by the clinician to be performed correctly.

Mechanical traction is performed through two methods—static and intermittent. With static traction, the same amount of force is applied through the treatment session. Intermittent traction differs in that there are set periods of traction and relaxation throughout the treatment. One main advantage that mechanical traction has over manual traction is that the force of traction and the time of treatment are well controlled. However, mechanical traction has some drawbacks as well. Mechanical traction is very time-consuming to set up. In addition, the harnesses may not be comfortable for the patient, and multiple joint segments are mobilized, not just the one that is being treated.

Clinical Effects

The clinical effects of traction include:

- stretching of soft tissue
- muscle relaxation
- joint mobilization
- disk protrusion reduction

Indications

Traction indications include:

- vertebral disc herniation
- nerve root impingement
- joint hypomobility
- subacute joint inflammation
- muscle spasms
- degenerative joint disease
- stenosis

- facet impingement
- radicular symptoms

Contraindications

Traction is contraindicated in the following cases:

- unstable fractures
- spinal cord compression
- acute inflammation
- joint hypermobility or instability
- when it may not specifically address the target symptoms
- bilateral neurological signs
- over areas where the harness or corset pressures may be harmful
- advanced degenerative joint disease
- cancer
- when motion is contraindicated
- osteoporosis

Patient Setup: Lumbar

The PTA follows specific procedures when utilizing traction interventions:

1. Question the patient regarding contraindications and precautions for treatment.
2. Explain the treatment procedure to the patient, the rationale for treatment relating to the patient's condition, how traction works, what the patient should and should not feel, and what the patient should and should not do during treatment.
3. Inspect the skin prior to initiating treatment.
4. Apply the thoracic and lumbar harness to patient.
5. Position the patient prone or supine on the traction table based upon the treatment goals. The treatment area should be over the portion of the traction it separates.
6. Attach the harnesses to the table and unit.
7. Select the appropriate treatment parameters:

- traction force: at least one-quarter to one-half the patient's body weight

- duration: 10 to 20 minutes
- static or intermittent
- hold/relax time

8. Provide the patient with a call bell and traction safety switch.
9. Turn on the unit and release the table.
10. Monitor the patient's response during treatment for several cycles, and adjust the treatment as necessary and appropriate.
11. At the end of treatment, turn off the machine, lock the table, release the tension on the traction, and remove the harnesses.
12. Assess the patient's response to the treatment.
13. Allow the patient to rest for several minutes before rising.
14. Document the treatment by noting the type of traction used, the patient's position, the maximum and the relaxation forces, hold/relax times, treatment time, and the patient's response to treatment.

Patient Setup: Cervical Traction

The PTA follows specific procedures when utilizing traction interventions:

1. Explain the procedure for the treatment to the patient, the duration of treatment, the rationale for treatment relating to patient's condition, how the treatment should feel, and what the patient should and should not do during treatment.
2. Inspect the treatment area, and ask the patient to remove any jewelry or restrictive clothing.
3. Make sure all settings on the machine are off or set to zero.
4. Have the patient lie supine, with knees bent, on the traction table, and fit the cervical harness properly.
5. Connect the unit rope to the cervical harness.
6. Give the patient the cutoff switch, and explain how to use it.

7. Correctly set parameters on the unit, including the mode (static or intermittent), poundage for on and off cycles, and the treatment time.
8. Turn on the machine, and stay with the patient for several cycles.
9. Obtain feedback about the treatment from the patient.
10. At the end of the treatment, turn off the machine, disconnect the rope from the harness, and remove the harness.
11. Allow the patient to rest for several minutes, and assist the patient to sit up.
12. Inspect the treatment area, and document the treatment. Be sure to include information about the type of traction used, the patient's position, the maximum force/relaxation force, hold/relax times, treatment time, and the patient's response to treatment.

Ultraviolet Light

This is a modality that is used to treat mainly skin conditions. Ultraviolet is at one end of the visible light spectrum of the electromagnetic spectrum. Infrared is found at the opposite end on the spectrum. The use of this modality for physical therapy is not common today because many skin conditions traditionally treated with ultraviolet are now treated with medications. Ultraviolet light uses radiant energy in the wavelength band of 180 to 400 nanometers (nm). There are three types of ultraviolet light. Each has a different wavelength band:

1. Ultraviolet A (UVA): 320 to 400 nm
2. Ultraviolet B (UVB): 290 to 320 nm
3. Ultraviolet C (UVC): 180 to 290 nm

The physiological effects of ultraviolet are influenced by the wavelength of the radiation, intensity of the light reaching the skin, and the depth of penetration of the ultraviolet light. The depth of penetration of ultraviolet light is influenced by the intensity of the radiation reaching the skin, the wavelength and power of the radiation source, the thickness of the pigmentation of the skin, and the duration of treatment. Similar to ultrasound, the absorption of ultraviolet light is inversely related to penetration. This means that the more energy that is absorbed, the more superficial the penetration. In contrast, the less energy that is absorbed, the deeper the penetration. This is related to the frequency of the ultraviolet light. The wavelength of the light is inversely proportionate to the frequency. The shorter the wavelength of the light, the higher the frequency of the wavelength. The shorter the wavelength, the quicker the energy is absorbed.

When performing ultraviolet treatment, there are two laws of physics that must be considered—the inverse square and the cosine laws. The inverse square law states that the intensity of waves from a source varies inversely with the square of the distance from the source. An example of this is if the distance of the lamp is increased from one to three feet from the patient, the area irradiated is nine times as large as the original. Therefore, the same area at three feet distance receives one-ninth the energy, making the treatment much less intense. Conversely, if the distance of the lamp is decreased from three feet to one foot, then the treatment becomes much more intense. The cosine law states that the absorption of rays is optimal when they strike the surface on a perpendicular angle. At a zero degree angle, the energy is at its strongest. As the angle between the energy beam and the perpendicular angle increases, the intensity of the energy is decreased in proportion to the cosine of the angle.

The local effects of ultraviolet light are:

- erythema
- stimulation of new cell production
- sloughing of the epidermis
- bacteria destruction
- formation of vitamin D

Indications

The indications for the use of ultraviolet light include:

- acne
- psoriasis
- decubitis ulcers
- reddening or tanning of the skin

Contraindications

Ultraviolet light is contraindicated in the following cases:

- fever
- systemic lupus erythematosus
- cardiac, kidney, or liver disease
- skin cancer
- pulmonary tuberculosis
- should not be used over eyes

Precautions

When using ultraviolet interventions, precautions should be taken in the following cases:

- use of photosensitizing medication
- photosensitivity
- recent X-ray therapy

Adverse Effects

These are among the adverse effects of ultraviolet interventions:

- burning
- premature aging of the skin
- carcinogenesis
- eye damage (cataracts)

Prior to performing ultraviolet treatment, the PTA must first determine how long a treatment should last. This is called dosimetry. In order to do this, the minimal erythemal dose (MED) must be determined. An MED produces redness of the skin, but it fades within 24 hours. This procedure is performed at least one day before beginning formal ultraviolet treatment. This test determines the length of the ultraviolet treatment. Besides the MED, there are three therapeutic doses that are used with ultraviolet treatment—first erythemal dose (E1), second erythemal dose (E2), and third erythemal dose (E3). An E1 dose is considered 2.5 times the MED. The erythema lasts two to three days before it fades. The maximal size of the treatment area is 20% of the body. When a patient receives an E2 dose, it is equivalent to five times the MED. This dosage produces intense erythema, edema, peeling, and pigmentation. The treatment should not be larger than 250 cm^2. The most intense treatment dose is an E3. This intensity is equal to ten times the MED. It produces severe blistering, peeling, and exudates. The maximum size of the treatment area is 25 cm^2, roughly four square inches.

Patient Setup

The PTA follows specific procedures when utilizing ultraviolet interventions:

1. Perform the treatment in a well-ventilated room.
2. Explain the procedure to the patient. Also, explain the responsibilities of the patient during treatment.
3. Allow the lamp to warm up.
4. Provide the patient with a pair of protective goggles, and instruct the patient to keep his or her eyes closed during the treatment.
5. Wash the treatment.
6. Position and drape the patient appropriately.
7. Measure the distance (one inch) and angle (preferably zero degrees) of the lamp to the patient.
8. Keep the treatment area covered, except for the prescribed length of time of exposure.
9. Expose the treatment area and open the shutters of the lamp.
10. Perform the procedure for the appropriate length of time, and close the shutters of the lamp.
11. Turn off the unit.
12. Inspect the skin.
13. Allow the patient to dress.
14. Document the treatment. Be sure to include information about the patient's skin response to the treatment, which specific ultraviolet lamp was used, the distance of the lamp from the patient, angle of incidence of the lamp to the patient, draping procedures, and exposure time.

Biofeedback

Biofeedback is a modality that measures muscle signals that are picked up, amplified, and translated into an audible and/or visible signal. These signals then specify motor recruitment, the inhibition of spasticity, and the promotion of muscle relaxation. Biofeedback differs from electrical stimulation. Whereas electrical stimulation delivers an electrical impulse to the body, biofeedback measures the electrical activity produced by a muscle. In biofeedback, there is no electrical sensation perceived by the patient.

One main advantage of biofeedback is that it provides the patient with the opportunity to make appropriate small changes in performance, which are noted immediately. It is an objective way to assess muscular activity without invading the body. Another advantage of the use of biofeedback is that it can be started early in the rehabilitation process.

Indications

Biofeedback is indicated for:

- muscle reeducation
- spasticity inhibition
- muscle relaxation
- incontinence

Contraindications

Biofeedback is contraindicated for:

- any condition in which a muscle contraction is contraindicated
- skin sensitivity to the adhesives or gels used with the electrodes

Biofeedback is not a specific modality used for the purpose of decreasing pain. Rather, it is a teaching tool used to facilitate muscle contractions or relaxation. As muscular activity becomes more efficient, the value of biofeedback becomes decreased because the patient will rely less on feedback from the unit.

Patient Setup

The PTA follows specific procedures when utilizing biofeedback interventions.

1. Explain the procedure to the patient and the patient's responsibilities during treatment.
2. Prepare the skin for electrode placement by removing any oil or dead skin. (Shaving hair may be required.)
3. Place the electrode as close as possible to the muscle being monitored.
4. If the goal of treatment is muscle reeducation, instruct the patient to contract the desired muscle, so that an audio-visual signal is produced.
5. Once a threshold level is determined, set the machine to signal when the patient contracts the muscle with enough force to reproduce the audio-visual signal.
6. The unit will not respond until the patient reaches the threshold.
7. Have the patient perform the prescribed number of sets and repetitions of muscle contractions.
8. If the goal of treatment is muscle relaxation, the first three sets remain the same. For relaxation,

the goal is to decrease muscle tension. With this procedure, the unit will produce an audio-visual signal until the muscle tension decreases below the set threshold. This will teach the patient how to relax his or her muscle.

9. Instruct the patient to try to relax the muscle for a set amount of time without producing the audio-visual signal.
10. At the end of treatment, remove the electrode and inspect the skin.
11. Document the treatment.

Continuous Passive Motion Machine

Continuous passive motion (CPM) machines are units that slowly and passively move joints through their ranges of motion for uninterrupted and extended periods of time. Research supports that joints that are moved passively are less likely to become stiff or have joint contractures as compared to joints that are immobilized. In addition, collagen fibers are well organized, and there is a significantly smaller chance of adhesions.

As CPM units are manufactured by a variety of companies, each company has developed its own specific protocol for operation. The units are designed to be easily adjustable and controlled and to be portable. Often, they are prescribed for home use for patients.

Effects

The effects of CPM units include:

- improved and promoted connective tissue strength, size, and shape
- decreased joint effusion
- enhanced joint nutrition
- minimized joint adhesions
- facilitated normal joint kinematics
- decreased articular cartilage changes
- minimized negative effects of immobilization
- improved range of motion
- reduced joint swelling
- allowing for earlier ambulation

- decreased postoperative pain
- improved synovial fluid nutrition
- improved rate of joint cartilage healing and regeneration

Indications

CPM is indicated for:

- joint contractions
- post-joint surgery
- post-immobilization of fractures
- joint arthrosis
- total joint replacements

CPM is often used in combination with other interventions to decrease pain and swelling. Interventions that may be combined with CPM include ice packs, anti-inflammatory medications, joint compression bandages, transcutaneous electrical nerve stimulation, and oral or intravenous analgesic medications.

Patient Setup

In using CPM, the PTA follows certain procedures:

1. Explain the procedure to the patient as well as his or her expectations and responsibilities during treatment.
2. Make sure the patient is in a comfortable position and drape properly.
3. Place the patient's extremity in the CPM unit.
4. Appropriately secure the body part.
5. Set the unit for the prescribed range of motion.
6. If available with the unit, provide the patient with a shutoff button.
7. Set the unit for the prescribed cycles per minute (usually one cycle per minute).
8. Turn on the unit, and stay with the patient for several cycles; adjust the settings as needed.
9. Length of treatment: CPM can be used for up to 24 hours per day for up to one month.
10. At the end of treatment, turn off the unit and remove the patient's extremity.
11. Document the treatment.

Electrical Stimulation

Electrical stimulation (ES) is a common modality used in physical therapy. It helps relieve pain, reeducate muscles, heal tissue, and relax muscle spasms. Electrical stimulation currents have the longest wavelength (clinically: 1 Hz to 4,000 Hz), lowest frequency, and the greatest depth of penetration of all modalities. ES provides nerve and muscle stimulation currents that are capable of pain modulation, production of muscle contractions and relaxation, soft tissue and bone healing, and the production of movement of ions through use of continuous direct current (DC) that produces chemical change within tissues.

Electricity Basics

All matter is made up of atoms. An atom is always neutrally charged and contains an equal number of proton and electrons. When an atom is not neutral, it is called an ion. An atom becomes charged through the addition or loss of an electron. Negative ions try to lose electrons and positive ions try to gain them. When an electron is free, it is capable of moving from one atom to another.

All electricity flows through circuits. The current flow of electricity is produced when there is a concentration difference or an electrical potential. In a closed circuit, the electrons are flowing; in an open circuit, the electron flow is stopped. There are two forms of circuits used with electricity. In a series circuit, there is only one path for the current to get from one terminal to another. The resistance to current flow in this type of circuit is equal to the resistance of all the components in the circuit added together. A visible representation is ($RT = R1 + R2 + R3$). Series circuits are not common in rehabilitation. A parallel circuit is a circuit that has two or more existing routes for the current to pass between the two terminals. The component resistors are placed side by side, and each of the resistors receives the same voltage ($VT = V1 = V2 = V3$). Parallel circuits are more common in rehabilitation.

Therapeutic Goals of Electrical Stimulation

Treatment goals of electrical stimulation include:

- decreasing pain
- improving motor control
- increasing strength of innervated muscle
- preventing atrophy
- delivering medicine

There are several forms of electrical stimulation used in therapy:

- Electrical muscle stimulation is used to stimulate denervated muscle in order to maintain muscle viability.
- Electrical stimulation for tissue repair (ESTR) is indicated for edema reduction, promotion of circulation, and wound care.
- Neuromuscular electrical stimulation (NMES) uses stimulation of innervated muscle for restoring muscle function, muscle strengthening, spasm reduction, atrophy prevention, and muscle reeducation.
- Functional electrical stimulation (FES) is used to activate muscles in order to perform functional activities.
- Transcutaneous electrical nerve stimulation is used for pain management.
- Ultrasound with electrical stimulation uses the effects of ultrasound along with those of ES.
- Iontophoresis uses electricity to drive charged ions through the skin.

The three types of current used with electrical stimulation are direct current (DC), alternating current (AC), and pulsatile currents. With direct current, there is a continuous, unidirectional flow of electricity. The electricity is received by one electrode and returns to the machine by the other. DC is also sometimes called galvanic or monophasic current. Alternating current is the uninterrupted, bidirectional flow of electricity changing direction at least one time per second. Pulsed current is the unidirectional or bidirectional flow of charged particles that periodically cease for a period of at least one second before the next electrical event. It can be either monophasic or biphasic. Interferential and Russian currents are examples of pulsed currents.

Compared to alternating current, direct current is perceived to be more uncomfortable to tolerate. Direct current is most often used for wound healing and iontophoresis.

Responses to Electrical Stimulation

Electrical stimulation produces three excitatory responses: sensory, motor, and pain (noxious). With sensory stimulation, the patient feels a tingling sensation. This is appropriate for acute conditions or when a muscle contraction is not desired. A motor response is used when either a muscle twitch or strong tetanic contraction is desired. This is more appropriate for subacute and chronic conditions. Noxious stimulation is used for pain relief. Subsensory stimulation is also a treatment approach used with ES, in the form of low-intensity stimulation. The strength of the stimulus response elicited by ES for treatment is dependent on the specific problem of the patient, the muscle group being treated, the type of electrode used during treatment, the intended treatment goal, and patient tolerance.

One of the main determinants that dictate tissue response is pulse frequency, which defines the quality of muscle response. Pulse frequency has a rate range of 1 to 120 pulses per second (pps). In ranges below 15 pps, the body can differentiate between the individual pulses. Above that range, it cannot. In order to get a strong, tetanic contraction, a pulse rate of 15 pps to 50 pps is needed.

Correct Use of Electrodes

Electrical stimulation is delivered through electrodes. Electrodes serve two functions: They apply stimulating current to the body tissue, and they record or detect the presence of electrical signals in the body (biofeedback). Electrodes can be either transcutaneous (above the skin), or subcutaneous (below the skin). The current density under the electrodes increases as the electrode size decreases. If the muscle being treated is small, the PTA should use smaller electrodes, and if large muscles are being treated, larger electrodes should be used. Electrode placement plays an important role in treatment. The closer the electrodes are placed, the more superficial the penetration of the current. The farther electrodes are apart, the deeper the penetration of the current.

The efficacy of using electrical stimulation to stimulate denervated muscles has been questioned. Currently, most clinicians do not recommend stimulating denervated muscles with direct current. In addition, although direct current electrical stimulation has traditionally been used to treat Bell's palsy, a placebo has been found to be just as effective.

Indications

The purpose of using electrical stimulation is to prevent muscle atrophy and to maintain muscle status. Its treatment goals are to limit edema, retard atrophy, and maintain flexibility. It is indicated for:

- painful conditions
- incontinence
- muscle reeducation
- decrease swelling
- muscle spasms
- functional activities

Contraindications

Contraindications of ES include:

- pregnancy
- pacemaker
- electrical stimulators
- cancer
- thrombophlebitis.
- active tuberculosis

- active bleeding
- over the carotid sinus
- in the area of the head of patients with epilepsy
- across the chest of patients with cardiac disease
- over the eyes
- mucosal surfaces
- impaired or absent sensation
- over areas where active movement must be avoided
- on or directly over superficial metals

Precautions

Precautions must be taken with the following situations:

- obesity
- absence or diminished sensation
- thin, fragile skin
- internal or external metal fixation devices
- skin conditions such as eczema, psoriasis, acne, or dermatitis

Rules

For ES units, the following rules apply:

- All electrical stimulation units must be plugged into a ground fault interrupter (GFI) outlet.
- Always instruct the patient regarding touching controls and changing body position during treatment. Advise about goals and expected outcomes of treatment and treatment time. In addition, instruct the patient to call the PTA with any problems during treatment.
- Inspect the patient's skin before and after treatment.
- Position the patient so that there is optimal patient comfort and electrode contact.
- Ask the patient what he or she feels and where he or she feels the stimulation.
- Stay with the patient for several minutes to monitor his or her reaction and tolerance to the level of amplitude of the electrical stimulation.

- Document the skin status pre- and post-treatment, the number of electrodes and their placement and size, which electrical stimulation machine was used, treatment parameters, and the patient's response to treatment.

Neuromuscular Electrical Stimulation

The use of electrical stimulation to facilitate muscular contractions requires an intact, or at least a partially intact, peripheral nerve to respond to the stimulation. Patients may not like neuromuscular electrical stimulation because it tends to be uncomfortable. While NMES is beneficial, a voluntary muscle contraction with electrical stimulation is superior to using electrical stimulation only. The pulse rate for treatment should be low (between 35 pps and 50 pps). The duty cycle (on/off cycle) should be a 1 to 3 or 1 to 5 (on/off ratio). The muscle contraction should be held long enough to sufficiently work the muscle. Therefore, the on-time should be between 2 and 10 seconds. The on/off interval allows for replenishment of adenotriphosphate (ATP). When ATP is replenished, the muscle is less likely to fatigue. Commonly accepted on/off intervals are on-times of 6 to 10 seconds and off-times of 50 to 120 seconds. The interval time depends on patient fatigue.

Patient positioning is also very important with this type of treatment. The patient must be positioned so that he or she is comfortable and able to see the muscle contraction. This will lead to patient cooperation with the treatment. In addition, the PTA should try to position the involved limb with a mild stretch. This allows for a stronger muscle contraction. When starting the patient with this stimulation program, the amplitude (intensity) must be gradually increased. An appropriate treatment time is 10 to 15 minutes, with the patient performing a minimum of ten repetitions per treatment session. It should be noted that if the treatment goal is to relieve muscle spasms, it is desired to fatigue the muscle. For this goal, the on/off interval should be equal. This will not allow the muscle to replenish its ATP.

The Uses of NMES

Neuromuscular electrical stimulation can be used for a variety of different treatment purposes. Uses of NMES include:

- increasing range of motion (e.g., to increase quadriceps strength for an individual with an extension lag)
- facilitating or retraining muscles
- management of muscle spasms to try to break pain-spasm cycle
- edema reduction
- orthotic substitution

When considering using NMES, the PTA must understand that certain current waveforms are more effective than others. For example, with muscle strengthening interventions, Russian (medium frequency burst) and biphasic symmetrical waveform currents are more effective than high-volt pulsed currents and interferential currents.

The placement of electrodes for NMES treatment is particularly important. Electrode placement should be parallel to superior muscle fibers. For large muscles, two channels with four electrodes are most appropriate. When stimulating small muscles, one channel with two electrodes is effective.

Patient Setup

For safety, the PTA follows these procedures:

1. Explain the treatment to the patient, and tell the patient that ES is used for muscle strengthening, endurance, reeducation, or decreasing edema or spasm.
2. Explain that the stimulation should feel like an intense tingling, but strong enough to produce a muscle contraction, and that it will go on and off. When the stimulation is on, the patient should not fight it, but rather work with it by performing an isometric contraction.

3. Tell the patient not to touch or remove the electrodes when the unit is on.

4. Instruct the patient of the duration of treatment (10 to 20 minutes).

5. Position the patient comfortably in order to facilitate a muscle contraction.

6. Drape the patient appropriately.

7. Inspect the skin.

8. Place the electrode as close to a motor point on the desired muscle as possible.

9. Make sure the unit is off.

10. Set the unit for the appropriate parameters (35 pps to 50 pps; 1:5 on/off ratio).

11. Slowly turn up the intensity.

12. When the muscle contraction is strong enough, set the unit so that the on/off intervals begin.

13. Give the patient a call bell.

14. Monitor the patient through several cycles.

15. At the end of the treatment, turn off the unit, remove the electrodes, assess the patient, and inspect the skin.

16. Document the treatment.

Electrical Stimulation for Tissue Repair

Electrical stimulation is useful for promoting tissue healing. This method of electrical stimulation entails the management of open wounds, transcutaneous drug delivery (iontophoresis), and decreasing edema. When performing ESTR, the desired current is direct because the use of a certain polarity is more beneficial than others. The use of a negative polarity promotes increased collagen production and inhibition of bacteria growth. In contrast, a positive polarity attracts white blood cells and promotes epithelial cell growth and vasoconstriction.

Uses

Electrical stimulation for tissue repair can be used for a variety of different treatment purposes. Uses of ESTR include:

- accelerating the rate of chronic wound healing
- debriding necrotic material
- attracting white blood cells
- increasing blood flow
- inhibiting bacteria growth

Benefits of ESTR

Electrical stimulation for tissue repair is beneficial to patients in a variety of ways and promotes many types of healing. Benefits of ESTR include:

- skin healing
- chronic wound healing (no adverse effects, less debridement is needed, and the wounds become less contaminated)
- normalization of tensile strength and structure of fibrous tissue

Indications

ESTR is indicated for chronic wounds due to:

- venous insufficiency
- pressure
- arterial insufficiency
- diabetes

It is also indicated for edema control.

Contraindications

ESTR is contraindicated in the following cases:

- malignancy
- potential osteomyelitis
- demand pacemakers
- over the carotid sinus
- thrombophlebitis
- medications that influence ionic balance
- over areas vulnerable to hemorrhage or hematoma
- over the eyes
- over areas of decreased sensation
- on the thoracic area of small patients (do not use in this area)

Precautions

Precautions are taken in the cases of skin irritations, poorly nurtured skin, and pregnancy.

Patient safety during this type of treatment is of utmost importance. For this reason, there should be one set of electrodes for each patient. After each treatment, the leads (cables) must be cleansed with an appropriate solution.

Documentation for ESTR

Documentation should include:

- the size of electrodes used
- the space between the electrodes
- the polarity of active electrodes
- the type of current used
- the amplitude (intensity) of the current
- the duration of treatment

Iontophoresis

Iontophoresis is the introduction of ions into the skin by use of direct current that is deposited subcutaneously. Parameters for treatment are based upon time or milliamps. The rate at which an ion may be delivered is determined by the concentration of the ion used, the pH of the solution, the molecular size of the solute, the current density, and the duration of treatment.

The advantages of iontophoresis are that the medication does not have to be absorbed by the gastrointestinal (GI) tract and that it is safer than an injection. The strength of the electrical field is determined by the current density under the electrode. This can be changed by increasing or decreasing the current intensity or by changing the size of the electrode. Because smaller electrodes have more current density at the same intensity, the electrical stimulus will feel more intense than it would if a larger electrode were used. To make the treatment more comfortable, the spacing between the electrodes can be increased. This will decrease the current density in superficial tissue.

The depth of ion penetration reaches 1 mm to 3 mm during treatment, and a maximum of 1.5 cm 12 to 24 hours post-treatment. In addition, the quantity of ions transferred into the tissue is determined by the intensity of current, the current density at the active electrode, the duration of current flow, and the concentration of current flow.

Because iontophoresis treatment can be uncomfortable and there is a risk of skin irritation to the patient, a low-voltage output iontophoresis has been developed. It decreases the risk of skin irritation and it improves comfort because it gives a prolonged drug delivery. The low current is given for a long period of time (1 to 24 hours) at a dose of 0.1 to 0.3 mA (milliamps). While low-voltage output iontophoresis is more comfortable, there may be a decrease in drug delivery because of high skin resistance.

Indications

Indications for iontophoresis include:

- athlete's foot
- post-traumatic edema
- plantar warts
- trigger points
- acute and subacute inflammatory conditions
- gout analgesia
- muscle spasm
- ischemia
- edema
- calcium deposits
- scar tissue
- hyperhydrosis
- herpes

Contraindications

Contraindications for iontophoresis include:

- skin sensitivity reactions to medication
- anesthetic skin

- recent scars
- metal embedded close to skin
- active bleeding
- cardiac pacemakers
- over skin with any damage

Treatment Tips

When administering iontophoresis interventions to a patient, the PTA should be sure to do the following:

- Know the polarity of substance being used for treatment, and be aware of the fact that like charges repel each other and opposite charges are attracted to one another.
- Thoroughly clean the treatment area to decrease skin resistance.
- Do not use two medications in the same treatment.
- Be careful with heating modalities prior to iontophoresis treatment.

Patient Setup

The PTA follows specific procedures when utilizing iontophoresis interventions:

1. Explain the treatment procedure to the patient, including the reason for using it, and describe the sensation the patient should feel (intense tingling to stinging feeling). Explain to the patient not to touch or remove the electrodes when the unit is on, what he or she should report to the PTA, and what the treatment duration will be.
2. Rule out any drug allergy.
3. Position the patient comfortably, and drape him or her appropriately.
4. Inspect the skin, and palpate the skin to determine any tenderness or tightness for electrode placement.
5. Clean the electrode placement site with alcohol.
6. Place the substance on the active electrode.
7. Make sure the unit is off, and then place the electrodes correctly so that the active and dispersive electrodes are in the appropriate areas and are the correct distance apart.
8. Place the correct leads to the appropriate electrodes. (The positive lead should go to the active electrode if a positively charged ion substance is being used, and vice versa.)
9. Set the unit for the appropriate parameters.
10. Turn on the unit and increase the intensity to the patient's tolerance.
11. Stay with the patient for several minutes to monitor his or her response to treatment.
12. Give the patient a call bell.
13. At the end of the treatment, turn off the machine, remove the electrodes, and inspect the skin.
14. Instruct the patient about any skin reactions (redness should fade within 10 to 12 hours after treatment and, any adverse reactions should be reported).
15. Document the treatment.

Electrical Stimulation for Pain Relief

When using electrical stimulation for relieving pain via sensory analgesia, the analgesia produces a tingling sensation. This affects the gating mechanism at the spinal cord level, and pain impulses are not transmitted to higher levels of the brain. When using this method of pain control, the electrodes should go directly over the pain site. One advantage of using sensory stimulation for pain relief is that the treatment can be performed 24 hours per day. This mode of stimulation is used on acute pain, but it can also be appropriate for subacute and chronic pain.

Stimulation of the opiate system can cause pain relief by producing a muscle twitch. It relieves pain by using a low pulse rate at an intense enough level to produce a muscle contraction. This contraction releases endorphins and enkephalins in the body which mimic the action of narcotic drugs to decrease pain. This method is indicated for intense or chronic pain. For this method, electrode placement should be on a motor point, a trigger point, or an acupuncture point. Parameters for treatment are determined by the type, location, and characteristics of the pain.

Pain Control Methods

Subsensory stimulation uses a current that is below the threshold of nerve depolarization. Therefore, the patient will not feel it. Sensory level stimulation uses the gate control theory. With this method, the decrease in pain is quick. However, the carryover is very limited after the unit is turned off. In addition, adaptation to the current is common with this method. Common parameters for this method are:

- pulse frequency—50 to 200
- intensity—sensory
- modulation of parameters—if needed
- amplitude—strong, but comfortable (no muscle contraction)
- treatment time—varies depending on patient tolerance and treatment goals

Because motor level stimulation uses the opiate release theory, it works better with chronic pain than acute pain. Common treatment parameters for this method are:

- low frequency (muscle twitch; no tetanic contraction)
- amplitude—maximum tolerable by the patient
- on/off—two to ten seconds
- treatment time—15 to 60 minutes

Similar to motor level stimulation, noxious level stimulation uses the opiate release method for pain relief. Noxious level stimulation tends to be better for chronic pain and is used when other methods have not worked. Like sensory level stimulation, the onset of pain relief is rapid. However, like motor level, there is more of a carryover than there is with sensory level stimulation. Common treatment parameters for noxious level stimulation are:

- amplitude—increased to a level of tolerable discomfort
- duration—varies depending whether the response is sensory or motor

Pain Control Theories

The gate control theory works on the premise that a vibration travels through type A-beta afferents faster than pain impulses. Because of this, the pain signals are blocked from going to the brain. In addition, this theory hypothesizes that gate control also helps break the pain-spasm-pain cycle.

The opiate mediated control theory states that electrical stimulation can decrease pain because it has been shown to release endorphins (opiates) that are produced by the body. These opiates bind to sites in the central nervous system and decrease pain perception. Different modes of electrical stimulation base the ability to decrease pain on one of these theories.

Rationale for Electrode Placement for Pain Relief

- For diffuse sensory analgesia (generalized pain relief), use four electrodes in a crossed pattern.
- For pain relief using a muscle twitch, put the electrode over a motor point.
- To produce analgesia for performing a painful procedure, use transcutaneous electrical nerve stimulation.
- For opiate release, use a low pulse rate electrical stimulation.

When a physical therapist is developing treatment goals and prescribes electrical stimulation for pain relief, the decision for which method to use is based upon the evaluation findings, the cause of the disabling condition, the previous activity level of the patient, the patient's psychological condition, the patient's prognosis, the current stage (phase) of healing, and the patient's motivation.

During the acute phase of healing, the patient will have pain at rest. For this reason, electrical stimulation is used to break up the pain-spasm-pain cycle because the treatment goal is to decrease this constant pain. Treatment time in the clinical setting is usually 20 to 30 minutes. If the treatment is effective, then the patient may be a candidate for a home unit, and the stimulation can be used up to 24 hours a day.

During the subacute phase of healing, the patient will tend to have pain at the end of the normal range of motion of a joint and will no longer have pain when the joint is at rest. At this time, the treatment goal for using electrical stimulation for pain relief is to decrease the pain resulting from the rehabilitation intervention. Therefore, stimulation is performed at the end of the treatment session.

When a patient is in the chronic phase of healing, he or she will have pain in the end range of motion, when overpressure is applied to the body part. As with the subacute phase healing, electrical stimulation is used to decrease the pain resulting from the rehabilitation intervention. If a patient has chronic pain, then electrical stimulation is used to decrease the intensity of pain at rest and the pain associated from the rehabilitation intervention. The treatment is performed to treat exacerbations in pain and to achieve the treatment goal of maintaining the patient's functional ability. The most common and effective electrical stimulation machines used to treat pain are transcutaneous neuromuscular stimulation, interferential stimulation, and high-volt pulsed current (HVPC).

Transcutaneous Electrical Nerve Stimulation

Three common modes of TENS are conventional, low rate, and burst. Conventional mode TENS decreases pain through the gating effect. The pulses per second for treatment range from 100 to 150. The patient should feel a tingling sensation (sensory). Because of this, conventional mode TENS is appropriate for acute pain and can be worn for up to 24 hours per day. However, although conventional mode TENS produces pain relief quickly, once the unit is turned off, the lasting effects are short-term. Another drawback of this mode is that adaptation to the stimulus is common.

Low rate, or acupuncture-like, mode TENS incorporates repetitive muscle (twitching) contractions using a rate of 2 to 10 pps for 20 to 30 minutes per treatment. Pain relief is brought about through the endorphin release theory. Once the unit is turned off, the lasting effects are longer than conventional TENS. Because this method relies on a muscle contraction, it is not appropriate for acute conditions.

Burst mode TENS uses the same mechanism as low rate TENS. Like low rate TENS, pain relief is brought about using the endorphin release theory. Also, once the unit is turned off, the effects last longer than conventional TENS. This treatment is not appropriate for acute conditions because it relies on a muscle contraction.

Ultrasound with Electrical Stimulation

Ultrasound with electrical stimulation is used to produce pain relief and for facilitating muscle contractions. The transducer of the ultrasound head serves as one electrode while the dispersive electrode of the high-volt machine serves as the other. With this treatment, the effects are the same as ultrasound and electrical stimulation.

Indications

Ultrasound with ES is indicated for:

- muscle spasm
- trigger points

Because this treatment combines both electrical stimulation and ultrasound, the contraindications include all those for both ultrasound and electrical stimulation as previously listed.

Precautions

Precautions mirror the individual ultrasound and electrical stimulation interventions. It has been proposed that the use of ultrasound and electrical stimulation together may be hazardous because this treatment combines high and low frequency currents.

Patient Setup

The PTA follows these specific procedures when utilizing ultrasound with electrical stimulation interventions:

1. Explain the treatment to the patient. Explain why this modality is being used, what sensations the patient should feel, what the patient should and should not do during the treatment, and the duration of the treatment.
2. Position the patient and drape him or her appropriately.
3. Inspect the treatment area.
4. Apply the coupling agent, and secure the dispersive electrode.
5. Set the unit for the appropriate parameters.
6. Place the ultrasound head on the patient and begin to move it.
7. Turn on the ultrasound intensity to the prescribed level.
8. Turn up the intensity of the electrical stimulation to a tolerable level.
9. Continue with the treatment monitoring the patient's response.
10. At the end of the treatment, turn off the machine, clean off the patient and ultrasound head, and remove the dispersive electrode.
11. Inspect the treatment area.
12. Document the treatment.

Interferential Current

Interferential current employs the use of two slightly different frequencies to create an interface. As a result, this blending of waves occurs through constructive and destructive interference. This difference between the two produces a beat frequency (for example 3,300 and 3,200, or 100 beat frequency). The variation in frequency prevents adaptation that is observed in other methods of electrical stimulation. In order to produce the beat frequency, the four electrodes must be crossed.

High-Volt Pulsed Current

HVPC (i.e.; monophasic pulsatile current) is one of the most versatile modes of electrical stimulation. It is effective in treating pain, edema, and muscle guarding; in promoting wound healing; and in muscle reeducation. Contraindications for HVPC are the same as those for other forms of electrical stimulation. The frequency is dictated by the treatment goals. For pain, edema reduction, and exercise, one to two times per day is appropriate. Wound healing can be performed up to four times per day.

Patient Setup

The PTA follows specific procedures when utilizing HVPC interventions:

1. Explain the treatment to the patient, including the rationale for using the modality, the sensations the patient will feel, and the mode of current.
2. Instruct the patient about what and what not to do during the treatment and to tell the PTA if the electrical current is too intense or not strong enough.
3. Tell the patient about the duration of the treatment.
4. Position the patient and drape him or her appropriately.
5. Palpate the treatment area.

6. Place treatment electrodes correctly, confirming that there is good skin contact, appropriate electrode spacing, appropriate number of channels, and that the unit is set at the appropriate parameters.
7. Slowly increase intensity of the unit to the desired level and patient tolerance.
8. Monitor the patient for several minutes, and provide a call bell.
9. At the end of the treatment, turn off the unit, remove the electrodes, and inspect the skin.
10. Attain feedback from the patient regarding the treatment.
11. Document the treatment.

Low-Intensity Stimulators (LIS)

Low-intensity stimulators are also known as micro-current electrical neuromuscular stimulators (MENS). This form of electrical stimulation is delivered at the sub-sensory level, so the patient will not feel the current. This treatment is not designed to elicit a muscle contraction. LIS currents are delivered below one milliamp or 1,000 microamps. Research has demonstrated LIS to be very effective in facilitating bone formation in delayed or non-union fractures in long bones. Other indications include pain management, wound healing, and tendon and ligament healing. Because of its efficacy in patient care, this modality is not common in the clinical setting.

Commonly Used Currents

The table below is a summary of the currents discussed and the indications for the use of each.

CURRENT	INDICATION
Direct	Stimulation of denervated muscle Iontophoresis Wound healing (very low intensity)
High-volt pulsed (monophasic pulsatile current)	Wound healing Pain modulation Acute pain Muscle re-education
Interferential	Pain modulation Chronic edema (muscle pump)
Russian	Muscle strengthening Neuromuscular electrical stimulation
Biphasic pulsatile	Muscle strengthening Neuromuscular electrical stimulation Pain relief

Practice 8

1. Ice massage treatment is an example of heat energy transferred from direct contact with a hot surface to a cooler surface. Which of the following terms correctly identifies this type of heat transfer?
   a. conduction
   b. convection
   c. conversion
   d. radiation

2. Which of the following signs is NOT an example of acute inflammation?
   a. cool skin
   b. dysfunction
   c. edema
   d. redness

3. For which of the following conditions would superficial heat treatment be contraindicated?
   a. acute injury
   b. chronic pain
   c. muscle guarding
   d. muscle spasms

4. Which of the following modalities is an example of conversion heat transfer?
   a. contrast bath
   b. diathermy
   c. hot packs
   d. whirlpool

5. Which of the following effects is one advantage that fluidotherapy has over moist heat and paraffin bath?
   a. decreases pain
   b. desensitization of tissue
   c. promotes tissue healing
   d. vasodilation

6. Which treatment objective below would NOT be accomplished by using cold packs on an involved extremity?
   a. decreased metabolism
   b. decreased nerve conduction velocity
   c. temporary reduction of spasticity
   d. vasodilation

7. A PTA is treating a patient with a diagnosis of left ankle sprain with swelling. The orders are for contrast bath. The PTA should use caution when performing this treatment on this patient because
   a. the injury is in the chronic stage of inflammation.
   b. the patient has edema.
   c. the patient has impaired venous circulation.
   d. the patient has Raynaud's phenomenon.

8. For which modality is 118°F to 126°F considered the proper temperature?
   a. cryotherapy
   b. fluidotherapy
   c. paraffin bath
   d. whirlpool

9. In which type of electrical stimulation must the four electrodes be in a crossed pattern?
   a. interferential current
   b. high-volt pulsed stimulation
   c. low-volt electrical stimulation
   d. Russian stimulation

10. When designing a pain relief treatment plan for a patient, which of the following is the primary consideration when selecting the mode of electrical stimulation to administer?
    a. patient's insurance
    b. patient's motivation
    c. prognosis
    d. stage (phase) of healing

11. A PTA is treating a patient with acute low back pain. For a patient in this phase of the injury, which of the following choices would be the most appropriate rationale for using electrical stimulation?
    a. to decrease pain
    b. to improve function
    c. to increase range of motion
    d. to increase muscle strength

12. A PTA places a patient on Russian current as a part of the treatment program. Which of the following is most likely to be the treatment goal?
    a. to decrease edema
    b. to decrease pain
    c. to increase range of motion
    d. to increase muscle strength

13. Individuals with arthritis tend to benefit from _____ temperatures in hydrotherapy.
    a. cold
    b. cool
    c. neutral
    d. warm

14. A patient is diagnosed with multiple sclerosis, and the plan of care includes hydrotherapy. When trying to decide the temperature of the water, the PTA remembers that patients with multiple sclerosis tend to benefit from which type of temperatures in hydrotherapy?
    a. cool
    b. hot
    c. very cold
    d. warm

15. Which of the following conditions is a contraindication for warm to hot whirlpools?
    a. arthritis
    b. generalized edema
    c. maceration (softening) around wound
    d. subacute inflammation

16. Which of the following modalities would be indicated for a 10-year-old patient who has an acute injury (24 hours since injury) to the left ankle?
    a. continuous ultrasound
    b. ice
    c. Russian stimulation
    d. warm whirlpool

17. The use of electricity to introduce ions into the tissues is
    a. interferential stimulation.
    b. iontophoresis.
    c. phonophoresis.
    d. transcutaneous electrical nerve stimulation.

18. In treatments with ultrasound energy, a coupling medium is used because ultrasonic energy
    a. diminishes the hazard of deep-tissue heating.
    b. reduces the force of the vibrations of energy.
    c. reduces the patient's sensitivity to the passage of energy.
    d. travels better through a medium than it does through air.

19. Which of the following modalities would be most effective in decreasing edema in a patient with a subacute left ankle sprain?
    a. high-voltage electrical stimulation
    b. infrared
    c. intermittent compression
    d. ultrasound

20. A PTA is treating a patient with low back pain with continuous ultrasound. In order to facilitate treatment effectiveness and prevent burns, the PTA should
    a. concentrate on moving the sound head over the bony prominences.
    b. keep the sound head stationary.
    c. remove all air bubbles from the sound head.
    d. treat as large an area of the body as possible.

21. A PTA is treating a patient, and the referral from the physician is for mechanical cervical traction. The PTA and the evaluating physical therapists decide not to perform this treatment on this patient because the patient has a condition that is a contraindication for this modality. Which of the following choices is a contraindication for this modality?
a. chronic herniated disc
b. muscle spasms
c. temporomandibular dysfunction
d. unhealed cervical fracture

22. To ensure their safe operation, whirlpool motors must be connected to which of the following instruments?
a. circuit breaker
b. ground fault interrupter
c. parallel circuit
d. three-prong outlet

23. A PTA is treating an elderly patient with the diagnosis of low back pain and diabetes. The orders are for a moist heat pack to the low back for 20 minutes. Which of the following actions would be most appropriate for treating this patient?
a. Assess the patient to determine whether or not the patient has the ability to differentiate between warmth and cold at the low back region.
b. As hot pack treatment is contraindicated for this patient, the PTA should not perform the treatment.
c. Perform the treatment with the patient in the prone position.
d. Use additional towels between the patient and the hot pack.

24. Which of the following conditions is considered a contraindication to the use of electrical stimulation treatment?
a. acute pain
b. postsurgical pain
c. chronic pain
d. pain that is undiagnosed

25. During the initial phase of a rehabilitation program following an injury, modalities are primarily used in physical therapy in order to achieve which of the following objectives?
a. facilitate muscular strength
b. promote tissue healing
c. restore passive range of motion
d. restore neuromuscular function

26. When performing a paraffin treatment, which of the following steps below must be performed prior to the start of every treatment?
a. Apply plastic wrap to the involved body part.
b. Perform friction massage to the body part.
c. Take girth measurements of the body part.
d. Wash and clean the body part.

27. Which of the following forms of electrical stimulation is used exclusively for pain management?
a. high-volt pulsed stimulation
b. iontophoresis
c. neuromuscular electrical stimulation
d. transcutaneous electrical nerve stimulation

Practice 8 Answers

1. a. The ice is in direct contact with the skin; therefore, the best answer is conduction. As the medium (water) is not moving, it is not convection. Conversion and radiation are not taking place during this treatment.

2. a. Cool skin is not an example of acute inflammation. Skin that is warm to the touch is a sign of acute inflammation, but cool skin is not. Dysfunction, edema, and redness are all signs of acute inflammation.

3. a. Superficial heat treatment is contraindicated for acute injury because heat increases circulation and metabolism. This is not a desired effect during the acute phase of healing. Superficial heat is indicated for chronic pain, muscle guarding, and muscle spasms.

4. b. Diathermy is an example of conversion heat transfer. Contrast baths and hot pack are examples of conduction heat transfer. Whirlpool is an example of both conduction and conversion.

5. b. One advantage that fluidotherapy has over moist heat and paraffin is that fluidotherapy helps to desensitize the tissue. Fluidotherapy, moist heat, and paraffin are all superficial heat modalities that decrease pain, promote tissue healing, and cause vasodilation. However, because the cellulose in the fluidotherapy is moving and making contact with the involved body part, it also helps with desensitization of tissue.

6. d. Vasodilation would not be accomplished by using cold packs on an involved extremity. When cold is applied to tissue, it causes decreased metabolism and nerve conduction velocity, as well as a temporary decrease in spasticity. However, it causes vasoconstriction, not vasodilation.

7. d. The PTA should use caution when performing this treatment on this patient because the patient has Raynaud's phenomenon. Chronic inflammation, edema, and impaired venous circulation are all indications for contrast baths. Raynaud's phenomenon is a precaution for cryotherapy. Therefore, it is a precaution for this modality.

8. c. The temperature for paraffin bath treatment is 118°F to 126°F. This temperature is too high for fluidotherapy and whirlpool. Cryotherapy uses temperatures that are below normal body temperature.

9. a. For interferential current, in order to achieve the beat frequency (interference), the four electrodes must be placed in a crossed pattern. The other forms of electrical stimulation do not require four electrodes or require that they be in a crossed pattern.

10. d. The stage of healing that the patient is in dictates which type of electrical stimulation and treatment parameters to use. The patient's motivation and prognosis are not primary reasons indicating which type of electrical stimulation and treatment parameters to use. The patient's insurance also should not be a guideline for which type of electrical stimulation and treatment parameters to use.

11. a. The main treatment goal during the acute phase is to decrease pain. In the acute phase of inflammation, movement of the body part should be minimized. This is why improving function and increasing range of motion are not appropriate choices during the acute phase. While a patient may be able to do submaximal isometric contractions during the acute phase, increasing strength is not a treatment goal during the acute phase.

12. d. Russian current is used to increase muscle strength and is most likely to be the treatment goal. It is not indicated for decreasing edema and pain or for increasing range of motion. Because of this, Russian current is not appropriate in the acute phase of healing.

13. d. As a rule, individuals with arthritis find warmer water more comfortable than cooler temperatures for treatment and aquatic exercise.

14. a. As a rule, patients with multiple sclerosis find cooler water more comfortable than warmer water for treatment and aquatic exercise.

15. c. Maceration (softening) around a wound is a contraindication for warm to hot whirlpools. Arthritis, generalized edema, and subacute inflammation are indications for warm to hot whirlpools.

16. b. Ice would be indicated for a 10-year-old patient who has an acute injury (24 hours since injury) to the left ankle. Only ice should be used for treatment during the acute phase of inflammation. Continuous ultrasound produces heat, and it is questionable whether or not it should be used with patients with open growth plates. Russian stimulation is indicated for increasing muscular strength, so it should not be used in the acute phase. As heat is contraindicated in the acute phase, a warm whirlpool is not an appropriate treatment.

17. b. The use of electricity to introduce ions into the tissues is called iontophoresis. Iontophoresis uses electricity to drive ions through the skin. Interferential current and transcutaneous electrical nerve stimulation are forms of electrical stimulation but do not drive ions through the skin. Phonophoresis is ultrasound that drives medicated molecules into the tissue.

18. d. In treatments with ultrasound energy, a coupling medium is used because ultrasonic energy travels better through a medium than it does through air. Sound travels faster and more efficiently through denser substances. A coupling medium, such as ultrasound gel, is denser than air.

19. c. Intermittent compression would be the most effective of the modalities listed in decreasing edema in a patient with a subacute left ankle sprain. High-voltage electrical stimulation can be used to treat edema, but it is more effective when used with another modality, such as intermittent compression. Infrared and ultrasound are not indicated for edema.

20. c. In order to facilitate treatment effectiveness of continuous ultrasound and prevent burns in a patient with low back pain, the PTA should remove all air bubbles from the sound head during treatment. Keeping the sound head stationary or moving it on bony prominences with continuous ultrasound can cause burning. Ultrasound treatment on small, localized areas is most effective.

21. d. Unhealed fractures are a contraindication for cervical traction. Temporomandibular dysfunction is a precaution, depending on the harness used. Chronic herniated disc and muscles spasms are indications for traction.

22. b. All electrical equipment that is used with or near water must be plugged into a ground-fault interrupter outlet.

23. a. The PTA should determine whether or not the patient has the ability to differentiate between warmth and cold at the low back region. The PTA should always assess a patient's ability to tell the differences between temperatures. Placing additional towels between the patient and the hot pack is appropriate, but assessing temperature differences still takes priority. Treatment in the prone position is an appropriate action because there is less weight on the hot pack, and the transfer of heat may be less intense. The treatment is not contraindicated. However, caution must be taken when treating this patient.

24. d. Pain that is undiagnosed is a contraindication to the use of electrical stimulation. Acute pain, postsurgical pain, and chronic pain are all indications for the use of electrical stimulation for treatment.

25. b. During the initial phase of a rehabilitation program following an injury, modalities are primarily used in physical therapy in order to promote tissue healing. Facilitating muscular strength, passive range of motion, and neuromuscular control are important treatment goals for later phases of rehabilitation. However, they are not the primary goals early in therapy, and modalities are not the best intervention to achieve them.

26. d. Prior to performing a paraffin bath treatment, the PTA should wash and clean the body part being treated.

27. d. Transcutaneous electrical nerve stimulation is used exclusively for pain management. While all forms of electrical stimulation listed are effective in decreasing pain, transcutaneous electrical nerve stimulation is only used for pain management. The other forms listed are also used for other treatment goals.

Standards of Care Review

CHAPTER SUMMARY

If you have been through a PTA curriculum, or just while reading this book, it should be obvious to you that the PTA must know an incredible amount of information about the human body. The PTA must understand how the musculoskeletal, neuromuscular, cardiovascular, and pulmonary systems all work together to produce normal movement. In addition, the PTA must be able to measure aspects of these systems to collect meaningful data. Also, he or she must be able to apply skilled physical therapy treatments to help the patient develop or restore the ability to move. However, there is one last domain of learning that is critical to review: the standards of proper care.

Safety and Protection

Without knowledge of the standards of care, even a person with a perfect understanding of the body's movement systems and how to apply physical therapy principles would be an abject failure as a PTA. A PTA cannot function in a safe and effective manner without a thorough understanding of patient safety and protection, legal and ethical standards of practice, teaching and learning principles, and evidence-based practice.

Patient Confidentiality

Confidentiality is defined as dealing with private affairs that are not available to those not needing to know, in other words, being entrusted with somebody's personal or private matters. Healthcare professionals have a clear legal and moral obligation to protect the privacy of those entrusted to their care. All those who have access to medical records have an ethical, moral, and legal obligation to protect the confidentiality of that information. The therapist assistant–patient privilege imposes an obligation to maintain the privacy of each patient's communications and personal medical information. Respect for this privacy is a central aspect of the inherent trust placed upon caregivers in the health professions.

The Standards

The Standards of Ethical Conduct for the Physical Therapist Assistant provides a foundation of conduct expected by all physical therapist assistants (not just those who are members of the APTA, as is commonly thought). These standards require the PTA to both maintain confidential information and report others who violate confidentiality. Specifically, standard 2 states that PTAs shall be trustworthy and compassionate in addressing the rights and needs of patients/clients; that PTAs shall protect confidential patient/client information and, in collaboration with the PT, may disclose confidential information to appropriate authorities only when allowed or as required by law. Standard 5 states that PTAs shall fulfill their legal and ethical obligations and that PTAs shall comply with applicable local, state, and federal laws and regulations. In many states, the physical therapy practice acts include language requiring physical therapist assistants to maintain confidentiality and to report any infraction to the practice act and code/standards of ethical conduct by licensed colleagues to the proper authorities.

Violations

The Health Insurance Portability and Accountability Act of 1996 is a federal law, administered through the U.S. Department of Health and Human Services, which regulates the use and disclosure of individuals' health information. Any patient's identifiable information is protected, including name, address, telephone, date of birth, and Social Security number. Violations involving disclosure of personal identifying information, even if accidental, can result in large fines. Knowingly releasing information without proper authorization can lead to charges being brought against the healthcare provider and institution. HIPAA does not allow disclosure of patient information without proper consent—even if the information is disclosed to another health provider for treatment purposes or when a patient puts a healthcare issue in a lawsuit; even then, proper consent must be obtained.

Complaints for violation of HIPAA laws must be filed within 180 days of the violation at www.hhs.gov to the Office of Civil Rights.

INFORMATION IN ACTION

A PTA lives in a city of 7,500 people and works at the local hospital. She is checking out at the grocery store when the clerk with whom she is acquainted says with true concern, "Oh, I heard Bill Smith had a stroke last week and is in the hospital. I hope he's doing okay?" The PTA actually treated Bill that morning and, despite wanting to assure the friend that Bill is doing fine, simply replies that she can't really say but that she knows Bill's wife would appreciate a note or a call.

Informed Consent

Consent is a voluntary agreement by a person with the mental capacity to make an intelligent choice to allow something suggested by another person to be performed on him or her. Informed consent is a legal concept regarding a person's right to be a fully informed participant in all aspects of his or her own healthcare. A patient has a right to understand the potential risks, benefits, and alternatives regarding procedures and treatment plans. Courts in the United States have emphasized and upheld that a competent adult has the right to decline any and all forms of medical intervention, including lifesaving or life-prolonging choices.

The Standards of Ethical Conduct for the Physical Therapist Assistant reflects the standard of care that the physical therapy profession embraces—the duty to respect a patient's, or client's right to self-determination and informed consent. Specifically, standard 2 states that PTAs shall be trustworthy and compassionate in addressing the rights and needs of patients or clients and that PTAs shall provide patients or clients with information regarding the interventions that they provide.

While the PT has the responsibility of providing information to the patient about the physical therapy plan of care and obtaining informed consent, the PTA participates in this every time he or she provides an intervention to the patient. PTAs meet the requirements of informed consent by clearly introducing themselves to the patient as physical therapist assistants, fully explaining the purpose and rationale for all treatments provided, describing what the patient will feel, and detailing the expected response the patient will have to the treatment. In this way, the patient is kept involved and invested in their physical therapy care.

INFORMATION IN ACTION

Rob, a PTA, greets his first patient of the day. "Good morning, Mrs. Jones. My name is Rob Maddox, and I'm a physical therapist assistant. I'll be working with you today. The PT wants us to start with a hot pack application prior to doing stretching exercises for your hamstring strain. The hot pack is a form of moist heat that will be applied directly to the back of your leg for about 20 minutes while you are lying on your stomach. The heat will make your tissues more pliable so the stretching is more effective. The heat should feel very pleasant. The stretch we are going to do involves your lying on your back while I lift your leg straight up for 30–60 seconds at a time. We'll repeat that two to three times. You'll feel a good stretch but no pain. Improving the hamstring flexibility will allow you to return to your gardening activities with more ease. Do you have any questions? Does this sound okay with you?"

The concepts of confidentiality and informed consent exemplify the duality between ethics and law. Providers of physical therapy services are to respect patients' or clients' autonomy by giving the patient or client the information they need to make informed decisions and to protect their privacy in all aspects of care.

Required Reporting

Patient abuse is the mistreatment or neglect of an individual under the care of a healthcare entity. Child abuse is the intentional mental, emotional, sexual, and/or physical injury inflicted by a parent or other person entrusted to care for a minor. Abuse may occur in an institution or in a person's home. Each state has a division responsible for receiving and investigating suspected or confirmed cases of child or elder abuse or neglect. All states have enacted laws to protect abused children. Most states protect healthcare workers reporting with a good-faith belief that the facts being reported are true. The criminal and civil risks for healthcare workers lie in failing to report suspected incidents of elder and/or child abuse.

It is the healthcare worker's responsibility to be aware of the regulations that affect the types of patients or clients in the setting in which he or she works. Failure to comply with the time frames and completion of the necessary forms when reporting abuse can result in fines to the healthcare agency, the provider, and in certain cases, can result in a reprimand on the healthcare worker's license.

Indications of Abuse

Abuse can be physical, psychological, medical, or financial and also includes neglect. Signs of abuse relating to domestic violence and the elderly include:

- broken bones
- bruises
- welts
- discoloration or burns
- absence of hair
- sudden, unexpected outbursts
- agitation or withdrawal not consistent with medical conditions
- a hesitation to speak openly
- implausible stories
- unusual or inappropriate bank account or other financial activity

Many of the physical signs/symptoms are the same in child abuse. Additionally, the abuse may appear as part of a pattern. The PTA may be in a position to identify signs of physical abuse or neglect due to viewing parts of the body exposed for treatment. However, abuse and neglect may be difficult to identify at times because the cause of the injury, behavior, or situation can often be attributed to other causes. For example, an elderly patient with balance problems may have bruising on the hips or buttocks due to falls.

When Abuse Is Suspected

What should the PTA do if abuse is suspected? The first step is to work together with the patient's physical therapist of record and follow facility guidelines. If the patient is a child, most states require reporting if abuse is suspected (not proven). The proper state agency must be contacted and a report made. If the patient is an adult and intimate partner abuse is suspected, the PT and PTA should provide information on where the person can obtain counseling, shelter, and assistance. Because the patient is an adult, she or he has the legal responsibility of reporting the abuse. The best support the PT and PTA can provide is to assure the patient that she or he has done nothing wrong and that no one deserves to be abused. As difficult as it may be for the PT and PTA to accept, the patient will have to decide on any further action to be taken. Finally, if the PTA suspects an elderly person is being abused, the reporting requirements vary state by state and will need to be determined.

While it may personally be very difficult for a PTA to get involved with a domestic violence issue, professionally there is no choice. The PTA has a responsibility to serve as an advocate for the patient. Signs of abuse or neglect must be addressed.

Cultural Competence

The Agency for Healthcare Research and Quality (AHRQ) states that there is no one definition for *culture* that is uniformly referenced. Culture is often defined as the integrated patterns of human behavior that include thoughts, communications, actions, beliefs, customs, as well as institutions of racial, ethnic, religious, or social groups. Cultural competence is the process by which the PTA continually strives to effectively work within the cultural context of the patient. The APTA recommends that students develop cultural competence by:

- assessing their own knowledge and values about diversity
- learning about diverse viewpoints that can influence health positively and negatively
- recognizing the need for a patient-centered approach to delivery of culturally competent physical therapy services
- valuing effective communication between the patient and the therapist
- applying core knowledge about culture, belief systems, and traditions to enhance the patient-therapist interaction

The LEARN Model

The process of attaining cultural competence is an ongoing one and certainly won't be mastered only by reading this review section. However, the LEARN model is a framework that can help promote culturally effective communication.

Listen: Identify and greet family or friends of the patient; ask the English as a second language patient if she would like an interpreter; start interview with an open-ended question; do not interrupt the patient as s/he speaks.

Elicit: The patient's health beliefs are elicited as they pertain to the health condition and the reason for the visit, as well as expectations.

Assess: Determine potential attributes and problems in the person's life that may have an impact on health and health behaviors.

Recommend: A plan of action is recommended with an explanation for your rationale.

Negotiate: A plan of action is negotiated with the patient after you have made your recommendations.

The goal of providing culturally competent care is simply to foster an environment in which each patient can meet therapy goals within the dimensions of his or her own value system.

Emergency Response

Despite strict adherence to safety guidelines, it is likely that a patient may experience a life-threatening emergency in the presence of the physical therapist assistant. Effectively responding to a patient or client and to environmental emergencies in one's practice setting is a competency expectation for PTAs. Advanced planning and careful observance of facility policies and procedures for emergencies in the practice setting are essential to minimizing risk and enhancing optimal patient safety.

Effective emergency preparedness includes:

- understanding policies/procedures and staying up-to-date as changes are enacted
- indentifying that an emergency exists in a timely manner
- taking necessary action, which may require seeking assistance in order to minimize potential negative results of the emergency
- competently using emergency management procedures to protect and save patients or clients and others (for example, the use of fire, tornado, hurricane, or disaster evacuation measures or the use of seizure precautions)
- providing emergency care including cardiopulmonary resuscitation (CPR) and basic first aid

The physical therapist assistant should communicate all pertinent information to the supervising physical therapist and/or therapist of record as well as to the facility manager in the event of a need for emergent care. The PTA should document the incident according to facility policies.

Employee Rights

Most of the rights and responsibilities of physical therapist assistants in the healthcare setting are regulated by both state and federal laws. Employment practice matters include but are not limited to wages, hours, working conditions, union activity, worker's compensation laws, occupational safety and health laws, and employment discrimination laws.

Historically, labor issues have been a source of discrimination often requiring court action to resolve. A variety of federal and state laws have been enacted to protect employees from unfair treatment at work. An example is the Equal Pay Act (EPA) of 1963, which prohibits gender discrimination regarding compensation. The Equal Employment Opportunity Commission (EEOC) enforces this and other laws related to fair employment practices.

Employee rights include:

- equal pay for equal work
- refusing to participate in care that contradicts one's fundamental beliefs, such as abortions or assisted suicide
- questioning a patient's care when harm to the patient is imminent
- being free from sexual harassment and intimidation
- being treated with dignity and respect
- employment at will
- fair treatment

Responsibility and Accountability

Healthcare providers hold special privileges with respect to the inherent trust placed in them by those they serve. With privilege comes great responsibility and accountability.

With every healthcare worker right comes a corresponding duty. These duties include:

- being a patient advocate
- honoring the patient's right to be an informed participant in all aspects of his or her care (patient autonomy)
- adherence to the Standards of Conduct for the PTA (Code of Ethics)
- maintaining confidentiality and following HIPAA regulations
- exercising good judgment
- practicing patient/client-centered care—putting the client's or patient's interest first and foremost
- adherence to safe practices
- displaying professionalism
- reporting unethical behavior and/or suspected patient abuse
- whistle-blowing if necessary (Whistle-blowing is defined as an act of someone who believes the public interest overrides the interest of the organization and contacts authorities if the company is involved in corrupt, illegal, fraudulent, or harmful activity.)

Administrative Law and Risk Management

Administrative law is an extensive body of public law which controls the operations of federal and state governments. Administrative agencies direct the implementation and oversight of laws created by Congress and state legislatures. Administrative laws deal with the enforcement and punishment of violations of rules and regulations that govern professions and services. Every licensed individual of a profession has a corresponding law that outlines the expectations and rules that must be followed by all those licensed in that profession. Physical therapists, physical therapist assistants, and students must abide by the state practice act in order to comply with administrative law. A violation of the rules and regulations set forth in the state-specific practice act could lead to an individual having a complaint filed against his or her license.

Physical therapy state practice acts vary greatly. It is imperative that each licensed PTA thoroughly understand and comply with the specific regulations in the state(s) in which he or she practices.

Risk management related to physical therapy practice is the process of identifying liability risks and ways to reduce them. Every lawsuit will involve an employee. The application process, ongoing competency training, and adherence to policy and procedures are areas of personnel management linked to litigation outcomes.

The Hiring Process

The hiring process must be consistent and completed for each employee with the goal of verifying that the person is qualified for the position and that there is no reason for exclusion. Gaps in work history, background checks, drug screens, and reference checks are frequent requirements when seeking employment as a PTA.

Essential Documentation

An initial orientation checklist, a copy of the specific job description, and the department's policy and procedure manual need to be completed, signed, and dated and kept in the employee's file. Ongoing training updates as dictated by the company or by federal or state law must be implemented to demonstrate continued competency. The physical therapist assistant must track and document completion of the minimal hours of continued education as dictated by the state practice act for re-licensure or credentialing.

Performance Reviews

Performance reviews for PTAs usually include explicit documentation that the clinician is competent to perform the job duties specific to employment. The PTAs plans to enhance proficiency in any given area of practice should be completed at least annually and documented in his or her file.

Incidents Reports

Due to the inherent risk involved in the practice of physical therapy, it is prudent to abide conscientiously by the policies, procedures, and risk management strategies set forth by one's employer. However, in the event that something considered out of the ordinary or unexpected occurs, the PTA should write an incident report, regardless of whether or not the incident resulted in a negative outcome. An incident report provides a place to document the circumstances of the event and an opportunity for an internal investigation surrounding the what, how, and why, as well as what can be done to reduce the risk of it happening again. Documents (such as incident reports) created in anticipation of litigation are typically not required to be submitted to the other party.

Practice 1

1. The legal term for a patient's right to be a fully informed participant in his or her own care is
  a. confidentiality.
  b. informed consent.
  c. coercion.
  d. incident reporting.

2. Which of the following is NOT specifically related to reducing risk of infection in the healthcare environment?
  a. providing all patients with a call light or call bell
  b. ensuring a clear work space
  c. using bar soap for hand washing
  d. stopping to wipe up a wet area on the tile floor

3. The approach to infection control in which all blood and bodily fluids are considered contaminated is called
  a. universal precaution.
  b. standard precaution.
  c. universal barrier.
  d. standard barrier.

4. True or false: The PTA should wear personal protective equipment (PPE) when treating every patient in the bone marrow transplant unit.
  a. true because the patients might infect the PTA
  b. true because the PTA might infect the patients
  c. false unless the patients in the transplant unit have a transmissible infection
  d. false unless the PTA has a transmissible infections

5. If a PTA is being sexually harassed by her employer, what specifically is this PTA's responsibility as a healthcare worker and member of the physical therapy profession?
  a. quit this job
  b. blow the whistle on this company to the EEOC
  c. put this on Facebook® so no one else will unknowingly accept employment from this company
  d. submit a complaint to the state licensing board

6. A breech of which document is illegal for all physical therapists and physical therapist assistants?
  a. core values
  b. company policy
  c. generic abilities
  d. practice act

7. Which of the following is the responsibility of the PTA in reducing liability risk in providing patient care?
  a. participating in the annual performance evaluation
  b. hiring a competent attorney
  c. avoiding the need for a drug test
  d. having personal liability insurance

8. Which of the following is NOT considered among the accepted roles of the PTA?
  a. measuring the active flexion of a patient following total knee arthroplasty
  b. teaching body mechanics to all new employees at a long-term care facility as a part of the facility's orientation program
  c. assessing a home and recommending modifications needed for a patient following a CVA
  d. documenting the medical record following a patient treatment session

9. Which of the following statements is true once the PTA has experience and specialization in an area?
a. General supervision may occur.
b. The number of PTAs that a PT can supervise can increase.
c. The PTA can do spinal mobilization.
d. The PT may delegate more readily.

Practice 1 Answers

1. b. The legal term for a patient's right to be a fully informed participant in all aspects of his or her own healthcare is informed consent. A patient has a right to understand the potential risks, benefits, and alternatives available regarding procedures and treatment plans.

2. c. Using bar soap for hand washing is not specifically related to reducing risk of infection in the healthcare environment. In order to reduce risk of infection in a healthcare environment, hand washing must be done with water, 3 to 5 mL of liquid soap, and friction for at least 10 to 15 seconds using a consistent technique that includes all surfaces of the wrists, hands, and fingers. The safety of each patient or client is of utmost importance to every member of the healthcare team. Creating and abiding by policy and procedures related to risk management activities and a commitment of every employee to maintain equipment that functions properly in a safe environment is required.

3. a. Universal precaution is an approach to infection control in which all blood and body fluids are managed as though they are contaminated.

4. b. When a patient's immune system is not working properly (when the patient is immunosupressed), the purpose of PPE is to protect the patient from the caregiver, whose body carries microorganisms that would not normally create an infection.

5. d. If a PTA is being sexually harassed by her employer, it is the PTA's responsibility as a healthcare worker and member of the physical therapy profession to submit a complaint to the state licensing board.

6. d. A breach of the practice act is illegal for all physical therapists and physical therapist assistants. Physical therapists, physical therapist assistants, and students studying to become physical therapists or physical therapist assistants must abide by the state practice act in order to comply with administrative law.

7. a. Performance evaluations, including explicit documentation that the clinician is competent to perform the job duties specific to employment and plans to enhance proficiency in any given area of practice, should be completed at least annually.

8. c. It is beyond the scope of the PTA to assess a home and recommend modifications needed for a patient following a CVA. Instead, the physical therapist would be responsible for assessing a home and recommending modifications needed for a patient following a CVA. It is the PT's responsibility to direct the course and progression of the patient's or client's plan of care.

9. d. Regardless of what, if any, aspects of care the PT chooses to involve the PTA in, the PT is ultimately responsible for and must be involved in each person's care. Delegation is a matter of deciding which parts of a patient or client's care will be performed by whom. In order to establish the trust needed for the PT to confidently share the responsibility of patient care with the PTA, the PTA must demonstrate competence, including an accurate self-assessment of limitations; the ability to make proper judgments; and communicating accurately and in a timely manner.

Roles and Responsibilities of the PTA

Physical therapist assistants are graduates of programs that are accredited by the Commission on Accreditation for Physical Therapy Education. Most, but not all, states require licensure or credentialing to work as a physical therapist assistant. PTAs provide physical therapy services only under the direction and supervision of physical therapists.

Role of the Physical Therapist Assistant

The roles of the physical therapist and the physical therapist assistant continue to evolve as radical changes in the healthcare delivery system unfold and as the profession of physical therapy becomes more autonomous and proactive. The specific limitations and expectations of the physical therapist assistant, within the clinical setting, are dictated by the practice act of each state.

PTAs assist PTs in the following ways:

- assisting with data collection
- implementing patient interventions
- making appropriate judgments
- modifying interventions within the PT's established plan of care
- participating in discharge planning and follow-up care
- documenting the care provided
- educating and interacting with PT and PTA students, aides, volunteers, patients, families, and caregivers
- demonstrating an understanding of the significance and impact of cultural and individual differences

Scope of Work

The scope of work of the PTA is determined by the supervising PT on the basis of federal and state laws and regulations, ethical standards, competency and skill levels, standards of practice established by the profession, and current workplace expectations. Differences of opinion regarding the appropriate role and utilization of PTAs have existed since the early 1960s, with the inception of the PTA profession. While profession-wide consensus regarding the educational preparation, accreditation requirements, and state laws concerning minimal standards have mostly been built, the specific job duties and supervision of the physical therapist assistant in the clinic or at the bedside remain controversial and vary greatly state to state.

The American Physical Therapy Association delineates the clinical relationship and practice requirements concerning support personnel in a variety of policies, positions, and standards. (To review these specific core documents, see www.apta.org/governance/HOD.) Regardless of state or practice setting, the PT is legally and ethically responsible for the physical therapy provided to the patient, whether or not any of the care has been delegated to a PTA.

Physical therapists have a responsibility to deliver services in ways that protect the public safety and maximize the availability of their services. They do this through direct delivery of services in conjunction with responsible utilization of physical therapist assistants, who assist with selected components of intervention. The physical therapist assistant is the only individual permitted to assist a physical therapist in selected interventions under the direction and supervision of a physical therapist.

Direction and Supervision by the PT

Direction and supervision are essential in the provision of quality physical therapy services. The degree of direction and supervision necessary for assuring quality physical therapy services is dependent upon many factors, including the education, experiences, and responsibilities of the parties involved, as well as the organizational structure in which the physical therapy services are provided.

Regardless of the setting in which the physical therapy service is provided, the following responsibilities must be borne solely by the physical therapist:

1. Interpretation of referrals when available
2. Initial examination, evaluation, diagnosis, and prognosis
3. Development or modification of a plan of care that is based on the initial examination or reexamination and that includes the physical therapy goals and outcomes
4. Determination of when the expertise and decision-making capability of the physical therapist requires personally rendering physical therapy interventions and when it may be appropriate to utilize the physical therapist assistant. A physical therapist should determine the most appropriate utilization of the physical therapist assistant, which provides for the delivery of service that is safe, effective, and efficient.
5. Reexamination of the patient or client in light of the patient's goals and revision of the plan of care when indicated
6. Establishment of the discharge plan and documentation of discharge summary or status
7. Oversight of all documentation for services rendered to each patient or client

The physical therapist remains responsible for the physical therapy services provided when the PT's plan of care involves the PTA assisting with selected interventions. The determination to utilize physical therapist assistants for selected interventions requires the education, expertise, and professional judgment of a physical therapist as described by the Standards of Practice, Guide to Professional Conduct, and Code of Ethics.

In determining the appropriate extent of assistance from the physical therapist assistant, the physical therapist should consider the following:

- the PTA's education, training, experience, and skill level
- patient or client criticality, acuity, stability, and complexity
- the predictability of the consequences
- the setting in which the care is being delivered
- federal and state statutes
- liability and risk management concerns
- the mission of physical therapy services for the setting
- the needed frequency of reexamination

The physical therapist assistant is a technically educated healthcare provider who assists the physical therapist in the provision of physical therapy. The physical therapist assistant is a graduate of a physical therapist assistant program accredited by the Commission on Accreditation in Physical Therapy Education.

The physical therapist is directly responsible for the actions of the physical therapist assistant related to patient or client management. The PTA may perform selected physical therapy interventions under the direction and at least general supervision of the physical therapist. In general supervision, the physical therapist is not required to be on-site for direction and supervision, but he or she must be available at least by telecommunications. The ability of the PTA to perform the selected interventions as directed should be assessed on an ongoing basis by the supervising physical therapist. The PTA makes modifications to selected interventions either to progress the patient or client as directed by the physical therapist or to ensure patient or client safety and comfort.

In all practice settings, the performance of selected interventions by the PTA must be consistent with safe and legal physical therapy practice and should be predicated on the complexity and acuity of the patient's or client's needs, proximity and accessibility to the physical therapist, supervision available in the event of emergencies or critical events, and the type of setting in which the service is provided. When a physical therapist is supervising a physical therapist assistant in any off-site setting, the following requirements must be observed:

- A physical therapist must be accessible by telecommunications to the physical therapist assistant at all times while the PTA is treating patients or clients.
- There must be regularly scheduled and documented conferences with the PTA regarding patients or clients, the frequency of which is determined by the needs of the patient or client and the needs of the physical therapist assistant.
- In those situations in which the PTA is involved in the care of a patient or client, a supervisory visit by the physical therapist must be made upon the PTA's request for a reexamination when a change is required in the plan of care, prior to any planned discharge, or in response to a change in the patient's or client's medical status. A visit should occur at least once a month (or at a higher frequency when established by the PT) in accordance with the needs of the patient or client.

A supervisory visit should include an on-site reexamination of the patient or client, an on-site review of the plan of care with appropriate revision or termination, and an evaluation of need and recommendation for utilization of outside resources.

Supervision, Direction, and Delegation

Supervision is a mutual responsibility between the PT and the PTA. Regardless of philosophy, competency, experience, reimbursement guidelines, or clinical setting, the minimally acceptable level of supervision of the PTA by the PT is as outlined in the state practice act. Levels of supervision required vary state to state but often include:

- **General supervision.** General supervision allows the PTA to practice without a PT continuously on the premises. The supervising PT must be readily available by telecommunications.
- **Periodic on-site supervision.** In periodic on-site supervision, the specific frequencies in which the PT must be physically present are defined. State requirements vary from 50% of the PTA's workweek to a specific number of patient encounters to once every two weeks.
- **Full on-site supervision.** In full on-site supervision, the supervising PT must be on the premises at all times when the PTA is providing patient-related care.

Many states limit the number of PTAs that one PT may supervise at any one time. There are also specific limits and requirements imposed by payer sources about utilization and PT supervision. It is imperative for the PTA to know and understand the laws for the state(s) in which he or she provides services, as well as for the various insurance companies that will be billed for these services. Failure to comply with these laws can lead to fines and the loss of the ability to practice.

Extent of PTA Involvement

It is the PT's responsibility to direct the course and progression of the patient or client's plan of care. Delegation is a matter of deciding who will perform which parts of a patient's or client's care. In order to establish the trust needed for the PT to confidently share the responsibility of patient care, the PTA must demonstrate competence (including accurate self-assessment of limitations); make proper judgments; and communicate accurately and in a timely manner.

The trust and rapport between the PT and PTA is very important because the PT must trust the PTA enough to delegate work to him or her. Effective delegation strategies were proposed as a taxonomy by Nancy Watts in a landmark article in 1971. Within this systematic approach for the division of responsibility, tasks are analyzed in terms of the process of decision making ("deciding" behaviors) versus delivering an intervention ("doing" behaviors) required in the practice of physical therapy. Factors to be considered specifically related to patient care include:

- **Predictability of consequence.** How uncertain is the situation?
- **Stability of the situation.** How much and how quickly is change likely to occur?
- **Observability of basic indicators.** How easy or difficult is it to elicit a response in order to detect a change in the patient's condition?
- **Ambiguity of basic indicators.** How difficult is it to interpret the changes occurring or to confuse changes with something else?
- **Criticality of results.** How serious is a consequence of a poor choice or inadequate recognition of an untoward change in condition?

Legal and Ethical Parameters

Laws are created to prevent harm to others while protecting individual rights. Regulations are laws that have to do with the fair distribution of goods and services which, in healthcare, relates to service delivery and reimbursement. There are four sources of law in the United States:

- **Constitutional law.** Guarantees personal rights and liberties in the Bill of Rights; typically takes precedence over all other laws.
- **Statutory law.** Established through state or federal legislatures. The physical therapy practice acts are examples of state statutes which is that differ in each state.
- **Common law.** Legal precedent which is created from judicial decisions that have not yet been enacted through a statute.

- **Administrative law.** State and/or federal agencies created to oversee the rules and regulations governing many aspects of healthcare delivery and those who provide it. As previously mentioned in this chapter (under Risk Management), licensure requirements to practice as a physical therapist assistant serve as examples of state administrative law. The regulations by which the Medicare system operates are examples of federal administrative law.

The laws and regulations that healthcare providers must follow are increasing and becoming more complex. Because of this, physical therapist assistants must be vigilant about remaining up-to-date and following the various laws, regulations, and standards of practice that apply to the profession and the specific practice setting. Medicare, for example, holds each provider responsible for any claim that is billed. It is considered fraud if billing is submitted that is not in compliance with Medicare regulations.

Accreditation and Standards

In addition to government authorities, external accrediting agencies establish standards and processes to monitor aspects of healthcare delivery in order to achieve and maintain accreditation status. Accreditation then serves as a benchmark of quality which often becomes required in order to remain in operation. The Joint Commission on Accreditation of Healthcare Organizations (JCAHO), for example, establishes expectations for acute care institutions that are required in order for the hospital to be eligible to participate in federal government reimbursement. The American Physical Therapy Association defines the standards of practice for physical therapy, which in turn define the acceptable standards of care for the profession. Although these standards are not laws themselves, various federal and state laws refer to and uphold them. The standards of care for physical therapy delivery are included in state physical therapy practice acts.

Ethical Behavior

Ethical behavior is how one chooses to conduct oneself in personal and professional endeavors. Ethical behavior involves doing the best or right thing in a given situation. Ethical standards dictate conduct and moral choices, as defined by specific professions, societies, religions, and cultures. Professions establish their own explicit codes of conduct, which serve to protect the public and provide standards for professional behavior. The APTA Code of Ethics and Guide for Conduct for the Physical Therapist Assistant protects the rights of patients or clients, establishes standards of autonomy and supervision, defines standards for peer review and reimbursement, and outlines expectations and responsibilities for members of the profession. Although only members of the APTA can be subjected to disciplinary processes regarding purely ethical violations, most state practice acts include language that holds each physical therapist and physical therapist assistant bound to the ethical standards set forth by the professional association. Indeed, if one is deemed unethical, a violation of the law may have occurred as well.

Fundamental Ethical Principles for PTAs

TERM	DEFINITION
Autonomy	To make one's own choices; be an informed participant in all aspects of one's own care
Beneficence	To promote good
Confidentiality	Keeping sensitive patient information in confidence; upholding HIPAA
Duty	Obligation to another individual/society
Fidelity	To keep promises and commitments; loyalty to patients or clients as well as to colleagues
Informed consent	To present benefits and risks of planned interventions to patients
Justice	To distribute benefits and burdens fairly
Non-maleficence	To "do no harm" (even in some cases when one cannot do good)
Paternalism	Failure to respect the autonomy of another person
Veracity	To speak and act truthfully

Each of the principles in the Standards of Ethical Conduct for the PTA represents one or more fundamental ethical principles for PTAs.

An ethical dilemma is a situation in which one must make performance decisions between unfavorable options. When there are two viable alternatives, however, there is usually no clear immediate answer due to conflicting values and factors. This circumstance requires careful reflection and moral reasoning based on the specific people and issues at hand. Various types of decision-making models exist to serve as a way to determine plausible options for resolution. Who is the recipient of an organ transplant when there are multiple people on a transplant list? This is a classical example of an ethical dilemma involving distributive justice. Metaethics takes place when the right thing to do exists but may be clouded by temptation and/or pressures to act differently. Cutting short a patient's treatment time because it is close to quitting time and everyone else is finished for the day is an example of metaethics. The morally acceptable or right thing to do is to stay to treat the patient instead of doing what is popular and convenient.

In addition to carrying out clinical responsibilities consistent with all elements of the state practice act and regulatory agencies as well as the Standards of Ethical Conduct for the PTA, it is imperative that effective communication and ongoing collaboration with each therapist of record and supervising physical therapist occur throughout the provision of services. It is essential that the PTA be aware of the standards of the profession.

Teaching and Learning

As more Americans reach retirement age and live longer, with many likely to be obese, strategies for health promotion and prevention of disease and disability become an even more important aspect of physical therapy management. Similarly, as healthcare costs continue to escalate, cost containment strategies have influenced and will continue to influence length of stay at in-patient facilities and number of visits allowed for therapy services. Accordingly, the provision of effective patient- or client-related instruction takes on an increasingly important role in achieving successful patient/client outcomes. Excellent communication and teaching skills are critical for the PTA when participating in various aspects of patient/client education.

Learning is defined as a relatively permanent change in performance or behavior. Performance is defined as a temporary change in ability or behavior. Typically, the goal for successful patient or client outcomes involves learning a movement, skill, or behavioral modification versus only performing one in the presence of the PT or the PTA.

The physical therapist assistant must incorporate principles of learning and apply effective teaching strategies when instructing a patient. While there are many theories related to teaching and learning principles, the following are central tenets that are essential for the (PTA) teacher:

- demonstrating genuine concern and respect for the learner
- recognizing and matching the learning style of the learner
- actively engaging the learner (making the instructions meaningful)
- success begets success: providing opportunities for the person to be successful at some aspect of the activity so he or she can build upon that success
- utilizing feedback and practice schedules consistent with the PT's plan of care and current research findings
- providing ample practice recognizing that "practice only makes perfect if what is being practiced is correct"
- recognizing that the learner must be interested and motivated to learn.
- showing (demonstrate), telling (explain step by step), doing (learner practices), and reflecting (the learner critiques self or others)

Evidence-Based Practice (EBP)

Evidence-based practice is the "integration of the best possible research evidence with clinical expertise and patient/client values, to optimize patient/client outcomes and quality of life and to achieve the highest level of excellence in the provision of physical therapy services. Evidence includes randomized or nonrandomized controlled trials; testimony or theory; meta-analysis; case reports and anecdotes; observational studies; narrative review article; case series in decision making for clinical practice and policy; effectiveness research for guidelines development; patient outcomes research; and coverage decisions by healthcare plans."

Physical therapists utilize critical thinking processes (such as utilizing the best available evidence and making objective judgments on the basis of well-supported reasons) in order to perform the five elements of the patient/client management model: examination, evaluation, diagnosis, prognosis (including plan of care), and intervention. Physical therapist assistants work closely with the PT in clinical problem-solving activities including the following:

- participating in patient status judgments by reporting changes to the therapist of record and requesting patient reexamination or revisions to intervention options within the established plan of care
- adjusting or withholding interventions based on patient status as determined through observation, data collection, and interpretive processes within the PT's established plan of care
- possessing the requisite knowledge to identify the situation, weigh alternatives, and select appropriate responses within the plan of care established by the PT
- identifying potential consequences of those solutions

Evidence that justifies physical therapy interventions and more accurately predicts what the patient/client can expect within a particular timeframe (prognosis) is increasingly expected by more savvy consumers and third-party payers with higher accountability expectations. Evaluating outcomes, with regard to whether the patient improved and/or met his or her goals, is also expected, and if attained, how effectively these goals were met. For example, "What did the therapy cost—in terms of time and resources?" "How cost-effective is a particular intervention or strategy over another?" These questions represent evidence-based practices that the PTA, working in conjunction with the PT, must consider.

PTAs add value in contributing their skills and observations in gathering and communicating vital information to support the clinical judgment of PTs. The PTA is expected to review and use the professional literature related to diagnosis, conditions, and therapy interventions. The APTA Standards of Care, the Standards of Ethical Conduct for the PTA, and various administrative laws include continued competency as a requirement for the physical therapist assistant as a member of the healthcare team.

Standardized Tests and Measures and Methodology

Obtaining measurements is an integral part of the physical therapist's practice. The PT synthesizes information collected during the initial examination (and subsequent examinations) in order to establish the diagnosis, prognosis, and plan of care. The use of tests and measures provides information used to determine goals and anticipated outcomes. Subsequent examinations (reexaminations) at regular intervals provide data to document changes in patient or client status and the progress the patient or client is making toward functional goals and expected outcomes.

The physical therapist assistant assists in the collection of data as directed by the PT. The *Guide to Physical Therapist Practice* lists 24 categories of tests and measures utilized in physical therapist management. Measurement and outcomes whose reliability and validity have been documented in peer-reviewed literature are increasingly important aspects of practice. Reliability is the extent to which a measurement is consistent time after time with as little variation as possible. Validity is the degree to which something measures what it intends or claims to measure.

There are multiple forms of reliability and validity described within the professional literature. A myriad of articles investigating the reliability and validity related to the measurement of impairment, functional limitation, and disability have been and continue to be published. It is imperative that the physical therapist assistant be competent in knowing how to administer every aspect of a standardized test or measure as directed by the physical therapist. The PTA must also understand the meaning of the results of each measure related to interventions and to the aspects of care to which they are assigned.

Standards of Ethical Conduct for the Physical Therapist Assistant

Effective July 1, 2010. www.apta.org/ethics

Preamble

The Standards of Ethical Conduct for the Physical Therapist Assistant (Standards of Ethical Conduct) delineate the ethical obligations of all physical therapist assistants as determined by the House of Delegates of the American Physical Therapy Association (APTA). The Standards of Ethical Conduct provide a foundation for conduct to which all physical therapist assistants shall adhere. Fundamental to the Standards of Ethical Conduct is the special obligation of physical therapist assistants to enable patients/clients to achieve greater independence, health and wellness, and enhanced quality of life.

No document that delineates ethical standards can address every situation. Physical therapist assistants are encouraged to seek additional advice or consultation in instances where the guidance of the Standards of Ethical Conduct may not be definitive.

Standards

Standard 1: Physical therapist assistants shall respect the inherent dignity and rights, of all individuals.

1A. Physical therapist assistants shall act in a respectful manner toward each person regardless of age, gender, race, nationality, religion, ethnicity, social or economic status, sexual orientation, health condition, or disability.

1B. Physical therapist assistants shall recognize their personal biases and shall not discriminate against others in the provision of physical therapy services.

Standard 2: Physical therapist assistants shall be trustworthy and compassionate in addressing the rights and needs of patients/clients.

2A. Physical therapist assistants shall act in the best interests of patients/clients over the interests of the physical therapist assistant.

2B. Physical therapist assistants shall provide physical therapy interventions with compassionate and caring behaviors that incorporate the individual and cultural differences of patients/clients.

2C. Physical therapist assistants shall provide patients/clients with information regarding the interventions they provide.

2D. Physical therapist assistants shall protect confidential patient/client information and, in collaboration with the physical therapist, may disclose confidential information to appropriate authorities only when allowed or as required by law.

Standard 3: Physical therapist assistants shall make sound decisions in collaboration with the physical therapist and within the boundaries established by laws and regulations.

3A. Physical therapist assistants shall make objective decisions in the patient's/client's best interest in all practice settings.

3B. Physical therapist assistants shall be guided by information about best practice regarding physical therapy interventions.

3C. Physical therapist assistants shall make decisions based upon their level of competence and consistent with patient/client values.

3D. Physical therapist assistants shall not engage in conflicts of interest that interfere with making sound decisions.

3E. Physical therapist assistants shall provide physical therapy services under the direction and supervision of a physical therapist and shall communicate with the physical therapist when patient/client status requires modifications to the established plan of care.

Standard 4: Physical therapist assistants shall demonstrate integrity in their relationships with patients/clients, families, colleagues, students, other healthcare providers, employers, payers, and the public.

4A. Physical therapist assistants shall provide truthful, accurate, and relevant information and shall not make misleading representations.

4B. Physical therapist assistants shall not exploit persons over whom they have supervisory, evaluative, or other authority (e.g., patients/clients, students, supervisees, research participants, or employees).

4C. Physical therapist assistants shall discourage misconduct by healthcare professionals and report illegal or unethical acts to the relevant authority, when appropriate.

4D. Physical therapist assistants shall report suspected cases of abuse involving children or vulnerable adults to the supervising physical therapist and the appropriate authority, subject to law.

4E. Physical therapist assistants shall not engage in any sexual relationship with any of their patients/clients, supervisees, or students.

4F. Physical therapist assistants shall not harass anyone verbally, physically, emotionally, or sexually.

Standard 5: Physical therapist assistants shall fulfill their legal and ethical obligations.

5A. Physical therapist assistants shall comply with applicable local, state, and federal laws and regulations.

5B. Physical therapist assistants shall support the supervisory role of the physical therapist to ensure quality care and promote patient/client safety.

5C. Physical therapist assistants involved in research shall abide by accepted standards governing protection of research participants.

5D. Physical therapist assistants shall encourage colleagues with physical, psychological, or substance related impairments that may adversely impact their professional responsibilities to seek assistance or counsel.

5E. Physical therapist assistants who have knowledge that a colleague is unable to perform their professional responsibilities with reasonable skill and safety shall report this information to the appropriate authority.

Standard 6: Physical therapist assistants shall enhance their competence through the lifelong acquisition and refinement of knowledge, skills, and abilities.

6A. Physical therapist assistants shall achieve and maintain clinical competence.

6B. Physical therapist assistants shall engage in lifelong learning consistent with changes in their roles and responsibilities and advances in the practice of physical therapy.

6C. Physical therapist assistants shall support practice environments that support career development and lifelong learning.

Standard 7: Physical therapist assistants shall support organizational behaviors and business practices that benefit patients/clients and society.

7A. Physical therapist assistants shall promote work environments that support ethical and accountable decision making.

7B. Physical therapist assistants shall not accept gifts or other considerations that influence or give an appearance of influencing their decisions.

7C. Physical therapist assistants shall fully disclose any financial interest they have in products or services that they recommend to patients/clients.

7D. Physical therapist assistants shall ensure that documentation for their interventions accurately reflects the nature and extent of the services provided.

7E. Physical therapist assistants shall refrain from employment arrangements or other arrangements that prevent them from fulfilling ethical obligations to patients/clients.

Standard 8: Physical therapist assistants shall participate in efforts to meet the health needs of people locally, nationally, or globally.

8A. Physical therapist assistants shall support organizations that meet the health needs of people who are economically disadvantaged, uninsured, and underinsured.

8B. Physical therapist assistants shall advocate for people with impairments, activity limitations, participation restrictions, and disabilities in order to promote their participation in community and society.

8C. Physical therapist assistants shall be responsible stewards of healthcare resources by collaborating with physical therapists in order to avoid over-utilization or under-utilization of physical therapy services.

8D. Physical therapist assistants shall educate members of the public about the benefits of physical therapy.

Proviso: The Standards of Ethical Conduct for the Physical Therapist Assistant as substituted will take effect July 1, 2010, to allow for education of APTA members and nonmembers.

Practice 2

1. The specific expectations and limitations of the physical therapist assistant in clinical practice are
   a. dictated by the Standards of Conduct of the PTA.
   b. set forth by the Commission on Physical Therapy Education.
   c. dictated by the state practice act.
   d. determined by the company's policies.

2. All of the following are within the purview of the PTA as directed by the PT EXCEPT
   a. assisting with data collection.
   b. modifying interventions within the established plan of care.
   c. documenting care provided.
   d. performing systems review.

3. Who is responsible for directing the course and progression of the patient's or client's plan of care?
   a. physical therapist
   b. PTA once the patient or client is delegated to the PTA
   c. this follows company policy because it depends on setting
   d. referring physician

4. Which of the following statements is false concerning the scope of work of the PTA?
   a. The PTA's scope of work is partially determined by federal and state laws.
   b. The PTA's scope of work has achieved profession-wide consensus.
   c. The PTA's scope of work is partially determined by the competency and skill levels of the PT and the PTA.
   d. The PTA's scope of work remains controversial.

5. Which of the following statements defines general supervision per state practice acts?
   a. The PT must be on the premises when the PTA is providing patient-related care.
   b. The PT is on-site at specified frequencies as stipulated within the law.
   c. The PTA can practice without the PT's being directly on premises, but the PT must be available through telecommunications.
   d. The PT must be within the line of sight while the PTA works.

6. Which of the following statements defines full on-site supervision per state practice acts?
   a. The PT must be on the premises when the PTA is providing patient-related care.
   b. The PT is on-site at specified frequencies as stipulated within the law.
   c. The PTA can practice without the PT's being directly on premises, but the PT must be available through telecommunications.
   d. The PT must be within the line of sight while the PTA works.

7. Delegation strategies considered to be "deciding" behaviors are within the purview of
   a. the physical therapist.
   b. the physical therapist assistant.
   c. both the physical therapist and the physical therapist assistant.
   d. neither the physical therapist nor the physical therapist assistant.

8. Factors to be considered by the PT when directing or delegating patient care to the PTA include all of the following EXCEPT
   a. length of experience of the PTA.
   b. ambiguity of basic indicators.
   c. predictability of consequences.
   d. criticality of results.

9. The physical therapy state practice act is an example of which type of law?
   a. constitutional law
   b. statutory law
   c. common law
   d. civil law

10. The external accrediting agency that serves as a benchmark of quality for acute care hospitals is called
    a. Commission on Acute Care Facilities.
    b. Accreditation for Acute Care Standards.
    c. Joint Commission on Accreditation of Healthcare Organizations.
    d. American Quality Standards Board.

11. Which of the following statements is NOT true about healthcare ethics?
    a. All healthcare professions share the same code of ethics.
    b. Ethics is about doing the best or right thing in a given situation.
    c. The code of ethics serves to protect the public.
    d. Each profession establishes its own code of ethics.

12. The federal law HIPAA is based upon which of the following ethical tenets?
    a. duty
    b. justice
    c. confidentiality
    d. beneficence

13. If a PTA cuts the ultrasound treatment for a patient just a little bit short in order to have time to complete paperwork, this would be an example of
    a. autonomy.
    b. veracity.
    c. an ethical dilemma.
    d. a metaethical decision.

14. While working on a weekend at a large hospital, a PTA encounters a patient on her assignment list that is tied to the bed, being restrained. The patient begs the PTA to untie him and says he has no idea who tied him up or why. The PTA notices that the patient follows instructions and appears alert and oriented throughout the treatment session. What should the PTA do?
   a. Leave the patient tied up because this is someone else's responsibility.
   b. Untie the patient because this is inhumane.
   c. Leave the patient as he was found and contact the PT of record to discuss the situation.
   d. Untie the patient and go find the nurse.

15. Due to escalating healthcare costs and often reduced coverage for PT visits, _____ requires even more attention by the PT and by the PTA.
   a. meticulous billing
   b. effective patient/client-related instruction
   c. attending more continuing education courses
   d. specialization

16. Which of the following terms is defined as a temporary change in ability or behavior?
   a. facilitation
   b. inhibition
   c. learning
   d. performance

17. What is a more desirable outcome as a result of patient/client instruction?
   a. facilitation
   b. inhibition
   c. learning
   d. performance

18. Breaking down a motor task into segments so that the patient can perform the segment correctly before moving on is a specific example of which teaching tenet?
   a. utilizing feedback that is consistent with the PT's plan of care
   b. taking less time to perform tasks
   c. success begets success
   d. taking more time to perform tasks

19. Which of the following is NOT an example of an acceptable use of clinical problem-solving by the PTA?
   a. notifying the PT of record that the patient has met the goals established
   b. increasing the time on the upper cycle to eight minutes
   c. recommending an AFO to the patient's family
   d. moving the patient following TKA from a walker to a quad cane

20. Membership in the APTA, attendance at workshops, and reading current journal articles related to frequently utilized interventions are strategies for the PTA to maintain which of the following?
   a. continued competency
   b. merit pay
   c. career laddering
   d. licensure

21. Which of the following aspects of the patient/client management model pertains to the PTA's scope of work?
   a. synthesizing the results of the examination
   b. collecting data using standardized tests or measures
   c. choosing outcome measurement tools
   d. establishing the plan of care

22. Which of the following terms is defined as the extent to which a measurement is consistent time after time with little variation?
   a. vigor
   b. predictability
   c. reliability
   d. validity

23. Which of the following terms is defined as the degree to which something measures what it intends or claims to measure?
   a. vigor
   b. predictability
   c. reliability
   d. validity

24. The Standards of Practice for Physical Therapy as set forth by the American Physical Therapy Association are required of
   a. all members of the professional association.
   b. all members of the profession.
   c. all physical therapists.
   d. all physical therapist members of the professional association.

25. The Standards of Ethical Conduct for the PTA as set forth by the American Physical Therapy Association are required of
   a. all members of the professional association.
   b. all members of the profession.
   c. all physical therapist assistants.
   d. all physical therapist assistant members of the professional association.

Practice 2 Answers

1. c. The specific limitations and expectations of the physical therapist assistant within the clinical setting are dictated by the practice act of that particular state.

2. d. Performing systems review is not within the purview of the PTA as directed by the PT. Systems review is a component of the examination element of the patient/client management model of physical therapy. Regardless of practice setting, this aspect of the physical therapy management model is performed by the physical therapist.

3. a. It is the physical therapist's responsibility to direct the course and progression of the patient's or client's plan of care.

4. b. The PTA's scope of work has not yet achieved profession-wide consensus. It is determined by the supervising PT on the basis of federal and state laws and regulations, ethical standards, competency and skill levels, standards of practice established by the profession, and current expectations in the workplace. Differences of opinion regarding the appropriate role and utilization of the PTA have existed since the early 1960s with the inception of the profession. While profession-wide consensus regarding the educational preparation, accreditation requirements, and state laws concerning minimal standards of competency for PTAs has nearly been built, the specific job duties and level of supervision by the physical therapist in the clinic or at the bedside remains controversial and varies greatly state to state.

5. c. General supervision allows the PTA to practice without a PT continuously on the premises. The supervising PT must be readily available by telecommunications. Levels of supervision for PTAs vary from state to state. Periodic on-site supervision defines the specific frequency in which the PT must be physically present. State requirements vary from having the PT present for 50% of the PTA's workweek to a specific number of patient encounters to once every two weeks. With full on-site supervision, the supervising PT must be on the premises at all times when the PTA is providing patient-related care.

6. a. With full on-site supervision, the supervising PT must be on the premises at all times when the PTA is providing patient-related care.

7. a. Delegation strategies considered to be "deciding" behaviors are within the purview of the physical therapist. Effective delegation strategies were proposed as a taxonomy by Nancy Watts in a landmark article in 1971. Within this systematic approach for the division of responsibility, tasks are analyzed in terms of the process of decision making ("deciding" behaviors) versus delivering an intervention ("doing" behaviors) required in the practice of physical therapy.

8. a. The length of experience of the PTA should not be considered by the PT when directing or delegating patient care. The following factors should, however, be considered: Predictability of consequences—how uncertain is the situation? Stability of the situation—how much and how quickly is change likely to occur? Observability of basic indicators—how easy or difficult is it to elicit a response in order to detect a change in patient's condition? Ambiguity of basic indicators—how difficult is it to interpret the changes occurring or confuse the changes with something else? Criticality of results—how serious are the consequences of a poor choice or inadequate recognition of an untoward change in condition?

9. b. The physical therapy state practice act is an example of statutory law, which is law established through state or federal legislatures. The physical therapy practice act is an example of state statute that differs in each state. Constitutional law is based on the U.S. Constitution; it guarantees personal rights and liberties in the Bill of Rights and typically takes precedence over all other laws in the United States. Common law consists of legal precedent created from judicial decisions that have not yet been enacted through statute. Civil and administrative law relating to healthcare consists of state and/or federal agencies created to oversee the rules and regulations governing many aspects of healthcare delivery and those who provide it. Licensure requirements to practice as a physical therapist assistant are examples of state administrative law. The regulations by which the Medicare system operates are examples of federal administrative law.

10. c. The external accrediting agency that serves as a benchmark of quality for acute care hospitals is called the Joint Commission on Accreditation of Healthcare Organizations (JCAHO). External accrediting agencies establish standards and processes to monitor aspects of healthcare delivery in order to achieve and maintain accreditation status. Accreditation then serves as a benchmark of quality which often becomes required in order to remain in operation. The JCAHO establishes expectations for acute care institutions that are required in order for the hospital to be eligible to participate in federal government reimbursement.

11. a. Not all healthcare professions share the same code of ethics. Ethical behavior is the manner in which one chooses to conduct oneself in personal and professional endeavors. Ethical behavior is about doing the best or right thing in a given situation. Ethical standards dictate conduct and moral choices as defined by specific professions, societies, religions, and cultures. Each profession establishes its own explicit code of conduct or code of ethics, which serves to protect the public and provides standards for professional behavior. The APTA Code of Ethics and Guide to Conduct for the Physical Therapist Assistant protects the rights of patients and clients, establishes standards of autonomy and supervision for PTAs, defines standards for peer review and reimbursement for PTAs, and outlines expectations and responsibilities for PTAs.

12. c. The Health Insurance Portability and Accountability Act of 1996 is a federal law that is based upon confidentiality and regulates the use and disclosure of an individual's health information.

13. d. If a PTA cuts the ultrasound treatment for a patient just a little bit short in order to have time to complete paperwork, this is an example of a metaethical decision. Metaethical decisions are decisions made when the right thing to do exists but may be clouded by temptation and/ or pressures to act differently. Cutting a patient's treatment time short because the PTA wants to have time to finish his or her paperwork is an example of a metaethical situation. It is a case in which the morally acceptable or right thing to do is to stay to treat the patient, but the PTA has chosen to do what is convenient even though it is not right.

14. c. The PTA should leave the patient as he was found and contact the PT of record to discuss the situation. In addition to carrying out clinical responsibilities consistent with all elements of the state practice act, regulatory agencies, and Standards of Ethical Conduct for the PTA, it is imperative that effective communication and ongoing collaboration with each physical therapist of record or supervising physical therapist occur throughout the provision of services.

15. b. Due to escalating healthcare costs and often reduced coverage for PT visits, effective patient/client-related instruction requires even more attention by the PT and the PTA.

16. d. Performance is defined as a temporary change in ability or behavior. Learning is defined as a relatively permanent change in performance or behavior. Inhibition is defined as an impediment to free activity. Facilitation is defined as the act of making something easier.

17. c. Learning is a more desirable outcome as a result of patient/client instruction. Typically, the goal for successful patient/client outcomes involves learning a movement, skill, or behavioral modification versus only performing them in the presence of the PT or the PTA.

18. c. While there are many theories related to teaching/learning principles, the following are central tenets that are essential for the PTA when teaching patients or clients:

- Demonstrate genuine concern and respect for the learner.
- Recognize and match the learning style of the learner.
- Actively engage the learner in order to make the instructions meaningful.
- Success begets success—create opportunities in which the patient or client can be successful and upon which the patient or client can build.
- Utilize feedback and practice schedules consistent with the PT's plan of care and current research findings.
- Provide ample practice recognizing that "practice only makes perfect if what is being practiced is correct."
- Recognize that the learner must be interested and motivated in order to learn.

- Show (demonstrate), tell (explain step by step), do (learner practices), reflect (learner critiques self or others).

19. c. Physical therapist assistants work closely with physical therapists in clinical problem-solving activities, including:

- participating in patient status judgments by reporting changes to the physical therapist of record and requesting patient reexamination or revisions to intervention options within the established plan of care
- adjusting or withholding interventions based on patient status as determined through observation, data collection, and interpretive processes within the physical therapist's established plan of care
- possessing the requisite knowledge to identify the situation, weigh alternatives, and select appropriate responses within the plan of care established by the physical therapist
- identifying potential consequences of those responses

20. a. Membership in the APTA, attendance at workshops, and reading current journal articles related to frequently utilized interventions are strategies for the PTA to use to maintain continued competency. The APTA Standards of Care and Standards of Ethical Conduct for the PTA and various administrative laws include continued competency as a requirement.

21. b. Collecting data using standardized tests or measures pertains to the PTA's scope of work. The physical therapist synthesizes information collected during the initial examination (and subsequent examinations) in order to establish the diagnosis, prognosis, and plan of care. The use of tests and measures provides information used to determine goals and anticipated outcomes. Subsequent examination (reexamination) at regular intervals provides

data to document changes in patient/client status and to document the progress that the patient/client is making toward functional goals and expected outcomes. The physical therapist assistant helps in the collection of data as directed by the physical therapist.

22. c. Reliability is the extent to which a measurement is consistent time after time, with as little variation as possible. There are multiple forms of reliability and validity described within the professional literature. A myriad of articles investigating the reliability and validity related to the measurement of impairment, functional limitation, and disability have been and continue to be published.

23. d. Validity is the degree to which something measures what it intends or claims to measure. There are multiple forms of reliability and validity described within the professional literature. A myriad of articles investigating the reliability and validity related to the measurement of impairment, functional limitation, and disability have been and continue to be published.

24. b. The American Physical Therapy Association sets forth the Standards of Practice for Physical Therapy which defines acceptable standards of care for all members of the profession. Although these standards are not laws themselves, various federal and state laws ensure that the standards are indeed upheld. The standards of care for physical therapy delivery are included in state physical therapy practice acts.

25. c. Although only members of the APTA can be subjected to disciplinary processes regarding purely ethical violations, most state practice acts include language that holds each physical therapist and physical therapist assistant bound to the ethical standards set forth by the professional association. Indeed, if one is deemed unethical, a violation of the law may have occurred as well.

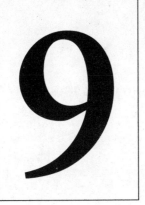
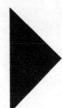

Practice Exam 1

CHAPTER SUMMARY

This practice exam should be taken after completing the Diagnostic Test in Chapter 4 and studying the subject areas you have identified in which you need more review. It is designed to help you practice for the national exam by including questions in academic and clinical areas in which you will need to recall important information and may need more review. Because the format mimics that of the NPTE for PTAs, taking it will help you familiarize yourself with the actual exam. You will be able to practice answering the types of questions that are on the exam as you review the content areas.

In addition to getting more practice in answering the kinds of questions on the NPTE for PTAs, this practice exam will help identify your strengths and weaknesses. Make a note of the types of questions you miss and the topics on which you need to further concentrate your study time. Do not neglect any subject area unless you have an almost perfect score in that area.

LEARNINGEXPRESS ANSWER SHEET

Part I

1. ⓐ ⓑ ⓒ ⓓ
2. ⓐ ⓑ ⓒ ⓓ
3. ⓐ ⓑ ⓒ ⓓ
4. ⓐ ⓑ ⓒ ⓓ
5. ⓐ ⓑ ⓒ ⓓ
6. ⓐ ⓑ ⓒ ⓓ
7. ⓐ ⓑ ⓒ ⓓ
8. ⓐ ⓑ ⓒ ⓓ
9. ⓐ ⓑ ⓒ ⓓ
10. ⓐ ⓑ ⓒ ⓓ
11. ⓐ ⓑ ⓒ ⓓ
12. ⓐ ⓑ ⓒ ⓓ
13. ⓐ ⓑ ⓒ ⓓ
14. ⓐ ⓑ ⓒ ⓓ
15. ⓐ ⓑ ⓒ ⓓ
16. ⓐ ⓑ ⓒ ⓓ
17. ⓐ ⓑ ⓒ ⓓ
18. ⓐ ⓑ ⓒ ⓓ
19. ⓐ ⓑ ⓒ ⓓ
20. ⓐ ⓑ ⓒ ⓓ
21. ⓐ ⓑ ⓒ ⓓ
22. ⓐ ⓑ ⓒ ⓓ
23. ⓐ ⓑ ⓒ ⓓ
24. ⓐ ⓑ ⓒ ⓓ
25. ⓐ ⓑ ⓒ ⓓ
26. ⓐ ⓑ ⓒ ⓓ
27. ⓐ ⓑ ⓒ ⓓ
28. ⓐ ⓑ ⓒ ⓓ
29. ⓐ ⓑ ⓒ ⓓ
30. ⓐ ⓑ ⓒ ⓓ
31. ⓐ ⓑ ⓒ ⓓ
32. ⓐ ⓑ ⓒ ⓓ
33. ⓐ ⓑ ⓒ ⓓ
34. ⓐ ⓑ ⓒ ⓓ
35. ⓐ ⓑ ⓒ ⓓ
36. ⓐ ⓑ ⓒ ⓓ
37. ⓐ ⓑ ⓒ ⓓ
38. ⓐ ⓑ ⓒ ⓓ
39. ⓐ ⓑ ⓒ ⓓ
40. ⓐ ⓑ ⓒ ⓓ
41. ⓐ ⓑ ⓒ ⓓ
42. ⓐ ⓑ ⓒ ⓓ
43. ⓐ ⓑ ⓒ ⓓ
44. ⓐ ⓑ ⓒ ⓓ
45. ⓐ ⓑ ⓒ ⓓ
46. ⓐ ⓑ ⓒ ⓓ
47. ⓐ ⓑ ⓒ ⓓ
48. ⓐ ⓑ ⓒ ⓓ
49. ⓐ ⓑ ⓒ ⓓ
50. ⓐ ⓑ ⓒ ⓓ

Part II

51. ⓐ ⓑ ⓒ ⓓ
52. ⓐ ⓑ ⓒ ⓓ
53. ⓐ ⓑ ⓒ ⓓ
54. ⓐ ⓑ ⓒ ⓓ
55. ⓐ ⓑ ⓒ ⓓ
56. ⓐ ⓑ ⓒ ⓓ
57. ⓐ ⓑ ⓒ ⓓ
58. ⓐ ⓑ ⓒ ⓓ
59. ⓐ ⓑ ⓒ ⓓ
60. ⓐ ⓑ ⓒ ⓓ
61. ⓐ ⓑ ⓒ ⓓ
62. ⓐ ⓑ ⓒ ⓓ
63. ⓐ ⓑ ⓒ ⓓ
64. ⓐ ⓑ ⓒ ⓓ
65. ⓐ ⓑ ⓒ ⓓ
66. ⓐ ⓑ ⓒ ⓓ
67. ⓐ ⓑ ⓒ ⓓ
68. ⓐ ⓑ ⓒ ⓓ
69. ⓐ ⓑ ⓒ ⓓ
70. ⓐ ⓑ ⓒ ⓓ
71. ⓐ ⓑ ⓒ ⓓ
72. ⓐ ⓑ ⓒ ⓓ
73. ⓐ ⓑ ⓒ ⓓ
74. ⓐ ⓑ ⓒ ⓓ
75. ⓐ ⓑ ⓒ ⓓ
76. ⓐ ⓑ ⓒ ⓓ
77. ⓐ ⓑ ⓒ ⓓ
78. ⓐ ⓑ ⓒ ⓓ
79. ⓐ ⓑ ⓒ ⓓ
80. ⓐ ⓑ ⓒ ⓓ
81. ⓐ ⓑ ⓒ ⓓ
82. ⓐ ⓑ ⓒ ⓓ
83. ⓐ ⓑ ⓒ ⓓ
84. ⓐ ⓑ ⓒ ⓓ
85. ⓐ ⓑ ⓒ ⓓ
86. ⓐ ⓑ ⓒ ⓓ
87. ⓐ ⓑ ⓒ ⓓ
88. ⓐ ⓑ ⓒ ⓓ
89. ⓐ ⓑ ⓒ ⓓ
90. ⓐ ⓑ ⓒ ⓓ
91. ⓐ ⓑ ⓒ ⓓ
92. ⓐ ⓑ ⓒ ⓓ
93. ⓐ ⓑ ⓒ ⓓ
94. ⓐ ⓑ ⓒ ⓓ
95. ⓐ ⓑ ⓒ ⓓ
96. ⓐ ⓑ ⓒ ⓓ
97. ⓐ ⓑ ⓒ ⓓ
98. ⓐ ⓑ ⓒ ⓓ
99. ⓐ ⓑ ⓒ ⓓ
100. ⓐ ⓑ ⓒ ⓓ

Part III

101. ⓐ ⓑ ⓒ ⓓ
102. ⓐ ⓑ ⓒ ⓓ
103. ⓐ ⓑ ⓒ ⓓ
104. ⓐ ⓑ ⓒ ⓓ
105. ⓐ ⓑ ⓒ ⓓ
106. ⓐ ⓑ ⓒ ⓓ
107. ⓐ ⓑ ⓒ ⓓ
108. ⓐ ⓑ ⓒ ⓓ
109. ⓐ ⓑ ⓒ ⓓ
110. ⓐ ⓑ ⓒ ⓓ
111. ⓐ ⓑ ⓒ ⓓ
112. ⓐ ⓑ ⓒ ⓓ
113. ⓐ ⓑ ⓒ ⓓ
114. ⓐ ⓑ ⓒ ⓓ
115. ⓐ ⓑ ⓒ ⓓ
116. ⓐ ⓑ ⓒ ⓓ
117. ⓐ ⓑ ⓒ ⓓ
118. ⓐ ⓑ ⓒ ⓓ
119. ⓐ ⓑ ⓒ ⓓ
120. ⓐ ⓑ ⓒ ⓓ
121. ⓐ ⓑ ⓒ ⓓ
122. ⓐ ⓑ ⓒ ⓓ
123. ⓐ ⓑ ⓒ ⓓ
124. ⓐ ⓑ ⓒ ⓓ
125. ⓐ ⓑ ⓒ ⓓ
126. ⓐ ⓑ ⓒ ⓓ
127. ⓐ ⓑ ⓒ ⓓ
128. ⓐ ⓑ ⓒ ⓓ
129. ⓐ ⓑ ⓒ ⓓ
130. ⓐ ⓑ ⓒ ⓓ
131. ⓐ ⓑ ⓒ ⓓ
132. ⓐ ⓑ ⓒ ⓓ
133. ⓐ ⓑ ⓒ ⓓ
134. ⓐ ⓑ ⓒ ⓓ
135. ⓐ ⓑ ⓒ ⓓ
136. ⓐ ⓑ ⓒ ⓓ
137. ⓐ ⓑ ⓒ ⓓ
138. ⓐ ⓑ ⓒ ⓓ
139. ⓐ ⓑ ⓒ ⓓ
140. ⓐ ⓑ ⓒ ⓓ
141. ⓐ ⓑ ⓒ ⓓ
142. ⓐ ⓑ ⓒ ⓓ
143. ⓐ ⓑ ⓒ ⓓ
144. ⓐ ⓑ ⓒ ⓓ
145. ⓐ ⓑ ⓒ ⓓ
146. ⓐ ⓑ ⓒ ⓓ
147. ⓐ ⓑ ⓒ ⓓ
148. ⓐ ⓑ ⓒ ⓓ
149. ⓐ ⓑ ⓒ ⓓ
150. ⓐ ⓑ ⓒ ⓓ

Part I

1. Which of the following positions typically results from a sling seat in a wheelchair?
   a. anterior pelvic tilt
   b. internal rotation and adduction of the lower extremities
   c. external rotation and abduction of the lower extremities
   d. adduction and internal rotation of one lower extremity and abduction and external rotation of the other lower extremity

2. Which of the following is most characteristic of a right cerebrovascular accident?
   a. weakness/paralysis on the right side of the body
   b. impaired right left discrimination
   c. impulsive behavior
   d. speech and language impairments

3. A patient exhibits a loss of vibratory and position sense with paralysis on one side of the body and loss of pain and temperature sensation on the other side of the body. What type of spinal cord injury is this most characteristic of?
   a. anterior cord syndrome
   b. cauda equina injuries
   c. central cord syndrome
   d. Brown-Sequard syndrome

4. In a SOAP note, after treatment, the physical therapist assistant documents the presence of trigger points in the paraspinal musculature at the base of the spine of the scapula. Anatomically, this corresponds with what vertebral level?
   a. T2
   b. T3
   c. T6
   d. T7

5. A physical therapist assistant places a small object in the patient's hand and asks her to identify the object with her vision occluded. This test assesses
   a. stereognosis.
   b. barognosis.
   c. graphesthesia.
   d. light touch.

6. Your patient requires a ramp to be built at his house to negotiate a height of four feet. What is the minimum acceptable length for this ramp?
   a. 12 feet
   b. 24 feet
   c. 48 feet
   d. 96 feet

7. Your patient has a pressure ulcer on the sacrum that extends through the epidermis to the dermis. It is painful with a reddened base. In what stage is this ulcer?
   a. stage I
   b. stage II
   c. stage III
   d. stage IV

8. Two clinicians, using standard procedure, take the same goniometric measurement on a patient and attain markedly different results. This is an example of poor
   a. objectivity.
   b. validity.
   c. intrarater reliability.
   d. interrater reliability.

9. A Cheyne-Stokes breathing pattern is an abnormal breathing pattern characterized by
   a. rapid breathing for 10 to 60 seconds followed by a period of apnea.
   b. rapid shallow breathing.
   c. slow breathing.
   d. prolonged expiration.

10. A patient's blood pressure is normally slightly higher in
   a. high fowler's position.
   b. standing.
   c. sitting.
   d. supine.

11. A patient has muscle tightness in the biceps resulting in a contracture at the elbow joint. A stretching technique is performed in which the patient's elbow is extended to end range. The patient performs an isometric contraction of the biceps and then relaxes. The PTA again stretches the elbow into extension and holds it for 15 to 30 seconds. This sequence is repeated until no further gains in range are attained. This is a description of what technique?
   a. hold-relax
   b. hold-relax-contract
   c. agonist contraction
   d. repeated contractions

12. In standing during the up phase of a squat, as the knee approaches full extension, the
   a. femur externally rotates on the tibia.
   b. femur internally rotates on the tibia.
   c. tibia externally rotates on the femur.
   d. tibia internally rotates on the femur.

13. The lowest manual muscle testing grade that can be given to a patient who can tolerate resistance in an antigravity position is
   a. 4/5.
   b. 4–/5.
   c. 3+/5.
   d. 3/5.

14. Your patient presents with acute onset of motor weakness starting distally in the lower extremities and moving proximally. The weakness has now progressed to the upper extremities, and distal sensory disturbances are also present. This is the typical presentation of
   a. multiple sclerosis.
   b. amyotrophic lateral sclerosis.
   c. Guillain-Barré syndrome.
   d. Huntington's disease.

15. Your patient is in the Thomas test position. In this position, on the involved lower extremity, the patient's thigh is level with the plinth and his or her knee is flexed 50 degrees. This would indicate tightness of the
   a. hamstrings.
   b. hip adductors.
   c. iliopsoas.
   d. rectus femoris.

16. Your patient experienced an inversion ankle sprain with severe loss of ligamentous stability, severe pain, swelling, and ecchymosis with loss of joint function. What grade sprain is described?
   a. grade I
   b. grade II
   c. grade III
   d. grade IV

17. Your patient is an 86-year-old woman who is one day status post total hip replacement involving a cemented prosthesis. Which of the following best describes the most likely weight-bearing status?

a. limited early weight-bearing progressing to full weight-bearing by 12 weeks

b. weight-bearing as tolerated increasing to full weight-bearing as able

c. non-weight-bearing for four weeks, then increase to full weight-bearing as able

d. non-weight-bearing for 12 weeks, then increase to full weight-bearing as able

18. Your patient is a long distance bicyclist. He presents with atrophy of the hypothenar eminence. Which nerve is most likely involved?

a. median

b. ulnar

c. radial

d. musculocutaneous

19. Your patient demonstrates excessive tone in all four extremities, which is resistant to active and passive movements. As you perform passive range of motion, you feel that the muscles catch and then release. Which term best describes this condition?

a. flaccidity

b. hypertonicity

c. spasticity

d. cog wheel rigidity

20. You are instructing a patient on descending stairs using bilateral axillary crutches. The patient is partial weight-bearing on the right. Which of the following describes the most appropriate sequence?

a. right lower extremity, then crutches

b. left lower extremity, then crutches

c. crutches, then right lower extremity

d. crutches, then left lower extremity

21. You are working with an infant who experienced a brachial plexus injury during birth. The C5 and C6 nerve roots were involved. Findings would include

a. claw hand.

b. waiter's tip deformity.

c. scapula winging.

d. paralysis of the hand intrinsics and wrist flexors.

22. The physical therapist asks you to initiate activities at the level of two metabolic equivalents with your cardiac patient. Which of the following would be appropriate?

a. raking leaves

b. cycling 8 mph

c. walking 4 mph

d. lifting 1 to 2 lb. weights

23. You are working with a 30-year-old woman three days post–Cesarean section. Which of the following exercises would NOT be appropriate?

a. pelvic floor exercises

b. straight leg raises

c. heel slides

d. diaphragmatic breathing

24. Your patient has spasmodic torticollis of the right sternocleidomastoid. ROM should stress

a. lateral flexion and rotation to the left.

b. lateral flexion and rotation to the right.

c. lateral flexion to the left and rotation to the right.

d. lateral flexion to the right and rotation to the left.

25. Which of the following would be the most appropriate treatment for an acute severe slipped capital femoral epiphysis?
   a. no treatment
   b. ROM and strengthening exercises
   c. bracing with limited weight-bearing
   d. surgery

26. You are developing a program to increase cardiovascular endurance for a 40-year-old male patient who is slightly overweight but otherwise in good health. An appropriate target heart rate would be
   a. 100 bpm.
   b. 120 bpm.
   c. 170 bpm.
   d. 180 bpm.

27. A physical therapist assistant is treating a patient who had arthroscopic surgery to his right knee. Post-op the patient developed a DVT in his right calf. He is currently on anticoagulants. At today's session, the patient complains of sharp pain under his right scapula. He denies pain when moving the right upper extremity. What should the PTA do?
   a. Continue treatment since this is probably not a significant event.
   b. Discontinue treatment and document the patient's complaints in the "O" section of the SOAP note.
   c. Discontinue treatment and contact the patient's physician.
   d. Continue treatment, document the patient's complaints in the "O" section of the SOAP note, and follow up at the next treatment session.

28. A normal two-and-a-half-year-old should be able to perform all of the following EXCEPT
   a. run.
   b. stair climb reciprocally.
   c. jump in place.
   d. hop repeatedly.

29. As you move your elderly patient from supine to sitting on the edge of the bed, she complains of lightheadedness. Most likely, she is experiencing
   a. autonomic dysreflexia.
   b. orthostatic hypertension.
   c. orthostatic hypotension.
   d. tachycardia.

30. When assessing your patient's posture, you note that he has pectus excavatum. Which of the following best describes this condition?
   a. sternum displaced anteriorly increasing the A-P diameter of the rib cage
   b. sternum displaced posteriorly decreasing the A-P diameter of the rib cage
   c. sternum displaced posteriorly increasing the A-P diameter of the rib cage
   d. increase in the medial-lateral diameter of the rib cage

31. The physical therapist asks you to test a patient for dysmetria. Which of the following would be an appropriate test?
   a. rapid alternating toe tapping
   b. minimal balance challenges in sitting
   c. manual muscle test the knee extensors
   d. pointing and past pointing

32. A physical therapist assistant measures the angle, labeled *x*, as illustrated in the figure.

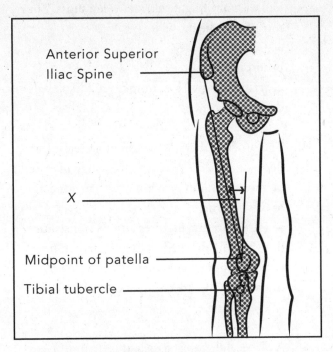

Anterior Superior
Iliac Spine

X

Midpoint of patella

Tibial tubercle

This measurement represents
a. a varus deformity.
b. the Q angle.
c. genu recurvatum.
d. genu varus.

33. You are checking the vital signs of an infant. Which of the following would NOT be indicative of a normal heart rate?
a. 60 bpm
b. 80 bpm
c. 120 bpm
d. 140 bpm

34. All of the following are characteristic of left-sided heart failure EXCEPT
a. dependent edema.
b. pulmonary edema.
c. dyspnea.
d. cough.

35. The physical therapist has instructed you to measure a patient's chest excursion. What anatomical landmark would you use for consistency of results?
a. the nipple line
b. the xiphoid process
c. the lowest palpable edge of the rib cage
d. the area on the rib cage that appears to expand the most during premeasurement trials

36. The property of water that allows patients to move more freely in the water than they can on land is
a. buoyancy.
b. hydrostatic pressure.
c. viscosity.
d. thermal effects.

37. The first stage in evidence-based practice is to
a. perform a literature review.
b. develop a clear, concise clinical question.
c. identify a problem.
d. gather clinical evidence.

38. The main line of defense in preventing nosocomial infections is
a. hand washing.
b. gloves and gowns.
c. masks.
d. gloves, gowns, and masks.

39. The physical therapist assistant writes, "The patient will ambulate 50 feet × 2 with a standard walker with contact guard of one in one week." This statement would be placed in which part of the SOAP note?
a. subjective
b. objective
c. assessment
d. plan

40. The term *quadrilateral socket* refers to the traditional shape of the socket of a
a. transtibial prosthesis.
b. transfemoral prosthesis.
c. Syme's prosthesis.
d. hip disarticulation prosthesis.

41. The physical therapist assistant is treating a 55-year-old accountant who experienced a fall while bicycling, resulting in a fracture of the right hip. The patient had a right total hip replacement and is currently receiving treatment in a short-term rehabilitation facility. According to the Nagi Model of Disability, which of the following is a disability?
a. inability to work
b. impaired ambulation
c. pain, decreased ROM, and decreased strength in the right hip
d. fracture in the right hip

42. A physical therapist assistant is treating a patient with post-polio syndrome. Interventions would probably include all of the following EXCEPT
a. energy conservation techniques.
b. pain management.
c. sensory retraining.
d. muscle strengthening.

43. Metabolic syndrome includes all of the following EXCEPT
a. hypertension.
b. insulin resistance.
c. hip/thigh obesity.
d. abdominal obesity.

44. Your patient presented to the hospital with the following symptoms: rectal bleeding, diarrhea, nausea, vomiting, fever, and weight loss. The most likely diagnosis is
a. Crohn's disease.
b. ulcerative colitis.
c. irritable bowel syndrome.
d. appendicitis.

45. The physical therapist assistant is treating an illiterate patient. Which of the following would be most useful in providing patient education to this patient?
a. incorporating pictures and demonstrations
b. providing detailed written instructions
c. using appropriate medical terminology
d. having a literate family member explain everything

46. A physical therapist assistant is treating a 72-year-old male patient with peripheral vascular disease. Which of the following would be least useful as part of the treatment program?
a. lower extremity stationary cycling
b. an aquatic therapy program
c. ambulation until pain is felt, rest until pain is relieved, and then repeat
d. low level plyometrics

47. A physical therapist assistant is treating a patient with a knee flexion contracture that developed after a knife injury. The original injury was approximately 12 months ago. Which of the following would be the most appropriate parameters for using ultrasound to treat the soft tissue shortening?
a. 3 MHz, 0.5–1.0 w/cm^2, pulsed 20%
b. 3 MHz, 0.15–0.25 w/cm^2, pulsed 20%
c. 1 MHz, 1.0–2.0 w/cm^2, continuous
d. 1 MHZ, 0.5–1.0 w/cm^2, continuous

48. You are treating a 60-year-old woman with Bell's palsy. She is exhibiting a total reaction of degeneration, resulting in complete denervation of the facial nerve. Which type of electrical stimulation would be most beneficial for this patient?

a. Russian stimulation to the motor points

b. interrupted DC to the motor points

c. high-volt pulsed DC to the motor points

d. transcutaneous electrical nerve stimulation

49. A physical therapist is treating a patient with an acromioclavicular joint separation. Which of the following is the most likely mechanism of injury?

a. a classic FOOSH injury, or fall on outstretched hand

b. a distraction injury where there was a pull on the arm

c. a direct blow to the shoulder in upright, for example being blocked in football

d. a fall landing directly on the tip of the shoulder

50. A physical therapist assistant is treating a patient with scleroderma. Which of the following activities would be least likely to be included in the plan of care?

a. range of motion and stretching exercises

b. orthotics

c. core strengthening exercises

d. skin care

Part II

51. A 24-year-old male was working on a car engine when there was a fire that resulted in burns to his groin, anterior lower extremities from the thighs to the toes, and posterior lower extremities from the knees to the soles of his feet. According to the rule of nines, what percentage of the patient's body is involved?

a. 27%

b. 28%

c. 36%

d. 37%

52. The physical therapist assistant is reading the SOAP note from the previous treatment session for a patient. It states that the patient requires moderate assistance with sit-to-stand transfers. How much assistance does this patient require?

a. The clinician must maintain contact with the patient for the patient to complete the transfer.

b. The clinician must provide at most 25% assist for the patient to complete the transfer.

c. The clinician must provide at most 50% assist for the patient to complete the transfer.

d. The clinician must provide at least 75% assist for the patient to complete the transfer.

53. A lever system where the resistance is between the axis and the force is classified as a
a. first class lever.
b. second class lever.
c. third class lever.
d. does not illustrate any existing lever system.

54. A physical therapist assistant is treating an 18-year-old woman who experienced a crush injury to her foot. Subsequently, she developed complex regional pain syndrome. Which of the following would be most appropriate to utilize during stage I complex regional pain syndrome?
a. closed-chain exercises
b. progressive resistive exercises
c. eccentric activities
d. electrical stimulation

55. Your 14-year-old female patient has a structural C-shaped scoliosis of the thoracic spine, with the convexity to the right. Which of the following would be the most likely postural deviation present?
a. fixed rotation of the vertebral bodies to the left
b. compression of the ribs on the right
c. waist space larger on the right
d. posterior rib hump on the right

56. Your patient has a positive modified Ober's test. What muscle(s) would you teach the patient to stretch?
a. tensor fascia latae
b. hamstrings
c. rectus femoris
d. iliopsoas

57. The physical therapist has asked you to stretch a patient. The chart indicates that the patient's PROM right knee is 25 to 150 degrees. What muscle(s) would you stretch?
a. gluteus maximus
b. hamstrings
c. quadriceps
d. gastrocnemius

58. You are treating a newborn, and the physician is concerned that the child might have developmental dysplasia of the hip. All of the following are tests for developmental dysplasia of the hip EXCEPT
a. apprehension sign.
b. Barlow maneuver.
c. Ortolani's click.
d. X-ray.

59. A physical therapist assistant, while assessing a patient's balance, has the patient with her feet together and her arms crossed over her chest.

   The patient remains in this position for 20 seconds with her eyes open, and then for 20 seconds with her eyes closed. This is a description of which test?

   a. Tinetti
   b. Berg Balance Scale
   c. Romberg
   d. Sharpened Romberg

60. The physical therapist has asked you to perform an MMT of a patient's quadriceps. Which of the following positions would be most appropriate?
   a. short sitting with the trunk erect
   b. long sitting
   c. short sitting with the trunk leaning slightly backward
   d. short sitting with the trunk leaning slightly forward

61. A physical therapist assistant is assessing a patient's wheelchair for proper fit. The PTA notes that the patient fits snugly between both sides of the wheelchair. Which of the following is true?
   a. This is the normal fit for wheelchair width so that the patient doesn't slide.
   b. There should be a half-inch clearance on each side.
   c. There should be a one-inch clearance on each side.
   d. There should be a two-inch clearance on each side.

62. A physical therapist assistant is treating a patient with pneumonia. What type of precaution level should be in place?
   a. isolation precautions

b. airborne precautions
c. droplet precautions
d. no precautions necessary

63. Which of the following orthoses would best limit all ankle and foot motion?
   a. posterior leaf spring AFO
   b. spiral AFO
   c. solid AFO
   d. a metal and leather orthosis with a valgus strap

64. Your 60-year-old male patient has a resting heart rate of 56 bpm. This heart rate is
   a. normal for this age.
   b. an indication of an arrhythmia.
   c. an example of tachycardia.
   d. an example of bradycardia.

65. The physical therapist assistant is instructing a patient with ankylosing spondylitis in breathing exercises in conjunction with chest mobilization exercises. Which of the following exercises would be most beneficial?
   a. bilateral upper extremity D2 flexion and extension
   b. bilateral upper extremity D1 flexion and extension
   c. pursed lip breathing
   d. trunk passive extension exercises

66. All of the following would be placed in the objective section of the SOAP note EXCEPT
   a. girth measurements.
   b. list of exercises performed during that session.
   c. problem list.
   d. current ambulatory status.

67. Your patient has a blood pressure of 120/80. This is considered to be
   a. normal.
   b. prehypertension.
   c. stage I hypertension.
   d. stage II hypertension.

68. Hypotonic cerebral palsy is characterized by all of the following EXCEPT
   a. floppy rag doll presentation.
   b. excessive range of motion.
   c. open mouth and protruding tongue.
   d. strong deep tendon reflexes.

69. Rheumatoid arthritis is characterized by all of the following EXCEPT
   a. may be either sudden or gradual in onset.
   b. initially low grade fever, fatigue, and general malaise.
   c. morning stiffness.
   d. being diagnosed in those over age 50.

70. Your patient is a 65-year-old male recently diagnosed with hemochromatosis. Treatment for this condition would likely include all of the following EXCEPT
   a. phlebotomy.
   b. blood transfusions.
   c. chelatin therapy if phlebotomy is not possible.
   d. avoiding iron pills and multivitamins with iron.

71. Selective debridement of a wound includes all of the following EXCEPT
   a. sharp debridement.
   b. wet to dry dressings.
   c. enzymatic debridement.
   d. autolytic debridement.

72. A physical therapist assistant is treating an 18-year-old male patient with a traumatic brain injury. Balance activities are being performed in the high kneel position. According to the developmental sequence, the PTA would next progress the patient to
  a. half kneel.
  b. modified plantigrade.
  c. plantigrade.
  d. parallel bar activities.

73. A physical therapist assistant has been treating a patient who is two weeks status post arthroscopic surgery to the right knee. Today, the patient complains of pain in her calf. Her calf is sensitive, warm to touch, and slightly swollen. The physical therapist assistant should
  a. discontinue treatment, ace wrap the calf, and check with the patient on the next day to see if the symptoms have resolved.
  b. discontinue treatment and contact the medical doctor.
  c. discontinue treatment and check with the patient on the next day to see if the symptoms have resolved.
  d. continue treatment but document the symptoms and check with the patient the next day to see if the symptoms have resolved.

74. A physical therapist assistant is treating a patient with diabetes with a neuropathic vascular ulcer on the sole of her foot. The PT has included whirlpool as part of the treatment plan. Which of the following would be an appropriate temperature for the whirlpool?
  a. 88 degrees F
  b. 92 degrees F
  c. 98 degrees F
  d. 100 degrees F

75. A physical therapist assistant is working with a patient performing gait training. The patient has advanced to uneven surfaces so the physical therapist assistant has taken the patient outside to the parking lot. It is summer and the PTA is concerned that the patient is experiencing signs of heatstroke. All of the following are signs of heatstroke EXCEPT
  a. skin cool and clammy.
  b. headache.
  c. increased heart rate.
  d. increased body temperature.

76. A physical therapist assistant is reviewing a videotape of a patient's gait. The physical therapist assistant notices that the patient has difficulty decelerating the swing leg just prior to initial contact. Which of the following muscles should be strengthened to control this deviation?
  a. quadriceps
  b. gastrocnemius
  c. hamstrings
  d. anterior tibialis

77. According to the concave-convex law, during the movement of a concave surface on a stable convex surface, the
  a. concave surface will move in the same direction that the body part is moving.
  b. concave surface will move in the opposite direction that the body part is moving.
  c. convex surface will move in the same direction that the body part is moving.
  d. convex surface will move in the opposite direction that the body part is moving.

78. A physical therapist assistant is treating a patient with a resolving peripheral nerve injury to the peroneal nerve. Which of the following exercises would be most beneficial in strengthening the affected muscles?
a. patient long sitting performing ankle plantarflexion with Thera-Band
b. patient standing performing heel raises
c. patient long sitting performing resisted eversion with Thera-Band
d. patient long sitting performing resisted inversion with Thera-Band

79. A physical therapist assistant is treating a patient who has a stage III pressure ulcer over her greater trochanter. Which of the following would be the most appropriate treatment parameters for using ultrasound to promote healing in this area?
a. 3 MHz, 0.5 w/cm^2, pulsed 20%
b. 3 MHz, 0.5 w/cm^2, continuous
c. 1 MHz, 0.5 w/cm^2, pulsed 20%
d. 1 MHz, 0.5 w/cm^2, continuous

80. A physical therapist assistant is working with a patient with a complete C6 quadriplegia. Which of the following pieces of equipment would be most useful in improving this patient's ability to perform activities of daily living?
a. elastic shoelaces
b. tenodesis splint
c. overhead trapeze
d. power wheelchair

81. A physical therapist assistant is treating a patient with diabetes mellitus. During the session, the PTA continually monitors the patient for signs of exercise-induced hypoglycemia. All of the following are signs of hypoglycemia EXCEPT
a. sweating.
b. excessive thirst.
c. confusion.
d. shallow respirations.

82. A physical therapist assistant is treating a 55-year-old male patient with gastroesophageal reflux disease. Which of the following positions would be the least likely to produce symptoms?
a. lying supine
b. lying in Trendelenburg position
c. left side-lying
d. right side-lying

83. A physical therapist assistant is treating a three-month-old infant. All of the following activities would be age appropriate for a three-month-old infant EXCEPT
a. prone on elbows.
b. tracks past midline.
c. smiles at mother.
d. hands fisted.

84. A physical therapist assistant is treating a child with cerebral palsy who has difficulty rolling. Which of the following reflexes would interfere the most with the ability to roll?
a. flexor withdrawal
b. Moro
c. asymmetrical tonic neck reflex
d. symmetrical tonic neck reflex

85. A physical therapist assistant is assessing a patient's proprioception. Which of the following tests would be most appropriate?
a. stereognosis
b. kinesthetic awareness
c. two point discrimination
d. barognosis

86. A physical therapist assistant has been instructed to assess a patient's functional status. All of the following are functional assessment tools EXCEPT
a. Barthel Index.
b. McGill Pain Questionnaire.
c. Functional Independence Measure.
d. Tinetti Performance Oriented Mobility Assessment.

87. A physical therapist assistant is treating a patient who developed lymphedema in her right upper extremity after undergoing a right mastectomy for the treatment of breast cancer. Which of the following would be the least effective in treating this condition?
a. manual lymphatic drainage
b. custom fitted pressure garment
c. external compression pump
d. elevating the extremity

88. All of the following are important functions of the skin EXCEPT
a. temperature control.
b. providing sensory information.
c. synthesizing of vitamin C.
d. maintaining fluid balance.

89. A physical therapist assistant is treating a child with pervasive developmental disorder. Which of the following would be least beneficial when treating this child?
a. alternating between a wide variety of activities
b. using familiar objects during treatment
c. following a set routine each and every session
d. using daily activities to improve strength and function

90. A physical therapist assistant is treating a patient with thoracic outlet syndrome. Which of the following is least likely to be included in the plan of care?
a. strengthening the trapezius and rhomboids
b. stretching the pectoralis major
c. postural exercises
d. passive extension exercises

91. A physical therapist assistant is gait training a patient with Parkinson's disease. Which of the following would be least useful in assisting with this activity?
a. making marks or footprints on the floor and having the patient step on them
b. weighting the lower extremities with one-pound cuff weights
c. using a mirror for visual feedback
d. using walking poles

92. A physical therapist assistant is wrapping the residual limb of a patient who had a below knee amputation. Which of the following is the least appropriate method of securing the bandage?
a. metal clips
b. velcro
c. tape
d. safety pins

93. A physical therapist assistant is treating a patient who had a total knee replacement. The physician has ordered a continuous passive motion machine for this patient. A continuous passive motion machine can assist with all of the following EXCEPT
a. preventing adhesions.
b. decreasing pain.
c. enhancing synovial fluid movement.
d. increasing strength.

94. A physical therapist assistant is instructing a patient in a series of movements where the patient short sits, turns their head 45 degrees to one side, and then quickly lies down on the opposite side. The patient maintains this position for approximately 30 seconds, then returns to the upright, seated posture (maintaining the head rotation) and repeats in the opposite direction. This is a treatment for which of the following conditions?
a. Meniere's disease
b. a type of benign paroxysmal positional vertigo
c. cervical vertigo
d. vertigo associated with multiple sclerosis

95. A physical therapist assistant is working with a 24-year-old patient who experienced a traumatic brain injury. Which of the following proprioceptive neuromuscular facilitation techniques would be least useful in developing core strength and stability with this patient?
a. rhythmic initiation
b. alternating isometrics
c. rhythmic stabilization
d. repeated contractions

96. A physical therapist assistant is working with a patient who experienced a CVA and is also depressed. Which of the following would be least helpful in motivating this patient?
a. offering positive feedback
b. emphasizing the patient's strengths
c. providing frequent encouragement
d. providing choices about the patient's treatment

97. A physical therapist assistant is treating a patient with emphysema. The patient takes multiple medications. Which of the following medications is least likely to be part of this patient's drug regime?
a. bronchodilators
b. anticoagulants
c. anti-inflammatory agents
d. antihistamines

98. A physical therapist assistant is treating a patient who had a coronary artery bypass graft. Which of the following would be the least likely activity included in early physical therapy sessions?
a. transfers and early ambulation
b. postural training
c. protective coughing
d. PREs with light weights for the upper extremities

99. Fibromyalgia syndrome is characterized by all of the following EXCEPT
   a. pain—usually concentrated on one side of the body.
   b. tender points in muscles, ligaments, and tendons.
   c. that it occurs more frequently in women.
   d. headaches, anxiety, and depression.

100. A physical therapist assistant is treating a patient with a rotator cuff tear. Which of the following is a test for a rotator cuff tear?
   a. apprehension test
   b. drop arm test
   c. Yergason's test
   d. Adson maneuver

Part III

101. The articulation between the distal ends of the fibula and tibia is classified as a(n)
   a. synarthrodial joint.
   b. amphiarthrodial joint.
   c. diarthrodial joint.
   d. gomphosis.

102. A physical therapist assistant is treating a child with spina bifida. Both feet are in a supinated position. Supination of the foot is a combination of what movements?
   a. dorsiflexion, eversion, and forefoot abduction
   b. plantar flexion, inversion, and forefoot adduction
   c. dorsiflexion, inversion, and forefoot adduction
   d. plantar flexion, eversion, and forefoot abduction

103. A patient with complete quadriplegia at the level of C5 is referred to your rehabilitation facility. Which of the following is NOT a realistic goal for this patient?
   a. able to complete lower extremity self-stretching in bed independently
   b. able to feed self independently with adaptive equipment
   c. able to self-propel a manual wheelchair with projections
   d. able to assist in transfers

104. You are treating a 55-year-old woman with progressive systemic sclerosis. The primary focus of your treatment program would be
   a. strengthening.
   b. aerobic conditioning.
   c. stretching and flexibility.
   d. isokinetic training.

105. Your patient is an eight-year-old boy who fell while skateboarding. He experienced an incomplete fracture characteristic of children. What is the name for this type of fracture?
   a. open fracture
   b. closed fracture
   c. comminuted fracture
   d. greenstick fracture

106. A physical therapist assistant is working with a patient who is supine on a mat. The patient has a SCI with a complete transaction at T5. The patient experiences an episode of autonomic dysreflexia. The PTA should

a. call for help, check the catheter, and give the appropriate drugs.

b. call for help, loosen the patient's clothing, and give the appropriate drugs.

c. call for help, sit the patient up, and check the catheter.

d. call for help, keep patient in supine, and check the catheter.

107. Your patient is receiving intermittent pelvic traction supine with the hips and knees flexed. This is the appropriate position for all of the following conditions EXCEPT

a. paraspinal muscle spasms.

b. facet joint hypomobility.

c. tightness in the posterior longitudinal ligament.

d. posterior lateral disc bulge.

108. Which of the following reflexes would NOT interfere with crawling?

a. palmar grasp

b. positive support

c. symmetrical tonic neck reflex

d. asymmetrical tonic neck reflex

109. The physical therapist has asked you to develop an exercise program for a patient concentrating on the shoulder internal rotators. Which of the following muscles comprise that group?

a. pectoralis major, anterior deltoid, subscapularis, teres major, and latissimus dorsi

b. pectoralis major, anterior deltoid, subscapularis, teres minor, and latissimus dorsi

c. infraspinatus, teres minor, and posterior deltoid

d. infraspinatus, teres major, and posterior deltoid

110. A patient has a decreased quadriceps reflex. A physical therapist assistant might also expect decreased sensation in what area(s)?

a. medial aspect of the lower leg

b. anterior upper thigh

c. lateral aspect of the lower leg

d. posterior thigh

111. A physical therapist assistant working in a cardiac rehab unit receives a new patient in phase I of cardiac rehab. The phase I program would include all of the following EXCEPT

a. active range of motion, ambulation, and self-care activities.

b. a maximal symptom limited exercise test.

c. patient and family education.

d. constant monitoring of vital signs.

112. All of the following are medications that a patient with cystic fibrosis is likely to utilize EXCEPT
  a. pancreatic enzymes.
  b. bronchodilators.
  c. antibiotics.
  d. antihistamines.

113. When transferring a patient between two surfaces of differing heights which of the following transfers would be the best choice?
  a. three-person lift
  b. two-person lift
  c. dependent squat pivot transfer
  d. sliding board transfer

114. Stage I, the cognitive stage of motor learning, includes all of the following EXCEPT
  a. learning a new skill.
  b. transfer of a skill to different settings.
  c. relearning an old skill.
  d. frequent practice and self correction.

115. The physical therapist assistant assesses a patient who experienced a right cerebrovasular accident. The PTA has the patient sitting with her hands on her thighs palms down. The PTA instructs the patient to quickly turn the palms up and down repeatedly. This is a test for which of the following coordination deficits?
  a. asthenia
  b. athetosis
  c. dysmetria
  d. dysdiadochokinesia

116. The physical therapist assistant is instructing a patient in the proper method to transfer sit to stand from a wheelchair with bilateral axillary crutches. The patient is NWB on the left lower extremity. Where does the PTA instruct the patient to hold the crutches?
  a. both on the left side
  b. both on the right side
  c. one on the left side and one on the right side
  d. both in front

117. A physical therapist assistant gently pinches the skin on the dorsal surface of a patient's hand and assesses how quickly the skin returns to place. What is the physical therapist assistant assessing?
  a. skin turgor
  b. skin texture
  c. skin mobility
  d. skin compressibility

118. A physical therapist assistant may perform all of the following duties EXCEPT
   a. data collection during a treatment session.
   b. make modifications to selected interventions within the scope of the plan of care.
   c. document the patient's progress.
   d. perform the discharge examination.

119. The physical therapist assistant is instructing a patient in postural exercises. Which of the following would be the least useful form of feedback?
   a. summary feedback
   b. visual feedback
   c. tactile feedback
   d. verbal feedback

120. The physical therapist assistant is treating a patient who had a right cerebrovascular accident. Spasticity is beginning to decline and the patient exhibits some out of synergy movements. Which Brunnstrom stage of recovery does this best illustrate?
   a. stage II
   b. stage III
   c. stage IV
   d. stage V

121. A physical therapist assistant is treating a patient with type II diabetes mellitus. Which of the following is least likely to be part of the plan of care?
   a. aerobic activities
   b. postural retraining
   c. compensatory techniques for sensory impairments
   d. skin care

122. A physical therapist assistant is treating a woman and notes that her skin is somewhat bronze in color. This bronze color could be indicative of all of the following EXCEPT
   a. Addison's disease.
   b. cirrhosis of the liver.
   c. carbon monoxide poisoning.
   d. hemochromatosis.

123. A physical therapist assistant is treating a 67-year-old male patient who is recovering from a surgical manipulation of his total knee replacement. The patient is receiving Demerol to help control his pain. The physical therapist assistant should be aware of the adverse effects of an opioid analgesic like Demerol, as these side effects could have a detrimental effect on the patient's rehabilitation. All of the following are adverse effects of opioid analgesics EXCEPT
   a. increased excitability.
   b. sedation.
   c. nausea and vomiting.
   d. dependence.

124. A physical therapist assistant is using aquatic therapy as part of a stretching program for a patient. To best stretch the hamstrings, the physical therapist assistant should use
   a. a buoyancy assisted position.
   b. a buoyancy supported position.
   c. a buoyancy resisted position.
   d. a buoyancy super-resisted activity.

125. The physical therapist assistant is using infrared to the low back of a patient with low back pain. If the PTA decreases the distance between the lamp and the patient by one-half (for example, from 30 inches to 15 inches), the dosage of radiation reaching the patient is
a. doubled.
b. halved.
c. quadrupled.
d. quartered.

126. According to the hierarchy of evidence, which of the following usually provides the strongest evidence for the effectiveness of a treatment?
a. a single case study
b. a meta-analysis
c. a cohort study
d. a randomized, controlled trial

127. A physical therapist assistant is treating a patient with lateral epicondylitis using iontophoresis. To attain the same dosage as prior sessions, if the physical therapist assistant increases the intensity compared to the last session, the physical therapist assistant must
a. decrease the concentration of the drug.
b. decrease the size of the active electrode.
c. decrease the treatment time.
d. increase the treatment time.

128. The physical therapist assistant is treating a patient by utilizing a cool whirlpool to the lower leg. Which of the following would be the most appropriate reason to apply this treatment?
a. acute conditions
b. active bleeding
c. cancer
d. deep venous thrombosis

129. A physical therapist assistant is treating a 10-year-old girl status post ACL repair. Which of the following would be contraindicated at the site of the repair?
a. hot pack
b. whirlpool
c. ultrasound
d. electrical stimulation

130. A physical therapist assistant is treating a patient who is six months post skin graft to the anterior elbow region. The area is well healed, but the patient has a moderate flexion contracture. Prior to stretching his elbow, which massage stroke would be most appropriate to loosen soft tissue adhesions?
a. effleurage
b. petrissage
c. tapotement
d. friction

131. Use of the concept of "uncorking the bottle" would be important when treating a patient with which of the following conditions?
a. Bell's palsy
b. muscle spasm of the levator scapulae
c. myositis ossificans
d. lymphedema

132. A physical therapist assistant is assessing a patient with increased anteversion at the hip. Which of the following would be the most common hip range of motion limitations in a patient with this condition?
a. increased hip external rotation and decreased hip internal rotation
b. increased hip internal rotation and decreased hip external rotation
c. increased hip abduction and decreased hip adduction
d. increased hip adduction and decreased hip abduction

133. A physical therapist assistant is assessing a patient with a hand injury. The physical therapist assistant notes atrophy of the web space and very prominent metacarpals. Which nerve is most likely injured?
    a. median nerve
    b. ulnar nerve
    c. radial nerve
    d. axillary nerve

134. A physical therapist assistant goes to the local deli for lunch with another healthcare professional. The other healthcare professional starts talking about a patient he had treated that morning, a patient the PTA is not treating and will not be treating. The PTA is very uncomfortable, as the other person is discussing the patient by name and providing other identifying information. The PTA knows this is a violation of which of the following regulations?
    a. ADA
    b. OSHA
    c. HIPAA
    d. IDEA

135. A physical therapist assistant is treating a patient with a venous ulcer on her lower leg. All of the following are characteristic of venous ulcers EXCEPT
    a. normal skin temperature.
    b. brownish skin color.
    c. edema present.
    d. pedal pulses decreased or absent.

136. Several muscles in the body have dual nerve innervation. Which of the following muscles does NOT have dual nerve innervation?
    a. flexor digitorum superficialis
    b. pectoralis major
    c. adductor magnus
    d. lumbricals

137. A physical therapist assistant is treating a patient with a disease that is characterized by a progressive degeneration and loss of motor neurons in the motor cortex, brain stem, and spinal cord. It is usually fatal in three to five years. The etiology is unknown, though it is familial in 5 to 10% of all cases. This is a description of which of the following diseases?
    a. multiple sclerosis
    b. peroneal muscular atrophy
    c. amyotrophic lateral sclerosis
    d. Guillain-Barré

138. A physical therapist assistant is treating a patient who experienced a myocardial infarction followed by a CVA. The patient is doing well in rehab but is still exhibiting difficulty with instrumental activities of daily living. All of the following would be examples of instrumental activities of daily living EXCEPT
    a. dressing.
    b. cooking.
    c. shopping.
    d. driving a car.

139. A physical therapist assistant is treating an infant. In the patient's chart it lists an Apgar score of eight at five minutes. All of the following are tested on an Apgar EXCEPT
    a. pupil response.
    b. muscle tone.
    c. heart rate.
    d. color.

140. The major cause of lower extremity amputation is
    a. trauma.
    b. peripheral vascular disease.
    c. infection.
    d. diabetes.

141. A physical therapist assistant is treating a patient with a suspected Achilles tendon rupture. All of the following would be useful in making the diagnosis EXCEPT
   a. magnetic resonance imaging.
   b. positive Thompson test.
   c. physical examination and palpation of the tendon.
   d. positive Thomas test.

142. A physical therapist assistant is assessing the drainage from an ulcer. The drainage is thin, watery, and red in color. This drainage would be classified as a
   a. sanguinous exudate.
   b. serous exudate.
   c. seropurulent exudate.
   d. purulent exudate.

143. A physical therapist assistant is treating an 18-year-old woman who initially presented to her doctor with complaints of general malaise, slight fever, joint pain, and a rash across her checks and nose. Blood tests were positive for high levels of antinuclear antibodies. The most likely diagnosis is
   a. rheumatoid arthritis.
   b. scleroderma.
   c. systemic lupus erythematosus.
   d. Lyme disease.

144. A physical therapist assistant is treating a patient with chronic restrictive lung disease. When the physical therapist assistant checks the results of pulmonary function testing on this patient, he or she would expect all of the following to be decreased EXCEPT
   a. vital capacity.
   b. functional residual capacity.
   c. total lung capacity.
   d. residual volume.

145. An exercise tolerance test (stress test) was ordered for a patient prior to initiating a physical therapy program. All of the following would be contraindications for an exercise tolerance test EXCEPT
   a. acute congestive heart failure.
   b. demand type pacemaker.
   c. unstable angina.
   d. dissecting aneurysm.

146. Which of the following cardiac arrhythmias is lethal?
   a. atrial fibrillation
   b. premature ventricular contraction
   c. ventricular tachycardia
   d. ventricular fibrillation

147. A physical therapist assistant is treating a patient who has a Swan-Ganz catheter in place. The purpose of this catheter is to easily
   a. provide nutrition.
   b. monitor pulmonary artery pressure.
   c. give fluids or medications.
   d. take blood samples.

148. A physical therapist assistant is treating a patient who is receiving chemotherapy for the treatment of breast cancer. All of the following are side effects of chemotherapy EXCEPT
   a. neuropathy.
   b. nausea and vomiting.
   c. hair loss.
   d. dermatitis.

149. A physical therapist assistant is treating a patient with medial epicondylitis. All of the following would probably increase the patient's pain EXCEPT
  a. palpation over the medial epicondyle.
  b. resisted wrist extension and passive wrist flexion.
  c. resisted wrist flexion and passive extension.
  d. golfing.

150. A physical therapist assistant is working with a patient who experienced a cerebrovascular accident. In order to elicit information about what goals the patient would like to attain throughout the course of treatment, the physical therapist assistant should use
  a. open-ended questions.
  b. closed-ended questions.
  c. the FIM.
  d. screening questions.

Answers and Explanations

1. b. The center of a sling seat will be the lowest point causing the thighs to fall inward into adduction and internal rotation. (O'Sullivan 2007, page 1,293)

2. c. Impulsive behavior is characteristic of a right cerebrovascular accident. (O'Sullivan 2007, page 349)

3. d. Brown-Sequard syndrome is a hemisection of the cord. This results in loss of vibration and position sense and movement on the same side due to damage to the dorsal columns and the corticospinal tract, as well as loss of pain and temperature sensations on the opposite side due to damage of the anterior lateral spinal thalamic tract. (O'Sullivan 2007, page 941)

4. b. The scapula lies on the thorax between T2 and T7 with the base of the spine at T3. (Lippert 2006, page 94)

5. a. Stereognosis is the ability to recognize culturally familiar objects by touch with the vision occluded. (O'Sullivan 2007, page 145)

6. c. The standard rise:run for a ramp is 1:12. A four foot high ramp would require a length of 48 feet. 1:12 = 4:48. (O'Sullivan 2007, page 404)

7. b. Stage II ulcers extend through the epidermis into the dermis (and may involve the dermis) and are painful due to the exposure of nerve endings in the dermis. (O'Sullivan 2007, page 662)

8. d. Interrater reliability refers to the consistency between repeated measurements of the same variable by different raters. (O'Sullivan 2007, page 383)

9. a. Cheyne-Stokes breathing is characterized by rapid breathing for 10 to 60 seconds followed by a period of apnea. (Dreeben 2008, page 351)

10. d. Blood pressure is normally slightly higher in supine due to the increased venous return in this position. (O'Sullivan 2007, page 601)

11. a. This is a description of hold-relax where the patient contracts the tight muscle, resulting in autogenic inhibition of the tight muscle. This allows the clinician to then further passively elongate the muscle, thereby increasing range of motion. (Kisner 2007, page 85)

12. b. This is a closed-chain activity so the femur will move on the tibia. The femur will internally rotate to lock the knee. This is called the screw home mechanism. (Lippert 2006, page 252)

13. c. For a grade of 3+/5, the patient moves the body part through the range against gravity and can tolerate minimal resistance in the static test position. (O'Sullivan 2007, page 181)

14. c. This description is the classic presentation of Guillain-Barré, which is an acute ascending polyneuropathy. (Goodman and Fuller 2007, page 1,622)

15. d. In the Thomas test position, the knee should flex at least 80 degrees; anything less indicates tightness in the rectus femoris. (Norkin 2009, page 214)

16. c. This is a typical description of a grade III ligamentous sprain. (Kisner 2007, page 779)

17. b. With a cemented prosthesis, the patient can usually bear weight as tolerated starting at the initiation of ambulation. (Kisner 2007, page 653)

18. b. The hypothenar eminence is the muscle mass found on the ulnar side of the palm and is innervated by the ulnar nerve. (Lippert 2006, pages 26 and 28)

19. d. Cog wheel rigidity is a specific type of spasticity characteristic of Parkinson's disease. The clinician will meet resistance during PROM, but with persistence the area will then give. (O'Sullivan 2007, page 856)

20. c. When descending stairs with axillary crutches, the crutches must go down first followed by the involved lower extremity. This allows the patient to balance and then lower himself or herself with the uninvolved lower extremity. Lastly, the patient moves the uninvolved extremity to the step. The crutches should always stay with the involved leg to protect it from excessive weight-bearing. (Minor 2006, page 336)

21. b. C5 innervates the deltoid and teres minor, resulting in a position of shoulder adduction and internal rotation. It also innervates the biceps, which would produce a position of elbow extension. C6 innervates the wrist extensors, resulting in a position of wrist flexion. With the elbow extended and wrist flexed and the shoulder in adduction and internal rotation, this produces a position much like a waiter requesting a tip. (Goodman and Fuller 2007, pages 1,148 and 1,150)

22. d. Activities at two metabolic equivalents, such as knitting or dusting furniture, are considered low-level activities. Exercise with 1 to 2 lb. weights would also fall into this level. Raking leaves and cycling at 8 mph are at 4–5 METS. Walking 4 mph is at 5–6 METs. (O'Sullivan 2007, page 607)

23. b. Straight leg raises would not be appropriate. To perform straight leg raises, the patient needs her abdominals to stabilize, and this is too soon after her surgery for this type of activity. (Kisner 2007, page 818)

24. c. To stretch, one moves in the opposite direction of that muscle's action. The right sternocleidomastoid produces lateral neck flexion to the right with neck rotation to the left. To stretch the right sternocleidomastoid, one moves in the opposite direction into left lateral flexion with right rotation. (Kisner 2007, page 90)

25. d. Acute slipped capital femoral epiphysis is a medical emergency often requiring surgery. (Drnach 2008, page 75)

26. b. Maximal heart rate equals 220 minus the patient's age and target heart rate; for an endurance type program, it is 60–90 % of MHR. For this patient, that means MHR = 220 – 40 = 180 and THR = 180 (60–90%) = 108–162. So 120 is within this range. (O'Sullivan 2007, page 96)

27. c. With this patient's history, he or she could have a pulmonary embolus. The physician should be notified; the physician can determine the need for further testing. (Goodman and Fuller 2007, page 626)

28. d. A two-and-a-half-year-old cannot hop. This skill develops near age four. A two-and-a-half-year-old should be able to run, stair climb reciprocally, or jump in place. (Drnach 2008, page 48)

29. c. A change from supine to sitting can cause a drop in blood pressure called orthostatic hypotension. (O'Sullivan 2007, page 110)

30. b. The term *pectus* refers to chest, and *excavatum* refers to a depression. *Pectus excavatum* would mean that the sternum moves posteriorly (depressed), and this would decrease the A-P diameter of the rib cage. (Kisner 2007, page 857)

31. d. Dysmetria refers to difficulty judging the distance or range of a movement. During the pointing and past pointing test, the therapist would judge the accuracy with which the patient is able to line up his fingertips with the therapist's. (O'Sullivan 2007, page 214)

32. b. This is a measure of the Q-angle, which is considered to be the line of pull of the quadriceps. (Magee 2008, page 800)

33. a. Normal heart rate for a newborn is 70 to 190 bpm. A heart rate of 60 bpm is below this range. (O'Sullivan 2007, page 82)

34. a. Dependent edema is characteristic of right-sided heart failure. Pulmonary edema, dyspnea, and cough are all characteristic of left-sided heart failure. Failure of the right ventricle causes a backup into the right atria and the venous circulation. Failure of the left ventricle causes a backup into the left atria and the pulmonary circulation. (Goodman and Snyder 2007, page 293)

35. b. The xiphoid process is used as the landmark for measuring rib cage excursion. (O'Sullivan 2007, page 109)

36. a. Buoyancy creates an upward thrust on the body, holding the body up and making it easier to move in water than on land. (Kisner 2007, page 275)

37. c. The first stage in evidence-based practice is to identify a problem. The researcher must then develop a clinical question based on the problem. (O'Sullivan 2007, page 16)

38. a. Hand washing is the main factor in limiting nosocomial (hospital acquired) infections. (Goodman and Fuller 2009, page 1,673)

39. c. This is a short-term goal, and goals are usually placed in the assessment area of the note. (Minor 2006, page 11)

40. b. The traditional transfemoral socket shape is quadrilateral. (O'Sullivan 2007, page 1,263)

41. a. According to the Nagi Model of Disability, inability to work is a disability. According to the Nagi Model, a disability is defined as difficulty in performing social roles due to an impairment. Impaired ambulation is a functional limitation. Pain, decreased ROM, and decreased strength are impairments. (O'Sullivan 2007, page 8)

42. c. Interventions for a patient with post-polio syndrome would probably not include sensory retraining, because sensation is usually not affected in post-polio syndrome. However, fatigue, pain, and muscle weakness are hallmark symptoms of the pathology. (Goodman and Fuller 2009, page 1,625)

43. c. Metabolic syndrome is a group of signs and symptoms characterized by insulin resistance and strongly associated with heart disease and type II diabetes. Hypertension, insulin resistance, and apple-shaped/abdominal obesity are three major characteristics of metabolic syndrome. Pear-shaped/hip/thigh obesity is not characteristic of metabolic syndrome. (Goodman and Snyder 2007, page 497)

44. b. The symptoms listed, especially rectal bleeding, are characteristic of ulcerative colitis. (Goodman and Snyder 2007, page 393)

45. a. The patient cannot read. Therefore, pictures and demonstrations would be the most useful approach. (Dreeben 2008, pages 8 and 12)

46. d. There is no rationale for this patient to perform plyometrics. Plyometrics exercises involve an eccentric loading of the muscle followed by a strong concentric contraction. They are useful for patients who will be performing activities that require rapid starting and stopping movements. (Kisner 2007, page 208)

47. c. This tissue is healthy, thick, and needs to be stretched. Therefore, 1 MHz continuous and 1.0–2.0 w/cm^2 would provide the proper depth and heating prior to stretching. (Prentice 2005, page 385)

48. b. Interrupted DC to the motor points is the type of stimulation that would be most beneficial for this patient. Totally denervated muscles need long duration interrupted DC to attain an action potential right at the muscle since there will be no reaction at the nerve. (Prentice 2005, page 135)

49. d. Landing directly on the tip of the shoulder is the usual mechanism of injury for an acromioclavicular, or AC, separation. (Magee 2008, page 235)

50. c. Scleroderma is a progressive connective tissue disease characterized by hardening of the connective tissue and excessive connective tissue. This leads to contractures, skin ulcerations, and damage to internal organs. It would be unlikely that this patient would require core strengthening exercises. However, the patient would require the other techniques listed to limit contractures and ulcers. (Dreeben 2008, page 462)

51. b. According to the rule of nines, both anterior lower extremities are 9% each, half of the posterior lower extremities are 4.5% each, and the groin is 1%. This would total 28%. (O'Sullivan 2007, page 1,098)

52. c. Moderate assist means that the patient can perform at least 50% of the task, requiring at most 50% assist from the clinician. (Minor 2006, page 198)

53. b. In a first class lever system, the axis is between the force and the resistance. In a second class lever system, the resistance is between the axis and the force. In a third class lever system, the force is between the resistance and the axis. (Lippert 2006, page 81)

54. a. Early weight-bearing activities can help prevent the progression of complex regional pain syndrome. Therefore, closed chain activities would be most appropriate to utilize during stage I CRPS. (Kisner 2007, page 380)

55. d. In the thoracic spine, vertebral rotation occurs opposite of lateral flexion. Since the concavity, or lateral flexion, is to the left, the vertebral bodies will be rotated to the right, and the ribs will be drawn back on that side. (Kisner 2007, page 396)

56. a. The modified Ober test is a test for flexibility of the tensor fascia latae. (Norkin 2009, page 228)

57. b. A range of 25 to 150 degrees indicates that the patient cannot fully extend the knee. Therefore, the flexors (hamstrings) are tight and should be stretched. (Norkin 2009, page 246)

58. a. The Barlow Maneuver, Ortaloni's Click, and X-ray are all tests for DDH. The apprehension sign is a test for anterior shoulder dislocation or for a dislocation of the patella. (Magee 2008, page 279)

59. c. This is a description of the Romberg test. The Sharpened Romberg test takes place with one foot in front of the other. The Tinetti and the Berg tests are standardized balance assessments that contain a number of items. (O'Sullivan 2007, page 254)

60. c. The patient would short sit leaning backward slightly to prevent active insufficiency of the rectus femoris and passive insufficiency of the hamstrings. (Hislop 2007, page 224)

61. c. When measuring for a wheelchair, the widest area across the patient's buttocks, hips, or thighs is measured, and then two inches are added for comfort, clothing, and to prevent pressure on the greater trochanters. This would allow one inch on each side. (Minor 2006, page 190)

62. c. Droplet precautions are sufficient since this type of infection does not suspend in the air, and the droplets carry less than three feet. (Minor 2006, page 56)

63. c. A solid AFO would support the weak dorsiflexors while providing medial-lateral stability. (O'Sullivan 2007, page 1,219)

64. d. A resting heart rate less than 60 bpm is considered slow for a male patient of 60 years old. The professional term for this is bradycardia. (O'Sullivan 2007, page 95)

65. a. Bilateral upper extremity D2 flexion and extension would allow the patient to combine inspiration with D2 flexion, thereby increasing the elevation of the rib cage and expiration with D2 extension, returning the rib cage to its original shape and size. Since the D2 flexion pattern includes abduction, doing it bilaterally will open up the anterior chest area. (Kisner 2007, page 199 and 867)

66. c. The problem list goes in the assessment section of a SOAP note. Girth measurements, the list of exercises performed during that session, and current ambulatory status all go in the objective section of a SOAP note. (Minor 2006, page 11)

67. b. New guidelines consider a blood pressure of 120/80 in the prehypertension stage. (Minor 2006, page 87)

68. d. Hypotonic cerebral palsy is characterized by low tone resulting in a rag doll floppy presentation, excessive range of motion, and tongue protrusion. Strong deep tendon reflexes would not indicate hypotonicity. (Dreeben 2008, page 543)

69. d. Rheumatoid arthritis is most frequently diagnosed between the ages of 20 and 50. (Goodman and Fuller 2009, page 1,265)

70. b. This patient has too much iron in his or her blood, so you would not give blood, which would give the patient more iron. (Goodman and Snyder 2007, page 501)

71. b. Wet to dry dressings are nonselective and can remove healthy tissue as well as necrotic tissue. (O'Sullivan 2007, page 667)

72. a. Half kneel is the next step in the developmental sequence after high kneel. (O'Sullivan 2007, page 112)

73. b. These are classic signs of a deep vein thrombosis, and the physical therapist assistant should contact the MD so that further medical intervention can be determined. (Goodman and Fuller 2009, page 626)

74. b. A patient with diabetes and a neuropathic ulcer will have both sensory and vascular deficits. A whirlpool at the same temperature as the skin (92˚F or 93˚F) would be most appropriate since the patient's temperature regulating mechanisms may be faulty. (Prentice 2005, page 30)

75. a. Cool, clammy skin is not characteristic of heatstroke. It is characteristic of heat exhaustion. Dry, warm skin is characteristic of heatstroke. (Goodman and Fuller 2009, page 132)

76. c. The hamstrings are responsible for slowing the forward movement of the tibia in preparation for initial contact. (Magee 2008, page 951)

77. a. On a fixed convex surface, the concave surface will move in the same direction as the body segments movement. (O'Sullivan 2007, page 30)

78. c. The patient long sitting performing resisted eversion with Thera-Band would be most beneficial in strengthening the affected muscles. The peroneal nerve innervates the peroneus brevis and the peroneus longus whose primary action is eversion. It also innervates anterior tibialis, but inversion can be performed by posterior tibialis, so it would not need strengthening as much as the everters would. (Lippert 2006, page 282)

79. a. The tissue in this area is thin and in poor condition, so 3 MHz would be the appropriate depth since that frequency is used when applying ultrasound to superficial tissues. This means that 0.5w/cm^2 at 20% duty cycle will result in an average intensity of 0.1 w/cm^2. This will provide nonthermal benefits to promote healing without heating the tissues, which could promote inflammation. (Prentice 2005, page 370)

80. b. At C6, the wrist extensors are innervated, and the patient will demonstrate a weak tenodesis grasp. A tenodesis splint will increase the force of the grasp and improve the patient's ability to manipulate items to perform activities of daily living. (Lusardi 2000, page 287)

81. b. Excessive thirst is a sign of ketosis, not of hypoglycemia. (Dreeben 2008, page 43)

82. c. Of the positions listed, left side-lying is least likely to promote acid reflux into the esophagus because the stomach is on the left side of the body. This position keeps the stomach contents below the esophageal juncture. Lying supine would allow for reflux into the esophagus, and Trendelenburg(head down) and right side-lying would promote gastroesophageal reflux. (Goodman and Fuller 2009, page 836)

83. d. A three-month-old should have his or her hands open most of the time. (Dreeben 2008, page 527)

84. c. If a child had a persistent ATNR when the head was turned to one side, then the extremities on that side would extend and the child could not roll over the outstretched arm. (Dreeben 2008, page 521)

85. b. Proprioception is the awareness of our body in space movement of the body parts. Kinesthetic awareness is the awareness of movement, so this is a proprioception test. (O'Sullivan 2007, page 145)

86. b. The McGill Pain Questionnaire assesses the quality of pain, which is an assessment of an impairment, not of function. The Barthel Index, FIM, and Tinetti are functional assessment tools. (O'Sullivan 2007, page 1,146)

87. d. Elevation is effective for mild or acute swelling, but lymphedema doesn't usually respond to simple elevation. (O'Sullivan 2007, page 654)

88. c. The skin is important in vitamin D synthesis, not vitamin C synthesis. (Dreeben 2008, page 467)

89. a. It would not be useful to alternate between a wide variety of activities. Children with pervasive developmental disorder do best with simple, well-structured routines. (Dreeben 2008, page 567)

90. d. Thoracic outlet syndrome is often associated with a forward head and shoulders posture with weakness of the trapezius and rhomboids and tightness of the pectoralis major.

Therefore, passive extension exercises would be the least helpful of those activities listed. (Kisner 2007, page 373)

91. b. Weighting the extremities is often used when the patient has proprioceptive problems. That is not one of the major concerns with Parkinson's disease. The other activities would be more beneficial in addressing the rigidity and akinesia common to patients with Parkinson's disease. (O'Sullivan 2007, page 879)

92. a. Metal clips should not be used to secure the bandage, as they come off easily and can scratch the patient. (O'Sullivan 2007, page 1,043)

93. d. A continuous passive motion unit would not increase strength, as it is a passive activity and there is no active muscle contraction. (Kisner 2007, page 61)

94. b. This treatment is called the Brandt-Davoff treatment for posterior semi-circular canal benign paroxysmal positional vertigo (BPPV). (O'Sullivan 2007, page 1,017)

95. a. Rhythmic initiation is a proprioceptive neuromuscular facilitation technique to promote mobility, not stability, and is typically used on the extremities. This technique would therefore not be useful in developing core strength and stability with this patient. (Kisner 2007, page 202)

96. d. Choice might overwhelm a depressed patient and then it might be difficult to get anything done. (O'Sullivan 2007, page 47)

97. b. Anticoagulants are blood thinners and would not be needed by a patient with emphysema unless another condition is also present. (Ciccone 2002, page 375)

98. d. In the early physical therapy sessions following a coronary artery bypass graft, the physical therapy assistant would not be likely to use PREs with light weights for the upper extremities. It is too early for resisted upper extremity exercises. Some physicians will

even limit flexibility exercises for the upper extremities at the shoulders for the first four to six weeks following a coronary artery bypass graft. (O'Sullivan 2007, page 622)

99. a. Fibromyalgia syndrome is usually characterized by pain present in all four quadrants of the body. (Goodman and Snyder 2007, page 527)

100. b. The drop arm test is a test for a possible rotator cuff tear. The patient's arm is placed in 90 degrees of abduction, and the patient is asked to slowly lower the arm. If the patient struggles with lowering the arm or the arm suddenly drops to the side, the test is positive for a possible rotator cuff tear. (Magee 2008, page 311)

101. a. The fibula and the tibia are joined at their distal ends by a strong fibrous membrane, which allows little to no movement. This is characteristic of a synarthrodial joint. (Lippert 2006, page 18)

102. b. Supination of the foot is a combination movement including plantar flexion at the talotibial joint, inversion at the subtalar joint, and forefoot adduction. (Lippert 2006, page 268)

103. a. The patient will not have the upper extremity strength and manipulation skills or the balance necessary to complete self-stretching independently in bed. Since the deltoid and rhomboids are innervated, the shoulder function will allow the patient to perform the other activities with adaptive equipment and/or assistance. (O'Sullivan 2007, page 962)

104. c. Progressive systemic sclerosis is a connective tissue disease resulting in loss of flexibility of connective tissue. Therefore, stretching and flexibility are the areas of concentration for physical therapy. (Dreeben 2008, page 462)

105. d. In a greenstick fracture in a child, the bone is fractured on the tension, or convex, side while the cortex and periosteum remain intact on the compression, or concave, side. This is similar to a young branch splintering when bent; hence the name greenstick fracture. (Kisner 2007, page 322)

106. c. Characteristic of autonomic dysreflexia is an increase in blood pressure. Call for help first because this is a medical emergency. Sitting the patient up if he or she is lying down would help lower the blood pressure. Check the catheter to make sure it is not blocked, which can lead to autonomic dysreflexia. (O'Sullivan 2007, page 943)

107. d. Intermittent pelvic traction supine with the hips and knees flexed is the appropriate position for paraspinal muscle spasms, facet joint hypomobility, or tightness in the posterior longitudinal ligament. If a patient has a posterior lateral disc bulge, traction should be performed with the spine in extension to load the posterior area and open the anterior area, allowing the bulge to relocate centrally. The position described would place the lumbar spine into flexion. (Prentice 2005, page 469)

108. b. The stimulus for the positive support reflex is pressure on the plantar aspect of the foot. Since during crawling, the soles of the feet are not in contact with the ground, the positive support reflex will not be elicited. Positive support would not interfere with crawling. (Dreeben 2008, page 523)

109. a. The shoulder internal rotators are composed of the pectoralis major, anterior deltoid, subscapularis, teres major, and latissimus dorsi muscles. These are the muscles that produce internal rotation. Infraspinatus, teres minor, and posterior deltoid all produce external shoulder rotation. (Lippert 2006, page 118)

110. a. A decreased quadriceps deep tendon reflex would indicate impairment of nerve roots L3 and L4. The cutaneous area of innervation for L3 and L4 is the medial aspect of the lower leg. (O'Sullivan 2007, page 124)

111. b. The goals of phase I are to prevent deconditioning and post-op complications, to assess response to activity, and to provide patient and family education. A maximal symptom limited exercise test is part of the phase II cardiac rehab program and would not be included in phase I cardiac rehab. (Kisner 2007, page 243)

112. d. Cystic fibrosis is a common hereditary disease affecting all major exocrine glands and resulting in thick secretions. These secretions form mucus plugs that can then block lung passages and other passages like the pancreatic and bile duct. This results in respiratory problems including frequent infections and digestive problems. Patients with cystic fibrosis frequently need pancreatic enzymes, bronchodilators, and antibiotics because of the above. Antihistamines are used to treat allergic responses and would not be necessary unless another condition was present. (Ciccone 2002, page 412)

113. b. A two-person lift is used to transfer a patient between areas of different heights, for example from the floor to a chair. (Minor 2006, page 216)

114. b. Transfer of a skill to different settings is part of stage III of motor learning, the autonomous/retention stage. (Umphred 2006, page 30)

115. d. This is a test for impaired rapid alternating movements; the professional term for impaired rapid alternating movements is dysdiadochokinesia. (O'Sullivan 2007, page 214)

116. b. The patient would hold the crutches on the right to balance the NWB status on the left and to allow the patient to push off on the left from the more stable wheelchair. (Minor 2006, page 316)

117. a. This is a test for skin turgor/skin hydration. If it takes longer than five seconds for the skin to return to place, the patient may be dehydrated. (Goodman and Snyder 2007, page 200)

118. **d.** The physical therapist assistant can not perform the discharge examination. The physical therapist can delegate the task of gathering some of the data for the discharge examination to the physical therapist assistant, but the physical therapist will evaluate the data and make the discharge decision. (Dreeben 2008, page 5)

119. **a.** Summary feedback, feedback provided at the end of the session or after a number of trials, would be the least useful type of feedback, as it would not allow the patient to self correct and reinforce the correction. (Umphred 2006, page 32)

120. **c.** This best illustrates stage IV. Stage IV is characterized by a decline in spasticity and the beginning of out-of-pattern movements. (O'Sullivan 2007, page 719)

121. **b.** Unless other conditions are present, postural retraining is not likely to be part of the plan of care for this patient. Postural problems are not a main area of concern for patients with diabetes. (Goodman and Fuller 2009, page 492)

122. **c.** Cherry red skin is characteristic of carbon monoxide poisoning. (Goodman and Fuller 2009, page 124)

123. **a.** Opioid analgesics depress the central nervous system. Therefore, an increase in excitability is not a characteristic side effect of opioid analgesics. Opioids can cause gastrointestinal upset and physical and/or psychological dependence. An increase in excitability is not a characteristic side effect of opioid analgesics such as Demerol. (Ciccone 2002, page 199)

124. **a.** A bouyancy assisted position would allow the buoyancy to help raise the limb while stretching. (Kisner 2007, page 282)

125. **c.** The inverse square law states that the intensity of radiant energy is inversely proportional to the distance squared. Therefore, if you decrease the distance by one-half, you will increase the intensity by a factor of four. (Prentice 2005, page 441)

126. **d.** A randomized controlled trial tests a specific variable. Two groups are randomized so that they are considered identical. One group receives the intervention and the other does not. The results are then evaluated. This provides the best evidence for the effectiveness of a treatment. A single case study describes the diagnosis and treatment of a single patient. With a case study, there is no comparison. A meta-analysis combines the results of a number of randomized controlled trials. A researcher may choose which studies to include and which studies to eliminate so they could choose studies favorable to their own viewpoint. A cohort study is a study where a group of subjects receiving a specific treatment or with a specific diagnosis are compared to a group without the diagnosis or not receiving the treatment. Since the groups are not randomized, cohort studies are not as reliable as randomized controlled trials. (O'Sullivan 2007, page 17)

127. **c.** In iontophoresis, the dosage is measured in milliamp-minutes so if one increases the intensity, he or she must decrease the time to attain the same dosage. For example, 4 mA for ten minutes equals 40 mA-minutes. If the intensity is increased to 5 mA, then the time would have to be decreased to eight minutes to attain a total dosage of 40 mA-minutes. (Prentice 2005, page 170)

128. **a.** If the temperature is manipulated, whirlpool can be used for some acute conditions. For example, a cool whirlpool may be applied for an acute ankle sprain. (Prentice 2005, page 303)

129. **c.** Ultrasound is contraindicated over the epiphyseal plates in a patient who is still growing. (Prentice 2005, page 47)

130. d. Cross-fiber friction will help release adhesions. Effleurage may be done during the stretching along the length of the fibers. (Prentice 2005, page 518)

131. d. Use of the concept of uncorking would be important when treating a patient with lymphedema. Uncorking is a concept from massage, which relates to the need to clear the proximal area first before moving to the distal area. Therefore, in an extremity, you would massage the proximal segment first (working distal to proximal within that segment) before moving to the next distal segment and following the same pattern. (Prentice 2005, page 507)

132. b. With increased anteversion at the hip, the lower extremity assumes a posture of increased internal rotation with decreased external rotation. (Lippert 2006, page 237)

133. b. The ulnar nerve innervates the interossei and lumbricals three and four. An injury to this nerve resulting in atrophy of these muscles would result in atrophy of the web space and very prominent metacarpals since these muscles are found between the metacarpals. (Lippert 2006, page 157)

134. c. Discussing a patient by name and providing other identifying information about a patient with a person who is not and will not be treating that patient is a violation of provisions of HIPAA, which protects the personal health information of patients. (Dreeben 2008, page 76)

135. d. Decreased pedal pulses are characteristic of arterial ulcers. Pulses are usually normal with venous ulcers. (O'Sullivan 2007, page 651)

136. a. Flexor digitorum superficialis has a single innervation, the median nerve. (Lippert 2006, page 149)

137. c. This is a description of amyotrophic lateral sclerosis. (Goodman and Fuller 2009, page 1,403)

138. a. Dressing is a basic activity of daily living. All of the other activities listed are instrumental activities of daily living. Instrumental activities of daily living are advanced skills that are necessary for a person to live independently in a community setting. (O'Sullivan 2007, page 8)

139. a. A pupil response is not tested during an Apgar. (Dreeben 2008, page 518)

140. b. Peripheral vascular disease, often associated with diabetes and smoking, is the major cause of lower extremity amputations. (O'Sullivan 2007, page 1,031)

141. d. The Thomas test is a test for hip flexor tightness and would not be useful in making the diagnosis of an Achilles tendon rupture. (Norkin 2009, page 212)

142. a. *Sanguinous* is the professional term for thin, red, watery discharge. (Dreeben 2008, page 430)

143. c. The signs and symptoms listed are characteristic of systemic lupus erythematosus. (Goodman and Fuller 2009, page 284)

144. d. Residual volume is usually normal in a patient with chronic restrictive lung disease. The problem is getting air in, not getting it out. Residual volume is often increased in patients with emphysema, which is a chronic obstructive pulmonary disease. (O'Sullivan 2007, page 568)

145. b. A demand type pacemaker is not a contraindication for an exercise tolerance test. (O'Sullivan 2007, page 608)

146. d. When the heart is in ventricular fibrillation, the ventricles are not actually contracting. This will be fatal if not resolved. (O'Sullivan 2007, page 631)

147. b. A Swan-Ganz catheter is placed in the pulmonary artery to monitor pressure there. (O'Sullivan 2007, page 605)

148. **c.** Dermatitis is a side effect of radiation therapy but not chemotherapy. (Goodman and Fuller 2009, page 169)

149. **b.** Medial epicondylitis is tendinitis of the wrist flexors at their origin on or near the lateral epicondyle of the humerus; also known as golfer's elbow. All the activities listed would increase pain except resisted wrist extension and passive flexion, which would increase pain in a patient with lateral epicondylitis. (Magee 2008, page 379)

150. **a.** Open-ended questions would provide a large amount of information in a short amount of time. Closed-ended questions are simple yes or no questions that would not yield as much information as open-ended questions. (Goodman and Snyder 2007, page 42)

10 ▶ Practice Exam 2

This practice exam should be taken after completing both the Diagnostic Test and Practice Exam 1. Like those exams, it is designed to help you practice for the national exam by including questions in academic and clinical areas in which you will need to recall important information and may need more review.

Part I

1. ⓐ ⓑ ⓒ ⓓ
2. ⓐ ⓑ ⓒ ⓓ
3. ⓐ ⓑ ⓒ ⓓ
4. ⓐ ⓑ ⓒ ⓓ
5. ⓐ ⓑ ⓒ ⓓ
6. ⓐ ⓑ ⓒ ⓓ
7. ⓐ ⓑ ⓒ ⓓ
8. ⓐ ⓑ ⓒ ⓓ
9. ⓐ ⓑ ⓒ ⓓ
10. ⓐ ⓑ ⓒ ⓓ
11. ⓐ ⓑ ⓒ ⓓ
12. ⓐ ⓑ ⓒ ⓓ
13. ⓐ ⓑ ⓒ ⓓ
14. ⓐ ⓑ ⓒ ⓓ
15. ⓐ ⓑ ⓒ ⓓ
16. ⓐ ⓑ ⓒ ⓓ
17. ⓐ ⓑ ⓒ ⓓ
18. ⓐ ⓑ ⓒ ⓓ
19. ⓐ ⓑ ⓒ ⓓ
20. ⓐ ⓑ ⓒ ⓓ
21. ⓐ ⓑ ⓒ ⓓ
22. ⓐ ⓑ ⓒ ⓓ
23. ⓐ ⓑ ⓒ ⓓ
24. ⓐ ⓑ ⓒ ⓓ
25. ⓐ ⓑ ⓒ ⓓ
26. ⓐ ⓑ ⓒ ⓓ
27. ⓐ ⓑ ⓒ ⓓ
28. ⓐ ⓑ ⓒ ⓓ
29. ⓐ ⓑ ⓒ ⓓ
30. ⓐ ⓑ ⓒ ⓓ
31. ⓐ ⓑ ⓒ ⓓ
32. ⓐ ⓑ ⓒ ⓓ
33. ⓐ ⓑ ⓒ ⓓ
34. ⓐ ⓑ ⓒ ⓓ
35. ⓐ ⓑ ⓒ ⓓ
36. ⓐ ⓑ ⓒ ⓓ
37. ⓐ ⓑ ⓒ ⓓ
38. ⓐ ⓑ ⓒ ⓓ
39. ⓐ ⓑ ⓒ ⓓ
40. ⓐ ⓑ ⓒ ⓓ
41. ⓐ ⓑ ⓒ ⓓ
42. ⓐ ⓑ ⓒ ⓓ
43. ⓐ ⓑ ⓒ ⓓ
44. ⓐ ⓑ ⓒ ⓓ
45. ⓐ ⓑ ⓒ ⓓ
46. ⓐ ⓑ ⓒ ⓓ
47. ⓐ ⓑ ⓒ ⓓ
48. ⓐ ⓑ ⓒ ⓓ
49. ⓐ ⓑ ⓒ ⓓ
50. ⓐ ⓑ ⓒ ⓓ

Part II

51. ⓐ ⓑ ⓒ ⓓ
52. ⓐ ⓑ ⓒ ⓓ
53. ⓐ ⓑ ⓒ ⓓ
54. ⓐ ⓑ ⓒ ⓓ
55. ⓐ ⓑ ⓒ ⓓ
56. ⓐ ⓑ ⓒ ⓓ
57. ⓐ ⓑ ⓒ ⓓ
58. ⓐ ⓑ ⓒ ⓓ
59. ⓐ ⓑ ⓒ ⓓ
60. ⓐ ⓑ ⓒ ⓓ
61. ⓐ ⓑ ⓒ ⓓ
62. ⓐ ⓑ ⓒ ⓓ
63. ⓐ ⓑ ⓒ ⓓ
64. ⓐ ⓑ ⓒ ⓓ
65. ⓐ ⓑ ⓒ ⓓ
66. ⓐ ⓑ ⓒ ⓓ
67. ⓐ ⓑ ⓒ ⓓ
68. ⓐ ⓑ ⓒ ⓓ
69. ⓐ ⓑ ⓒ ⓓ
70. ⓐ ⓑ ⓒ ⓓ
71. ⓐ ⓑ ⓒ ⓓ
72. ⓐ ⓑ ⓒ ⓓ
73. ⓐ ⓑ ⓒ ⓓ
74. ⓐ ⓑ ⓒ ⓓ
75. ⓐ ⓑ ⓒ ⓓ
76. ⓐ ⓑ ⓒ ⓓ
77. ⓐ ⓑ ⓒ ⓓ
78. ⓐ ⓑ ⓒ ⓓ
79. ⓐ ⓑ ⓒ ⓓ
80. ⓐ ⓑ ⓒ ⓓ
81. ⓐ ⓑ ⓒ ⓓ
82. ⓐ ⓑ ⓒ ⓓ
83. ⓐ ⓑ ⓒ ⓓ
84. ⓐ ⓑ ⓒ ⓓ
85. ⓐ ⓑ ⓒ ⓓ
86. ⓐ ⓑ ⓒ ⓓ
87. ⓐ ⓑ ⓒ ⓓ
88. ⓐ ⓑ ⓒ ⓓ
89. ⓐ ⓑ ⓒ ⓓ
90. ⓐ ⓑ ⓒ ⓓ
91. ⓐ ⓑ ⓒ ⓓ
92. ⓐ ⓑ ⓒ ⓓ
93. ⓐ ⓑ ⓒ ⓓ
94. ⓐ ⓑ ⓒ ⓓ
95. ⓐ ⓑ ⓒ ⓓ
96. ⓐ ⓑ ⓒ ⓓ
97. ⓐ ⓑ ⓒ ⓓ
98. ⓐ ⓑ ⓒ ⓓ
99. ⓐ ⓑ ⓒ ⓓ
100. ⓐ ⓑ ⓒ ⓓ

Part III

101. ⓐ ⓑ ⓒ ⓓ
102. ⓐ ⓑ ⓒ ⓓ
103. ⓐ ⓑ ⓒ ⓓ
104. ⓐ ⓑ ⓒ ⓓ
105. ⓐ ⓑ ⓒ ⓓ
106. ⓐ ⓑ ⓒ ⓓ
107. ⓐ ⓑ ⓒ ⓓ
108. ⓐ ⓑ ⓒ ⓓ
109. ⓐ ⓑ ⓒ ⓓ
110. ⓐ ⓑ ⓒ ⓓ
111. ⓐ ⓑ ⓒ ⓓ
112. ⓐ ⓑ ⓒ ⓓ
113. ⓐ ⓑ ⓒ ⓓ
114. ⓐ ⓑ ⓒ ⓓ
115. ⓐ ⓑ ⓒ ⓓ
116. ⓐ ⓑ ⓒ ⓓ
117. ⓐ ⓑ ⓒ ⓓ
118. ⓐ ⓑ ⓒ ⓓ
119. ⓐ ⓑ ⓒ ⓓ
120. ⓐ ⓑ ⓒ ⓓ
121. ⓐ ⓑ ⓒ ⓓ
122. ⓐ ⓑ ⓒ ⓓ
123. ⓐ ⓑ ⓒ ⓓ
124. ⓐ ⓑ ⓒ ⓓ
125. ⓐ ⓑ ⓒ ⓓ
126. ⓐ ⓑ ⓒ ⓓ
127. ⓐ ⓑ ⓒ ⓓ
128. ⓐ ⓑ ⓒ ⓓ
129. ⓐ ⓑ ⓒ ⓓ
130. ⓐ ⓑ ⓒ ⓓ
131. ⓐ ⓑ ⓒ ⓓ
132. ⓐ ⓑ ⓒ ⓓ
133. ⓐ ⓑ ⓒ ⓓ
134. ⓐ ⓑ ⓒ ⓓ
135. ⓐ ⓑ ⓒ ⓓ
136. ⓐ ⓑ ⓒ ⓓ
137. ⓐ ⓑ ⓒ ⓓ
138. ⓐ ⓑ ⓒ ⓓ
139. ⓐ ⓑ ⓒ ⓓ
140. ⓐ ⓑ ⓒ ⓓ
141. ⓐ ⓑ ⓒ ⓓ
142. ⓐ ⓑ ⓒ ⓓ
143. ⓐ ⓑ ⓒ ⓓ
144. ⓐ ⓑ ⓒ ⓓ
145. ⓐ ⓑ ⓒ ⓓ
146. ⓐ ⓑ ⓒ ⓓ
147. ⓐ ⓑ ⓒ ⓓ
148. ⓐ ⓑ ⓒ ⓓ
149. ⓐ ⓑ ⓒ ⓓ
150. ⓐ ⓑ ⓒ ⓓ

Part I

1. Refer to the figure below. Which muscle is being assessed by placing the patient in the position illustrated?

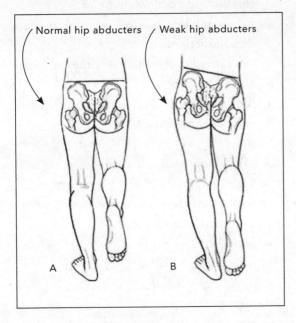

Normal hip abducters   Weak hip abducters

A   B

    a. gluteus medius
    b. gluteus maximus
    c. quadriceps
    d. hamstrings

2. What levels of myotome involvement should be suspected by the PTA when a patient is unable to perform toe walking?
    a. L2–L3
    b. L3–L4
    c. L4–L5
    d. S1–S2

3. A physical therapist requests that a PTA perform sharp debridement. Which one of the following references will best determine whether a PTA will legally perform sharp debridement?
    a. laws of the state
    b. insurance reimbursement guide
    c. patient plan of care
    d. patient pain tolerance

4. During unassisted ambulation to a treatment room, a PTA observes a new patient with back pain exhibiting foot drop. This can be a result of a pathology to which of the following structures?
    a. tibialis anterior muscle
    b. deep peroneal nerve
    c. L3 nerve root lesion
    d. deep fibular nerve

5. A PTA would utilize which of the following movements to accurately assess a patient's shoulder joint end feel?
    a. resisted isometric
    b. active-assistive range of motion
    c. active range of motion
    d. passive range of motion

6. What is the best way to open an unresponsive person's airway when a cervical injury is not suspected?
    a. Give abdominal thrusts and then sweep out the mouth.
    b. Use the head tilt/chin lift.
    c. Use the tongue lift/finger sweep.
    d. Use a mask while giving breaths to the victim.

7. Weakness in which muscle is most likely the cause of the postural fault known as scapular winging?
  a. upper trapezius
  b. serratus anterior
  c. rhomboid
  d. pectoralis minor

8. A PTA is creating a home program for a patient treated for a frozen shoulder. What key element of this program is used to help the patient maintain ROM during daily activities?
  a. self-stretching
  b. contract-relax
  c. PNF
  d. plyometrics

9. A PTA is using the daily adjustable progressive resistance exercise (DAPRE) technique to provide resistance training for a patient. Based on the information, the patient performed eight repetitions on set number three (which was the last set of the day). Would the PTA increase or decrease the amount of weight for this patient on the next day?
  a. increase 10–15 pounds
  b. increase 5–10 pounds
  c. decrease 0–5 pounds
  d. decrease 5–10 pounds

10. A PTA is providing education for a patient who just received a total hip replacement with a posterolateral approach. What motions would the PTA stress that this patient avoid?
  a. hip flexion greater than 90°, internal rotation, and adduction
  b. hip flexion less than 90°, internal rotation, and abduction
  c. hip extension less than 90°, internal rotation, and adduction
  d. hip extension greater than 90°, internal rotation, and abduction

11. A PTA is employed in an outpatient physical therapy private practice. What type of supervision is required for a PTA to treat a patient with Medicare Part B?
  a. periodic supervision
  b. indirect supervision
  c. direct supervision
  d. no supervision

12. A PTA witnesses a car hit a pedestrian in the hospital parking lot. After initial assessment, the PTA determines that the person is not breathing, but the PTA suspects a neck injury. How should the PTA open the airway?
  a. jaw thrust
  b. head tilt/chin lift
  c. head lift/chin tilt
  d. abdominal thrust

13. In which shoulder range of motion activity should a PTA monitor patient performance, prohibiting patient substitution with trunk side bending, toe raising, or abduction?
  a. wand performed in supine
  b. wall climbing performed in standing
  c. overhead pulleys performed in sitting
  d. Thera-Band performed in standing

14. A PTA is providing rehabilitation for a frail 78-year-old deconditioned female patient with a negative history of other pathologies. What would be the best exercise program for this patient?
   a. endurance exercise
   b. high intensity isotonic resistance exercise
   c. isometric exercise
   d. low to moderate intensity exercise

15. A patient with a history of decreased physical activity secondary to hypertension and coronary artery disease reports that her shoes are so tight she cannot wear them. What medical condition does the PTA suspect is causing this problem?
   a. hypothyroidism
   b. congestive heart failure
   c. peripheral neuropathy
   d. gout

16. While attending a parent-teacher conference, the teacher, knowing the student's mother is a PTA, tells her about the gradual onset over the past several months of visual disturbances, progressive lower limb weakness, spasticity, and incontinence. What should the PTA suspect?
   a. phlebitis
   b. multiple sclerosis
   c. hyperthyroidism
   d. congestive heart failure

17. During a gait training session, a PTA observes the midstance phase of gait from the anterior (front) view of the left lower extremity. The pelvis has an exaggerated downward tilt on the right side, and the right lower extremity is in swing phase. What muscle would the PTA assess for adequate strength?
   a. right hip abductor
   b. left hip adductor
   c. right hip adductor
   d. left hip abductor

18. A PTA using the Karvonen Method to calculate 40% to 60% target heart rate range for a 78-year-old patient with a resting pulse rate of 66 would arrive at what range?
   a. 80–92
   b. 90–106
   c. 96–112
   d. 116–128

19. A PTA explains the treatment plan to a patient, but the patient does not consent to it. What is the best course of action for the PTA?
   a. Provide care and inform the physical therapist.
   b. Provide care and schedule the next appointment.
   c. Call the patient's identified emergency contact for consent.
   d. Do not give care and inform the physical therapist.

20. A PTA is assisting the physical therapist performing a preseason screening of a local high school basketball team. What is the purpose of the preseason screening?
   a. assisting the coach in identifying injuries
   b. helping to identify existing musculoskeletal imbalances that could lead to injury
   c. providing patients for physical therapy
   d. identifying the best athlete on the team

21. A child is attending a physical therapy session with her mother and accidentally eats some ultrasound gel with 10% hydrocortisone mixture. What action should the PTA take?
   a. Call occupational health.
   b. Call internal medicine.
   c. Call the poison control center.
   d. Call the child's father.

22. A PTA wants to check the muscle strength of a patient's brachioradialis muscle. What position is the forearm placed in?
   a. supinate
   b. pronated
   c. anatomical position
   d. neutral

23. A PTA is working with a patient to strengthen the rotator cuff. Which muscle will NOT be included in the exercise program?
   a. infraspinatus
   b. subscapularis
   c. teres minor
   d. pectoralis minor

24. A PTA is working to teach a patient scapular stabilization exercises prior to surgery. What muscle(s) will the program feature?
   a. teres major and teres minor
   b. rhomboid major and rhomboid minor
   c. pectoralis major and pectoralis minor
   d. sternocleidomastoid

25. A PTA observes a PT perform the drop arm test. What does a positive test indicate?
   a. biceps tendonitis
   b. triceps tear
   c. pronator teres tear
   d. rotator cuff tear

26. A PTA must ensure that a patient authorization form, informed consent form, and release form are signed and part of the patient's chart prior to releasing any information to the patient's attorney due to what federal regulation?
   a. Taft Act
   b. Health Insurance Portability and Accountability Act
   c. Buckley Amendment
   d. Freedom of Information Act

27. A PTA is providing intermittent compression pump treatment for a patient with venous insufficiency. What is the best parameter for pressure (mm Hg) setting?
   a. 5–25 mm Hg
   b. 50–75 mm Hg
   c. 30–60 mm Hg
   d. 75–90 mm Hg

28. A PTA is performing monofilament testing at several sites on a patient's foot, and the patient is unable to sense the 5.07 size monofilament. What information does this provide?
   a. Protective sensation is absent.
   b. Normal sensation is present.
   c. Plantar ulcers are present.
   d. Dorsalis pedis pulse is absent.

29. A PTA is performing palpation on a patient's edematous ankle that presents with a deep indentation when pressure is applied and returns to normal within 30 seconds. What is the correct scale number to assign the patient?
   a. 4+
   b. 3+
   c. 1+
   d. 2+

30. A PTA is instructing a patient to perform a posterior pelvic tilt. What mucles(s) would be involved in the training?
    a. intercostal
    b. gluteus medius
    c. adductor magnus
    d. gluteus maximus

31. A PTA is instructing a patient pre-op in open chain lower extremity exercise. Which of the following is an appropriate open-chain kinetic activity?
    a. step-ups
    b. wall slides
    c. straight leg raise
    d. jogging

32. A PTA is working in a nursing home and wants to screen an elderly patient for possible balance and gait problems. Which of the following is the best test to use?
    a. Tinetti Performance Orientated Mobility Assessment scale
    b. functional reach test
    c. slump test
    d. Visual Analog Scale

33. A PTA is observing a patient perform progressive resistive exercise. During the patient exercise, which is the most dangerous practice which the PTA must safeguard against?
    a. patient groaning
    b. patient holding breath
    c. patient mottling
    d. diaphragmatic breathing

34. A PTA is treating a hospital inpatient at bedside and notices a sign on the patient's bed that reads "DNR" (do not resuscitate). What advance directive, completed by the patient, requires the posting of this sign?
    a. living will
    b. power of attorney
    c. informed consent
    d. elder care

35. What is the number one cause of a lower limb amputation that a PTA may encounter in rehabilitation?
    a. infections
    b. trauma
    c. peripheral vascular disease (PVD)
    d. tumors

36. A PTA is reading a patient's history and notes the patient sustained a traction injury to the upper brachial plexus (Erb's palsy) as a newborn. What nerve levels does this involve?
    a. C3 and C4
    b. C5 and C6
    c. C7 and C8
    d. C8 and T1

37. A PTA is working with a pediatric patient. What are the stages of motor control in the order of occurrence?
    a. stability, mobility, skill, controlled mobility
    b. stability, mobility, controlled mobility, skill
    c. mobility, controlled mobility, stability, skill
    d. mobility, stability, controlled mobility, skill

38. What is the best method for a PTA to measure the depth of a deep tracking wound?
  a. clear piece of acetate with a calibrated grid
  b. exposed radiographic film
  c. the end of a sterile cotton-tipped applicator
  d. photography

39. A PTA is taking a position in an acute-care hospital that treats burns, trauma, or organ transplants. What vaccine is available for protection from occupational exposure?
  a. HBV
  b. HIV
  c. TB
  d. MRSA

40. A PTA is observing a head trauma patient for gait deviations and notes the occurrence and timing of each deviation of a special form. What is the most common observational gait analysis (OGA) system being used by the PTA?
  a. Trendelenburg test
  b. functional reach test
  c. Ranchos Los Amigos OGA system
  d. Tinetti Performance Oriented Mobility Assessment

41. A PTA is performing a home health visit on a patient whose status is two weeks post a total hip replacement. The patient is reporting calf pain and mild warmth. What would the PTA suspect?
  a. lymph edema
  b. peripheral neuropathy
  c. early onset multiple sclerosis
  d. deep vein thrombosis

42. A patient presents a lumbar scoliosis with the convexity of the curve on the left side of the spine and the concavity on the right side of the spine. Which would be the most beneficial course of action?
  a. convex and concave strengthening exercise
  b. concave strengthening exercise
  c. convex strengthening exercise
  d. cervical dorsal glide exercise

43. A PTA is selecting a therapeutic heat modality for a patient with hand pain. Which is the best therapeutic heat choice to prevent rebound vasoconstriction?
  a. fluidotherapy
  b. infrared lamp
  c. paraffin bath
  d. moist heat packs

44. What is the best way for a PTA to prevent transient cavitation when performing ultrasound?
  a. Avoid excessive intensity.
  b. Perform a stationary technique.
  c. Use pulsed ultrasound.
  d. Perform an alternative treatment.

45. A PTA would withhold intermittent compression pump treatment on a patient with which of the following medical problems?
  a. post-sprain effusion
  b. lymphedema
  c. gangrene
  d. postmastectomy

46. A PTA is working with a patient who is one week post arthroscopic knee surgery and is unable to perform a straight leg raise. What is the best means of treatment to improve the problem presented?
  a. intermittent compression
  b. biofeedback
  c. TENS
  d. ultrasound

47. A PTA is treating a patient with a cold pack to the forearm and wrist. At the conclusion of the treatment, the PTA inspects the patient's hand and finds it is discolored, appearing white and blue. What should the PTA suspect is causing the discoloration?
  a. Raynaud's phenomenon
  b. mottling
  c. modeling
  d. erythema

48. The primary difference between voluntary muscle contraction and electrical stimulation supplemented muscle contraction is recruitment. What is recruited first in a muscle contraction utilizing electrical stimulation?
  a. type I muscle fibers
  b. type II muscle fibers
  c. smaller type I motor nerves
  d. larger type I motor nerves

49. Using the clock method, which numbers would a PTA use to measure the length of a wound?
  a. 12 o'clock (left) to 6 o'clock (right)
  b. 9 o'clock (head) to 3 o'clock (foot)
  c. 12 o'clock (head) to 6 o'clock (foot)
  d. 9 o'clock (left) to 3 o'clock (right)

50. A PTA is giving a patient a contrast bath. What is the temperature range for hot and cold phases of the contrast bath?
  a. hot 102–110°F and cold 50–66°F
  b. hot 96–100°F and cold 66–72°F
  c. hot 90–96°F and cold 72–80°F
  d. hot 112–120°F and cold 42–48°F

Part II

51. A PTA can utilize which of the following techniques to examine static balance and predict the likelihood of falling?
  a. slump test
  b. functional reach test
  c. Tinetti Performance Oriented Mobility Assessment
  d. gait abnormality rating scale

52. What is the most effective means for a PTA to reduce cross contamination and the spread of many infections from one person to another?
  a. immunization
  b. hand washing
  c. protective isolation
  d. gown and gloves

53. Which of the following is an example of upper extremity open kinetic chain activity?
  a. a person executing plyometric throws
  b. a person performing bench press exercises
  c. a person performing prone press ups
  d. a person completing Cod man's pendulum exercises

54. A PTA is supervising the treadmill workout of a patient with cardiac problems and periodically checks the patient's blood pressure, respiration, and pulse. What other important physical information should be monitored?
a. perspiration rate
b. rating of perceived exertion
c. speed of the treadmill
d. elevation of the treadmill

55. What is being described if a patient report indicates that the patient has no pain to 95°, pain to 120°, and is pain-free through the remainder of the range while performing shoulder abduction?
a. muscle spasm
b. hypermobile
c. painful arc
d. hypomobile

56. A PTA observes during the heel-strike phase of a gait training session from the lateral (side) view that the right foot is being placed flat on the floor in plantar flexion accompanied with the slapping of the forefoot. With this information, what muscle action would the PTA closely examine?
a. ankle dorsiflexors
b. knee extensors
c. knee flexors
d. ankle plantar flexors

57. Prior to the application of electrical stimulation, the PTA examines the skin and observes that it is very dry. What is the best technique to apply to enhance the treatment?
a. application of an ice pack
b. application of skin lotion
c. application of rubbing alcohol
d. application of a moist heat pack

58. What type of activity would a PTA select for a high-intensity and high-velocity exercise to develop coordination and muscle power?
a. flexibility exercises
b. resistance training
c. plyometric training
d. manual stretching

59. Which of the following exercise regimens provides reduced amount of weight per RM on the first set of the exercise?
a. Oxford regimen
b. DAPRE regimen
c. circuit training
d. DeLorme regimen

60. A patient with low-back pain is unable to perform heel walking. What myotome involvement should the PTA expect?
a. L2
b. S1
c. S2
d. L4

61. A PTA is instructing a patient to perform an anterior pelvic tilt. Which muscle(s) would be involved in the training?
a. quadratus lumborum
b. iliopsoas
c. gluteus maximus
d. biceps femoris

62. A patient reports that her ankle buckled under her, turning in as she stepped off the curb. Which ligament would likely sustain injury from this movement?
a. deltoid ligament
b. alar ligament
c. annular ligament
d. anterior talofibular ligament

63. After a week of performing seated overhead pulleys at the physical therapy clinic and at home, the patient complains of anterolateral shoulder pain. What anatomical structures should the PTA suspect are affected?
a. clavicle and sternum
b. acromion and humerus
c. scapula and ribs
d. clavicle and acromion

64. What is the appropriate course of action to relieve severe choking in a responsive infant?
a. Start basic life support measures.
b. Initiate cycles of five back slaps followed by five chest thrusts.
c. Perform the Heimlich maneuver.
d. Give two rescue breaths.

65. A patient reports to a PTA during a scheduled outpatient visit, stating that she awoke that morning to find severe joint pain and swelling in both knees. What medical condition should the PTA suspect?
a. multiple sclerosis
b. peripheral neuropathy
c. gout
d. Baker's cyst

66. A PTA is treating a patient who is four weeks status post left knee arthroscopic surgery. The patient presents on Monday with a warm, painful, and extremely tender left gastrocnemius. What should the PTA suspect?
a. phlebitis
b. Baker's cyst
c. multiple sclerosis
d. hyperthyroidism

67. A patient is referred to physical therapy for treatment of pes anserinus bursitis. Over what area will the PTA provide ultrasound to accomplish the correct treatment of the prescribed tissue?
a. proximal to the lateral femoral condyle
b. inferior to the medial tibial condyle
c. superior to the lateral tibial condyle
d. proximal to the medial femoral condyle

68. While cleaning the whirlpool, a co-worker accidentally gets some cleaning agent splashed in his eyes. In addition to helping the person to the eye wash station, how should the PTA determine the potential hazards of the agent?
a. Consult internal medicine.
b. Consult material safety data sheet.
c. Consult occupational health safety administration.
d. Consult occupational health guidelines.

69. A PTA observes a male pedestrian collapse in front of the door to the outpatient clinic, and upon checking the person for unconsciousness, he does not respond. What should the PTA do next?
a. Check for signs of life.
b. Drive the patient to the hospital.
c. Call or have someone call 911 or the local emergency number.
d. Give two rescue breaths.

70. A five-year-old child presents in the physical therapy clinic with a complaint of pain in the proximal forearm. On a field trip, the child was holding hands with a classmate who pulled very hard to get the child to follow him, causing dislocation of the radial head. What structure was injured?
   a. medial collateral
   b. lateral collateral
   c. anterior cruciate
   d. annular ligament

71. What is the best way for a PTA to determine if a patient is unresponsive?
   a. Give the patient CPR.
   b. Tap or gently shake the patient and shout, "Are you okay?"
   c. Lift the patient up to a sitting position.
   d. Look, listen, and feel for signs of breathing.

72. What test would a PTA use to look for hip flexion contracture on a below-knee amputee patient?
   a. Smith test
   b. Ober test
   c. Thomas test
   d. Oppenheim test

73. A PTA is instructing a patient in an exercise program to address the functional limitation of combing hair and putting on garments with sleeves. What motion would this program feature?
   a. adduction
   b. internal rotation
   c. external rotation
   d. flexion

74. A PTA is performing abdominal thrusts on a choking co-worker who became unresponsive. Another co-worker has called for help. What does the PTA do next?
   a. Continue the Heimlich maneuver until the object comes out of the person's airway, then begin the steps of CPR.
   b. Give chest thrusts for two minutes, then begin CPR.
   c. Begin CPR. When you open the airway, look for and remove the object (if seen) before giving rescue breaths.
   d. Perform a tongue-jaw lift and finger sweep.

75. A PTA observes a PT perform an anterior drawer test. What does a positive drawer test indicate?
   a. anterior cruciate ligament tear
   b. lateral collateral ligament tear
   c. annular ligament tear
   d. iliopubic ligament tear

76. A PTA is working on a patient to improve personal wellness. What does a Body Mass Index of 27.5 represent?
   a. underweight
   b. normal
   c. overweight
   d. obese

77. A PTA is using electrical stimulation for wound healing of a stage IV decubitus ulcer. What is the best waveform for this goal?
   a. low-voltage current
   b. high-voltage pulsatile current
   c. altenating current
   d. biphasic current

78. A PTA observes a physical therapist test hip joint pathology. What test did the physical therapist perform?
   a. Thomas test
   b. Ober test
   c. Fabere test
   d. Oppenheim test

79. It is afternoon, and a PTA is working in the gym with a patient on a back exercise program. After ten minutes of activity, the patient appears pale and sweating and complains that the room is very warm, although the temperature is 70 degrees. The patient has diabetes and reports skipping lunch to perform errands. What does the PTA suspect?
   a. hyperglycemia
   b. stroke
   c. hypoglycemia
   d. angina

80. A PTA is working with a patient who has a hypermobile glenohumeral shoulder joint. Which of the following treatment activities may the PTA safely perform?
   a. manipulation
   b. mobilization
   c. stabilization
   d. auto-mobilization

81. Which one of the following references will best determine whether or not a PT may legally delegate joint mobilization to a PTA?
   a. insurance reimbursement guide
   b. APTA white paper on PTA utilization
   c. laws of the state
   d. patient plan of care

82. A PTA may decide against using volumetric measurement technique in which type of patient problem?
   a. preoperative
   b. crush injuries
   c. post-immobilization
   d. open wounds

83. A PTA is teaching a patient recovering from a low back injury a safe lifting technique to get a coordinated contraction of the transversus abdominis, diaphragm, and pelvic floor musculature. What is the physiological effect of this activity when performed correctly?
   a. decreased intra-abdominal pressure
   b. decreased stability
   c. increased load on the spine
   d. increased intra-abdominal pressure

84. A PTA is applying electrical stimulation on a patient and has set the frequency at 50 pulses per second. What must the PTA do to obtain a sustained contraction of the muscle?
   a. set on/off cycle
   b. set time
   c. set amplitude
   d. set pressure mm Hg

85. A PTA is educating a patient with a below-knee amputation on proper positioning. What positions should the patient avoid to prevent contractures from developing on the lower extremity with the amputation?
   a. hip extension, adduction, and knee flexion
   b. hip adduction and knee extension
   c. hip extension and knee flexion
   d. hip flexion, abduction, and knee flexion

86. A PTA reports an ankle injury with moderate pain that requires stopping activity. When the PTA places stress on the ankle and palpates the tissue, pain is greatly increased. What grade of tissue injury should the PTA suspect?
    a. grade III
    b. grade I
    c. grade II
    d. grade IV

87. A PTA is working with a pediatric patient. At what month should creeping be present in normal development of a pediatric patient?
    a. 5 months
    b. 8 months
    c. 9 months
    d. 12 months

88. Using the pressure ulcer classification system adopted by the National Pressure Ulcer Advisory Panel (NPUAP), what classification would a PTA give a shallow ulcer with a blister and a red-pink wound bed?
    a. stage I
    b. stage II
    c. stage III
    d. stage IV

89. Which one of the four cardinal signs of inflammation is produced by distension of tissue spaces from swelling and pressure and by chemical irritation of tissue receptors?
    a. umor (swelling)
    b. dolor (pain)
    c. rubor (redness)
    d. calor (heat)

90. A PTA is inspecting a patient's lower extremity and observes tissue that is taut and moist on the dorsum of the foot. What type of lymphedema should the PTA suspect?
    a. pitting edema
    b. brawny edema
    c. weeping edema
    d. chronic edema

91. A PTA is selecting electrodes for a patient's electrical stimulation treatment. The PTA wants to maximize current passage. Which size electrode will best accomplish this goal?
    a. five square inches
    b. two square inches
    c. four square inches
    d. ten square inches

92. A PTA is treating a hand patient with De Quervain's syndrome. The tendons of which muscles are involved with this diagnosis?
    a. brachioradialis
    b. abductor pollicis longus and extensor pollicis brevis
    c. adductor pollicis longus and flexor pollicis brevis
    d. adductor pollicis brevis and longus

93. A PTA is trying to decide whether to use cold or heat on a patient injury. What is the most important consideration for making this decision?
    a. patient's insurance coverage
    b. patient preference
    c. predetermined time frame
    d. desired physiological effect

94. A PTA is performing electrical stimulation on a patient. Which nerve fibers would be the most difficult to stimulate?
   a. A-beta
   b. C fibers
   c. A-delta
   d. A-gamma

95. The PTA is applying intermittent cervical traction in an effort to reduce patient pain caused by what anatomical structure?
   a. annulus fibrosus pushing through the ligament
   b. annulus fibrosus protruding through the nucleus pulposus
   c. nucleus pulposus protruding through the annulus fibrosus
   d. nucleus pulposus pushing through the skin

96. A PTA is working with a patient who is lifting a heavy amount of weight for a six repetition maximum. Which type of skeletal muscle fiber is being trained?
   a. type III
   b. type II
   c. type I
   d. type IV

97. When a PTA is applying modalities of either hot or cold to a patient with pain, which of the following is most likely to be the treatment goal?
   a. reciprocal inhibition
   b. analgesia
   c. anesthesia
   d. counterirritant

98. A PTA seeks to obtain a sustained muscle tetany. What is the number of pulses per second required to achieve this goal?
   a. 50 pps
   b. 10 pps
   c. 5 pps
   d. 20 pps

99. A PTA is checking a patient's lower extremity for reflexes and sensation. The PTA runs the pointed end of a reflex hammer across the plantar surface of the foot from the calcaneus along the lateral border to the forefoot. The patient's great toe extends while the other toes are plantar, flexed, and splayed. What does this result signify?
   a. positive Thomas test
   b. positive Homan test
   c. positive Oppenheim test
   d. positive Babinski test

100. A PTA is providing ultrasound to the gastrocnemius muscle. What frequency should be used for the treatment?
   a. 3 MHz
   b. 2 MHz
   c. 1 MHz
   d. 4 MHz

Part III

101. A PTA is documenting a patient's response post-exercise. What is the most common type of rating method used when attempting to quantify a patient's complaint of pain?
   a. Waddell Inventory
   b. Roland Morris Disability Questionnaire
   c. Visual Analog Scale
   d. McGill Pain Questionnaire

102. A PTA notes a patient's inability to detect a 10 g Semmes-Weinstein nylon filament on the plantar aspect of the foot. This assists in identifying the patient's risk for developing which type of ulcer?
   a. arterial
   b. venous
   c. neurotrophic
   d. capillary

103. A PTA is checking adequate breathing before giving breaths to an adult victim who is unresponsive. This is done by looking for the chest rise and feeling airflow through the person's nose or mouth. What other signs should be assessed?
   a. counting the person's breaths for at least 15 seconds
   b. looking into the person's mouth to see if anything is blocking the airway
   c. listening for airflow from the person's nose or mouth
   d. listening carefully for gasps because they are signs of adequate breathing

104. A PTA is instructing a patient in a home exercise program. Which of the following is an appropriate lower extremity closed chain activity?
   a. step-ups
   b. heel slides
   c. straight leg raise
   d. knees to chest

105. A PTA would utilize which of the following treatment positions to initiate PROM for shoulder flexion and rotation following a total shoulder replacement?
   a. seated
   b. side-lying
   c. supine
   d. standing

106. During a home health visit, the patient's mother asks the PTA for the requirements for recommended ramp construction ratio to assist her child in a wheelchair. What is the correct ratio?
   a. 6:1
   b. 4:1
   c. 12:1
   d. 2:1

107. A PTA is monitoring an aquatic program. Prior to the start of the session, the PTA checks the pool water temperature. What is the safest temperature in which to conduct aquatic therapy?
   a. 26°C –37°C
   b. 26°C –33°C
   c. 24°C –34°C
   d. 27°C –37°C

108. A PTA is assigned to work with a runner who has tight hamstring muscles. What is the safest activity that can be used to increase flexibility for this patient?
   a. ballistic stretching
   b. static stretching
   c. cyclic stretching
   d. isometric stretching

109. Extra precaution should be used by the PTA when establishing a resistance training program for which of the following groups?
   a. teenagers who have stopped growing
   b. college athletes in competition
   c. young children who are still growing
   d. athletes who have been actively involved in lifelong competition

110. A PTA is providing physical therapy for a patient two days post-op knee surgery who also uses the continuous passive motion (CPM) unit. What activity does the PTA stress to prepare the patient during treatment sessions for ambulation?
  a. passive ROM
  b. quad sets
  c. wall slides
  d. step-ups

111. During a gait training session, a PTA observes a patient having difficulty lifting the lower extremity high enough to clear the surface during the swing phase of gait. Which muscles require examination to determine the cause of this difficulty?
  a. gluteus medius
  b. iliopsoas
  c. biceps femoris
  d. gluteus maximus

112. A patient reports to a PTA that he is having trouble performing the functional activity of putting a belt through his belt loops or reaching the back pocket of his pants. What shoulder motion would be addressed in treatment?
  a. abduction
  b. external rotation
  c. internal rotation
  d. flexion

113. A PTA is performing a bedside visit when he/she hears agonal gasps from the patient in the neighboring bed. What course of action should the PTA pursue?
  a. Call a code red and begin assessment.
  b. Complete the bedside therapy sessions.
  c. Give the patient oxygen.
  d. Give the patient two rescue breaths.

114. On a home health visit, a patient's spouse reports symptoms of confusion, blurred vision, arrhythmias, and gastrointestinal distress. What should the PTA suspect?
  a. vitamin C toxicity
  b. low sodium level
  c. digitalis toxicity
  d. hypotension

115. A PTA is having coffee with a neighbor who describes a mildly painful, unexplained swelling in the popliteal fossa of her right knee. What should the PTA suspect is the cause of the swelling?
  a. gout
  b. multiple sclerosis
  c. Baker's cyst
  d. congestive heart failure

116. At Thanksgiving dinner, a PTA observes his brother, whom he has not seen in a year, present with very noticeable weight loss, tremors, palpitations, and nervousness. The PTA takes his brother's blood pressure, which is 160/80, and resting pulse rate is 120. What should the PTA suspect?
  a. multiple sclerosis
  b. phlebitis
  c. gout
  d. hyperthyroidism

117. Which of the following responses will occur if an ice massage is applied to the gastrocnemius muscle with spasticity?
  a. decreased muscle spindle sensitivity
  b. decreased valsalva
  c. increased muscle metabolism
  d. increased muscle spindle sensitivity

118. A PTA was trained in Pennsylvania and has practiced in the state for five years, where PT to PTA supervision ratio is three to one. The PTA is moving to Florida. What will determine if the supervision ratio will stay the same?
a. APTA Code of Ethics
b. Florida Practice Act
c. APTA white paper on PTA supervision
d. APTA HOD number 168

119. A member of the maintenance department accidentally cuts his arm while installing a wall rack in the physical therapy gym. What emergency action does the PTA take?
a. Apply direct pressure with sterile or clean dressing.
b. Apply pressure at a pressure point.
c. Add a bulky dressing to reinforce original bandages.
d. Treat the victim for shock.

120. A PTA is working with a patient with emphysema who is performing circuit strengthening activities. What is the best breath activity to enhance the patient's exercise program?
a. involuntary breathing
b. oblique breathing
c. diaphragmatic breathing
d. accessory breathing

121. A PTA is using an AED on an adult victim and the AED signals "no shock indicated" or "no shock advised." What is the best course of action until advanced medical personnel arrive?
a. Place the patient in the recovery position.
b. Remove the pads from the patient's chest.
c. Leave pads on the patient's chest and continue CPR beginning with compressions.
d. Remove the pads from the patient's chest and continue CPR.

122. A PTA is working to improve the posture on a patient with rounded shoulders. Which of the following muscles would the PTA instruct the patient to stretch?
a. pectoralis minor
b. teres minor
c. supraspinatus
d. latissimus dorsi

123. A PTA is observing a patient with a frozen shoulder perform abduction. What does the PTA detect?
a. no sternoclavicular motion
b. no glenohumeral motion
c. no scapulothoracic motion
d. no scapuloclavicular motion

124. A PTA instructs a person new to using crutches not to lean on them to prevent injuring which nerve?
a. axillary
b. radial
c. medical
d. long thoracic

125. A PTA is treating a patient with osteoarthritis bilaterally at the hip joint. What phase of the Nagi Model of Disability would involve physical therapy for decreased ambulation?
a. active pathology
b. functional limitation
c. impairment
d. disability

126. A PTA is using ultrasound on a stage II venous ulcer for wound healing. What is the frequency and duty cycle for the treatment?
a. 1 MHz, pulsed
b. 3 MHz, continuous
c. 1 MHz, continuous
d. 3 MHz, pulsed

127. A PTA is instructing a patient in closed chain upper extremity exercise following shoulder surgery. Which of the following is an appropriate closed-chain kinetic activity?
a. finger ladder
b. wall pulley
c. pendulum
d. push-ups

128. A PTA observes a patient's lower extremity that presents as lymphostatic elephantiasis, hardening of dermal tissues, papillomas of the skin, and the appearance of skin is elephant-like. What is the correct stage of lymphedema?
a. stage II
b. stage III
c. stage I
d. subclinical

129. While a PTA is exercising a patient at home and the patient is speaking, the patient suddenly stops speaking and slumps to the right side. The PTA observes the patient's mouth is now lower on the right side and that the patient cannot sit upright without support. What should the PTA suspect?
a. stroke
b. seizure
c. shock
d. angina

130. A PTA includes a bridging activity in a patient's exercise program to strengthen which of the following muscles?
a. gluteus medius
b. gluteus maximus
c. biceps femoris
d. popliteus

131. What test would a PTA use to assess iliotibial band length?
a. Ober test
b. Drawer test
c. Thomas test
d. Oppenheim test

132. A PTA is instructing a class of pregnant women in techniques to assist them during labor and delivery. During the second stage of labor, what instruction and technique should be provided?
a. performing glut set
b. relaxing the abdominal wall
c. relaxing the pelvic floor
d. performing calf pumping

133. A PTA is providing a patient with educational instruction that includes removal of abnormal secretions and vigilant treatment of pulmonary infections. What medical condition is best characterized by these impairments?
a. hypoxic hypoxia
b. atelectasis
c. cystic fibrosis
d. pneuomothorax

134. A PTA is working with a patient who sustained a compression fracture of T12. Which type of brace would be most appropriate?
a. Boston brace
b. CASH brace
c. Charleston bending brace
d. Milwaukee brace

135. A PTA is performing gait training with a patient with an above-knee prosthesis and notices the patient is vaulting during the swing phase of gait. What should the PTA suspect is causing the problem?
a. The prosthesis is too long.
b. The prosthesis is too short.
c. The prosthesis is too tight.
d. The prosthesis is too loose.

136. A PTA is working with a patient with a C5-level spinal cord injury. Which muscle allows the patient to continue to breath independently?
a. abdominals
b. intercostal
c. diaphragm
d. serratus anterior

137. A PTA is instructing a patient who is primarily in bed and the patient's family on turning and positioning schedules to reduce the effects of shearing forces on superficial and deep structures. What is the best schedule to follow?
a. every two hours
b. every four hours
c. every six hours
d. every eight hours

138. Which of the following solutions is best used by a PTA to clean spills of body fluids on the exercise mat?
a. betadine solution
b. betadine scrub
c. ammonia solution
d. bleach and water

139. A PTA is observing a wound. Which of the following wound drainage color types would present an odor?
a. translucent
b. serosanguineous
c. serous
d. purulent

140. A PTA is applying a wet-to-dry dressing to a patient. Which type of wound debridement does this dressing method represent?
a. selective debridement
b. nonselective debridement
c. nonforceful irrigation
d. sharp debridement

141. A PTA is providing an exercise program for a patient with a diagnosis of spinal stenosis. What activities are best for this medical condition?
a. flexion
b. extension
c. side-bending
d. rotation

142. A patient receiving a hot pack reports unusual warmth in the area. Upon examination of the skin, the tissue is ghost-white in areas with beet-red splotches. What is this condition?
a. modeling
b. mottling
c. erythema
d. urticaria

143. At the conclusion of an ultrasound treatment, stretching of the tissue must begin within how many minutes to promote tissue extensibility?
a. 1 minute
b. 3 minutes
c. 10 minutes
d. 15 minutes

144. The PTA should not exceed what pressure setting on the intermittent compression pump to ensure patient safety during treatment?
a. resting heart rate
b. systolic blood pressure
c. target heart rate
d. diastolic blood pressure

145. A PTA is applying massage to remove edema from a limb. Which technique should the PTA use?
a. Initiate strokes proximal and work distally.
b. Initiate strokes peripherally and work distally.
c. Initiate treatment on the noninvolved extremity.
d. Initiate ipsilateral extremity treatment.

146. When a PTA applies hot or cold to a patient, which fibers detect the sensation?
a. A-charlie fibers
b. A-beta fibers
c. A-delta fibers
d. C fibers

147. The PTA is using electrical stimulation on a patient and desires a maximal contraction. What is the ideal phase duration to achieve patient muscle contraction?
a. 1 to 2 seconds
b. 25 microseconds
c. 300 to 500 microseconds
d. 30 seconds

148. The owner of an apartment wishes to make some upgrades and requests assistance to comply with the United States Access Board (USAB) recommended height for a toilet. What is the height range?
a. 21–22 inches
b. 14–16 inches
c. 18–20 inches
d. 17–19 inches

149. A PTA is working at a pro bono community outpatient physical therapy clinic where a patient presents with wrist drop. What nerve involvement should the PTA suspect is injured?
a. ulnar nerve
b. radial nerve
c. median nerve
d. palmar nerve

150. A PTA is treating a high school football player for an acute gastrocnemius contusion and strain. The patient complains of severe pain and swelling that developed since the last treatment. What should the PTA suspect is the cause of the pain and swelling?
a. lymphedema
b. compartment syndrome
c. Baker's cyst
d. inversion sprain

Answers and Explanations

1. a. The gluteus medius muscle on the stance limb functions to support the pelvis by keeping it parallel to the surface while the opposite limb is unsupported by either the unilateral (stork) stand or the swing phase of gait. (Hoppenfeld 1976, page 164)

2. d. The gastrocnemius-soleus muscle is responsible for toe-off (push-off) from the stance phase of gait, presenting the appearance of flatfoot. The muscle is innervated by the tibial nerve, S1, S2. (Hoppenfeld 1976, page 229)

3. a. Jurisprudence, in this situation, is the state physical therapy practice act which defines appropriate activities for a physical therapist assistant in its rules and regulations. (Scott 1997, pages 10–11)

4. b. The tibialis anterior is innervated by the deep peroneal nerve (L4). (Hoppenfeld 1976, page 227) The action of the tibialis anterior muscle is dorsiflexion of the ankle joint. (Kendall 1983, page 141)

5. d. A PTA would utilize passive range of motion to accurately assess a patient's shoulder joint end feel. End feel is the sensation detected by the practitioner's hands as a joint is passively moved through a range of motion. (Cyriax 1982, page 53)

6. b. The head tilt/chin lift is the American Heart Association's recommended way to open the airway. This method relieves airway obstruction in the unresponsive victim, when the tongue and epiglottis can block the upper airway. Utilizing the head tilt/chin lift maneuver lifts the tongue and relieves airway obstruction. (American Heart Association, BLS for Healthcare Providers 2006, pages 5–8)

7. b. The serratus anterior is involved when weakness causes scapular winging. When the origin is fixed—for example, outer surfaces and superior borders of the upper eight or nine ribs—the medial border of the scapula firmly holds against the rib cage. (Hoppenfeld 1976, page 30)

8. a. Self stretching or flexibility exercises independently performed by a homebound, discharged patient, from a supervised program, are paramount to maintain ROM gained during treatment. Decreased movement results in shortening of tissue structures. (Kisner and Colby 2007, page 83)

9. b. The DAPRE system is based on a six RM working weight. The next session is determined by the maximum number of repetitions performed in set number three using the current working weight. (Kisner and Colby 2007, page 208)

10. a. The positions such as crossing the legs (adduction) or sitting on low chairs, beds, or toilets (hip flexion greater than 90°) may cause disarticulation of the femoral head and should be avoided by this patient. (Kisner and Colby 2007, page 659)

11. c. When providing care for Medicare Part B (private practice), direct supervision is required unless the state practice act is more stringent. (*PT Magazine*, January 2006, Volume 14, Issue 1)

12. a. When a neck injury is suspected, the head tilt/chin lift technique is not used, as it may lead to further neck injuries with extension. Instead, the jaw thrust is used to prevent neck flexion. (American Heart Association, BLS for Healthcare Providers 2005, page 69)

13. b. To perform the shoulder ROM activity of wall climbing properly and safely (which may be accomplished using a finger ladder), the patient should perform the flexion when facing the wall and in abduction. Careful attention should be maintained by the patient, and the PTA should monitor the exercise for extraneous motions. Wall climbing is performed in standing while overhead pulley is generally seated and wand is in supine. Thera-Band is a strengthening activity. (Kisner and Colby 2007, page 60)

14. d. Patients that are too weak to participate in a progressive resistive exercise, endurance training, or isometric exercise would begin with a supervised low-intensity exercise program that would include active range of motion of extremities at five to ten repetitions each. The program would be advanced with increased patient tolerance. Pulse rate should be monitored before and after exercise. (Kauffman 1999, pages 72–73)

15. b. Congestive heart failure may present clinically as fluid accumulation in dependent areas of the body, such as the feet. If untreated, this can become a medical emergency. (Kauffman 1999, pages 224–226) Peripheral neuropathy presents as muscle weakness, paresthesis, and impaired reflexes. (Taber 2001, page 1,447) Hypothyroidism results from inadequate levels of thyroid hormone in the body. Symptoms include intolerance of cold temperatures, fatigue, dry skin, and muscle aches. (Taber 2001, page 1,049) The clinical course of gout generally has four stages: asymptomatic, acute, intercritical, and chronic. The hallmark of the acute stage is that the patient awakes to unexplained joint pain and swelling. (Kauffman 1999, page 91)

16. b. Multiple sclerosis is a chronic central nervous system disease where the myelin on the brain stem and spinal cord is destroyed. Symptoms include visual disturbances, progressive limb weakness, spasticity, and incontinence. (Taber 2001, pages 1,935–1,936)

17. d. The gluteus medius muscle on the stance limb functions to support the pelvis by keeping it parallel to the surface while the opposite limb is unsupported by unilateral (stork) stand in the swing phase of gait. (Hoppenfeld

1976, page 164) and (Norkin and Levangie 1992, pages 449–495)

18. c. Calculation for Karvonen Method:
<u>40% TARGET HEART RANGE</u>
Maximal heart rate 220 minus age
$(220 - 78) = 142$
Subtract resting heart rate
$(142 - 66) = 76$ (heart rate reserve)
Multiply heart rate reserve
(76) by % intensity $(76 \times 40\%$ or $.40) = 30$
Add back resting heart rate
$(30 + 66) = 96$ bpm
<u>60% TARGET HEART RANGE</u>
Maximal heart rate 220 minus age
$(220 - 78) = 142$
Subtract resting heart rate
$(142 - 66) = 76$ (heart rate reserve)
Multiply heart rate reserve (76) by %
intensity $(76 \times 60\%$ or $.60) = 46$
Add back resting heart rate
$(46 + 66) = 112$ bpm
<u>RESULTS</u>
Target heart rate range
$40–60\% = 96–112$ bpm
(Kauffman 1999, page 200)

19. d. Prior to providing treatment, the provider should thoroughly explain the procedure, answer any patient questions related to the procedure, and obtain patient consent for treatment. If the patient does not consent to the treatment plan, the PTA may not give care and must inform the physical therapist. (Scott 1997, pages 113–140)

20. b. The preseason screen utilizes the principle of prehabilitation. Prehabilitation identifies potential musculoskeletal imbalance and attempts to prevent injuries before they occur through a preventative management program designed for the individual. (France 2004, page 97)

21. c. When the name of the potential poison is known, call the poison control center for instruction on giving first aid for poisoning. The telephone number of the poison control center should be prominently posted. (American Heart Association, Heartsaver First Aid 2006, pages 84–85)

22. d. The brachioradialis originates from the lateral supracondylar ridge of the humerus. The muscle becomes prominent by having the patient make a fist and place the forearm in neutral. The biceps brachii muscle is tested in the supinated position, and the brachialis is placed in a pronated position. (Hoppenfeld 1976, page 47)

23. d. The rotator cuff is comprised of the subscapularis, infraspinatus, teres minor, and supraspinatus. The acronym SITS may help you to remember the rotator cuff muscles. (Norkin and Levangie 1992, pages 225–226)

24. b. The rhomboid major and minor originate along C7–T5 of the spine and extend diagonally and laterally, attaching on the medial border of the scapula. The action of the rhomboid muscles is adduction and elevation of the scapula. (Hoppenfeld 1976, page 20)

25. d. The patient is asked to abduct the arm to 90° and slowly and smoothly lower the arm. If the patient is unable to perform this task, the indication is a tear of the supraspinatus. (Hoppenfeld 1976, page 33)

26. b. Effective April 2002, HIPAA requires protection and confidentiality of patient medical information and records. (Minor and Minor 2010, page 32)

27. c. An intermittent pressure below 30 mm Hg provides minimal compression while pressure in excess of 60 mm Hg may occlude blood flow in some patients. (Guccione 2000, page 390)

28. a. The thinner the monofilament, the lower the number and the lower the amount of force needed to induce filament buckling. Protective sensation of the foot is considered absent if the patient is unable to feel the 5.07 monofilament. An individual has normal sensation when a 4.17 (1 g of force) monofilament can be detected. (Gucionne 2000, page 387)

29. b. The examiner applies pressure to the area with the fingertips and scores the pitting using the following scale:

   1+   Indentation is barely detectable.

   2+   Slight indentation is visible when skin is depressed and returns to normal in 15 seconds.

   3+   Deeper indentation occurs when pressed and returns to normal within 30 seconds.

   4+   Indentation lasts for more than 30 seconds.

The presence of pitting edema may indicate liver disease, renal disease, or congestive heart failure. (O'Sullivan and Schmitz 2007, page 659)

30. d. The posterior pelvis flattens the lumbar spine and decreases the lumbar lordosis, placing the spine in a stable position. The anterior superior iliac spine of the pelvis is moved in a superior direction while the posterior superior iliac spine moves in an inferior direction. The hip extensors (gluteus maximus) and trunk flexors (rectus abdominis) create this motion. (Kisner and Colby 2007, page 646)

31. c. The straight leg raise exercise is performed with a patient in a supine (gravity lessened) position. The patient is unable to load the lower extremity in this position, making the activity open chain. The descriptive exercise terms, open and closed chain, originate from the science of biometrics. The reference is to whether or not the extremity is fixed at the distal end during an exercise. (Donatelli and Wooten 1994, page 620)

32. a. The performance oriented mobility assessmen developed by Tinetti provides a means to measure static and dynamic balance. The balance test items include sitting balance, sit-to-stand, standing balance, and stand-to-sit. The gait test items include initiation of gait, path missed step, turning, and timed walk. (Guccione 2000, page 448)

33. b. A patient holding his or her breath causes the glottis, nose, and mouth to close. This results in an increased intrathoracic pressure accompanied by a collapse of the veins of the chest wall. Additionally, there is a decrease in blood return and a drop in arterial blood pressure. The sudden drop in blood pressure due to the Valsalva maneuver may result in seeing black dots and the feeling of dizziness. In extreme situations where a patient has hypertension, hypotension, or cardiac disease, a medical emergency could develop. (O'Sullivan and Schmitz 2007, page 110)

34. a. A living will, also known as a "directive to physicians" or a "natural death act instrument," is a legal document whereby an individual indicates personal preferences for treatment. An individual has the right to refuse a treatment, even if doing so may lead to his or her death. (Guccione 1999, page 436)

35. c. The majority of amputations in adults occur from peripheral vascular disease. PVD affects peripheral blood vessels, and it may result from embolism, thrombosis, trauma, vasospasm, inflammation, or arteriosclerosis. The significance of PVD is that clinical postoperative rehabilitation will present with a medical history which may delay rehab efforts. (Cameron 1999, pages 10–11)

36. b. Erb's or Erb-Duchenne paralysis affects the shoulder and proximal arm. The arm presents in a position of internal rotation and adduction. There is visual asymmetry with noticeable space in the axilla region. (Hollinshead 1974, page 189, and Hoppenfeld 1976, page 2)

37. d. Motor development is the physiological process resulting in motor behavior changes related to age. During the first 12 months after birth, significant motor milestones occur. The order of occurrence is mobility, stability, controlled mobility, and skill. (Tecklin 1999, pages 1–30)

38. c. A deep tracking wound may contain a sinus track. This canal or passage may lead to an abscess or any cavity having a relatively narrow opening. The end of a sterile cotton-tipped applicator is the best method to measure depth. Acetate grid, radiographic filmed photography will measure width. (McCulloch, Kloth, and Feedar 1995, pages 118 and 420)

39. a. The Centers for Disease Control (CDC) indentifies hepatitis B virus (HBV) transmission through body fluids and waste products. In addition to handling precautions, an HBV vaccine is available. HIV transmission has not been documented after exposure to body fluids including feces, nasal secretions, sputum, sweat, tears, urine, or vomitus. (Pierson 1999, pages 311–312)

40. c. The Rancho Los Amigos OGA system is the most commonly used due to the organized review of 48 descriptors of gait deviations that may occur during the gait cycle. The OGA method involves a systemic examination of the movement patterns of a body. Segments at each point in the gait cycle include ankle, foot, knee, hip, pelvis, and trunk. (O'Sullivan and Schmitz 2007, page 320)

41. d. Research has shown deep vein thrombosis may arise several days or months post injury, trauma, or surgery. DVT is due to a formation of a blood clot in the deep venous system which occurs most frequently in the lower extremities. The clinical symptoms include warmth, pain, and swelling in the affected extremity. (O'Sullivan and Schmitz 2007, page 1,331)

42. c. In scoliosis cases, the muscles on the convex side of the curve are stretched and weakened, whereas the muscles on the concave side of the curve are strong and tight. The convex side would benefit from lumber extensor muscle strengthening, while the concave side would benefit from stretching exercises. (Kisner and Colby 2007, page 471)

43. d. During a therapeutic heat application, maximal vasodilation occurs, and if the intensity of the treatment remains constant or increases, the vessels begin to constrict. This response is called rebound vasoconstriction, which occurs around 20 minutes of treatment time. Physiologically, the body begins to sacrifice the superficial tissue layer in an attempt to save the deeper tissues. Moist heat packs lose heat while infrared lamp, paraffin bath, and fluidotherapy stay constant during the treatment. (Starkey 1999, pages 125–126)

44. a. Transient (unstable) cavitation is an unwanted effect caused when ultrasound is applied with an intensity that is too high. This preventable side effect can damage immobile tissue, free-floating blood cells, and other structures in the area. (Starkey 1999, page 287)

45. c. Intermittent compression contraindication includes fractures, compartment syndrome, peripheral vascular disease, gangrene, dermatitis, deep vein thrombosis, and thrombophlebitis. (Starkey 1999, page 310)

46. b. Biofeedback detects and amplifies the body's electrical activity, which is converted into an auditory and/or visual signal. The signals can be used to teach the patient relaxation, education, and strengthening. In the situation provided, a patient needs to recruit many motor units in the quad muscle group to perform a straight leg raise. Biofeedback can train recruitment. (Starkey 1999, pages 315–316)

47. a. Raynaud's phenomenon is a benign condition that is caused by a vascular reaction to cold application, which presents as white, red, or blue discoloration of the extremities. The distal areas such as toes and fingers are affected first. (Starkey 1999, page 113)

48. b. Muscle strength gains achieved by electrical stimulation are based on two factors: (1) a response to the placement of an increased load on the muscle (overload principle) and (2) recruitment of type II muscle fibers. Electrical stimulation depolarizes large diameter nerves first (A-beta), which brings type II muscle contractions earlier. (Starkey 1999, page 209)

49. c. To assess length and width wound dimensions, length measurements are made along a line from 12 o'clock (head) to 6 o'clock (foot), while width measurements are made from 9 o'clock (left) to 3 o'clock (right). (Pierson 1999, page 298)

50. a. A temperature contrast of 50–60°F exists between hot cycle temperature of 102 to 110°F and cold cycle temperature of 50 to 60°F. (France 2004, pages 218–219)

51. b. The functional reach test provides a quick screen of balance problems. If a problem is identified, additional tests may be performed to gain more specific information. (O'Sullivan and Schmitz 2007, page 257) The slump test is a lower extremity neural tension test. With the patient seated, the examiner flexes the patient's neck, thorax, and lower back while extending the knee and dorsiflexing the ankle to the point of tissue resistance in an attempt to reproduce symptoms. (Kisner and Colby 2007, page 369) The performance oriented mobility assessment developed by Tinetti provides a means to measure static and dynamic balance. The balance test items include sitting balance, sit-to-stand, standing balance, and stand-to-sit. The gait test items include initiation of gait, path missed step, turning, and timed walk. (Guccione 2000, page 448)

52. b. According to the Centers for Disease Control, despite its simplicity, hand washing remains the most effective measure to reduce cross contamination and the spread of infection. (Pierson 1994, page 219)

53. c. Push-ups are an example of closed-chain exercise. The descriptive exercise terms—open-and closed-chain—originate from the science of biometrics. The reference is to whether or not the extremity is fixed at the distal end during an exercise. When the hand or foot stays in contact with a stable surface it is a closed kinemation chain. (Donatelli and Wooten 1994, page 620)

54. b. Perceived exertion is how hard you feel your body working. While it is a subjective measure, a person's exertion rating may provide a good estimate of the actual heart rate during physical activity. (Guccione 2000, pages 249–250)

55. c. A painful arc is described as pain felt during a portion of the range of motion. Common causes include bursitis, tendonitis, or soft tissue impingement. (Cyriax 1982, page 51)

56. a. The tibialis anterior supports the foot in the ankle dorsiflexion (or neutral) phase, during and after the heel strike phase of gait. A tibialis anterior with a fair minus (3–/5) muscle grade or weaker cannot perform this function. (Norkin and Levangie 1992, pages 448–497)

57. d. Dry skin increases resistance to electrical stimulation. Applying a moist heat pack decreases skin resistance and thereby improves the effectiveness of electrical stimulation. (Starkey 1999, page 195)

58. c. Plyometric training incorporates activities to create relative bursts of force in specific functional movement patterns. This is an advanced rehabilitation technique used on selected patients, such as athletes, with the intent to train the neuromuscular system. (Kisner and Colby 2007, page 208)

59. d. The DeLorme technique utilizes a graduated or progressive load during strength training work from half to full weight over the ten RM (three sets). In contrast, the Oxford system starts at the maximum load and is regressive. It reduces from the full weight to half of the amount over the ten RM (three sets). (Kisner and Colby 2007, page 207)

60. d. The tibialis anterior muscle dorsiflexes the foot and is innervated by the deep peroneal nerve (L4). The ability to hold a sustained contraction of the tibialis anterior muscle is required to perform heel walking activity. (Hoppenfeld 1976, pages 227 and 250)

61. b. Muscles with anterior origins on the pelvis and femur would shorten when contracted and pull the anterior superior iliac spine in an inferior direction. Muscles performing this action include iliopsoas and rectus femoris. (Kendall 2005, pages 65–66)

62. d. More than 90% of ankle sprains are inversion sprains involving the lateral ligament structures: anterior talofibular, calcanofibular, and posterior talofibular. Eversion ankle sprains occur infrequently due to foot anatomy and the broad, thick medical deltoid (spring) ligament. (Hoppenfeld 1976, pages 213 and 217)

63. b. Overhead pulleys provide ROM gains in shoulder flexion and abduction when used appropriately. However, if the patient becomes too aggressive (for example, by forcefully raising his or her arm or performing too many repetitions), shoulder pain and decreased function may occur. Improper patient technique can create compression of the humerus against the acromion process. (Kisner and Colby 2007, page 60)

64. b. The correct sequence for relieving choking in a responsive infant is to repeat a sequence of five back slaps followed by five chest thrusts until the object is removed or the infant becomes unresponsive. (American Heart Association, BLS for the Healthcare Provider 2005, pages 63–67)

65. c. The clinical course of gout generally has four stages: asymptomatic, acute, intercritical, and chronic. The hallmark of the acute stage is that the patient awakes to unexplained joint pain and swelling. (Kauffman 1999, page 91)

66. a. Phlebitis is an inflammation of a vein caused by chemical or mechanical irritation. Symptoms include pain, tender, red, or swollen veins. (Taber 2001, page 1,645)

67. b. The pes anserinus insertion and bursa is inferior to the medial tibial plateau and the medial tibial condyle. (Hoppenfeld 1976, pages 174–175)

68. b. Worksites should have material safety data sheets (MSDS) for any chemicals used in the facility. The MSDS provides a detailed description of the potential effects of the agent. A new employee should receive MSDS training during "right to know" orientation. (American Heart Association, Heartsaver First Aid 2006, pages 84–85)

69. c. The American Heart Association's adult chain of survival contains four links: (1) early recognition of the emergency and activation of the emergency response system, (2) early

CPR, (3) early defibrillation, (4) early advanced care. (American Heart Association, Heartsaver First Aid 2006, pages 10–11)

70. d. The injury is to the annular ligament that attaches anteriorly and posteriorly to the radial notch of the ulna holding the radial head in place. (Hoppenfeld 1976, page 48)

71. b. Upon arrival at the scene, check to make sure it is safe and look for signs of the cause of the problem. Check whether the victim responds. Tap the victim and shout, "Are you okay?" If the victim does not respond and does not move or react in any way when you tap him or her, get help. (American Heart Association, Heartsaver First Aid 2006, page 15)

72. c. The Thomas test is used to identify flexion contractures of the hip and measure hip flexion range of motion. The test is performed with the patient supine. When hip flexion contracture is present, the patient is unable to extend the leg straight without arching the thoracic spine. (Hoppenfeld 1976, page 155)

73. c. The motion of external rotation is required to perform functional activities such as hair combing or donning and doffing a shirt or jacket. (Norkin and Levangie 1992, page 226)

74. c. Choking is caused by a foreign object in the victim's pharynx. When a responsive choking victim becomes unresponsive, CPR is started. The rescuer must stop to look for the reed object in the mouth before giving each breath. If the object is present, it must be removed. (American Heart Association, BLS for Healthcare Providers 2006, page 62)

75. a. The anterior cruciate ligament prevents the femur from sliding off the tibia. The anterior drawer is performed with the patient supine and knees flexed to 90 degrees. The examiner clasps their hands around the knee joint (from anterior to posterior) and attempts to draw the tibia forward. Both knees are examined. The forward movement of the tibia is compared between involved and noninvolved sides. Excessive forward movement of the tibia suggests a tear of the ACL. (Hoppenfeld 1976, pages 186–187)

76. c. Body Mass Index is used to classify a person's weight and height. The classifications include:
Underweight—BMI of less than 18.5
Normal—BMI between 18.5 and 24.9
Overweight—BMI between 25.0 and 29.9
Obese—BMI greater than 30.0
(Minor and Minor 2010, page 132)

77. b. Kloth and Feedar demonstrated high-voltage pulsatile current can be used to heal stage IV decubitus ulcers. (Guccione 2000, page 389)

78. c. The Fabere or Patrick test can detect arthritis or tumors in the hip joint as well as sacroiliac joint problems. The patient is placed supine, and the patient's heel (on the extremity to be tested) is placed on the opposite knee, which positions the joint in a position of flexion, abduction, and external rotation. The examiner puts a hand on the opposite ASIS to stabilize the pelvis and applies a downward force on the knee; a positive test causes hip pain. (Hoppenfeld 1976, page 262)

79. c. Hypoglycemia (low blood sugar results when a person with diabetes doesn't eat enough sugar for the amount of insulin injected, causing the blood sugar level to drop. Exercise will speed up the process. Symptoms of low blood sugar may include: confusion, irritability, hunger, thirst, weakness, sweating, pale skin color, or seizures. If low blood sugar is suspected, give the person something with sugar and call for emergency response if the victim does not feel better after several minutes. (American Heart Association, Heartsaver First Aid 2006, pages 35–36)

80. c. The joints of patients with potential necrosis of the ligaments or capsules, due to hypermobility should not be stretched. (Kinser and Colby 2007, page 115)

81. c. Jurisprudence in this situation is the state physical therapy practice act which defines appropriate activities for a physical therapist assistant in the rules and regulations. (Scott 1997, pages 10–11)

82. d. The volumetric measurement technique is an accurate method for measuring changes in body dimensions from edema or effusion. The technique utilizes the Archimedes principle of fluid displacement. The potential risk of cross contamination exists when using this technique with open wounds. (O'Sullivan and Schmitz 2007, page 658)

83. d. A coordinated contraction of the transversus abdominis, diaphragm, and pelvic floor musculature increases intra-abdominal pressure, which unloads the spine and provides stability, aiding lift-related activities. (Kisner and Colby 2007, pages 392–393)

84. c. To obtain a sustained or fused tetanic muscle contraction, the amplitude must be turned to an intensity that is high enough to sustain the contraction in order to recruit sufficient motor units of the target muscle. A lesser intensity will result in muscle fasciculations. This is an application of the law of DuBois-Reymond (1818–1896). (Cameron 1999, page 367)

85. d. If the patient develops contractures of hip flexion, abduction or knee flexion, this will delay gait and rehabilitation. The use of pillows to elevate or abduct the hip should be avoided, as well as allowing the residual below-knee limb to dangle unsupported. (O'Sullivan and Schmitz 2007, pages 1,044–1,045)

86. c. Severity of tissue injury is as follows: grade I (first degree)—mild pain at the time of injury or within the first 24 hours. Mild swelling, local tenderness, and pain occur when the tissue is stressed. Grade II (second degree)—moderate pain that requires stopping the activity. Stress and palpation of the tissue greatly increase the pain. Ligament injuries with torn fibers increase joint mobility. Grade III (third degree)—near-complete or complete tear or avulsion of the tissue (tendon or ligament) with severe pain. Stress to the tissue is usually painless; palpation may reveal the defect. Increased ligament fiber tears result in instability of the joint. (Kisner and Colby 2007, page 297)

87. b. At eight months, creeping is the primary means of locomotion. The activity of creeping utilizes the same movement components as belly crawling. Progression to reciprocal creeping occurs when the trunk has gained sufficient control to support counter-rotation of the shoulder girdle and pelvis. (Bly 1983, page 17)

88. b. NPUAP descriptions are as follows: Stage I—intact skin with non-blanchable redness of a localized area usually over a bony prominence; darkly pigmented skin may not have visible blanching; its color may differ from the surrounding area. Stage II—partial thickness-loss of dermis presenting as a shallow open ulcer with a red-pink wound bed, without slough; may also present as an intact or open/ruptured serum-filled blister. Stage III—full-thickness tissue loss; subcutaneous fat may be visible, but bone, tendon, or muscle are not exposed; slough may be present but does not obscure the depth of tissue loss; may include undermining and tunneling. Stage IV—full-thickness tissue loss with exposed bone, tendon, or muscle; slough or eschar may be present on some parts of the wound bed; often includes undermining and tunneling. (McCulloch, Kloth, and Feedar 1995, page 196)

89. b. Dolor pain is produced by distention of tissue spaces from swelling and pressure by any chemical irritation of nociceptor receptors. The clinical significance of pain and swelling may lead to reduced or a total loss of function. (McCulloch, Kloth, and Feedar 1995, page 3)

90. c. Weeping edema is the most severe and long-duration form of lymphedema. Physiologically, fluid leaks from skin tissues, cuts, or sores. The fluid creates ischemia and impairs wound healing. Weeping edema occurs in the lower extremities. (Kisner and Colby 2007, page 835)

91. b. The size of an electrode inversely affects the density of the current. As the size of the electrode decreases, the current density increases. For example, current passes through two electrodes, one having a surface area of ten square inches and the other two square inches. The smaller electrode (two square inches) would have five times as much current passing through per square inch than the larger one. (Starkey 1999, pages 195–196)

92. b. De Quervain's disease is the stenosing tenosynovitis of the first dorsal compartment of the wrist. Anatomical structures involved include the abductor pollicis longus and the extensor pollicis brevis. (O'Sullivan and Schmitz 2007, page 1,331)

93. d. The consideration to use heat or cold should avoid references to predetermined time frames or patient preference. The decision should be based on the desired physiological responses at the given point in time in the treatment process. (Starkey 1999, pages 127–129)

94. b. C-nerve fibers are small in diameter and unmyelinated, whereas A-beta and A-delta are large and myelinated. Three criteria determine a nerve's response to electrical stimulation: (1) diameter of the nerve, (2) depth of the nerve in relationship to the electrode, and (3) duration of the pulse. (Starkey 1999, page 202)

95. c. The intervertebral disk is comprised of two anatomical portions. The outer area, the annulus fibrosus is ropelike and collagen-rich and surrounds the inner portion—the nucleus pulposus, which is comprised of a gelatinous shock-absorbing substance. When a disk herniation occurs, the nucleus pushes or protrudes through a weakened or torn area of the annulus fibrosus and places pressure on the nerve. (Starkey 1999, page 324)

96. c. Type I (slow-twitch) muscle fibers produce a low intensity contraction using aerobic energy; the contraction can be sustained for a long period of time in events such as distance running. Type II (fast-twitch) muscle fibers produce high intensity contraction using anaerobic energy; the contraction can be sustained for a short period of time in activities such as sprinting. (Starkey 1999, page 7)

97. d. Physiologically, a counterirritant (hot or cold) causes an irritation and stimulates large diameter, myelinated sensory nerve fibers (A-beta). In contrast, unmyelinated, small diameter nerve fibers that normally perceive pain are the last to respond to heat and cold. (Starkey 1999, pages 116–117)

98. a. Muscle tetany is defined as a total contraction of a muscle obtained by the recruitment and contraction of all motor units. A sustained tetany requires a pulse frequency of 50 pulses per second. (Benton, Baker, Bowman, and Waters 1981, page 23)

99. d. The positive Babinski reflex test indicates an upper motor neuron lesion usually associated with brain damage following trauma or an expanding brain tumor. A Babinski is positive in a newborn but disappears after birth. In a negative Babinski, the toes do not move or bunch up uniformly. (Hoppenfeld 1976, page 256)

100. c. The gastrocnemius muscle is a large muscle. Therefore, when utilizing ultrasound to treat deep muscle lesions or bursitis, 1 MHz frequency should be used because it penetrates up to 5 cm in depth. (France 2004, pages 220–221)

101. c. The Visual Analog Scale utilizes a 10 cm horizontal line to document a patient's self-reported (subjective) pain rating. The left of the line is 0 which is "no pain" while the right of the line is 10 which is "very severe pain." The patient marks a vertical line at the number that correlates with their pain level. The test is one dimensional and can be administered within seconds both pre- and post-treatment or activity. (Guccione 1999, page 354) The Roland Morris Disability Questionnaire is a disability index comprised of 24 items used on the Sickness Impact Profile (SIP). Each item has the phrase "because of my back" and is scaled as 0 or 1 with a range of scores from 0 to 24. (Rothstein, et al. 2005, pages 180–181) In Waddell's nonorganic physical signs in low back pain (1980), the examiner performs tenderness, simulation, and distraction tests and assesses regional disturbances and overcorrection. The examiner scores any individual sign as a positive sign for the type of assessment performed. A score of three or more of the five types of nonorganic physical signs is clinically significant. (Rothstein, et al. 2005, pages 178–179) The McGill Pain Questionnaire is a multidimensional tool for measuring pain. It includes a body diagram to map pain, a pain rating index using word descriptors, and a five-category pain intensity scale. The questionnaire exists in a short version that can be completed in two to five minutes or a longer version which takes ten minutes or longer. (Guccione 2000, page 354)

102. c. A neurotrophic ulcer often appears at increased pressure points on the bottom of the feet. This results from diminished afferent (sensory) sensation. (McCulloch, Kloth, and Feedar 1995, page 118)

103. c. When checking a person's breathing, the rescuer must look, listen, and feel for breaths. In addition to looking for chest rise and feeling for airflow, the rescuer must also listen through the person's nose or mouth. (American Heart Association, BLS for Healthcare Providers 2006, page 12)

104. a. To perform a step-up activity, the patient loads weight in the lower extremity, which fixes the distal end of the extremity. The descriptive exercise terms—open and closed chain—originate from the science of biometrics. The reference is to whether or not the extremity is fixed at the distal end during an exercise. (Donatelli and Wooten 1994, page 620)

105. c. In the supine position, the shoulder is supported in a gravity lessened position, and movement is controlled by the PT or the PTA. This would be the proper treatment position following a TSR. (Kisner and Colby 2007, pages 496–500)

106. c. The appropriate ratio for ramp elevation height is one foot of ramp (12 inches) for every 1 inch of elevation height. (Minor and Minor 2010, pages 19–20)

107. b. Water conducts temperature 25 times faster than air. Physiologically cooling or warming a patient occurs with exposure and physical activity. Adequate core temperature cannot be maintained at temperatures lower than 25°C. Temperatures at 37°C or higher significantly increase cardiac output at rest. This leaves only choice **b** as the correct answer. (Kisner and Colby 2007, page 276)

108. b. The safest activity that can be used to increase flexibility for this patient is static stretching. While research indicates that tension created in the muscle while performing a ballistic stretch is twice that of the static stretch, the static stretch is deemed safer. The static stretch technique holds targeted soft tissues in an elongated position just past the point in the range of tissue resistance for a period of time. A ballistic stretch is a high-speed and high-intensity stretch produced by quick bouncing movements. Cyclic stretch is a short-duration stretch held and released for multiple repetitions. (Kisner and Colby 2007, page 79)

109. c. Extra precaution should be used by the PTA when establishing a resistance training program for young children who are still growing. While the risks involved in resistance training are low, growth-plate and soft tissue injuries may occur if guidelines and precautions are absent or not followed carefully. (Kisner and Colby 2007, page 205)

110. b. The PTA stresses quad sets to prepare the patient during treatment sessions for ambulation. It is imperative that the patient develop motor control of the post-op lower extremity to avoid delays in post-op rehabilitation. The quadriceps muscles are used extensively in the gait cycle. (Kisner and Colby 2007, page 62)

111. b. During the swing phase of gait, hip flexion is required to allow the swing limb to move from the posterior position to the anterior position for heel strike. The iliopsoas contracts, causing hip flexion at the swing leg joint and allowing passage of the swing limb under the body from the posterior position to the anterior position. (Norkin and Levangie 2001, pages 457–465)

112. c. Functional activities such as drying the back with a towel, placing a belt in trousers, and reaching a back pocket requires the movement of internal rotation. (Hoppenfeld 1976, pages 21 and 28)

113. a. Agonal gasps may occur in the first few minutes following sudden cardiac arrest. Agonal gasps are not adequate breathing. If a victim is not breathing or presents agonal gasps, breaths must be provided. (American Heart Association, BLS for the Healthcare Provider 2005, pages 69 and 73)

114. c. A small margin for error exists with digitalis drugs, which have the potential to accumulate rapidly in the bloodstream causing toxicity in older patients. Digitalis drugs can induce fatal arrhythmias. Other symptoms include blurred vision, confusion, and gastrointestinal distress. (Kauffman 1999, page 62)

115. c. Baker's cyst is a synovial cyst arising from the synovial lining of the knee that occurs in the popliteal fossa. (Taber 2001, page 216)

116. d. Hyperthyroidism is a disease caused by excessive levels of thyroid hormone in the body. Symptoms include weight loss, tachycardia, tremors, increased systolic blood pressure, palpitations, nervousness, and anxiety. (Taber 2001, page 1,937)

117. a. The application of cold will physiologically decrease the muscle spindle sensitivity. Research reports a reduction or elimination of achilles tendon reflex (ATR) and clonus after cold application. (Michlovitz 1996, pages 82–83 and 97–100)

118. b. Jurisprudence, in this situation, is the state physical therapy practice act rules and regulations which define the required supervision ratio for a physical therapist supervising physical therapist assistants. (Scott 1997, pages 10–11)

119. a. In many cases, a rescuer can stop bleeding by applying firm pressure over the bleeding area with the fingers or the palm of the hand. If the bleeding does not stop, add a second dressing and press harder. A dressing can be a piece of gauze or a clean piece of cloth. If neither is available, use a gloved hand or hands. (American Heart Association, Heartsaver First Aid 2006, pages 48–49)

120. c. For a healthy person, breathing at rest requires minimal effort. However, a patient with emphysema struggles to breath at rest. The breathing effort intensifies with physical activity. Therefore, instruction in diaphragmatic breathing facilitates a controlled breathing pattern that can be adopted to improve breathing quality during physical activity. (Frownfelter and Dean 1996, pages 389–391)

121. c. If the AED does not detect a rhythm requiring a shock, the AED will prompt the rescuer to resume CPR, beginning with chest compressions. The pads should be left on the victim's chest. The AED may prompt the rescuer to clear the victim to allow analysis in about two minutes. The AED voice prompts should be followed. (American Heart Association, BLS for Healthcare Providers 2006, page 4)

122. a. The pectoralis minor originates from the superior margins—outer surfaces of third, fourth, and fifth ribs near the cartilages—and from the fasciae of corresponding intercostal muscles. The muscle inserts on the medial border, superior surface of the coracoid process of the scapula. When the pectoralis minor is shortened, it tilts the scapula anteriorly. (Kendall 2005, page 320)

123. b. During abduction of the shoulder, motion occurs in the glenohumeral joint and the scapulothoracic joint in a 2 to 1 ratio. With 180° abduction available, approximatley 120° occur in the glenohumeral joint and 60° in the scapulothoracic joint. Adhesive capsulitis occurs in the glenohumeral joint and significantly reduces the glenohumeral abduction motion. The patient with acute adhesive capsulitis would present less than 90° of abduction. (Hoppenfeld 1976, page 23)

124. **a.** The armpit or axilla contains axillary vessels and nerves. Improperly fit crutches that are too long or a patient resting on the crutch pads irritates these structures. (Pierson 1999, pages 194–198)

125. **b.** The Nagi Model of Disability describes four sequential phases: (1) active pathology, (2) impairment, (3) functional limitation, and (4) disability. Functional limitation involves decreased ability to independently perform activities of daily living. (Minor and Minor 2010, page 33)

126. **d.** Research reports a reduction in wound size by 33% using a 3 MHz, pulsed, nonthermal ultrasound at an intensity of 0.2 to 1 W/cm^2 for five to ten minutes, one to three times per week, over four weeks. (Guccione 2000, page 392)

127. **d.** The push-up is an example of an upper extremity closed-chain activity. The position to perform a push-up loads the distal upper extremity with the weight of the upper torso. By definition, closed-chain exercises involve activities where the body moves on a distal segment that is fixed or stabilized on a support surface. (Kisner and Colby 2007, page 176)

128. **b.** The following is a description of the stages: Subclinical: patient begins to feel heaviness in the limb; fibrotic changes and fluid accumulation occur before visible swelling or pitting; approximately 50% of patients with minimal edema report feeling heaviness or fullness in the extremity. Stage I: reversible lymphedema—accumulation of protein-rich fluid; elevation reduces swelling; pits on pressure. Stage II: spontaneously irreversible lymphedema—proteins stimulate fibroblast formation; connective and scar tissues

proliferate; minimal pitting even with moderate swelling. Stage III: lymphatic elephantiasis—hardening of dermal tissues; papillomas of the skin; appearance of skin is elephant-like. (O'Sullivan and Schmitz 2007, page 659)

129. **a.** Warning signs of stroke include: sudden numbness or weakness of the face, arm, or leg, especially on one side of the body; sudden confusion and/or trouble speaking; sudden trouble seeing in one or both eyes; sudden trouble walking, dizziness, loss of balance or coordination; or sudden, severe headache with no known cause. A stroke is a medical emergency and in this situation, the PTA should call for an emergency medical team. (American Heart Association, Heartsaver First Aid 2006, pages 38–39)

130. **b.** During the bridging exercise, the abdominals function with the gluteus maximus to control pelvic tilt, while the lumbar extensors stabilize the spine against the pull of the gluteus maximus. Holding the bridge position develops isometric control. (Kisner and Colby 2007, pages 474–475)

131. **a.** The Ober test is used to identify a tight iliotibial band. The patient is tested in the sidelying position, and the hip is abducted to the end range with the knee joint in 90 degrees of flexion. The extremity is left unsupported by the examiner. If the extremity does not drop to a position of adduction, the test is positive. (Hoppenfeld 1976, page 167)

132. **c.** Dilation of the cervix occurs in the second stage of labor. At this stage, the woman can assist the uterus during contraction to aid in pushing the baby down the birth canal. The proper instruction for her when bearing down is to take in a breath, contract the abdominal wall, and slowly breathe out. If followed correctly, this will increase pressure

on the abdomen and relax the pelvic floor. (Kisner and Colby 2007, page 816)

133. c. Cystic fibrosis affects the excretory glands of the body. The thickened secretions narrow or obstruct airways leading to infection, hyperinflation, and tissue destruction. Prompt removal of secretions and prevention of infection are important in the medical management of this disease. (O'Sullivan and Schmitz 2007, pages 567–568)

134. b. The cruciform anterior spinal hyperextension (CASH) orthosis is cruciform in shape and uses a three-point contact system to prevent forward flexion of the thoracic spine. The other braces listed are used in the management of scoliosis. (Seymour 2002, page 438)

135. a. Vaulting appears when a patient has difficulty bringing the prosthetic leg forward in swing and either flexes the knee excessively or raises the body up on the toe of the non-involved extremity to allow room for the elongated prosthetic foot to clear. (May 1996, page 155)

136. c. The diaphragm is a primary muscle of inspiration and is innervated by the phrenic nerve (C3, C4, C5). The intercostal muscles are innervated by T1 through T12 while the abdominal muscles are innervated by spinal cord levels T10 to T12. The serratus anterior muscle is innervated by the long thoracic nerve (C5, C6, C7, C8). (Kisner and Colby 2007, pages 852 and 853)

137. a. Research by Willams-Kretschmer and Majno (1969) determined that superficial dermis can withstand ischemia for two to six hours, but after eight hours of ischemia, necrotic tissue changes occur followed by tissue sloughing. Therefore, strict adherence to change of position schedules every two hours is important to ulcer prevention. (McCulloch, Kloth, and Feedar 1995, page 188)

138. d. Spills of body fluids require immediate attention and should be wiped up with one part 5.25% sodium hypochlorite (bleach) diluted with ten parts of water. The person cleaning the spill should wear gloves, and a gown should be considered. Towels and linen used to clean the spill should be disposed of properly. (Pierson 1999, page 314)

139. d. Purulent drainage (pus) appears creamy yellow to brown or other color and may give off several odors indicating wound infection. Serous drainage is clear in color, while sero-sanguineous drainage is clear with a tinge of blood. Translucent drainage is cloudy but permits the passage of light. (McCulloch, Kloth, and Feedar 1995, pages 71, 139, and 140)

140. b. The wet-to-dry dressing consists of wet gauze applied to the wound. When the dry dressing is removed, it functions to debride the wound pulling away necrotic tissue as well as fibrin and other cells critical to wound healing. (O'Sullivan and Schmitz 2007, pages 666–668)

141. a. Spinal stenosis is a degenerative narrowing of the spinal canal. Flexion widens the intervertebral foramina while extension decreases the size of the foramina. Extension, lateral bending, and rotation activities may additionally increase neurological symptoms and decrease mobility. (Kisner and Colby 2007, page 429)

142. b. Mottling of the skin is a warning sign that tissue temperatures are rising to a potentially dangerous level. Mottling of the skin appears as ghost-white and beet-red splotches. When mottling occurs, the treatment should be discontinued. (Starkey 1999, page 126)

143. b. Research reports that thermal heating effects must be initiated within three minutes after the conclusion of the treatment when utilizing a 3 MHz ultrasound. When using 1 MHz, effective stretching time initiation is slightly over three minutes. (Starkey 1999, page 291)

144. d. The intermittent compression ranges from 40 to 60 mm Hg for the upper extremity and 60 to 100 mm Hg for the lower extremity. The pressure should not exceed the diastolic blood pressure. (Starkey 1999, page 309)

145. a. To effectively reduce edema, the proximal tissue is treated first, which "uncorks the bottle" by removing proximally trapped edema. This technique opens the area for distal edema to follow when pressure is applied. (Starkey 1999, pages 335–336)

146. b. A-beta nerve fibers are large in diameter and covered with thick myelin, which aids in the quick transmission of sensations, such as hot, cold, touch, and pressure. (Starkey 1999, pages 81–82)

147. c. The optimal phase duration to elicit a maximal muscle contraction is between 300–500 microseconds. A muscle contraction is necessary to enhance strength or delay atrophy. A phase duration of less than 1,000 microseconds (1 millisecond) is unable to stimulate denervated muscle. (Starkey 1999, page 208)

148. d. The United States Access Board (USAB) recommended toilet height range to be 17 to 19 inches, measured from the floor to the top of the toilet seat. Standard toilet bowl heights range from 14 to 16 inches. The lower heights require increased hip and knee flexion which make it difficult for patients with various medical afflictions to rise or lower from sit to stand or stand to sit. (Minor and Minor 2010, page 22)

149. b. The brachioradialis, extensor carpi radialis longus, and extensor carpi radialis brevis are muscles that are innervated by the radial nerve (C7). (Hoppenfeld 1976, pages 93–94)

150. b. Compartment syndrome may develop after contusions, fractures, crush injuries, localized infection, excessive exercise, or overstretching. The symptoms include swelling and pain. The four lower extremity compartments where compartment syndrome may appear include anterior compartment, peroneal compartment, deep posterior compartment, and superficial posterior compartment. (France 2004, pages 360–361)

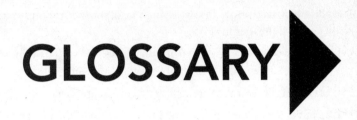

GLOSSARY

absolute refractory period   time when the nerve cannot be further excited

absorption energy   energy that stimulates a particular tissue to perform its normal function

accommodation   process of a nerve gradually becoming less responsive to stimulation

action potential   changing flow of ions across cell membrane. This produces an excitatory response. During the resting state (–60 to –90 mV (millivolts)), there is no response. When there is an action potential, depolarization and repolarization across the cell membrane occurs.

adrenal glands   govern the body's autonomic nervous system

adrenal medulla   the inner, reddish brown, soft part of the suprarenal gland

aerobic capacity   degree to which an individual uses up oxygen in the blood for respiration

afferent   conveying impulses toward the central nervous system

agonist-contraction technique   uses the principle of reciprocal inhibition to stretch the tight muscle. The tight muscle is first taken to its most elongated position. Then an isometric contraction of the agonist muscle (the muscle that produces the motion that is limited) occurs for three to five seconds; the patient is then asked to actively move to the new elongated position.

alternating current (AC)   periodic reversal of electron flow in a sinusoidal pattern

amplitude   the maximum current or voltage delivered in one phase of a pulse. It is measured in milliamperes or volts (intensity).

anabolism   constructive metabolic process by which organisms convert substances into other useable chemical components

anatomic dead space volume (VD)   volume of air occupying non-respiratory conducting airways

anode   positive electrode (negative ions migrate to it)

anterior cerebral arteries (ACA)   supply the brain with its arterial supply

arachnoid   spiderlike middle layer of the meninges

arterial insufficiency   condition in which the arteries are unable to supply adequate oxygen and nutrients to tissues to meet demand

aspiration   the removal of fluids or gases from a cavity by the application of suction

autograft   a skin graft taken from the patient's body, which provides permanent coverage of a burn

autonomic nervous system (ANS)   controls all involuntary activities, such as cardiovascular, respiratory, digestive, endocrine, urinary, and reproductive systems

ballistic stretching   involves a high load, short duration stretch, such as a bouncing movement while reaching to touch the toes in sitting

basal ganglia   part of the diencephalon section of the brain; responsible for the regulation of posture and muscle tone, with a role in the control of voluntary and automatic movement

basal metabolic rate   measurement of energy used when the body is at rest

basilar artery   an artery formed by the union of the two vertebral arteries that supplies blood to the cerebrum, the cerebellum, and the inner ear

Berg Balance Scale (BBS)   an assessment tool made up of 14 common functional activities that become progressively more difficult for the individual being tested. Each item is rated on a scale from zero to four, with a maximum score possible of 56. The BBS is a strong fall predictor, and it can be used to identify the functional areas in which instability or fear is present.

blood volume   the volume of blood circulated per minute is affected by arterial/venous pressure and peripheral resistance. Blood volume is usually 7% to 8% of the whole body weight.

Borg Rate of Perceived Exertion (RPE) Scale   a standardized way for the patient to measure how hard he or she is working

breathing strategies   are often helpful during an acute flare-up of symptoms. Calmly encouraging the patient to breathe in through the nose and out through the mouth or "smell the roses and blow out the candles" can help the patient separate him or herself from the situation until you can remove the noxious source of the symptoms.

brain stem   area of the brain that lies between the cerebral hemispheres and the spinal cord and which contains the medulla, pons, midbrain, and the 12 cranial nerves. It controls breathing, swallowing, seeing, hearing, facial expressions, eye and tongue movement, and salivation through the 12 cranial nerves.

burn shock   see hypovolemic shock.

cardiac index   provides a more complete assessment of a patient's cardiac output by looking at the amount of blood being pumped from the heart per minute per square meter of body mass. Normal CI range is 2.5 to 3.5 $L/min/m^2$.

cardiac output   the amount of blood that is pumped out of the heart and into the aorta per minute. Normal range is 4 to 6 L/min, with males being on the higher end and females lower. Determined by stroke volume × heart rate.

catabolism   destructive metabolic process by which organisms convert substances and excrete them

cathode   negative electrode (positive ions migrate to it)

central nervous system (CNS)   the brain and the spinal cord

cephalocaudal   pertaining to the long axis of the body, from the head to toe

cerebellum   portion of the brain that lies over the brain stem and rests just below the cerebral hemispheres. The cerebellum coordinates the action of voluntary muscles and coordinates contractions to provide smooth and accurate movements.

cerebral arteries (anterior, posterior, and middle)   arteries through which the brain receives its arterial supply

cerebral spinal fluid (CSF)   a barrier which, along with the blood brain, barrier, helps preserve the brain's safe status, provides nourisment, and physically protects the brain from trauma

cerebrum portion of the brain (the surface is the cortex) that initiates movement and thought processes. It consists of four major sections: the frontal lobe, the parietal lobe, the temporal lobe, and the occipital lobe.

charge number of free electrons flowing. It is measured in coulombs.

chronaxie the duration of a stimulus that is twice the rheobase that causes a minimal response (muscle twitch)

chronic long-lasting or incurable

circle of Willis a circle of arteries that supply blood to the brain

circuit the path of current from the generating power source through various components back to the generating source

closed circuit a circuit in which the electrons are flowing

compensated Trendelenburg gait gait pattern characterized by lateral lean over the stance leg; may be caused by gluteus medius weaknesss or hip pain

conductance the ease with which a current flows along a conducting medium

conductors materials that are composed of very reactive atoms with free moving and loosely bound electrons in the outer orbit

consent a voluntary agreement by a person with the mental capacity to make an intelligent choice to allow something suggested by another person to be performed on him or her

constant current stimulators a stimulator in which the current does not vary and is independent of resistance. The machine maintains the same current regardless of resistance. With this unit, the voltage increases or decreases in order to maintain constant current.

constant voltage stimulators a stimulator in which the voltage does not vary. The current increases or decreases depending on the changes in resistance.

continuous passive motion (CPM) machines that slowly and passively move joints through their ranges of motion for uninterrupted and extended periods of time

contrast bath thermal modality involving placement of the limb alternately into warm and cool water

current the rate at which free electrons flow. The rate of flow is measured in amperes (amps), with one amp equal to one coulomb/sec.

cyanotic characterized by bluish discoloration, applied especially to such discoloration of skin and mucous membranes due to reduced hemoglobin in the blood

decay time the time it takes for peak amplitude of a waveform to decrease back to zero

dependent rubor reddening of the skin when the limb is below the level of the heart

dermatome the area of skin innervated by neurons from a single spinal level

diagnosis physical therapy determination identifying problems associated with faulty biomechanical or neuromuscular actions

diaphoresis excessive sweating

diastole the dilation, or period of dilation, of the heart, especially at the ventricles

diathermy heating of the body tissues due to their resistance to the passage of high-frequency electromagnetic radiation

diencephalon portion of the brain that rests beneath the cortex in the center of the brain and contains the basal ganglia and related structures

direct current (DC) electrons flowing continuously in one direction

disability inability of a person to perform or participate in activities related to one's work, home, or community; inability to fulfill social roles

discharge   process of discontinuing intervention in a single episode of care

distal   see proximal-distal.

dura   tough outer layer of the meninges

duty cycle   on time period when current is delivered

Dynamic Gait Index (DGI)   an index used to assess the characteristics of gait in individuals with balance or vestibular deficits

edema   abnormally large amounts of fluid in the intercellular tissue spaces of the body

efferent   conveying nervous impulses away from the central nervous system

electrical muscle stimulation (EMS)   is used to stimulate denervated muscle in order to maintain muscle viability

electrical power   defined as watts = volts × amperage

electrical stimulation (ES)   a common modality used in physical therapy. It helps relieve pain, re-educate muscles, heal tissue, and relax muscle spasms.

electrical stimulation for tissue repair (ESTR)   indicated for edema reduction, promotion of circulation, and wound care

endocrine system   the system of ductless glands that regulate bodily functions through hormones secreted into the bloodstream; controls metabolic activity

endoneurium   connective tissue that surrounds the individual nerve fiber (with its myelin and neurilemma)

endurance testing   the body's ability to respond to increased oxygen demands

epinephrine   hormone secreted by the adrenal gland that increases blood pressure and stimulate the heart

epineurium   connective tissue that makes up the first outer layer of a nerve

epithelial tissue   outer layer of the skin; epidermis

eschar   brown or black necrotic tissue

escharotomy   an incision made into hard eschar to relieve the pressure on underlying, intact tissues

evaluation   dynamic process during which the PT makes clinical judgments based on patient data; results in determination of diagnosis, prognosis, and interventions

examination   process for gathering patient data leading to diagnostic classification; includes patient/client history, systems review, and tests and measures

expiratory reserve volume (ERV)   maximal volume expired after a normal expiration (1,000 mL)

facilitated stretching   involves the use of an inhibitory technique to relax and elongate tissue during static or ballistic stretching

fasciculus   a bundle of nerve fibers within each nerve, or muscle fibers within a muscle

Feldenkreis method   awareness through movement. Although many of the other aspects of relaxation are incorporated into this method, the focus is on identifying imbalance within the muscular system in order to self correct these imbalances and achieve harmony.

fluidotherapy   a dry heat modality that transfers heat by convection and is commonly used to treat the distal extremities

frequency   number of cycles or pulses per second (PPS or CPS)

frontal lobe   portion of the brain that initiates voluntary muscle movement, emotion, and cognition and which is known as the principle motor area. This area controls eye movements, personality, emotional IQ, and the motor portion of speech.

full-thickness graft   a skin graft that requires removing the epidermis and dermis

functional electrical stimulation (FES) used to activate muscles with electrical stimulation in order to perform functional activities

functional limitations inability of a patient to perform a task or activity in the expected manner

functional residual capacity (FRC) volume in the lungs after normal expiration

gate control theory a pain control theory that works on the premise that sensory inputs can block transmission of pain signals at the level of the spinal cord

glucagon a polypeptide hormone secreted in response to hypoglycemia

glucocorticoids class of steroid hormones that affects carbohydrate metabolism; most important one is cortisol, the hormone produced when under stress

granulation tissue healthy tissue that is beefy red, shiny, moist, and bumpy (granular) in appearance

gross-fine large movement of an extremity versus small hand or finger movement.

Gross Motor Function Measure (GMFM) a tool used to assess change in the gross motor function of children with cerebral palsy and Down syndrome. The GMFM assesses rolling, crawling, kneeling, sitting, standing, walking, running, and jumping.

Gross Motor Performance Measure (GMPM) a tool that was designed to be used with the Gross Motor Function Measure. It assesses body alignment in space, coordination, movement dissociation, postural stability, and weight shifting.

guided imagery uses techniques developed through self hypnosis to allow the patient to visualize a calm or peaceful scene. The patient is encouraged (through a series of cues) to use as many senses as possible to perceive the scene that he or she is imagining. Once he or she is deeply immersed in the scene, the patient is able to relax and become refreshed before returning to day-to-day activities.

hemosiderin an intracellular storage form of iron; the granules consist of an ill-defined complex of ferric hydroxides, polysaccharides,and proteins having an iron content of about 33 percent by weight

high-voltage current current in which waveform has an amplitude of greater than 150 V (volts)

hippocampus portion of the brain that is located in the temporal lobe; responsible for memory

hold-relax technique uses the principle of autogenic inhibition to stretch the tight muscle. The tight muscle is first taken to its most elongated position. An isometric contraction is performed with the tight muscle for three to five seconds, and then the muscle is passively repositioned to its new elongated position. This may be repeated three times and ends with a static stretch in the new elongated position for 15 to 60 seconds.

homeostasis the body's process of maintaining equilibrium of autonomic functions such as body temperature or blood pressure

homunculus pictoral representation of the areas of the body controlled by the sensory and motor cortices

hydrostatic pressure as an object is immersed deeper in water, the density of the liquid increases

hyperpolarization relative refractory period

hypoactive pertaining to or characterized by abnormally diminished activity

hypothalamus part of the diencephalon part of the brain. It is one of the master glands of the brain, which helps control homeostasis, blood pressure, heart rate, wake cycles, and endocrine function.

hypoxia decreased oxygen to tissues

hypovolemic shock (also called burn shock) evaporation of fluid which has leaked onto the skin out of capillaries, due to vessel damage and vasodilation after a burn and the loss of the protective barrier of the skin, resulting in a low circulating blood volume and decreased cardiac output

immediate memory register and recall of information after an interval of a few seconds

impairments   abnormalities or dysfunctions of the bones, joints, ligaments, tendons, muscles, nerves, skin, or problems with movement resulting from pathologies

impedance   resistance to electrical flow in biological tissues

informed consent   a legal concept regarding a person's right to be a fully informed participant in all aspects of his or her own healthcare

inspiratory capacity (IC)   amount of air that can be inspired after a normal expiration. Usually, IC is 75 to 80% of vital capacity or 55 to 60% of total lung capacity.

inspiratory reserve volume (IRV)   maximal volume inspired after normal inspiration

insulin   a protein that is essential for the regulation of glucose levels in the blood and the metabolism of carbohydrates; insufficient insulin production results in diabetes mellitus.

insulators   materials whose electrons are tightly bound in the outer shell

intermittent claudication   lower extremity pain after ambulation due to hypoxia; it is often experienced by patients with arterial insufficiency

internal carotid artery   the internal branch of the carotid artery that supplies blood to the brain and other structures in the head

interstitial fluid   fluid located between parts or in the interspaces of a tissue

intervention   skilled techniques and activities that make up a treatment plan

iontophoresis   the introduction of ions into the skin by use of direct current

ischemia   an insufficient flow of oxygenated blood to a certain part of the body

joint mobilization   a manual therapy technique used to increase mobility at a joint that is limited due to a tight capsule or ligament at the joint

Katz Index of activities of daily living (ADLs)   assesses assistance needed to perform six basic ADLs, including bathing, dressing, toileting, transferring, continence, and feeding

kinesthesia   the awareness of movement

lateralization   localization of function so that different hemispheres of the brain have more control of certain parts of the body than of other parts

light touch   a common sensory test for the perception of tactile sensation

long-term memory   recall of facts or events that occurred years before

low-intensity stimulators   (also known as micro-current electrical neuromuscular stimulators (MENS)) a form of electrical stimulation that is delivered at the subsensory level so that the patient will not feel the current

low load prolonged stretching (LLPS)   the application of a minimal force, or low load, to an elongated muscle in order to maintain the position of elongation over a prolonged period of time. This type of stretching can be maintained for different lengths of time—from 30 minutes at a time up to hours at a time.

low-voltage current   current in which waveform has an amplitude of less than 150 V (volts)

maceration   white, wrinkled, and fragile condition of skin after prolonged exposure to moisture

macrophage   any of the many forms of mononuclear phagocytes found in tissues

manual muscle testing (MMT)   an examination tool and grading system used to quantify muscle strength that can provide information on the function of peripheral nerves that innervate the muscles tested

melanocytes   cells on the bottom layer of the epidermis that produce the pigment melanin

meninges   membranes made of a tough connective tissue that cover and protect the brain tissue physically

metabolism   the body's physical and chemical process that breaks down substances to generate and use energy

mineralocorticoids   hormones that predominantly help to regulate the body's electrolyte and water balance

Mini Mental State Exam (MMSE)   a common measurement tool used to assess overall cognition

mirroring   a method in which the patient indicates the movement that the PTA is performing to one side of his or her body by moving the opposite side of the body to the same position

modulation   varying one or more of the electrical parameters (intensity, frequency) or currents as a whole over time while delivering the stimulus. This helps prevent accommodation.

motor cortex   portion of the frontal lobe of the brain which includes Broca's area, which controls the motor or expressive portion of speech. Damage to the motor cortex causes spastic paralysis.

motor impulses   efferent impulses that send messages toward the body from the cerebral hemisphere

motor point   the site of optimal excitability of an individual muscle because it is the point where the motor nerve enters muscle. Because of this, it requires less stimulation to elicit a response from the tissue.

multidirectional reach test   an assessment tool similar to the functional reach test that provides information about the risk of falling forward, backward, right, and left

muscle endurance   the ability of the muscle to repeatedly contract over a period of time and resist fatigue

muscle power   the ability of the muscle to perform a quick, powerful contraction. The goal of muscle power is to improve the contractility of the muscle over a shorter period of time.

muscle strength   the ability of the muscle to produce tension

neurological   pertaining to the nervous system

neuromuscular electrical stimulation (NMES)   stimulation of innervated muscle for restoring muscle function, muscle strengthening, spasm reduction, atrophy prevention, and muscle reeducation

neuron   a nerve cell; the basic unit of the nervous system

neuropathy   an injury affecting the peripheral nerve due to infection, a toxin, or a metabolic disorder

norepinephrine   a hormone, secreted by the adrenal gland, that gives the body sudden energy during stress. As a neurotransmitter, it gives a sense of fulfillment.

occipital lobe   portion of the brain that is the center of the visual perceptual system and which works with the visual cortex

off-time   period when electrical current flow stops

ohm   the unit of electrical resistance

one-legged stance test   a tool used to measure static control of posture. This test can also measure fall risk.

open circuit   a circuit in which the electron flow is stopped

opiate mediated control theory   a pain control theory that states that electrical stimulation can decrease pain because it has been shown to release endorphins (opiates) that are produced by the body

osteomyelitis   inflammation of bone caused by a pyogenic organism. It may remain localized or may spread through the bone to involve the marrow, cortex, cancellous tissue, and periosteum

ovaries   the female sexual glands in which the ova, or reproductive cells or eggs, are formed

pallor   paleness, absence of skin coloration

pancreas   gland that is subdivided into lobes. The endocrine part produces insulin and glucagons.

parallel circuit   a circuit that has two or more exciting routes for current to pass between the two terminals

parathyroid glands   small bodies apposed to the posterior surface of the thyroid gland

parietal lobe   portion of the brain responsible for sensation and perception, in addition to integration of sensory input. It works with the visual system in the occipital lobe for spatial coordination.

pathological   anything related to disease

patient confidentiality   rules and laws that deal with patient privacy with regard to medical information. Medical information should not be made available to those not needing to know without written authorization from the patient. All who have access to medical records have an ethical, moral, and legal obligation to protect the confidentiality of that information.

perineurium   a layer of connective tissue that surrounds nerve fibers

peripheral nervous system (PNS)   consists of the nerves leading to and from the central nervous system (CNS), including the cranial nerves exiting the brain stem and spinal roots exiting the spinal cord, many of which combine to form peripheral nerves

phonophoresis   the process of driving medicine through the skin and into deeper tissue using ultrasound

pia mater   the soft inner covering of the meninges

pineal gland   the site of synthesis of melatonin

pituitary gland   a small oval endocrine gland that lies at the base of the brain. It is sometimes called the master gland of the body because all of the other endocrine glands depend on its secretion for stimulation.

polyneuropathy   widespread, bilateral insults to the peripheral nerve

posterior cerebral arteries (PCA)   provide the brain with its arterial supply

postural (orthostatic) hypotension   abnormally low blood pressure when moving into an upright position

prognosis   judgment of the PT about the level of optimal improvement a patient may achieve and the amount of time needed for treatment

progressive relaxation   developed by Jacobson it uses systematic isometric contractions of muscles from distal to proximal to release voluntary control of tight muscles. By actively tightening the muscles, the patient receives feedback on what the muscle is like when contracted and then actively and consciously relaxes the muscles to reduce tension.

progressive resistance exercises (PREs)   strenghtening exercises that are quantitavely progressed over time.

proprioception   the awareness of a joint at rest and the position of a joint at rest

proximal-distal   nearest, as opposed to farther from the axial skeleton

pulse duration   the time period extended from beginning to end of one phase of a pulse

pulse frequency   the number of pulses delivered in one second. It is also known as pulses/sec, PPS, and pulse rate.

pulse oximetry   may be used to assess the amount of oxygen in the blood

pulse train   a continuous series of individual pulses delivered over a period of time

pulsed current   the unidirectional or bidirectional flow of charged particles periodically ceasing for a period of less than one second before the next electrical event

ramp time   how long it takes to go from zero to peak amplitude or reverse. Ramping can be ramped up and/or ramped down. Usually, two seconds is sufficient. When a ramp up is incorporated, it produces a smooth muscle contraction. When a ramp down is in place, it adds to patient comfort.

reactive hyperemia   reddening of the skin

reflection   the bending back of light or sound waves from a surface that the waves strike

relative refractory period   time when a greater than usual stimulus is applied in order to produce another action potential. This is also known as hyperpolarization.

residual volume (RV)   volume remaining in the lungs after maximal expiration

resistance   the ease or difficulty of current moving through a substance (measured in ohms)

reticular activating system (RAS)   part of the brain that is located in the medulla, pons, and midbrain which helps maintain arousal, filter many inputs, and regulate visceral functions

rheobase   the minimal strength of the stimulus needed to excite tissue

rise time   the time it takes for amplitude of a wave form to increase from zero to peak amplitude

rule of nines   a method of estimating how much of the body of a patient has been burned by dividing the body into areas of 9% of total body surface area or multiples thereof

Russian stimulation   a time-modulated alternating current that is used for muscle strengthening. Russian stimulation treatment is typically uncomfortable for the patient.

sensory impulses   afferent impulses that send messages toward the cerebral hemispheres from the peripheral part of the body

series circuit   a circuit in which there is only one path for the current to get from one terminal to another

sex hormones   chemical substances released by cells having estrogenic (female sex hormone) activity or androgenic (male sex hormone) activity

shear   force that is applied parallel to the soft tissues

short-term memory   retrieval of material after an interval of minutes, hours, or days

slough   stringy or mucous-like yellow or white necrotic tissue

somatic nervous system (SNS)   involves 12 pairs of cranial nerves located in the brain stem which can be sensory, motor, or mixed in function

somatosensory system   the body's system of sensation

sphygmomanometer   an instrument for measuring blood pressure in the arteries

split-thickness graft   a skin graft that requires removal of the epidermis and part of the dermis

spinal cord   part of the CNS that lies below the brain and extends from the brain stem to the lower back. It transmits motor and sensory messages.

steppage gait   gait pattern characterized by increased hip and knee flexion during swing phase to clear the toes

stereognosis   the ability to identify an object by touch

stroke volume   amount of blood that is ejected with each contraction of the heart per minute. Can be affected by preload (amount of blood in the ventricle), contractility (the ability of the ventricle to contract), and afterload (the force needed to overcome and open the aortic valve).

subcutaneous   beneath the skin

synthesis   artificial combining of chemical compounds or other substances

systole   the contraction of the heart, especially that of the ventricles

temporal lobe   portion of the brain that provides information for communication and sensation and which is the primary auditory area. It contains the hippocampus, which is responsible for memory.

testes   the male gonads, normally situated in the scrotum, wherein spermatozoa are produced

thalamus   part of the diencephalon part of the brain that is the inner room of the brain. It sorts and processes sensory information from all over the peripheral nervous system and central nervous system in order to fine-tune movements.

thyroid gland   an endocrine gland normally situated in the lower part of the front of the neck, which secretes the thyroid hormones needed to regulate metabolism

thyroxine   the major hormone produced by the thyroid for the purpose of increasing the rate of cell metabolism

tidal volume (TV)   total volume inspired and expired per breath (500 mL)

timed up and go (TUG) test   assesses an individual's basic mobility skills. It is made up of very functional activities, such as standing up from a chair and walking at a self-selected pace.

total lung capacity (TLC)   volume measured at the end of a maximal inspiration

transcutaneous   through or across the skin

transcutaneous electrical nerve stimulation (TENS)   used for pain management

transmission   propagation of energy through a particular biologic tissue into deeper tissues

trophic changes   pertaining to changes in nutrition

tunneling   the presence of a hole between the layers of fascia in tissue

two-point discrimination   a test that assesses the ability to perceive two points in contact with the skin at the same time

ultrasound   a technique in which high frequency sound waves are applied to the body to promote healing or provide deep heating

undermining   the separation of the intact epidermis and dermis at the periphery of a wound from the tissue below the dermis

vasodilation   dilation of a vessel, especially dilation of arterioles leading to increased blood flow to a part

vestibular system   proprioceptors in the inner ear that regulate the body's orientation to gravity

viscous   a thick liquid

vital capacity (VC)   maximal volume forcefully expired after a maximal inspiration (4,000 to 5,000 mL)

venous return   the amount of blood flowing back into the right atrium from the veins per minute. In a healthy system, this should be similar in volume to cardiac output.

venous stasis   a stoppage or diminution of the flow of blood to the veins

vertebral artery   either one of two arteries that branch off the subclavian artery and travel through the foramina of the transverse processes of the upper six cervical vertebrae to the foramen magnum and into the brain

voltage   flow of current. The flow can be from negative to positive or positive to negative. It is the force created by electrical potential which goes from one of high concentration to low concentration.

waveform   a visual representation of the pulse. The selection of which waveform used in treatment is based upon the equipment available and the treatment goal.

wavelength   distance from one point in a propagating wave to the same point in the next wave

Wolff's law   states that the body system adapts over time to the stresses placed upon it; usually used in reference to the skeletal system

ADDITIONAL ONLINE PRACTICE ▶

Whether you need help building basic skills or preparing for an exam, visit the LearningExpress Practice Center! On this site, you can access additional practice materials. Using the code below, you'll be able to log in and take an additional Physical Therapist Assistant Exam. This online practice will also provide you with:

- **Immediate scoring**
- **Detailed answer explanations**
- **Personalized recommendations for further practice and study**

Log in to the LearningExpress Practice Center by using this URL: **www.learnatest.com/practice**

This is your access code: **7540**

Follow the steps online to redeem your access code. After you've used your access code to register with the site, you will be prompted to create a username and password. For easy reference, record them here:

Username: _____ Password:_____

With your username and password, you can log in and answer these practice questions as many times as you like. If you have any questions or problems, please contact LearningExpress customer service at 1-800-295-9556 ext. 2, or e-mail us at **customerservice@learningexpressllc.com**.

NOTES

NOTES

NOTES

NOTES